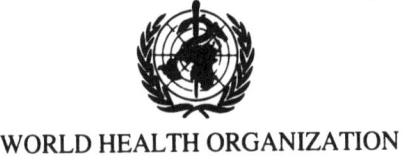

WORLD HEALTH ORGANIZATION

INTERNATIONAL AGENCY FOR RESEARCH ON CANCER

IARC MONOGRAPHS
ON THE
EVALUATION OF CARCINOGENIC RISKS TO HUMANS

Human Papillomaviruses

VOLUME 64

This publication represents the views and expert opinions
of an IARC Working Group on the
Evaluation of Carcinogenic Risks to Humans,
which met in Lyon,

6–13 June 1995

1995

IARC MONOGRAPHS

In 1969, the International Agency for Research on Cancer (IARC) initiated a programme on the evaluation of the carcinogenic risk of chemicals to humans involving the production of critically evaluated monographs on individual chemicals. In 1980 and 1986, the programme was expanded to include evaluations of carcinogenic risks associated with exposures to complex mixtures and other agents.

The objective of the programme is to elaborate and publish in the form of monographs critical reviews of data on carcinogenicity for agents to which humans are known to be exposed and on specific exposure situations; to evaluate these data in terms of human risk with the help of international working groups of experts in chemical carcinogenesis and related fields; and to indicate where additional research efforts are needed.

This project is supported by PHS Grant No. 5-UO1 CA33193-14 awarded by the United States National Cancer Institute, Department of Health and Human Services. Additional support has been provided since 1986 by the European Commission.

©International Agency for Research on Cancer 1995

IARC Library Cataloguing in Publication Data

IARC Working Group on the Evaluation of Carcinogenic Risks to
    Humans (1995 : Lyon, France)
Human papillomaviruses : views and expert opinions of an IARC Working
Group on the Evaluation of Carcinogenic Risks to Humans which met in
Lyon, 6–13 June 1995.

(IARC monographs on the evaluation of carcinogenic risks to humans ; 64)

1. Carcinogens – toxicity – congresses   2. Papillomavirus, human – congresses
I. Series

ISBN 92 832 1264 9   (NLM Classification: W1)
ISSN 0250-9555

Publications of the World Health Organization enjoy copyright protection in accordance with the provisions of Protocol 2 of the Universal Copyright Convention.

All rights reserved. Application for rights of reproduction or translation, in part or in toto, should be made to the International Agency for Research on Cancer.

Distributed by the International Agency for Research on Cancer

PRINTED IN THE UNITED KINGDOM

CONTENTS

NOTE TO THE READER 1

LIST OF PARTICIPANTS 3

PREAMBLE 9
    Background 9
    Objective and Scope 9
    Selection of Topics for Monographs 10
    Data for Monographs 11
    The Working Group 11
    Working Procedures 11
    Exposure Data 12
    Studies of Cancer in Humans 14
    Studies of Cancer in Experimental Animals 17
    Other Data Relevant to an Evaluation of Carcinogenicity and Its Mechanisms 19
    Summary of Data Reported 21
    Evaluation 22
    References 26

GENERAL REMARKS 31

THE MONOGRAPH

Human papillomaviruses
1. Human papillomavirus (HPV) infection 35
    1.1   Structure and molecular biology of human papillomaviruses 35
            1.1.1   Structure of the viruses 35
            1.1.2   Taxonomy 36
            1.1.3   Genomic variability 39
            1.1.4   Host range 39
            1.1.5   Related animal papillomaviruses 40
            1.1.6   Target tissues 40
            1.1.7   Genomic structure and properties of gene products 40
            1.1.8   Regulation of gene expression 43
            1.1.9   Replication 47
    1.2   Serological response 47
            1.2.1   Antigenic properties of HPVs 47

		1.2.2	Immune response to papillomavirus infections 49

1.2.2 Immune response to papillomavirus infections 49
    (a) Initial studies 49
    (b) Use of genetically engineered or synthetic viral antigens in
        serological assays 49
1.3 Methods for detection of HPV infections 52
    1.3.1 HPV diagnosis by morphology 52
    1.3.2 Detection of HPV proteins in infected tissues 53
    1.3.3 Detection of HPV genomic sequences 53
        (a) PCR-based methods 53
        (b) ViraPap™ and Hybrid Capture™ 55
        (c) Southern blot hybridization 56
        (d) In-situ hybridization 56
        (e) Filter in-situ hybridization 56
        (f) Comparison of HPV testing methods 57
    1.3.4 Detection of HPV infections and HPV-associated cancers by serological
           assays 57
1.4 Epidemiology of infection 58
    1.4.1 Transmission 58
    1.4.2 Incidence 60
    1.4.3 Prevalence 61
    1.4.4 Natural history 65
1.5 Pathology of HPV genital tract infection and evidence from pathology for
    progression to malignancy 66
    1.5.1 Terminology 67
        (a) Dysplasia and carcinoma *in situ* 67
        (b) Cervical intraepithelial neoplasia (CIN) 67
        (c) Squamous intraepithelial lesion (SIL) 69
        (d) Other organs in the male and female anogenital tract 70
    1.5.2 Temporal and spatial relationships between cervical cancer precursors
           and invasive cancer 70
        (a) Histological observations 70
        (b) Microinvasive and early invasive cervical cancers 70
        (c) Clinical observations 70
    1.5.3 Histological changes in HPV-related lesions of the lower female
           genital tract 71
        (a) Non-productive (latent) HPV infection 71
        (b) Low-grade CIN 71
        (c) High-grade CIN 74
        (d) Microinvasive and invasive squamous-cell cancer of the cervix 75
        (e) Vaginal intraepithelial neoplasia 76
        (f) Vulva 77
        (g) Vagina, anus and penis 78
        (h) Adenocarcinoma *in situ* and adenocarcinoma 78

		1.5.4	Pathology of non-melanoma skin cancer and cutaneous HPV infection 79
			(a) Cutaneous HPV infection 79
			(b) Non-melanoma skin cancer.. 79
		1.5.5	Pathology of HPV-induced changes in the nude mouse system and tissue culture studies 80
	1.6	Clinical disease of established HPV etiology (other than precancer and cancer)... 80
		1.6.1	Genital area 80
		1.6.2	Upper respiratory and digestive tract and conjunctiva.......................... 81
		1.6.3	Skin 82
	1.7	Therapy and vaccination 83
		1.7.1	Therapy of benign disease... 83
		1.7.2	Therapy of precancers 84
		1.7.3	Vaccination 86
2.	Studies of cancer in humans 87
	2.1	Descriptive studies of anogenital cancer.. 88
		2.1.1	Cancer of the uterine cervix 88
		2.1.2	Other anogenital cancers 89
	2.2	Case reports and case series 91
		2.2.1	Cancer of the uterine cervix 91
			(a) Pre-invasive cervical lesions 91
			(b) Squamous-cell carcinoma 91
			(c) Adenocarcinoma and adenosquamous carcinoma 99
			(d) Geographical and temporal variation... 99
		2.2.2	Anogenital cancers 103
			(a) Cancer of the vulva and vagina.. 103
			(b) Cancer of the penis.. 107
			(c) Cancer of the anus... 107
		2.2.3	Other cancers... 107
			(a) Oral cancer 114
			(b) Cancer of the pharynx and tonsil 114
			(c) Oesophageal cancer... 114
			(d) Cancer of the colon and rectum 114
			(e) Nasal/sinonasal cancer 114
			(f) Laryngeal cancer 114
			(g) Lung cancer... 121
			(h) Cancer of the skin 121
			(i) Breast cancer 123
			(j) Ovarian cancer 123
			(k) Cancer of the bladder and urethra 130
			(l) Prostate cancer 130
			(m) Cancer of the eye.. 130
	2.3	Cohort studies 130
		2.3.1	Following HPV DNA detection in normal women to cytological diagnosis of CIN 133

2.3.2 Following mild dysplasia/koilocytotic atypia to CIN III/invasive cancer 135
(a) Prospective studies of mild dysplasia/koilocytotic atypia without HPV DNA testing 135
(b) Prospective studies of mild dysplasia/koilocytotic atypia with HPV DNA testing 138
2.3.3 Prospective studies of HPV infection at body sites other than the cervix 141
2.4 Case–control studies 141
2.4.1 Cervical cancer 142
(a) HPV and CIN III 142
(b) HPV and invasive cancer of the uterine cervix 163
2.4.2 Other cancers 184
(a) Anogenital cancers 184
(b) Other cancers 189
2.4.3 Cofactors 194
2.5 Special populations 196
2.5.1 Skin cancer in patients with epidermodysplasia verruciformis (EV) 196
HPV types in warts and skin cancers in EV patients 197
2.5.2 Studies of cancer incidence in transplant patients 200
(a) HPV infection, CIN and invasive cervical and anogenital carcinoma in transplant recipients 200
(b) HPV DNA in transplant-associated skin lesions 204
(c) HPV infection and cancer at other sites 212
2.5.3 Studies in HIV-infected persons 212
(a) Studies of the uterine cervix 214
(b) Studies of the anorectal region 222
3. Molecular mechanisms of carcinogenesis 233
3.1 Experimental data supporting the carcinogenicity of specific HPV genotypes and analysing the mechanism of HPV-linked carcinogenesis 233
3.1.1 Low-risk and high-risk HPV infections 233
3.1.2 Chromosomal instability of high-risk HPV-infected cells 233
3.1.3 Immortalization and transformation of cells by HPVs 234
(a) Contribution of viral and cellular genes 234
(b) Chromosomal abnormalities in HPV-immortalized cells 235
(c) Transcriptional modulation by HPV oncoproteins 236
(d) Positive and negative transforming functions of HPV 236
(e) HPV-targeted cellular proteins in cervical carcinogenesis 240
3.1.4 Experimental evidence for a role of high-risk HPVs in malignant conversion and in human cervical cancers 242
(a) Requirement for HPV gene expression for invasive growth and the malignant phenotype 242
(b) Integration of HPV sequences 243
(c) Chromosomal abnormalities in HPV-associated cancers 244
(d) Alterations of specific proto-oncogenes 245

		3.1.5	Interactions between HPV and environmental agents 246

        3.1.5 Interactions between HPV and environmental agents 246
            (a) Interaction with other viruses 246
            (b) Hormones and antioestrogens 248
            (c) Chemicals 249
            (d) Radiation 250
        3.1.6 HPV in mice 251
            (a) HPV recombinant retrovirus 251
            (b) HPV transgenic mice 251
   3.2 Immune mechanisms and HPV-associated neoplasia 253
        3.2.1 Immunosuppression 253
        3.2.2 Histological studies 254
        3.2.3 Cell-mediated immunity 255
            (a) Helper T-cell responses 255
            (b) Cytotoxic T-cell responses 256
        3.2.4 Major histocompatibility complex (MHC) expression 257
            (a) MHC class I 257
            (b) MHC class II 258
        3.2.5 HLA polymorphisms: association with cervical cancer risk 259
4. Studies of cancer in animals 261
   4.1 Non-human primate papillomavirus 261
        Rhesus monkey genital papillomavirus 261
   4.2 Bovine papillomavirus 263
        4.2.1 Heterogeneity of bovine papillomavirus 263
        4.2.2 BPV-1 263
            (a) BPV-1 in hamsters 264
            (b) BPV-1 in transgenic mice 264
        4.2.3 BPV-2 264
            (a) BPV-2 in bladder cancers 264
            (b) BPV-2 latency 265
            (c) BPV-2 in hamsters 267
        4.2.4 BPV-3 267
        4.2.5 BPV-4 267
            (a) BPV-4 and alimentary tract cancer 267
            (b) BPV-4 in mouse xenografts 268
            (c) BPV-4 in hamsters 268
        4.2.6 BPV-5 and BPV-6 269
        4.2.7 Bovine ocular squamous-cell carcinoma (OSCC) 269
        4.2.8 Bovine skin carcinoma 269
        4.2.9 BPV in equine sarcoids 270
   4.3 Equine papillomavirus (EqPV) 271
   4.4 Papillomaviruses in cervidae 271
   4.5 Ovine papillomatosis 272
   4.6 Cottontail rabbit papillomavirus (CRPV) 273
        4.6.1 CRPV and co-carcinogens 273

		4.6.2 CRPV latency	274
		4.6.3 CRPV in transgenic rabbits	274
	4.7	Domestic rabbit oral papillomavirus	275
	4.8	*Mastomys natalensis* papillomavirus (MnPV)	275
	4.9	Mouse papillomavirus (MmPV)	275
	4.10	Canine oral papillomavirus (COPV)	276
	4.11	Feline papillomas	276
	4.12	Avian papillomavirus	276
5.	Summary of data reported and evaluation		277
	5.1	HPV infection	277
	5.2	Studies of cancer in humans	278
	5.3	Molecular mechanisms of carcinogenesis	280
	5.4	Studies of cancer in animals	281
	5.5	Evaluation	281
6.	References		283

SUPPLEMENTARY CORRIGENDA TO VOLUMES 1–63 379

CUMULATIVE INDEX TO THE *MONOGRAPHS* SERIES 381

NOTE TO THE READER

The term 'carcinogenic risk' in the *IARC Monographs* series is taken to mean the probability that exposure to an agent will lead to cancer in humans.

Inclusion of an agent in the *Monographs* does not imply that it is a carcinogen, only that the published data have been examined. Equally, the fact that an agent has not yet been evaluated in a monograph does not mean that it is not carcinogenic.

The evaluations of carcinogenic risk are made by international working groups of independent scientists and are qualitative in nature. No recommendation is given for regulation or legislation.

Anyone who is aware of published data that may alter the evaluation of the carcinogenic risk of an agent to humans is encouraged to make this information available to the Unit of Carcinogen Identification and Evaluation, International Agency for Research on Cancer, 150 cours Albert Thomas, 69372 Lyon Cedex 08, France, in order that the agent may be considered for re-evaluation by a future Working Group.

Although every effort is made to prepare the monographs as accurately as possible, mistakes may occur. Readers are requested to communicate any errors to the Unit of Carcinogen Identification and Evaluation, so that corrections can be reported in future volumes.

IARC WORKING GROUP ON THE EVALUATION OF CARCINOGENIC RISKS TO HUMANS: HUMAN PAPILLOMAVIRUSES

Lyon, 6–13 June 1995

LIST OF PARTICIPANTS

Members

H.-U. Bernard, Laboratory for Papillomavirus Biology, Institute of Molecular and Cell Biology, National University of Singapore, 10 Kent Ridge Crescent, Singapore 0511, Singapore

F.X. Bosch, Unit of Epidemiology and Cancer Registry, Hospital Duran i Reynals, Autovia Castellfels, km 2.7, 08907 L'Hospitalet del Llobregat, Spain

M.S. Campo, The Beatson Institute for Cancer Research, Wolfson Laboratory for Molecular Pathology, Garscube Estate, Switchback Road, Bearsden, Glasgow G61 1BD, United Kingdom

J. Cuzick, Department of Mathematics, Statistics and Epidemiology, Imperial Cancer Research Fund, PO Box 123, 61 Lincoln's Inn Fields, London WC2A 3PX, United Kingdom (*Chairman*)

L. Gissmann, Department of Obstetrics and Gynecology, Division of Research, Stritch School of Medicine, Loyola University Chicago Medical Center, 2160 South First Avenue, Maywood, IL 60153, USA

L.A. Koutsky, Center for AIDS and STDs, 1001 Broadway, Suite 205, Seattle, WA 98122, USA

S.K. Kjaer, Division for Cancer Epidemiology, Danish Cancer Society, Strandboulevarden 49, Box 839, 2100 Copenhagen Ø, Denmark

J.M. McGregor, Department of Photobiology, Institute of Dermatology, St John's Skin Center, St Thomas's Hospital, London SE1, United Kingdom

M. Melbye, Danish Epidemiology Science Centre, State Serum Institute, 2300 Copenhagen S, Denmark

K. Münger, Department of Pathology, Harvard Medical School, 200 Longwood Avenue, Boston, MA 02115, USA

R.M. Richart, Division of Obstetric/Gynaecological Pathology, The Sloane Hospital For Women, College of Physicians and Surgeons of Columbia University, 630 West 168th Street, New York, NY 10032, USA

A. Schneider, Department of Gynecology, Friedrich Schiller University Jena, Bachstrasse 18, 07743 Jena, Germany

M.H. Schiffman, Environmental Epidemiology Branch, National Cancer Institute, Executive Plaza North, Room 443, Bethesda, MD 20892-7374, USA

K.V. Shah, Department of Molecular Microbiology and Immunology, Johns' Hopkins University School of Hygiene and Public Health, 615 North Wolfe Street, Baltimore, MD 21205-2179, USA (*Vice-Chairman*)

M.A. Stanley, Division of Cellular Pathology, Department of Pathology, University of Cambridge, Tennis Court Road, Cambridge CB2 1QP, United Kingdom

L.L. Villa, Ludwig de Pesquisa Institute of Cancer, rua Prof. Antonio Prudente, 109-4° andar, 01509.010 Sao Paulo, SP, Brazil

K. Vousden, ABL-Basic Research Program, Frederick Cancer Research and Development Center, Building 539, Room 222A, PO Box B, Frederick, MD 21702-1201, USA

J.M.M. Walboomers, Institute of Pathology, Academisch Ziekenhuis Vrije Universiteit, De Boelelaan 1117, 1081 HV Amsterdam, The Netherlands

H. zur Hausen, German Cancer Research Center, Im Neuenheimer Feld 280, 69120 Heidelberg, Germany

IARC Secretariat

P. Boffetta, Unit of Environmental Cancer Epidemiology
A. Dufournet, Unit of Carcinogen Identification and Evaluation
S. Franceschi, Unit of Field and Intervention Studies
M.-J. Ghess, Unit of Carcinogen Identification and Evaluation
V. Krutovskikh, Unit of Multistage Carcinogenesis
D. McGregor, Unit of Carcinogen Identification and Evaluation
D. Mietton, Unit of Carcinogen Identification and Evaluation
H. Møller, Unit of Carcinogen Identification and Evaluation[1]
W.G. Morgan, Edinburgh, United Kingdom
N. Muñoz, Unit of Field and Intervention Studies
A. Mylvaganam, Programme of Radiation and Cancer[2]
H. Nakazawa, Unit of Multistage Carcinogenesis
C. Partensky, Unit of Carcinogen Identification and Evaluation
M. Plummer, Unit of Field and Intervention Studies
S. Ruiz, Unit of Carcinogen Identification and Evaluation
P. Webb, Unit of Carcinogen Identification and Evaluation[3]
J. Wilbourn, Unit of Carcinogen Identification and Evaluation

---

[1] Present address: Center for Registerbased Studies in Health and Society, Sejerøgade 11, DK-2100 Copenhagen Ø, Denmark
[2] Present address: 16/88 Albert Road, Strathfield, NSW 2135, Australia
[3] Present address: Department of Social and Preventive Medicine, University of Queensland, Medical School, Herston Road, Herston Qld 4006, Australia

Secretarial assistance

M. Lézère
J. Mitchell
S. Reynaud

PREAMBLE

IARC MONOGRAPHS PROGRAMME ON THE EVALUATION OF CARCINOGENIC RISKS TO HUMANS[1]

PREAMBLE

1. BACKGROUND

In 1969, the International Agency for Research on Cancer (IARC) initiated a programme to evaluate the carcinogenic risk of chemicals to humans and to produce monographs on individual chemicals. The *Monographs* programme has since been expanded to include consideration of exposures to complex mixtures of chemicals (which occur, for example, in some occupations and as a result of human habits) and of exposures to other agents, such as radiation and viruses. With Supplement 6 (IARC, 1987a), the title of the series was modified from *IARC Monographs on the Evaluation of the Carcinogenic Risk of Chemicals to Humans* to *IARC Monographs on the Evaluation of Carcinogenic Risks to Humans*, in order to reflect the widened scope of the programme.

The criteria established in 1971 to evaluate carcinogenic risk to humans were adopted by the working groups whose deliberations resulted in the first 16 volumes of the *IARC Monographs series*. Those criteria were subsequently updated by further ad-hoc working groups (IARC, 1977, 1978, 1979, 1982, 1983, 1987b, 1988, 1991a; Vainio *et al.*, 1992).

2. OBJECTIVE AND SCOPE

The objective of the programme is to prepare, with the help of international working groups of experts, and to publish in the form of monographs, critical reviews and evaluations of evidence on the carcinogenicity of a wide range of human exposures. The *Monographs* may also indicate where additional research efforts are needed.

The *Monographs* represent the first step in carcinogenic risk assessment, which involves examination of all relevant information in order to assess the strength of the available evidence that certain exposures could alter the incidence of cancer in humans. The second step is quantitative risk estimation. Detailed, quantitative evaluations of epidemiological data may be made in the *Monographs*, but without extrapolation beyond the range of the data available. Quantitative extrapolation from experimental data to the human situation is not undertaken.

---

[1]This project is supported by PHS Grant No. 5-UO1 CA33193-14 awarded by the United States National Cancer Institute, Department of Health and Human Services. Since 1986, the programme has also been supported by the European Commission.

The term 'carcinogen' is used in these monographs to denote an exposure that is capable of increasing the incidence of malignant neoplasms; the induction of benign neoplasms may in some circumstances (see p. 18) contribute to the judgement that the exposure is carcinogenic. The terms 'neoplasm' and 'tumour' are used interchangeably.

Some epidemiological and experimental studies indicate that different agents may act at different stages in the carcinogenic process, and several different mechanisms may be involved. The aim of the *Monographs* has been, from their inception, to evaluate evidence of carcinogenicity at any stage in the carcinogenesis process, independently of the underlying mechanisms. Information on mechanisms may, however, be used in making the overall evaluation (IARC, 1991a; Vainio *et al.*, 1992; see also pp. 25–26).

The *Monographs* may assist national and international authorities in making risk assessments and in formulating decisions concerning any necessary preventive measures. The evaluations of IARC working groups are scientific, qualitative judgements about the evidence for or against carcinogenicity provided by the available data. These evaluations represent only one part of the body of information on which regulatory measures may be based. Other components of regulatory decisions may vary from one situation to another and from country to country, responding to different socioeconomic and national priorities. **Therefore, no recommendation is given with regard to regulation or legislation, which are the responsibility of individual governments and/or other international organizations.**

The *IARC Monographs* are recognized as an authoritative source of information on the carcinogenicity of a wide range of human exposures. A users' survey, made in 1988, indicated that the *Monographs* are consulted by various agencies in 57 countries. Each volume is generally printed in 4000 copies for distribution to governments, regulatory bodies and interested scientists. The Monographs are also available from the International Agency for Research on Cancer in Lyon and via the Distribution and Sales Service of the World Health Organization.

3. SELECTION OF TOPICS FOR MONOGRAPHS

Topics are selected on the basis of two main criteria: (a) there is evidence of human exposure, and (b) there is some evidence or suspicion of carcinogenicity. The term 'agent' is used to include individual chemical compounds, groups of related chemical compounds, physical agents (such as radiation) and biological factors (such as viruses). Exposures to mixtures of agents may occur in occupational exposures and as a result of personal and cultural habits (like smoking and dietary practices). Chemical analogues and compounds with biological or physical characteristics similar to those of suspected carcinogens may also be considered, even in the absence of data on a possible carcinogenic effect in humans or experimental animals.

The scientific literature is surveyed for published data relevant to an assessment of carcinogenicity. The IARC information bulletins on agents being tested for carcinogenicity (IARC, 1973–1994) and directories of on-going research in cancer epidemiology (IARC, 1976–1994) often indicate those exposures that may be scheduled for future meetings. Ad-hoc working groups convened by IARC in 1984, 1989, 1991 and 1993 gave recommendations as to which agents should be evaluated in the IARC Monographs series (IARC, 1984, 1989, 1991b, 1993).

As significant new data on subjects on which monographs have already been prepared become available, re-evaluations are made at subsequent meetings, and revised monographs are published.

4. DATA FOR MONOGRAPHS

The *Monographs* do not necessarily cite all the literature concerning the subject of an evaluation. Only those data considered by the Working Group to be relevant to making the evaluation are included.

With regard to biological and epidemiological data, only reports that have been published or accepted for publication in the openly available scientific literature are reviewed by the working groups. In certain instances, government agency reports that have undergone peer review and are widely available are considered. Exceptions may be made on an ad-hoc basis to include unpublished reports that are in their final form and publicly available, if their inclusion is considered pertinent to making a final evaluation (see pp. 25–26). In the sections on chemical and physical properties, on analysis, on production and use and on occurrence, unpublished sources of information may be used.

5. THE WORKING GROUP

Reviews and evaluations are formulated by a working group of experts. The tasks of the group are: (i) to ascertain that all appropriate data have been collected; (ii) to select the data relevant for the evaluation on the basis of scientific merit; (iii) to prepare accurate summaries of the data to enable the reader to follow the reasoning of the Working Group; (iv) to evaluate the results of epidemiological and experimental studies on cancer; (v) to evaluate data relevant to the understanding of mechanism of action; and (vi) to make an overall evaluation of the carcinogenicity of the exposure to humans.

Working Group participants who contributed to the considerations and evaluations within a particular volume are listed, with their addresses, at the beginning of each publication. Each participant who is a member of a working group serves as an individual scientist and not as a representative of any organization, government or industry. In addition, nominees of national and international agencies and industrial associations may be invited as observers.

6. WORKING PROCEDURES

Approximately one year in advance of a meeting of a working group, the topics of the monographs are announced and participants are selected by IARC staff in consultation with other experts. Subsequently, relevant biological and epidemiological data are collected by IARC from recognized sources of information on carcinogenesis, including data storage and retrieval systems such as MEDLINE and TOXLINE, and EMIC and ETIC for data on genetic and related effects and reproductive and developmental effects, respectively.

For chemicals and some complex mixtures, the major collection of data and the preparation of first drafts of the sections on chemical and physical properties, on analysis, on production and use and on occurrence are carried out under a separate contract funded by the United States National Cancer Institute. Representatives from industrial associations may assist in the preparation of sections on production and use. Information on production and trade is obtained from governmental and trade publications and, in some cases, by direct contact with industries. Separate production data on some agents may not be available because their publication could disclose confidential information. Information on uses may be obtained from published sources but is often complemented by direct contact with manufacturers. Efforts are made to supplement this information with data from other national and international sources.

Six months before the meeting, the material obtained is sent to meeting participants, or is used by IARC staff, to prepare sections for the first drafts of monographs. The first drafts are compiled by IARC staff and sent, prior to the meeting, to all participants of the Working Group for review.

The Working Group meets in Lyon for seven to eight days to discuss and finalize the texts of the monographs and to formulate the evaluations. After the meeting, the master copy of each monograph is verified by consulting the original literature, edited and prepared for publication. The aim is to publish monographs within six months of the Working Group meeting.

The available studies are summarized by the Working Group, with particular regard to the qualitative aspects discussed below. In general, numerical findings are indicated as they appear in the original report; units are converted when necessary for easier comparison. The Working Group may conduct additional analyses of the published data and use them in their assessment of the evidence; the results of such supplementary analyses are given in square brackets. When an important aspect of a study, directly impinging on its interpretation, should be brought to the attention of the reader, a comment is given in square brackets.

7. EXPOSURE DATA

Sections that indicate the extent of past and present human exposure, the sources of exposure, the people most likely to be exposed and the factors that contribute to the exposure are included at the beginning of each monograph.

Most monographs on individual chemicals, groups of chemicals or complex mixtures include sections on chemical and physical data, on analysis, on production and use and on occurrence. In monographs on, for example, physical agents, occupational exposures and cultural habits, other sections may be included, such as: historical perspectives, description of an industry or habit, chemistry of the complex mixture or taxonomy. Monographs on biological agents have sections on structure and biology, methods of detection, epidemiology of infection and clinical disease other than cancer.

For chemical exposures, the Chemical Abstracts Services Registry Number, the latest Chemical Abstracts Primary Name and the IUPAC Systematic Name are recorded; other synonyms are given, but the list is not necessarily comprehensive. For biological agents, taxonomy and structure are described, and the degree of variability is given, when applicable.

Information on chemical and physical properties and, in particular, data relevant to identification, occurrence and biological activity are included. For biological agents, mode of replication, life cycle, target cells, persistence and latency and host response are given. A description of technical products of chemicals includes trades names, relevant specifications and available information on composition and impurities. Some of the trade names given may be those of mixtures in which the agent being evaluated is only one of the ingredients.

The purpose of the section on analysis or detection is to give the reader an overview of current methods, with emphasis on those widely used for regulatory purposes. Methods for monitoring human exposure are also given, when available. No critical evaluation or recommendation of any of the methods is meant or implied. The IARC publishes a series of volumes, *Environmental Carcinogens: Methods of Analysis and Exposure Measurement* (IARC, 1978–93), that describe validated methods for analysing a wide variety of chemicals and mixtures. For biological agents, methods of detection and exposure assessment are described, including their sensitivity, specificity and reproducibility.

The dates of first synthesis and of first commercial production of a chemical or mixture are provided; for agents which do not occur naturally, this information may allow a reasonable estimate to be made of the date before which no human exposure to the agent could have occurred. The dates of first reported occurrence of an exposure are also provided. In addition, methods of synthesis used in past and present commercial production and different methods of production which may give rise to different impurities are described.

Data on production, international trade and uses are obtained for representative regions, which usually include Europe, Japan and the United States of America. It should not, however, be inferred that those areas or nations are necessarily the sole or major sources or users of the agent. Some identified uses may not be current or major applications, and the coverage is not necessarily comprehensive. In the case of drugs, mention of their therapeutic uses does not necessarily represent current practice nor does it imply judgement as to their therapeutic efficacy.

Information on the occurrence of an agent or mixture in the environment is obtained from data derived from the monitoring and surveillance of levels in occupational environments, air, water, soil, foods and animal and human tissues. When available, data on the generation, persistence and bioaccumulation of the agent are also included. In the case of mixtures, industries, occupations or processes, information is given about all agents present. For processes, industries and occupations, a historical description is also given, noting variations in chemical composition, physical properties and levels of occupational exposure with time and place. For biological agents, the epidemiology of infection is described.

Statements concerning regulations and guidelines (e.g. pesticide registrations, maximal levels permitted in foods, occupational exposure limits) are included for some countries as indications of potential exposures, but they may not reflect the most recent situation, since such limits are continuously reviewed and modified. The absence of information on regulatory status for a country should not be taken to imply that that country does not have regulations with regard to the exposure. For biological agents, legislation and control, including vaccines and therapy, are described.

8. STUDIES OF CANCER IN HUMANS

(a) Types of studies considered

Three types of epidemiological studies of cancer contribute to the assessment of carcinogenicity in humans—cohort studies, case–control studies and correlation (or ecological) studies. Rarely, results from randomized trials may be available. Case series and case reports of cancer in humans may also be reviewed.

Cohort and case–control studies relate individual exposures under study to the occurrence of cancer in individuals and provide an estimate of relative risk (ratio of incidence or mortality in those exposed to incidence or mortality in those not exposed) as the main measure of association.

In correlation studies, the units of investigation are usually whole populations (e.g. in particular geographical areas or at particular times), and cancer frequency is related to a summary measure of the exposure of the population to the agent, mixture or exposure circumstance under study. Because individual exposure is not documented, however, a causal relationship is less easy to infer from correlation studies than from cohort and case–control studies. Case reports generally arise from a suspicion, based on clinical experience, that the concurrence of two events—that is, a particular exposure and occurrence of a cancer—has happened rather more frequently than would be expected by chance. Case reports usually lack complete ascertainment of cases in any population, definition or enumeration of the population at risk and estimation of the expected number of cases in the absence of exposure. The uncertainties surrounding interpretation of case reports and correlation studies make them inadequate, except in rare instances, to form the sole basis for inferring a causal relationship. When taken together with case–control and cohort studies, however, relevant case reports or correlation studies may add materially to the judgement that a causal relationship is present.

Epidemiological studies of benign neoplasms, presumed preneoplastic lesions and other end-points thought to be relevant to cancer are also reviewed by working groups. They may, in some instances, strengthen inferences drawn from studies of cancer itself.

(b) Quality of studies considered

The Monographs are not intended to summarize all published studies. Those that are judged to be inadequate or irrelevant to the evaluation are generally omitted. They may be mentioned briefly, particularly when the information is considered to be a useful supplement to that in other reports or when they provide the only data available. Their inclusion does not imply acceptance of the adequacy of the study design or of the analysis and interpretation of the results, and limitations are clearly outlined in square brackets at the end of the study description.

It is necessary to take into account the possible roles of bias, confounding and chance in the interpretation of epidemiological studies. By 'bias' is meant the operation of factors in study design or execution that lead erroneously to a stronger or weaker association than in fact exists between disease and an agent, mixture or exposure circumstance. By 'confounding' is meant a situation in which the relationship with disease is made to appear stronger or to appear weaker than it truly is as a result of an association between the apparent causal factor and another factor that is associated with either an increase or decrease in the incidence of the disease. In evaluating the extent to which these factors have been minimized in an individual study, working groups consider a number of aspects of design and analysis as described in the report of the study. Most of these considerations apply equally to case–control, cohort and correlation studies. Lack of clarity of any of these aspects in the reporting of a study can decrease its credibility and the weight given to it in the final evaluation of the exposure.

Firstly, the study population, disease (or diseases) and exposure should have been well defined by the authors. Cases of disease in the study population should have been identified in a way that was independent of the exposure of interest, and exposure should have been assessed in a way that was not related to disease status.

Secondly, the authors should have taken account in the study design and analysis of other variables that can influence the risk of disease and may have been related to the exposure of interest. Potential confounding by such variables should have been dealt with either in the design of the study, such as by matching, or in the analysis, by statistical adjustment. In cohort studies, comparisons with local rates of disease may be more appropriate than those with national rates. Internal comparisons of disease frequency among individuals at different levels of exposure should also have been made in the study.

Thirdly, the authors should have reported the basic data on which the conclusions are founded, even if sophisticated statistical analyses were employed. At the very least, they should have given the numbers of exposed and unexposed cases and controls in a case–control study and the numbers of cases observed and expected in a cohort study. Further tabulations by time since exposure began and other temporal factors are also important. In a cohort study, data on all cancer sites and all causes of death should have been given, to reveal the possibility of reporting bias. In a case–control study, the effects of investigated factors other than the exposure of interest should have been reported.

Finally, the statistical methods used to obtain estimates of relative risk, absolute rates of cancer, confidence intervals and significance tests, and to adjust for confounding should have been clearly stated by the authors. The methods used should preferably have been the generally accepted techniques that have been refined since the mid-1970s. These methods have been reviewed for case–control studies (Breslow & Day, 1980) and for cohort studies (Breslow & Day, 1987).

(c) *Inferences about mechanism of action*

Detailed analyses of both relative and absolute risks in relation to temporal variables, such as age at first exposure, time since first exposure, duration of exposure, cumulative exposure and time since exposure ceased, are reviewed and summarized when available. The analysis of temporal relationships can be useful in formulating models of carcinogenesis. In particular, such analyses may suggest whether a carcinogen acts early or late in the process of carcinogenesis, although at best they allow only indirect inferences about the mechanism of action. Special attention is given to measurements of biological markers of carcinogen exposure or action, such as DNA or protein adducts, as well as markers of early steps in the carcinogenic process, such as proto-oncogene mutation, when these are incorporated into epidemiological studies focused on cancer incidence or mortality. Such measurements may allow inferences to be made about putative mechanisms of action (IARC, 1991a; Vainio et al., 1992).

(d) Criteria for causality

After the quality of individual epidemiological studies of cancer has been summarized and assessed, a judgement is made concerning the strength of evidence that the agent, mixture or exposure circumstance in question is carcinogenic for humans. In making their judgement, the Working Group considers several criteria for causality. A strong association (i.e. a large relative risk) is more likely to indicate causality than a weak association, although it is recognized that relative risks of small magnitude do not imply lack of causality and may be important if the disease is common. Associations that are replicated in several studies of the same design or using different epidemiological approaches or under different circumstances of exposure are more likely to represent a causal relationship than isolated observations from single studies. If there are inconsistent results among investigations, possible reasons are sought (such as differences in amount of exposure), and results of studies judged to be of high quality are given more weight than those of studies judged to be methodologically less sound. When suspicion of carcinogenicity arises largely from a single study, these data are not combined with those from later studies in any subsequent reassessment of the strength of the evidence.

If the risk of the disease in question increases with the amount of exposure, this is considered to be a strong indication of causality, although absence of a graded response is not necessarily evidence against a causal relationship. Demonstration of a decline in risk after cessation of or reduction in exposure in individuals or in whole populations also supports a causal interpretation of the findings.

Although a carcinogen may act upon more than one target, the specificity of an association (i.e. an increased occurrence of cancer at one anatomical site or of one morphological type) adds plausibility to a causal relationship, particularly when excess cancer occurrence is limited to one morphological type within the same organ.

Although rarely available, results from randomized trials showing different rates among exposed and unexposed individuals provide particularly strong evidence for causality.

When several epidemiological studies show little or no indication of an association between an exposure and cancer, the judgement may be made that, in the aggregate, they show evidence of lack of carcinogenicity. Such a judgement requires first of all that the studies giving rise to it meet, to a sufficient degree, the standards of design and analysis described above. Specifically, the possibility that bias, confounding or misclassification of exposure or outcome could explain the observed results should be considered and excluded with reasonable certainty. In addition, all studies that are judged to be methodologically sound should be consistent with a relative risk of unity for any observed level of exposure and, when considered together, should provide a pooled estimate of relative risk which is at or near unity and has a narrow confidence interval, due to sufficient population size. Moreover, no individual study nor the pooled results of all the studies should show any consistent tendency for relative risk of cancer to increase with increasing level of exposure. It is important to note that evidence of lack of carcinogenicity obtained in this way from several epidemiological studies can apply only to the type(s) of cancer studied and to dose levels and intervals between first exposure and observation of disease that are the same as or less than those observed in all the studies. Experience with human cancer indicates that, in some cases, the period from first exposure to the development of clinical cancer is seldom less than 20 years; latent periods substantially shorter than 30 years cannot provide evidence for lack of carcinogenicity.

9. STUDIES OF CANCER IN EXPERIMENTAL ANIMALS

All known human carcinogens that have been studied adequately in experimental animals have produced positive results in one or more animal species (Wilbourn et al., 1986; Tomatis et al., 1989). For several agents (aflatoxins, 4-aminobiphenyl, azathioprine, betel quid with tobacco, BCME and CMME (technical grade), chlorambucil, chlornaphazine, ciclosporin, coal-tar pitches, coal-tars, combined oral contraceptives, cyclophosphamide, diethylstilboestrol, melphalan, 8-methoxypsoralen plus UVA, mustard gas, myleran, 2-naphthylamine, nonsteroidal oestrogens, oestrogen replacement therapy/steroidal oestrogens, solar radiation, thiotepa and vinyl chloride), carcinogenicity in experimental animals was established or highly suspected before epidemiological studies confirmed the carcinogenicity in humans (Vainio et al., 1995). Although this association cannot establish that all agents and mixtures that cause cancer in experimental animals also cause cancer in humans, nevertheless, **in the absence of adequate data on humans, it is biologically plausible and prudent to regard agents and mixtures for which there is sufficient evidence (see p. 24) of carcinogenicity in experimental animals as if they presented a carcinogenic risk to humans**. The possibility that a given agent may cause cancer through a species-specific mechanism which does not operate in humans (see p. 26) should also be taken into consideration.

The nature and extent of impurities or contaminants present in the chemical or mixture being evaluated are given when available. Animal strain, sex, numbers per group, age at start of treatment and survival are reported.

Other types of studies summarized include: experiments in which the agent or mixture was administered in conjunction with known carcinogens or factors that modify carcinogenic effects; studies in which the end-point was not cancer but a defined precancerous lesion; and experiments on the carcinogenicity of known metabolites and derivatives.

For experimental studies of mixtures, consideration is given to the possibility of changes in the physicochemical properties of the test substance during collection, storage, extraction, concentration and delivery. Chemical and toxicological interactions of the components of mixtures may result in nonlinear dose–response relationships.

An assessment is made as to the relevance to human exposure of samples tested in experimental animals, which may involve consideration of: (i) physical and chemical characteristics, (ii) constituent substances that indicate the presence of a class of substances, (iii) the results of tests for genetic and related effects, including genetic activity profiles, DNA adduct profiles, proto-oncogene mutation and expression and suppressor gene inactivation. The relevance of results obtained, for example, with animal viruses analogous to the virus being evaluated in the monograph must also be considered. They may provide biological and mechanistic information relevant to the understanding of the process of carcinogenesis in humans and may strengthen the plausibility of a conclusion that the biological agent that is being evaluated is carcinogenic in humans.

(a) *Qualitative aspects*

An assessment of carcinogenicity involves several considerations of qualitative importance, including (i) the experimental conditions under which the test was performed, including route and schedule of exposure, species, strain, sex, age, duration of follow-up; (ii) the consistency of the results, for example, across species and target organ(s); (iii) the spectrum of neoplastic response, from preneoplastic lesions and benign tumours to malignant neoplasms; and (iv) the possible role of modifying factors.

As mentioned earlier (p. 11), the *Monographs* are not intended to summarize all published studies. Those studies in experimental animals that are inadequate (e.g. too short a duration, too few animals, poor survival; see below) or are judged irrelevant to the evaluation are generally omitted. Guidelines for conducting adequate long-term carcinogenicity experiments have been outlined (e.g. Montesano *et al.*, 1986).

Considerations of importance to the Working Group in the interpretation and evaluation of a particular study include: (i) how clearly the agent was defined and, in the case of mixtures, how adequately the sample characterization was reported; (ii) whether the dose was adequately monitored, particularly in inhalation experiments; (iii) whether the doses and duration of treatment were appropriate and whether the survival of treated animals was similar to that of controls; (iv) whether there were adequate numbers of animals per group; (v) whether animals of both sexes were used; (vi) whether animals were allocated randomly to groups; (vii) whether the duration of observation was adequate; and (viii) whether the data were adequately reported. If available, recent data on the incidence of specific tumours in historical controls, as well as in concurrent controls, should be taken into account in the evaluation of tumour response.

When benign tumours occur together with and originate from the same cell type in an organ or tissue as malignant tumours in a particular study and appear to represent a stage in the progression to malignancy, it may be valid to combine them in assessing tumour incidence (Huff *et al.*, 1989). The occurrence of lesions presumed to be preneoplastic may in certain instances aid in assessing the biological plausibility of any neoplastic response observed. If an agent or mixture induces only benign neoplasms that appear to be end-points that do not readily undergo transition to malignancy, it should nevertheless be suspected of being a carcinogen and requires further investigation.

(b) *Quantitative aspects*

The probability that tumours will occur may depend on the species, sex, strain and age of the animal, the dose of the carcinogen and the route and length of exposure. Evidence of an increased incidence of neoplasms with increased level of exposure strengthens the inference of a causal association between the exposure and the development of neoplasms.

The form of the dose–response relationship can vary widely, depending on the particular agent under study and the target organ. Both DNA damage and increased cell division are important aspects of carcinogenesis, and cell proliferation is a strong determinant of dose–

response relationships for some carcinogens (Cohen & Ellwein, 1990). Since many chemicals require metabolic activation before being converted into their reactive intermediates, both metabolic and pharmacokinetic aspects are important in determining the dose–response pattern. Saturation of steps such as absorption, activation, inactivation and elimination may produce nonlinearity in the dose–response relationship, as could saturation of processes such as DNA repair (Hoel *et al.*, 1983; Gart *et al.*, 1986).

(c) Statistical analysis of long-term experiments in animals

Factors considered by the Working Group include the adequacy of the information given for each treatment group: (i) the number of animals studied and the number examined histologically, (ii) the number of animals with a given tumour type and (iii) length of survival. The statistical methods used should be clearly stated and should be the generally accepted techniques refined for this purpose (Peto *et al.*, 1980; Gart *et al.*, 1986). When there is no difference in survival between control and treatment groups, the Working Group usually compares the proportions of animals developing each tumour type in each of the groups. Otherwise, consideration is given as to whether or not appropriate adjustments have been made for differences in survival. These adjustments can include: comparisons of the proportions of tumour-bearing animals among the effective number of animals (alive at the time the first tumour is discovered), in the case where most differences in survival occur before tumours appear; life-table methods, when tumours are visible or when they may be considered 'fatal' because mortality rapidly follows tumour development; and the Mantel-Haenszel test or logistic regression, when occult tumours do not affect the animals' risk of dying but are 'incidental' findings at autopsy.

In practice, classifying tumours as fatal or incidental may be difficult. Several survival-adjusted methods have been developed that do not require this distinction (Gart *et al.*, 1986), although they have not been fully evaluated.

10. OTHER DATA RELEVANT TO AN EVALUATION OF CARCINOGENICITY AND ITS MECHANISMS

In coming to an overall evaluation of carcinogenicity in humans (see p. 25), the Working Group also considers related data. The nature of the information selected for the summary depends on the agent being considered.

For chemicals and complex mixtures of chemicals such as those in some occupational situations and involving cultural habits (e.g. tobacco smoking), the other data considered to be relevant are divided into those on absorption, distribution, metabolism and excretion; toxic effects; reproductive and developmental effects; and genetic and related effects.

Concise information is given on absorption, distribution (including placental transfer) and excretion in both humans and experimental animals. Kinetic factors that may affect the dose–response relationship, such as saturation of uptake, protein binding, metabolic activation, detoxification and DNA repair processes, are mentioned. Studies that indicate the metabolic fate of the agent in humans and in experimental animals are summarized briefly, and comparisons of data from humans and animals are made when possible. Comparative information on the relationship between exposure and the dose that reaches the target site may be of particular importance for extrapolation between species. Data are given on acute and chronic toxic effects (other than cancer), such as organ toxicity, increased cell proliferation, immunotoxicity and endocrine effects. The presence and toxicological significance of cellular receptors is described. Effects on reproduction, teratogenicity, fetotoxicity and embryotoxicity are also summarized briefly.

Tests of genetic and related effects are described in view of the relevance of gene mutation and chromosomal damage to carcinogenesis (Vainio et al., 1992). The adequacy of the reporting of sample characterization is considered and, where necessary, commented upon; with regard to complex mixtures, such comments are similar to those described for animal carcinogenicity tests on p. 17. The available data are interpreted critically by phylogenetic group according to the end-points detected, which may include DNA damage, gene mutation, sister chromatid exchange, micronucleus formation, chromosomal aberrations, aneuploidy and cell transformation. The concentrations employed are given, and mention is made of whether use of an exogenous metabolic system *in vitro* affected the test result. These data are given as listings of test systems, data and references; bar graphs (activity profiles) and corresponding summary tables with detailed information on the preparation of the profiles (Waters et al., 1987) are given in appendices.

Positive results in tests using prokaryotes, lower eukaryotes, plants, insects and cultured mammalian cells suggest that genetic and related effects could occur in mammals. Results from such tests may also give information about the types of genetic effect produced and about the involvement of metabolic activation. Some end-points described are clearly genetic in nature (e.g. gene mutations and chromosomal aberrations), while others are to a greater or lesser degree associated with genetic effects (e.g. unscheduled DNA synthesis). In-vitro tests for tumour-promoting activity and for cell transformation may be sensitive to changes that are not necessarily the result of genetic alterations but that may have specific relevance to the process of carcinogenesis. A critical appraisal of these tests has been published (Montesano et al., 1986).

Genetic or other activity manifest in experimental mammals and humans is regarded as being of greater relevance than that in other organisms. The demonstration that an agent or mixture can induce gene and chromosomal mutations in whole mammals indicates that it may have carcinogenic activity, although this activity may not be detectably expressed in any or all species. Relative potency in tests for mutagenicity and related effects is not a reliable indicator of carcinogenic potency. Negative results in tests for mutagenicity in selected tissues from animals treated *in vivo* provide less weight, partly because they do not exclude the possibility of an effect in tissues other than those examined. Moreover, negative results in short-term tests with genetic end-points cannot be considered to provide evidence to rule out carcinogenicity of agents or mixtures that act through other mechanisms (e.g. receptor-mediated effects, cellular toxicity with regenerative proliferation, peroxisome proliferation) (Vainio et al., 1992). Factors that may lead to misleading results in short-term tests have been discussed in detail elsewhere (Montesano et al., 1986).

When available, data relevant to mechanisms of carcinogenesis that do not involve structural changes at the level of the gene are also described.

The adequacy of epidemiological studies of reproductive outcome and genetic and related effects in humans is evaluated by the same criteria as are applied to epidemiological studies of cancer.

Structure–activity relationships that may be relevant to an evaluation of the carcinogenicity of an agent are also described.

For biological agents—viruses, bacteria and parasites—other data relevant to carcinogenicity include descriptions of the pathology of infection, molecular biology (integration and expression of viruses, and any genetic alterations seen in human tumours) and other observations, which might include cellular and tissue responses to infection, immune response and the presence of tumour markers.

11. SUMMARY OF DATA REPORTED

In this section, the relevant epidemiological and experimental data are summarized. Only reports, other than in abstract form, that meet the criteria outlined on p. 11 are considered for evaluating carcinogenicity. Inadequate studies are generally not summarized: such studies are usually identified by a square-bracketed comment in the preceding text.

(a) Exposures

Human exposure to chemicals and complex mixtures is summarized on the basis of elements such as production, use, occurrence in the environment and determinations in human tissues and body fluids. Quantitative data are given when available. Exposure to biological agents is described in terms of transmission, and prevalence of infection.

(b) Carcinogenicity in humans

Results of epidemiological studies that are considered to be pertinent to an assessment of human carcinogenicity are summarized. When relevant, case reports and correlation studies are also summarized.

(c) Carcinogenicity in experimental animals

Data relevant to an evaluation of carcinogenicity in animals are summarized. For each animal species and route of administration, it is stated whether an increased incidence of neoplasms or preneoplastic lesions was observed, and the tumour sites are indicated. If the agent or mixture produced tumours after prenatal exposure or in single-dose experiments, this is also indicated. Negative findings are also summarized. Dose–response and other quantitative data may be given when available.

(d) Other data relevant to an evaluation of carcinogenicity and its mechanisms

Data on biological effects in humans that are of particular relevance are summarized. These may include toxicological, kinetic and metabolic considerations and evidence of DNA binding, persistence of DNA lesions or genetic damage in exposed humans. Toxicological information, such as that on cytotoxicity and regeneration, receptor binding and hormonal and immunological effects, and data on kinetics and metabolism in experimental animals are given when considered relevant to the possible mechanism of the carcinogenic action of the agent. The results of tests for genetic and related effects are summarized for whole mammals, cultured mammalian cells and nonmammalian systems.

When available, comparisons of such data for humans and for animals, and particularly animals that have developed cancer, are described.

Structure–activity relationships are mentioned when relevant.

For the agent, mixture or exposure circumstance being evaluated, the available data on endpoints or other phenomena relevant to mechanisms of carcinogenesis from studies in humans, experimental animals and tissue and cell test systems are summarized within one or more of the following descriptive dimensions:

(i) Evidence of genotoxicity (i.e. structural changes at the level of the gene): for example, structure–activity considerations, adduct formation, mutagenicity (effect on specific genes), chromosomal mutation/aneuploidy

(ii) Evidence of effects on the expression of relevant genes (i.e. functional changes at the intracellular level): for example, alterations to the structure or quantity of the product of a proto-oncogene or tumour suppressor gene, alterations to metabolic activation/inactivation/DNA repair

(iii) Evidence of relevant effects on cell behaviour (i.e. morphological or behavioural changes at the cellular or tissue level): for example, induction of mitogenesis, compensatory cell proliferation, preneoplasia and hyperplasia, survival of premalignant or malignant cells (immortalization, immunosuppression), effects on metastatic potential

(iv) Evidence from dose and time relationships of carcinogenic effects and interactions between agents: for example, early/late stage, as inferred from epidemiological studies; initiation/promotion/progression/malignant conversion, as defined in animal carcinogenicity experiments; toxicokinetics

These dimensions are not mutually exclusive, and an agent may fall within more than one of them. Thus, for example, the action of an agent on the expression of relevant genes could be summarized under both the first and second dimension, even if it were known with reasonable certainty that those effects resulted from genotoxicity.

12. EVALUATION

Evaluations of the strength of the evidence for carcinogenicity arising from human and experimental animal data are made, using standard terms.

It is recognized that the criteria for these evaluations, described below, cannot encompass all of the factors that may be relevant to an evaluation of carcinogenicity. In considering all of the relevant scientific data, the Working Group may assign the agent, mixture or exposure circumstance to a higher or lower category than a strict interpretation of these criteria would indicate.

(a) *Degrees of evidence for carcinogenicity in humans and in experimental animals and supporting evidence*

These categories refer only to the strength of the evidence that an exposure is carcinogenic and not to the extent of its carcinogenic activity (potency) nor to the mechanisms involved. A classification may change as new information becomes available.

An evaluation of degree of evidence, whether for a single agent or a mixture, is limited to the materials tested, as defined physically, chemically or biologically. When the agents evaluated are considered by the Working Group to be sufficiently closely related, they may be grouped together for the purpose of a single evaluation of degree of evidence.

(i) *Carcinogenicity in humans*

The applicability of an evaluation of the carcinogenicity of a mixture, process, occupation or industry on the basis of evidence from epidemiological studies depends on the variability over time and place of the mixtures, processes, occupations and industries. The Working Group seeks to identify the specific exposure, process or activity which is considered most likely to be responsible for any excess risk. The evaluation is focused as narrowly as the available data on exposure and other aspects permit.

The evidence relevant to carcinogenicity from studies in humans is classified into one of the following categories:

Sufficient evidence of carcinogenicity: The Working Group considers that a causal relationship has been established between exposure to the agent, mixture or exposure circumstance and human cancer. That is, a positive relationship has been observed between the exposure and cancer in studies in which chance, bias and confounding could be ruled out with reasonable confidence.

Limited evidence of carcinogenicity: A positive association has been observed between exposure to the agent, mixture or exposure circumstance and cancer for which a causal interpretation is considered by the Working Group to be credible, but chance, bias or confounding could not be ruled out with reasonable confidence.

Inadequate evidence of carcinogenicity: The available studies are of insufficient quality, consistency or statistical power to permit a conclusion regarding the presence or absence of a causal association, or no data on cancer in humans are available.

Evidence suggesting lack of carcinogenicity: There are several adequate studies covering the full range of levels of exposure that human beings are known to encounter, which are mutually consistent in not showing a positive association between exposure to the agent, mixture or exposure circumstance and any studied cancer at any observed level of exposure. A conclusion of 'evidence suggesting lack of carcinogenicity' is inevitably limited to the cancer sites, conditions and levels of exposure and length of observation covered by the available studies. In addition, the possibility of a very small risk at the levels of exposure studied can never be excluded.

In some instances, the above categories may be used to classify the degree of evidence related to carcinogenicity in specific organs or tissues.

(ii) Carcinogenicity in experimental animals

The evidence relevant to carcinogenicity in experimental animals is classified into one of the following categories:

Sufficient evidence of carcinogenicity: The Working Group considers that a causal relationship has been established between the agent or mixture and an increased incidence of malignant neoplasms or of an appropriate combination of benign and malignant neoplasms in (a) two or more species of animals or (b) in two or more independent studies in one species carried out at different times or in different laboratories or under different protocols.

Exceptionally, a single study in one species might be considered to provide sufficient evidence of carcinogenicity when malignant neoplasms occur to an unusual degree with regard to incidence, site, type of tumour or age at onset.

Limited evidence of carcinogenicity: The data suggest a carcinogenic effect but are limited for making a definitive evaluation because, e.g. (a) the evidence of carcinogenicity is restricted to a single experiment; or (b) there are unresolved questions regarding the adequacy of the design, conduct or interpretation of the study; or (c) the agent or mixture increases the incidence only of benign neoplasms or lesions of uncertain neoplastic potential, or of certain neoplasms which may occur spontaneously in high incidences in certain strains.

Inadequate evidence of carcinogenicity: The studies cannot be interpreted as showing either the presence or absence of a carcinogenic effect because of major qualitative or quantitative limitations, or no data on cancer in experimental animals are available.

Evidence suggesting lack of carcinogenicity: Adequate studies involving at least two species are available which show that, within the limits of the tests used, the agent or mixture is not carcinogenic. A conclusion of evidence suggesting lack of carcinogenicity is inevitably limited to the species, tumour sites and levels of exposure studied.

(b) Other data relevant to the evaluation of carcinogenicity and its mechanisms

Other evidence judged to be relevant to an evaluation of carcinogenicity and of sufficient importance to affect the overall evaluation is then described. This may include data on preneoplastic lesions, tumour pathology, genetic and related effects, structure–activity relationships, metabolism and pharmacokinetics, physicochemical parameters and analogous biological agents.

Data relevant to mechanisms of the carcinogenic action are also evaluated. The strength of the evidence that any carcinogenic effect observed is due to a particular mechanism is assessed, using terms such as weak, moderate or strong. Then, the Working Group assesses if that particular mechanism is likely to be operative in humans. The strongest indications that a particular mechanism operates in humans come from data on humans or biological specimens obtained from exposed humans. The data may be considered to be especially relevant if they show that the agent in question has caused changes in exposed humans that are on the causal pathway to carcinogenesis. Such data may, however, never become available, because it is at least conceivable that certain compounds may be kept from human use solely on the basis of evidence of their toxicity and/or carcinogenicity in experimental systems.

For complex exposures, including occupational and industrial exposures, the chemical composition and the potential contribution of carcinogens known to be present are considered by the Working Group in its overall evaluation of human carcinogenicity. The Working Group also determines the extent to which the materials tested in experimental systems are related to those to which humans are exposed.

(c) Overall evaluation

Finally, the body of evidence is considered as a whole, in order to reach an overall evaluation of the carcinogenicity to humans of an agent, mixture or circumstance of exposure.

An evaluation may be made for a group of chemical compounds that have been evaluated by the Working Group. In addition, when supporting data indicate that other, related compounds for which there is no direct evidence of capacity to induce cancer in humans or in animals may also be carcinogenic, a statement describing the rationale for this conclusion is added to the evaluation narrative; an additional evaluation may be made for this broader group of compounds if the strength of the evidence warrants it.

The agent, mixture or exposure circumstance is described according to the wording of one of the following categories, and the designated group is given. The categorization of an agent, mixture or exposure circumstance is a matter of scientific judgement, reflecting the strength of the evidence derived from studies in humans and in experimental animals and from other relevant data.

Group 1—The agent (mixture) is carcinogenic to humans.
The exposure circumstance entails exposures that are carcinogenic to humans.

This category is used when there is *sufficient evidence* of carcinogenicity in humans. Exceptionally, an agent (mixture) may be placed in this category when evidence in humans is less than sufficient but there is *sufficient evidence* of carcinogenicity in experimental animals and strong evidence in exposed humans that the agent (mixture) acts through a relevant mechanism of carcinogenicity.

Group 2

This category includes agents, mixtures and exposure circumstances for which, at one extreme, the degree of evidence of carcinogenicity in humans is almost sufficient, as well as those for which, at the other extreme, there are no human data but for which there is evidence of carcinogenicity in experimental animals. Agents, mixtures and exposure circumstances are assigned to either group 2A (probably carcinogenic to humans) or group 2B (possibly carcinogenic to humans) on the basis of epidemiological and experimental evidence of carcinogenicity and other relevant data.

Group 2A—The agent (mixture) is probably carcinogenic to humans.
The exposure circumstance entails exposures that are probably carcinogenic to humans.

This category is used when there is *limited evidence* of carcinogenicity in humans and sufficient evidence of carcinogenicity in experimental animals. In some cases, an agent (mixture) may be classified in this category when there is inadequate evidence of carcinogenicity in humans and *sufficient evidence* of carcinogenicity in experimental animals and strong evidence that the carcinogenesis is mediated by a mechanism that also operates in humans. Exceptionally, an agent, mixture or exposure circumstance may be classified in this category solely on the basis of limited evidence of carcinogenicity in humans.

Group 2B—The agent (mixture) is possibly carcinogenic to humans.
The exposure circumstance entails exposures that are possibly carcinogenic to humans.

This category is used for agents, mixtures and exposure circumstances for which there is *limited evidence* of carcinogenicity in humans and less than *sufficient evidence* of carcinogenicity in experimental animals. It may also be used when there is *inadequate evidence* of carcinogenicity in humans but there is *sufficient evidence* of carcinogenicity in experimental animals. In some instances, an agent, mixture or exposure circumstance for which there is *inadequate evidence* of carcinogenicity in humans but *limited evidence* of carcinogenicity in experimental animals together with supporting evidence from other relevant data may be placed in this group.

Group 3—The agent (mixture or exposure circumstance) is not classifiable as to its carcinogenicity to humans.

This category is used most commonly for agents, mixtures and exposure circumstances for which the evidence of carcinogenicity is inadequate in humans and inadequate or limited in experimental animals.

Exceptionally, agents (mixtures) for which the evidence of carcinogenicity is inadequate in humans but sufficient in experimental animals may be placed in this category when there is strong evidence that the mechanism of carcinogenicity in experimental animals does not operate in humans.

Agents, mixtures and exposure circumstances that do not fall into any other group are also placed in this category.

Group 4—The agent (mixture) is probably not carcinogenic to humans.

This category is used for agents or mixtures for which there is *evidence suggesting lack of carcinogenicity* in humans and in experimental animals. In some instances, agents or mixtures for which there is *inadequate evidence* of carcinogenicity in humans but *evidence suggesting lack of carcinogenicity* in experimental animals, consistently and strongly supported by a broad range of other relevant data, may be classified in this group.

References

Breslow, N.E. & Day, N.E. (1980) *Statistical Methods in Cancer Research*, Vol. 1, *The Analysis of Case–Control Studies* (IARC Scientific Publications No. 32), Lyon, IARC

Breslow, N.E. & Day, N.E. (1987) *Statistical Methods in Cancer Research*, Vol. 2, *The Design and Analysis of Cohort Studies* (IARC Scientific Publications No. 82), Lyon, IARC

Cohen, S.M. & Ellwein, L.B. (1990) Cell proliferation in carcinogenesis. *Science*, **249**, 1007–1011

Gart, J.J., Krewski, D., Lee, P.N., Tarone, R.E. & Wahrendorf, J. (1986) *Statistical Methods in Cancer Research*, Vol. 3, *The Design and Analysis of Long-term Animal Experiments* (IARC Scientific Publications No. 79), Lyon, IARC

Hoel, D.G., Kaplan, N.L. & Anderson, M.W. (1983) Implication of nonlinear kinetics on risk estimation in carcinogenesis. *Science*, **219**, 1032–1037

Huff, J.E., Eustis, S.L. & Haseman, J.K. (1989) Occurrence and relevance of chemically induced benign neoplasms in long-term carcinogenicity studies. *Cancer Metastasis Rev.*, **8**, 1–21

IARC (1973–1994) *Information Bulletin on the Survey of Chemicals Being Tested for Carcinogenicity/Directory of Agents Being Tested for Carcinogenicity*, Numbers 1–16, Lyon

    Number 1 (1973)   52 pages
    Number 2 (1973)   77 pages
    Number 3 (1974)   67 pages
    Number 4 (1974)   97 pages
    Number 5 (1975)   8 pages
    Number 6 (1976)   360 pages
    Number 7 (1978)   460 pages
    Number 8 (1979)   604 pages
    Number 9 (1981)   294 pages
    Number 10 (1983) 326 pages
    Number 11 (1984) 370 pages
    Number 12 (1986) 385 pages
    Number 13 (1988) 404 pages
    Number 14 (1990) 369 pages
    Number 15 (1992) 317 pages
    Number 16 (1994) 293 pages

IARC (1976–1994)

Directory of On-going Research in Cancer Epidemiology 1976. Edited by C.S. Muir & G. Wagner, Lyon

Directory of On-going Research in Cancer Epidemiology 1977 (IARC Scientific Publications No. 17). Edited by C.S. Muir & G. Wagner, Lyon

Directory of On-going Research in Cancer Epidemiology 1978 (IARC Scientific Publications No. 26). Edited by C.S. Muir & G. Wagner, Lyon

Directory of On-going Research in Cancer Epidemiology 1979 (IARC Scientific Publications No. 28). Edited by C.S. Muir & G. Wagner, Lyon

Directory of On-going Research in Cancer Epidemiology 1980 (IARC Scientific Publications No. 35). Edited by C.S. Muir & G. Wagner, Lyon

Directory of On-going Research in Cancer Epidemiology 1981 (IARC Scientific Publications No. 38). Edited by C.S. Muir & G. Wagner, Lyon

Directory of On-going Research in Cancer Epidemiology 1982 (IARC Scientific Publications No. 46). Edited by C.S. Muir & G. Wagner, Lyon

Directory of On-going Research in Cancer Epidemiology 1983 (IARC Scientific Publications No. 50). Edited by C.S. Muir & G. Wagner, Lyon

Directory of On-going Research in Cancer Epidemiology 1984 (IARC Scientific Publications No. 62). Edited by C.S. Muir & G. Wagner, Lyon

Directory of On-going Research in Cancer Epidemiology 1985 (IARC Scientific Publications No. 69). Edited by C.S. Muir & G. Wagner, Lyon

Directory of On-going Research in Cancer Epidemiology 1986 (IARC Scientific Publications No. 80). Edited by C.S. Muir & G. Wagner, Lyon

Directory of On-going Research in Cancer Epidemiology 1987 (IARC Scientific Publications No. 86). Edited by D.M. Parkin & J. Wahrendorf, Lyon

Directory of On-going Research in Cancer Epidemiology 1988 (IARC Scientific Publications No. 93). Edited by M. Coleman & J. Wahrendorf, Lyon

Directory of On-going Research in Cancer Epidemiology 1989/90 (IARC Scientific Publications No. 101). Edited by M. Coleman & J. Wahrendorf, Lyon

Directory of On-going Research in Cancer Epidemiology 1991 (IARC Scientific Publications No.110). Edited by M. Coleman & J. Wahrendorf, Lyon

Directory of On-going Research in Cancer Epidemiology 1992 (IARC Scientific Publications No. 117). Edited by M. Coleman, J. Wahrendorf & E. Démaret, Lyon

Directory of On-going Research in Cancer Epidemiology 1994 (IARC Scientific Publications No. 130). Edited by R. Sankaranarayanan, J. Wahrendorf & E. Démaret, Lyon

IARC (1977) *IARC Monographs Programme on the Evaluation of the Carcinogenic Risk of Chemicals to Humans*. Preamble (IARC intern. tech. Rep. No. 77/002), Lyon

IARC (1978) *Chemicals with* Sufficient Evidence *of Carcinogenicity in Experimental Animals*—IARC Monographs *Volumes 1–17* (IARC intern. tech. Rep. No. 78/003), Lyon

IARC (1978–1993) *Environmental Carcinogens. Methods of Analysis and Exposure Measurement*:

Vol. 1. *Analysis of Volatile Nitrosamines in Food* (IARC Scientific Publications No. 18). Edited by R. Preussmann, M. Castegnaro, E.A. Walker & A.E. Wasserman (1978)

Vol. 2. *Methods for the Measurement of Vinyl Chloride in Poly(vinyl chloride), Air, Water and Foodstuffs* (IARC Scientific Publications No. 22). Edited by D.C.M. Squirrell & W. Thain (1978)

Vol. 3. Analysis of Polycyclic Aromatic Hydrocarbons in Environmental Samples (IARC Scientific Publications No. 29). Edited by M. Castegnaro, P. Bogovski, H. Kunte & E.A. Walker (1979)

Vol. 4. *Some Aromatic Amines and Azo Dyes in the General and Industrial Environment* (IARC Scientific Publications No. 40). Edited by L. Fishbein, M. Castegnaro, I.K. O'Neill & H. Bartsch (1981)

Vol. 5. *Some Mycotoxins* (IARC Scientific Publications No. 44). Edited by L. Stoloff, M. Castegnaro, P. Scott, I.K. O'Neill & H. Bartsch (1983)

Vol. 6. *N-Nitroso Compounds* (IARC Scientific Publications No. 45). Edited by R. Preussmann, I.K. O'Neill, G. Eisenbrand, B. Spiegelhalder & H. Bartsch (1983)

Vol. 7. *Some Volatile Halogenated Hydrocarbons* (IARC Scientific Publications No. 68). Edited by L. Fishbein & I.K. O'Neill (1985)

Vol. 8. *Some Metals: As, Be, Cd, Cr, Ni, Pb, Se, Zn* (IARC Scientific Publications No. 71). Edited by I.K. O'Neill, P. Schuller & L. Fishbein (1986)

Vol. 9. *Passive Smoking* (IARC Scientific Publications No. 81). Edited by I.K. O'Neill, K.D. Brunnemann, B. Dodet & D. Hoffmann (1987)

Vol. 10. *Benzene and Alkylated Benzenes* (IARC Scientific Publications No. 85). Edited by L. Fishbein & I.K. O'Neill (1988)

Vol. 11. *Polychlorinated Dioxins and Dibenzofurans)* (IARC Scientific Publications No. 108). Edited by C. Rappe, H.R. Buser, B. Dodet & I.K. O'Neill (1991)

Vol. 12. *Indoor Air* (IARC Scientific Publications No. 109). Edited by B. Seifert, H. van de Wiel, B. Dodet & I.K. O'Neill (1993)

IARC (1979) *Criteria to Select Chemicals for* IARC Monographs (IARC intern. tech. Rep. No. 79/003), Lyon

IARC (1982) *IARC Monographs on the Evaluation of the Carcinogenic Risk of Chemicals to Humans, Supplement 4, Chemicals, Industrial Processes and Industries Associated with Cancer in Humans* (IARC Monographs, Volumes 1 to 29), Lyon

IARC (1983) *Approaches to Classifying Chemical Carcinogens According to Mechanism of Action* (IARC intern. tech. Rep. No. 83/001), Lyon

IARC (1984) *Chemicals and Exposures to Complex Mixtures Recommended for Evaluation in IARC Monographs and Chemicals and Complex Mixtures Recommended for Long-term Carcinogenicity Testing* (IARC intern. tech. Rep. No. 84/002), Lyon

IARC (1987a) *IARC Monographs on the Evaluation of Carcinogenic Risks to Humans, Supplement 6, Genetic and Related Effects: An Updating of Selected* IARC Monographs *from Volumes 1 to 42*, Lyon

IARC (1987b) *IARC Monographs on the Evaluation of Carcinogenic Risks to Humans, Supplement 7, Overall Evaluations of Carcinogenicity: An Updating of* IARC Monographs *Volumes 1 to 42*, Lyon

IARC (1988) *Report of an IARC Working Group to Review the Approaches and Processes Used to Evaluate the Carcinogenicity of Mixtures and Groups of Chemicals* (IARC intern. tech. Rep.No. 88/002), Lyon

IARC (1989) *Chemicals, Groups of Chemicals, Mixtures and Exposure Circumstances to be Evaluated in Future IARC Monographs, Report of an ad hoc Working Group* (IARC intern. tech. Rep. No. 89/004), Lyon

IARC (1991a) *A Consensus Report of an IARC Monographs Working Group on the Use of Mechanisms of Carcinogenesis in Risk Identification* (IARC intern. tech. Rep. No. 91/002), Lyon

IARC (1991b) *Report of an Ad-hoc* IARC Monographs *Advisory Group on Viruses and Other Biological Agents Such as Parasites* (IARC intern. tech. Rep. No. 91/001), Lyon

IARC (1993) *Chemicals, Groups of Chemicals, Complex Mixtures, Physical and Biological Agents and Exposure Circumstances to be Evaluated in Future* IARC Monographs, *Report of an ad-hoc Working Group* (IARC intern. Rep. No. 93/005), Lyon

Montesano, R., Bartsch, H., Vainio, H., Wilbourn, J. & Yamasaki, H., eds (1986) *Long-term and Short-term Assays for Carcinogenesis—A Critical Appraisal* (IARC Scientific Publications No. 83), Lyon, IARC

Peto, R., Pike, M.C., Day, N.E., Gray, R.G., Lee, P.N., Parish, S., Peto, J., Richards, S. & Wahrendorf, J. (1980) Guidelines for simple, sensitive significance tests for carcinogenic effects in long-term animal experiments. In: *IARC Monographs on the Evaluation of the Carcinogenic Risk of Chemicals to Humans, Supplement 2, Long-term and Short-term Screening Assays for Carcinogens: A Critical Appraisal*, Lyon, pp. 311–426

Tomatis, L., Aitio, A., Wilbourn, J. & Shuker, L. (1989) Human carcinogens so far identified. *Jpn. J. Cancer Res.*, **80**, 795–807

Vainio, H., Magee, P., McGregor, D. & McMichael, A., eds (1992) *Mechanisms of Carcinogenesis in Risk Identification* (IARC Scientific Publications No. 116), Lyon, IARC

Vainio, H., Wilbourn, J.D., Sasco, A.J., Partensky, C., Gaudin, N., Heseltine, E. & Eragne, I. (1995) Identification of human carcinogenic risk in *IARC Monographs*. *Bull. Cancer*, **82**, 339–348 (in French)

Waters, M.D., Stack, H.F., Brady, A.L., Lohman, P.H.M., Haroun, L. & Vainio, H. (1987) Appendix 1. Activity profiles for genetic and related tests. In: *IARC Monographs on the Evaluation of Carcinogenic Risks to Humans*, Suppl. 6, *Genetic and Related Effects: An Updating of Selected IARC Monographs from Volumes 1 to 42*, Lyon, IARC, pp. 687–696

Wilbourn, J., Haroun, L., Heseltine, E., Kaldor, J., Partensky, C. & Vainio, H. (1986) Response of experimental animals to human carcinogens: an analysis based upon the IARC Monographs Programme. *Carcinogenesis*, **7**, 1853–1863

GENERAL REMARKS

This sixty-fourth volume of the *IARC Monographs on the Evaluation of Carcinogenic Risks to Humans* considers human papillomaviruses (HPVs).

Interest in the carcinogenicity of HPV first arose from studies of cervical cancer. Cervix cancer is the second most common cancer in women world-wide and there are about 400,000 new cases and 200,000 deaths from cervical cancer every year. It would probably be even more common if effective screening procedures for precursor lesions did not exist. HPV-16 was first isolated and characterized in 1983 from a cervical cancer specimen. To date, more than 70 HPV types have been identified and over 15 of them have been reported in cervical cancer biopsies.

These agents are unique in the *IARC Monographs* series for wealth of both epidemiological and mechanistic investigations. More than 100 epidemiological case–control or cohort studies have been reported and several more are still underway. In addition, a great deal of information is available on the molecular mechanisms employed by the virus and the host, and HPV is probably the best understood of any putative human carcinogen at the mechanistic level.

The findings in cervical cancer have led to studies of HPV at other anogenital sites and more remote sites. Of particular note are studies in skin cancer, for which a different range of types have been found. In addition, a number of closely related papillomaviruses infect animals and there is a large experimental literature for these viruses.

Improved screening, and ultimately vaccination, offer prospects for the eventual elimination of this cancer.

HUMAN PAPILLOMAVIRUSES

1. Human papillomavirus (HPV) infection

1.1 Structure and molecular biology of human papillomaviruses

1.1.1 Structure of the viruses

HPVs form icosahedral non-enveloped particles with a diameter of approximately 55 nm. They contain a double-stranded, circular and covalently closed DNA genome of 7500–8000 base pairs (bp) (about 4950–5280 kDa), which is complexed by cellular histones (Klug & Finch, 1965; Pfister, 1987; Baker *et al.*, 1991; Pfister & Fuchs, 1994). Papillomaviruses are resistant to organic solvents and to heating at 56 °C (Bonnez *et al.*, 1994a). Virus particles have a buoyant density of 1.34 g/ml in caesium chloride and a sedimentation coefficient ($S_{20,w}$) of 300 (Crawford & Crawford, 1963; Pfister *et al.*, 1977).

Since papillomaviruses cannot be grown efficiently in tissue culture, studies on the architecture of the virus particles were originally restricted to those viruses that can be obtained from naturally occurring tumours, such as bovine papillomavirus (BPV), human papillomavirus type 1 (HPV-1) and cotton-tail rabbit papillomavirus (CRPV) (Crawford & Crawford, 1963; Finch & Klug, 1965; Klug & Finch, 1965; Favre *et al.*, 1975; Pfister *et al.*, 1977). More recently, it was demonstrated that virus-like particles of BPV-1, CRPV, HPV-1, -6, -11, -16, -18 and -33 can be obtained by expression of the structural proteins in recombinant vectors such as vaccinia or baculoviruses (Zhou *et al.*, 1991a; Kirnbauer *et al.*, 1992; Hagensee *et al.*, 1993; Kirnbauer *et al.*, 1993; Rose *et al.*, 1993; Christensen *et al.*, 1994a; Le Cann *et al.*, 1994; Pfister & Fuchs, 1994; Rose *et al.*, 1994a; Volpers *et al.*, 1994). The major capsid protein, L1, appears to be sufficient for particle formation (Kirnbauer *et al.*, 1993). The antigenic and structural properties of virus-like particles were shown to be similar to those of virions (Hagensee *et al.*, 1993; Christensen *et al.*, 1994b; Rose *et al.*, 1994a,b).

The virus capsid is composed of 72 capsomeres, which are arranged on an icosahedral surface lattice. Sixty of the capsomeres are six-coordinated and the remaining 12 are five-coordinated (Finch & Klug, 1965; Klug & Finch, 1965; Pfister & Fuchs, 1994). Analysis by cryo-electron microscopy has been performed on BPV-1 and HPV-1 particles (Baker *et al.*, 1991). Capsomeres consist of a trunk with distal and proximal thickening. They associate at their base and project radially. Within each capsomere a central cylindrical channel can be visualized. Capsomeres exhibit a fivefold symmetry and, therefore, are composed of five identical molecules — most likely to be molecules of the L1 protein, which makes up about 90% of the total protein (Favre *et al.*, 1975; Doorbar & Gallimore, 1987; Pfister & Fuchs, 1994).

The L1 proteins have a molecular mass of about 55 000 and are highly conserved among all papillomaviruses. Glycosylation of L1 protein of BPV-1 and HPV-16 (expressed by a recombinant vaccinia virus) has been reported, but the role of this modification in particle formation is unclear as yet (Mose Larsen *et al.*, 1987; Browne *et al.*, 1988; Zhou *et al.*, 1993; Pfister & Fuchs, 1994).

The minor structural proteins, L2, have a molecular mass of about 75 kDa and are less-well conserved among papillomaviruses. Their position within the virus particle is not clear but their N-terminus has been shown to bind DNA in a sequence-independent manner, which suggests a role of L2 in packaging of the HPV genome (Komly et al., 1986; Pfister & Fuchs, 1994; Zhou et al., 1994).

1.1.2 Taxonomy

Papillomaviruses have been placed as a subfamily (Shah & Howley, 1992) together with polyomaviruses in the family Papovaviridae. Both groups of viruses have capsids with similar structure and double-stranded, circular, covalently closed DNA genomes. It is now known that the genome size and organization differ between the two virus groups and that there is no significant amount of nucleotide or amino acid sequence homology between individual viral genes, with the possible exception of some small protein domains (Clertant & Seif, 1984; Phelps et al., 1988). For these reasons the two groups should therefore be considered to be unrelated and placed in separate families (for a review, see Bernard et al., 1994a).

There have been several reviews of the classification of papillomaviruses, both by phenotypic aspects and sequence similarities (Chan et al., 1992a; Van Ranst et al., 1992a; Bernard et al., 1994a; Myers et al., 1994; de Villiers, 1994; Chan et al., 1995). Different papillomaviruses are classified as 'types'. HPV types are defined by genomic analyses and therefore represent genotypes. Currently they are not classified by serology, and, therefore, the term 'serotype' is inappropriate (see section 1.2). At present, a novel HPV genome is described as a new HPV type if the nucleotide sequences of its *E6*, *E7* and *L1* genes (i.e. about one-third of the genome) differ by more than 10% from those of any previously described HPV type (de Villiers, 1994). Although this definition was established arbitrarily, it appears to be sufficient to define the natural taxonomic units — most recent isolates have been either almost identical to previously described HPV types, differing by less than 2%, or novel. The former are referred to as 'variants' or 'subtypes' (Gissmann et al., 1983; Deau et al., 1993; Ho et al., 1993a,b; Ong et al., 1993), as defined by nucleotide sequence comparison rather than by phenotypic analyses (see below). Two pairs of HPV types (HPV-34/64, HPV-44/55) differ by less than 10% of their nucleotide sequences, but their historic taxonomic status has not been revised (Chan et al., 1995).

To date, 70 HPV types have been described (Table 1) and their clinical origins and genomic sequences have been reviewed (de Villiers, 1989; Delius & Hofmann, 1994; Van Ranst et al., 1994; de Villiers, 1994). The genomic sequences are available in EMBL (European Molecular and Biological Laboratory) and GenBank databases and are edited by the HPV Sequence Database at the National Laboratory at Los Alamos (Myers et al., 1994). Studies of partial genomic sequences predict the existence of additional HPV types (Bernard et al., 1994a,b; Shamanin et al., 1994a; Berkhout et al., 1995).

Taxonomic orders based on similarities in sequence of *E6*, *E7* and *L1* genes helped to identify groupings of related HPVs (Pfister & Fuchs, 1994). At the level of greatest diversity ('major branches'), five supergroups of papillomaviruses can be distinguished, of which three contain HPVs (supergroups A, B and E) (Chan et al., 1995). Figure 1 shows these relationships in the form of a phylogenetic tree. This tree is based on nucleotide sequence comparisons and, at least on the level of supergroups, does not strictly reflect phenotypic or pathogenic similarities or differences.

Table 1. Taxonomic association and origin of HPV types 1 to 70

HPV type	Taxonomic status (supergroup)[a]	Origin of cloned genome[b,c]	HPV type	Taxonomic status (supergroup)[a]	Origin of cloned genome[b,c]
HPV-1	E	Verruca plantaris	HPV-38	B	Malignant melanoma
HPV-2	A	Verruca vulgaris	HPV-39	A	PIN
HPV-3	A	Verruca plana	HPV-40	A	PIN
HPV-4	B	Verruca vulgaris	HPV-41	E	Disseminated warts
HPV-5	B	EV lesion	HPV-42	A	Vulvar papilloma
HPV-6	A	Condyloma acuminatum	HPV-43	A	Vulvar hyperplasia
HPV-7	A	Butcher's wart	HPV-44	A	Vulvar condyloma
HPV-8	B	EV lesion	HPV-45	A	CIN
HPV-9	B	EV lesion	HPV-46 (= HPV-20b) (not recognized as separate type)		
HPV-10	A	Verruca plana	HPV-47	B	EV lesion
HPV-11	A	Laryngeal papilloma	HPV-48	B	Cutaneous squamous-cell carcinoma
HPV-12	B	EV lesion			
HPV-13	A	Focal epithelial hyperplasia	HPV-49	B	Verruca plana
HPV-14	B	EV lesion	HPV-50	B	EV lesion
HPV-15	B	EV lesion	HPV-51	A	CIN
HPV-16	A	Cervical carcinoma	HPV-52	A	CIN
HPV-17	B	EV lesion	HPV-53	A	Normal cervical mucosa
HPV-18	A	Cervical carcinoma	HPV-54	A	Condyloma acuminatum
HPV-19	B	EV lesion	HPV-55	A	Bowenoid papulosis
HPV-20	B	EV lesion	HPV-56	A	CIN, cervical carcinoma
HPV-21	B	EV lesion	HPV-57	A	Inverted papilloma of the maxillary sinus
HPV-22	B	EV lesion			
HPV-23	B	EV lesion			
HPV-24	B	EV lesion	HPV-58	A	CIN
HPV-25	B	EV lesion	HPV-59	A	VIN
HPV-26	A	Verruca vulgaris	HPV-60	B	Epidermoid cyst
HPV-27	A	Verruca vulgaris	HPV-61	A	VaIN
HPV-28	A	Verruca plana	HPV-62	A	VaIN
HPV-29	A	Verruca vulgaris	HPV-63	E	Myrmecia
HPV-30	A	Laryngeal carcinoma	HPV-64	A	VaIN
HPV-31	A	CIN	HPV-65	B	Pigmented wart
HPV-32	A	Focal epithelial hyperplasia	HPV-66	A	Cervical carcinoma
HPV-33	A	Cervical carcinoma	HPV-67	A	VaIN
HPV-34	A	Bowen's disease	HPV-68	A	Genital lesion
HPV-35	A	Cervical carcinoma	HPV-69	A	CIN
HPV-36	B	Actinic keratosis	HPV-70	A	Vulvar papilloma
HPV-37	B	Keratoacanthoma			

[a] For details of the taxonomy, see section 1.1.2, Figure 1 and Chan et al. (1995)
[b] For references concerning the cloning of these HPV types, see de Villiers (1989, 1994)
[c] EV, epidermodysplasia verruciformis; CIN, cervical intraepithelial neoplasia; VIN, vulvar intraepithelial neoplasia; VaIN, vaginal intraepithelial neoplasia; PIN, penile intraepithelial neoplasia

Figure 1. Relationship among 95 human and animal papillomaviruses, in the form of a phylogenetic tree

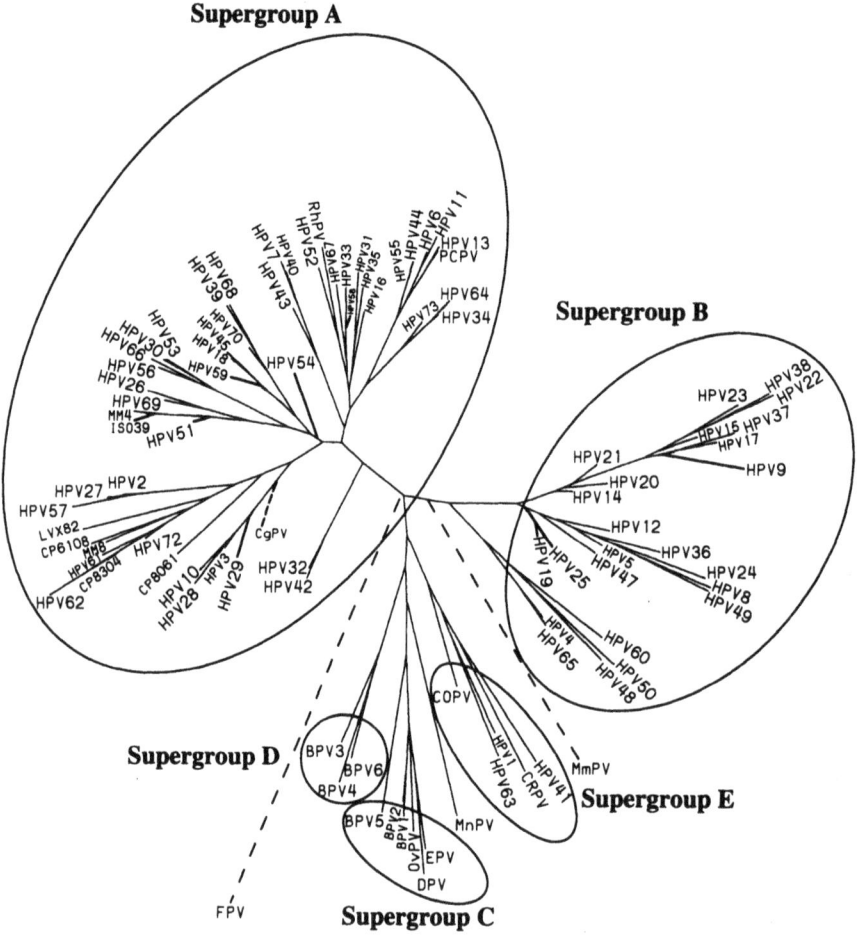

From Chan *et al.* (1995)

The largest supergroup, A, includes 44 HPV types and seven additional but untyped genomes (Chan *et al.*, 1995). These types are phenotypically heterogeneous. In addition to all the HPV types that are found mostly in genital lesions, supergroup A contains several HPV types (e.g. HPV-2), that are normally associated with non-genital lesions such as common warts. The supergroup also includes HPV-7, which is normally found in 'butcher's warts' (Orth *et al.*, 1981; Ostrow *et al.*, 1981). Eleven groups can be distinguished within supergroup A, most of which unite phenotypically and pathologically similar HPV types. One of these groups contains HPV-16, -31, -33 and -35 and another contains HPV-18 and -45, the HPV types most frequently reported in association with malignant genital lesions. Yet another group contains HPV-6 and -11, which induce genital warts and other benign genital lesions as well as laryngeal papillomas.

Supergroup B contains most of the HPV types associated with epidermodysplasia verruciformis (EV) such as HPV-5 and -8 (but with the exception of HPV-3 and -10, which are associated with verruca plana of EV-patients, although these viruses belong taxonomically to supergroup A). Phenotypically, this group is also not homogeneous as it includes several HPV types, such as HPV-4, that are found in cutaneous lesions of individuals not afflicted by EV. These HPV types are found on a separate branch remotely related to the other EV-HPVs. Recently, numerous novel HPV genomes, which also belong to the supergroup B, have been identified in squamous-cell carcinomas of immunosuppressed patients (Shamanin et al., 1994a; Berkhout et al., 1995).

1.1.3 Genomic variability

Genomic variability has been studied in detail in HPV-5 (Deau et al., 1993), HPV-6, -11 (Kitasato et al., 1994; Heinzel et al., 1995), HPV-8 (Deau et al., 1991), HPV-16 (Icenogle et al., 1991; Eschle et al., 1992; Ho et al., 1993a,b), HPV-18 and -45 (Ong et al., 1993). For these HPV types, the variability of the nucleotide sequence does not exceed 2% in coding and 5% in non-coding regions. The genomes of papillomaviruses evolve at rates at least five orders of magnitude slower than those of some RNA viruses, and 1% of genomic variability may originate over a period exceeding 100 000 years. Some particular genomic variants have been reported throughout the world and other variants appear to segregate according to ethnic groups. These findings strongly suggest that the known HPV types have existed in nearly identical molecular form since the beginning of the human species (Ong et al., 1993). Databases of genomic variation of HPV types are powerful tools for biomedical research because they allow for more refined studies of the epidemiology and pathology of HPV infection (Ho et al., 1993b).

Some nucleotide differences found in HPV-16 variants cause changes in amino acid codons (Icenogle et al., 1991; Chan et al., 1992b; Eschle et al., 1992). Examples of functional and antigenic alterations of L1 or L2 proteins of HPV-6 and -16 have been described (Kirnbauer et al., 1993; Yaegashi et al., 1993). Mutations altering binding sites for the transcription repressor YY1 have been recovered for HPV-16-associated cancers (May et al., 1994). Consistent variation in the HPV-16 E6 protein sequence has been observed in cervical cancers, which alters the peptide epitope for HLA-B7 in a way likely to influence immune recognition by cytological T cells (Ellis et al., 1995).

1.1.4 Host range

Papillomaviruses are highly specific for their respective hosts. No HPV type has been detected in any host other than humans, and, of the ~20 animal papillomaviruses described so far (one isolated from a bird, the others from different mammals; see section 4), most have been found in a single host species. Exceptions are the bovine papillomavirus types 1 and 2, which are also associated with equine sarcoids (see section 4). Hypotheses addressing specific interactions between viral and cellular proteins determining host specificity have been proposed (Shadan & Villarreal, 1993).

1.1.5 Related animal papillomaviruses

Phylogenetic studies suggest that papillomaviruses have co-evolved with their animal hosts. Lesions with a likely papillomavirus etiology are widespread among different taxa (Sundberg, 1987), but so far the genomes of only about 20 mammalian papillomaviruses have been cloned.

Four papillomavirus genomes have been cloned from monkeys and apes (O'Banion *et al.*, 1987; Kloster *et al.*, 1988; Ostrow *et al.*, 1991; Reszka *et al.*, 1991; Van Ranst *et al.*, 1992b), and, as each of them is related to an individual HPV type, they may form the basis for useful animal models for the pathogenicity of HPV (Ostrow *et al.*, 1991).

The molecular biology of two animal papillomaviruses, CRPV (Shope & Hurst, 1933) and BPV-1 (Lancaster & Olson, 1978) have been studied intensively. Methods developed in these studies have become powerful tools for the study of the molecular biology of HPVs (for a review, see Lambert *et al.*, 1988). Although sequence alignments show only a small residual degree of similarity, it is likely that most, if not all, genes of BPV-1 correspond to those of HPV-16 and other genital HPV types. Consequently, the biology of BPV-1 proteins, such as those encoded by the *E1, E2, E4, E5, L1* and *L2* genes, can be considered as a model to understand HPV proteins. Important phenotypic differences exist, however, with a particularly large divergence of the transforming proteins E6 and E7 and of *cis*-responsive elements.

1.1.6 Target tissues

All papillomaviruses infect epithelial cells and, with the exception of the ungulate-specific fibro-papillomaviruses (e.g. BPV-1) which also infect dermal fibroblasts, they are restricted to this target cell population. The mechanism for this restriction is not clear since papillomavirus particles attach to and are taken up by cells derived from different tissues and different species (Roden *et al.*, 1994a; Müller *et al.*, 1995a). Epithelial-specific transcription activation is likely to play an important role in the selection of epithelial target cells (Cripe *et al.*, 1987; Gloss *et al.*, 1987).

1.1.7 Genomic structure and properties of gene products

The circular DNA genome of all papillomaviruses can be divided into three segments of unequal size. The long control region (LCR), also called the upstream regulatory region (URR) or non-coding region (NCR), represents about 10% of the genome (see section 1.1.8). The early (*E*) and late (*L*) genes are coded by about 50 and 40% of the genome, respectively.

The terms 'early' and 'late' genes are used for historical reasons rather than meaning a strict sequential expression of genes. For example, the product of the *E4* gene seems to play a role late during the course of viral infection. The *L* genes both code for viral capsid proteins, whereas the *E* genes encode proteins with a variety of regulatory functions. The two *L* genes, *L1* and *L2*, each encode a single protein. Of the *E* genes, three, *E4, E5* and *E7*, apparently encode single polypeptide chains. The other three open reading frames, *E1, E2* and *E6*, give rise to more than one protein through differential splicing (at least in some papillomavirus types). Figure 2 is a schematic representation of a typical papillomavirus genome and indicates the functions of the encoded proteins (for review, see Galloway & McDougall, 1989).

Figure 2. Genome organization of papillomaviruses

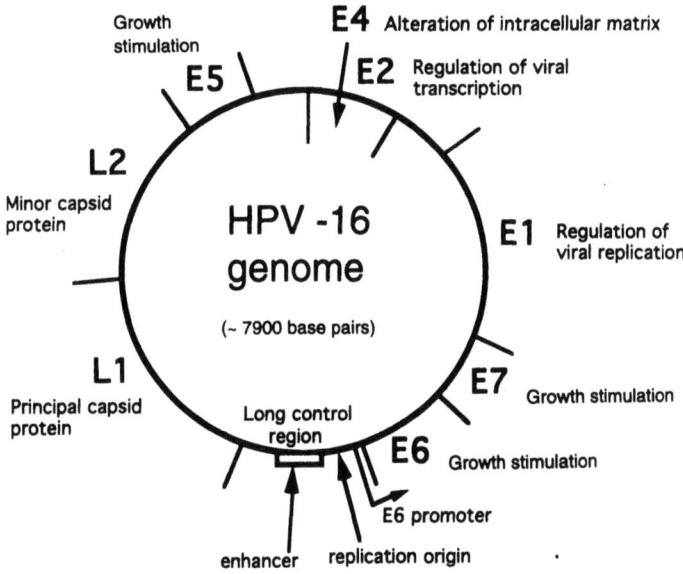

Genes *E5*, *E6* and *E7* encode proteins with growth-stimulating functions. The properties of these proteins, which are relevant for the carcinogenicity of the virus, are summarized briefly here and are discussed in detail in section 3.1.3.

The *E5* gene is located at the 3´ end of the early region, downstream from the *E2* gene, and is probably expressed through a polycistronic mRNA that also encodes E2. E5 proteins are small polypeptides, 44 amino acids in BPV-1 and nearly twice that size in genital HPVs. Although they lack extensive homology they are all extremely hydrophobic and are located within the lipid bilayer of the cellular membranes. They interact with transmembrane domains of receptor kinases, thereby altering their half-life and responses to ligands (Horwitz *et al.*, 1989; Martin *et al.*, 1989; Conrad *et al.*, 1993). E5 proteins bind specifically to a 16 kDa cellular protein, which is a component of vacuolar ATPases (Goldstein *et al.*, 1991; Conrad *et al.*, 1993). The diverse consequences of these interactions include changes in intracellular signalling, which may result in alterations similar to those brought about by mutations of *ras* genes in tumours that do not contain HPV genomes.

E6 and *E7* genes are positioned at the 5´ end of the early region and are expressed in the form of a polycistronic mRNA transcribed from the *E6/E7* promoter (P97 in HPV-16; Cripe *et al.*, 1987). The two reading frames are spaced by a short variable distance (2 bp in HPV-16, 8 bp in HPV-18, excluding the termination codon of *E6*).

E6 proteins of some genital HPVs (size: 158 amino acids in HPV-16) associate with the tumour suppressor protein p53, thereby inducing ubiquitin-dependent degradation of p53 (Werness *et al.*, 1990), which leads to elimination of the p53-dependent control of the cell cycle.

E6 proteins can also repress and activate transcription of heterologous and homologous promoters through interactions with p53 or with the basic transcription initiation complex (Lamberti et al., 1990; Desaintes et al., 1992; Lechner et al., 1992). E6 genes of HPV types involved in malignancy seem to be able to be spliced differentially to shorter proteins (E6*, E6**). The expression and function of E6* and E6** proteins *in vivo* are not understood, although the mRNAs are detectable and that for E6* is particularly abundant (for review, see Roggenbuck et al., 1991).

The properties of the HPV E7 protein have been reviewed (Münger & Phelps, 1993). The E7 protein of HPV-16 has 98 amino acids, forms a complex with the retinoblastoma tumour suppressor protein (pRB) and interferes with the binding of pRB to E2F transcription factors. A consequence of *E7* expression is the release of E2F transcription factors, which activate the expression of several genes involved in the cell cycle (described in section 3.1.3).

E1 proteins initiate the replication of the papillomavirus genome. The *E1* open-reading frame is transcribed into polycistronic RNAs that start at the *E6/E7* promoter. Additional *E1* transcripts of HPV-1, -6 and -11 start within the *E7* genes and, in BPV-1, within *E1* itself (Stenlund et al., 1985; Baker & Howley, 1987; Chow et al., 1987a,b; Rotenberg et al., 1989). In addition, experiments with BPV-1 point to the relevance of a promoter within the LCR for *E1* expression (Stenlund et al., 1987). In spite of this large amount of data, it has not yet been resolved which one of these transcripts serves as the principal mRNA for translation of E1 proteins.

E1 is the largest open-reading frame of papillomaviruses and encodes two known polypeptide products of about 68 and 27 kDa. The function of the smaller product is not known (Hubert & Lambert, 1993). The 68 kDa protein binds to a specific sequence within the replication origin and is functionally necessary for replication *in vivo* and *in vitro* (Blitz & Laimins, 1991; Wilson & Ludes-Meyers, 1991; Spalholz et al., 1993) (see section 1.1.9). These E1 proteins have similarities with the ATP-binding sites of SV40/polyoma T antigens and can function as ATPases and helicases (Clertant & Seif, 1984; Bream et al., 1993; Seo et al., 1993; Yang et al., 1993).

E2 proteins regulate transcription and replication of papillomavirus genomes. Expression of the *E2* gene is complex and probably occurs in several promoters in each papillomavirus. In BPV-1, the full-length E2 protein is derived from an mRNA initiating at the promoter P2443, a short distance 5′ of the *E2*-ATG. Two shorter transcripts include only the carboxyl-terminal part of *E2*. One of them starts at P3080, within the *E2* gene. The other one starts upstream of *E2* and includes, by differential splicing, an E8 leader peptide (for reviews, see Ham et al., 1991; McBride et al., 1991). The situation is less well understood in HPV-11 and -16, in which transcripts have been reported that initiate immediately upstream of *E2* but also internally of *E2*. Other transcripts originate from the *E6/E7* promoter or a promoter within *E7* and are spliced in a variety of ways to different parts of E2 (Chow et al., 1987a; Rotenberg et al., 1989; Sherman & Alloul, 1992). Most of these experiments aimed at qualitative rather than quantitative data and, because of this, it is not clear which E2 mRNAs are translated.

The properties of E2 proteins have been reviewed (Giri & Yaniv, 1988; Ham et al., 1991; McBride et al., 1991). *E2* genes of papillomaviruses encode proteins that differ in size from 410–430 amino acids in BPV-1, HPV-1 and EV-HPVs to about 370 amino acids in genital

HPVs. The proteins have highly conserved N-terminal transcription activation domains of about 200 amino acids and highly conserved carboxyl-terminal DNA binding domains of about 85 amino acids (Hegde et al., 1992). These two domains are linked by sequence-diverse hinge regions. E2 proteins form dimers through sequences of their carboxyl-terminal domain. E2 dimers are DNA-binding factors and their carboxyl-terminal domains have a high specificity for recognizing the sequence 5′-ACCGNNNNCGGT-3′ (Gauthier et al., 1991). Bound to DNA, E2 proteins can function as transcriptional activators and repressors or as modulators of replication (see sections 1.1.8 and 1.1.9). The two short forms of E2 proteins, which contain the carboxyl-terminal DNA-binding but not the N-terminal transcription-activation domain, function as repressors by competing for binding sites with the large E2 protein. These short E2 proteins are abundant in BPV-1 but are rare in HPV-infected cells.

E4 proteins seem to be involved in maturation and release of papillomavirus particles. In HPV-11-containing lesions, the *E4* gene is expressed from an abundant spliced transcript that includes the beginning of the *E1* open-reading frame (Nasseri et al., 1987; Stoler et al., 1989). *E4* genes overlap with the variable central part of *E2* genes, but E4 proteins differ from E2 protein sequences as they are encoded by a different reading frame. E4 proteins of different HPVs have little nucleotide sequence similarity but they share a high proline content (about 15%). E4 proteins form organized filamentous cytoplasmic networks that co-localize with cytokeratin filaments and, at least *in vitro* in the case of HPV-16, can induce the collapse of the cytokeratin network (Doorbar et al., 1991; Roberts et al., 1993).

L1 and L2 proteins are components of papillomavirus capsids. The late genes *L1* and *L2* are transcribed in BPV-1 and HPV-8 from a promoter in the LCR (Baker & Howley, 1987; Stubenrauch et al., 1992) and, during the generation of mRNAs, sequences corresponding to the early genes have to be spliced out from the primary transcript. An equivalent promoter has not yet been reported for genital HPVs. In HPV-6 and -11, transcripts starting 5′ of the *L2* gene have been detected together with other transcripts that use the *E6/E7* promoter or the *E7* internal promoter P847. These are spliced to E4 and include the genes *L2* and *L1* (Chow et al., 1987a). It is not yet clear whether any of these promoters gives rise to the majority of the in-vivo translated *L2* and *L1* mRNAs. Nuclear localization signals direct the transport of the capsid proteins into the nucleus (Zhou et al., 1991b) where the viral particles are assembled.

1.1.8 Regulation of gene expression

The regulation of gene expression in papillomaviruses is complex — it is controlled by different cellular and viral transcription factors, different promoter usage, differential splicing, differential transcription termination and mRNA stability. In spite of significant insight into the mechanisms operative *in vitro*, it is still largely unclear how they interplay *in vivo* and what their relevance is during the normal papillomavirus life cycle. In principle, the mechanisms have to achieve the following: (i) epithelial-specific transcription; (ii) differential expression of papillomavirus genes during the differentiation of squamous epithelia, in particular the switch from early to late genes; (iii) feedback control by papillomavirus gene products, which may play an important role in the persistence of papillomavirus infections; and (iv) response to physiological factors of the infected host on papillomavirus gene expression. Many or all of these phenomena are deregulated during malignant progression of papillomavirus lesions.

Most of these regulatory events are controlled by protein factors bound to *cis*-responsive elements in the LCR (see Figures 2 and 3). The LCRs of genital HPVs range in size from 800 to 900 bp and are much shorter in many other papillomaviruses, particularly in EV-HPVs. The LCRs of all genital HPVs have a similar organization of *cis*-responsive elements, which deviates from that of EV-HPVs, BPV-1 and CRPV. This diversity may reflect biologically distinct mechanisms. Most of the following discussion concentrates on genital HPVs.

Figure 3 is a schematic representation of the HPV-16 LCR. Four E2 binding sites, typical for the LCRs of all genital HPVs, serve as landmarks in its molecular organization. Counting from the 5´ side, the first and second E2 binding sites divide the LCR into three functionally distinct segments.

The 5´ segment is about 300 bp long and is bracketed by the translation termination codon of *L1* and the first E2 binding site (often referred to as E2 site No. 4, as it is most distal to the transcriptional start site). This segment contains transcription termination and polyadenylation sites for late transcripts as well as a negative regulatory element acting at the level of late mRNA stability (Kennedy *et al.*, 1991). Additional regulation exerted by this segment may include transcription modulation function (Auborn & Steinberg, 1991). The distal E2 binding site influences transcription from the *E6/E7* promoter (Romanczuk *et al.*, 1990) but may also have yet undetected functions.

The central segment of the LCR is about 400 bp long (Gloss *et al.*, 1987) and is flanked by two E2 binding sites. The properties of this segment have been studied in HPV-11, -16 and -18 and findings from these HPV types can probably be generalized to other genital HPV types. This LCR segment functions as an epithelial-specific transcription enhancer (Cripe *et al.*, 1987; Gloss *et al.*, 1987; Chin *et al.*, 1989; Cid *et al.*, 1993), which is probably an important mechanism for the epithelial tropism of HPVs. This enhancer is also modulated by physiological factors such as steroid hormones and by intracellular signalling pathways downstream of membrane-bound receptors. At least nine different cellular transcription factors have been reported to bind about 20 different sites in this part of the LCR in each of the three extensively studied genital HPVs. These factors are activator protein (AP1), papillomavirus enhancer binding factor (PEF1), glucocorticoid and progesterone receptors, nuclear factor (NFI), octamer binding factor 1 (Oct-1), transcriptional enhancer factors (TEF-1, TEF-2) and transcription repressor (YY1) (Gloss *et al.*, 1987; Chan *et al.*, 1989; Gloss *et al.*, 1989; Chan *et al.*, 1990; Chong *et al.*, 1990; Sibbet & Campo, 1990; Chong *et al.*, 1991; Bauknecht *et al.*, 1992; Ishiji *et al.*, 1992; Cuthill *et al.*, 1993; Sibbet *et al.*, 1995).

Several of these transcription factors induce epithelial-specific activation, although they occur in a similar form in cell types where no papillomavirus transcription can be measured *in vitro*. The enigma of this mechanism is that mutations in binding sites for these factors reduce transcription in epithelial cells, but occupation of the sites does not activate transcription in non-epithelial cells. The following observations may resolve this contradiction: two factors, NFI and AP1, are heterodimers and consist of subunits with antagonistic functions that are expressed differently in epithelial and non-epithelial cells (Thierry *et al.*, 1992; Apt *et al.*, 1993, 1994). In addition, the TEF-1 factor requires a cofactor, which is absent in some non-epithelial cells (Ishiji *et al.*, 1992).

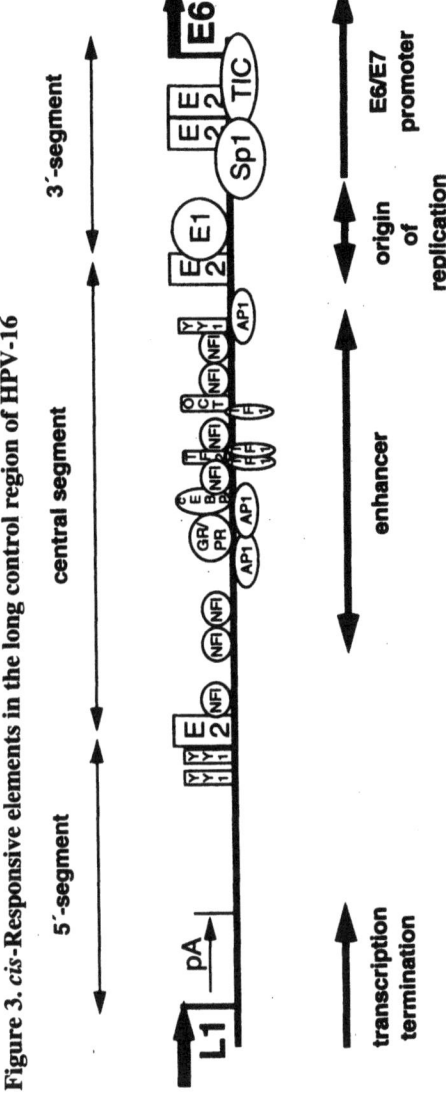

Figure 3. *cis*-Responsive elements in the long control region of HPV-16

The enhancers of many genital HPVs are activated by glucocorticoid and progesterone receptors (Gloss et al., 1987; Pater et al., 1988; Chan et al., 1989; Cid et al., 1993) with the consequence of increased expression of the *E6* and *E7* genes. Mechanistically, glucocorticoid and progesterone act through the same *cis*-responsive elements. Different elements that might mediate responses to oestrogen, testosterone or retinoids have not been found so far. A repressive effect of retinoids on HPV gene expression has been observed (Bartsch et al., 1992) and it is possible that this mechanism is mediated by AP1 binding sites, as AP1 and retinoids are molecular antagonists (Fanjul et al., 1994).

The AP1 transcription factor is a downstream target of intracellular signalling cascades initiated by receptors for extracellular ligands such as epidermal, keratinocyte or tumour growth factors, but it is not known which of these hormones may have effects on HPV gene expression *in vivo*. *E6* and *E7* gene expression is strongly stimulated by tumour promoting substances, such as phorbol esters, which mimic some signalling pathways (Chan et al., 1990).

The principal role of the E2 binding site at the 3′ side of the central segment of the LCR is in replication initiation (see below). However, *in vitro* it can also modulate transcription of the *E6* and *E7* genes (Thierry et al., 1992).

This E2 binding site and the translation start codon of the *E6* gene delineate the 3′ segment of the LCR, which is about 140 bp long. This segment contains a single E1 binding site, which identifies the origin of replication (see below). The transcription start site, which is only about 5 bp upstream of the ATG of *E6*, is located about 90 bp downstream of the E1 binding site. A segment of about 45 bp within these 90 bp contains a Sp1 transcription factor binding site, two E2 binding sites and a TATA box. These four sites provide a complex means for the modulation of *E6/E7* promoter activity. The TATA box is required to establish the basic transcription complex and the Sp1 factor for mediating the long-range effect of the enhancer. The E2 sites overlap with the TATA box and with the Sp1 site in such a way that occupancy by E2 proteins displaces the basic transcription complex and the Sp1 factor (Dostatni et al., 1991; Tan et al., 1994a). As the E2 proteins also have transcription stimulation functions, differential occupancy of the two E2 binding sites leads to modulation of *E6* promoter activity rather than to a simple switch. The interruption of negative regulation by E2 after chromosomal integration may play a role in progression of HPV-infected cells (Schwarz et al., 1985). However, integration does not seem to be a necessary prerequisite — many cancers contain episomal HPV copies (Fuchs et al., 1989; Matsukura et al., 1989; Cullen et al., 1991; Snijders et al., 1992a) and somatic cell hybridization of HPV-expressing cells with normal cells results in non-tumorigenic hybrids that continue to express *E6/E7* genes from integrated genomes (Saxon et al., 1986; Koi et al., 1989; Bartsch et al., 1992).

The factor YY1 can repress as well as stimulate promoters. Each of the three segments of the LCR of HPV-16 and -18, and possibly of all genital HPVs, has one or multiple YY1 binding sites (Bauknecht et al., 1992; May et al., 1994; Myers et al., 1994; Bauknecht et al., 1995). Some of these binding sites repress *E6/E7* transcription. Repression is relieved by mutational change of some YY1 sites *in vivo* resulting in mutant genomes with increased carcinogenicity (May et al., 1994).

Regulation of expression of the late genes is poorly understood in genital HPVs and, in spite of the cloning of late gene transcripts, no strong transcription start site for these genes has yet been identified. A promoter has been detected in HPV-8 that, *in vivo*, gives rise to transcripts encoding the late genes and, surprisingly, is stronger in transient transfections in tissue culture than the *E6/E7* promoter of this virus (Stubenrauch & Pfister, 1994). This promoter is located in the 5′ part of the LCR of HPV-8, in a region similar to a site where a late promoter has been found for BPV-1 (Baker & Howley, 1987). Since the structures of the LCRs of HPV-8 and BPV-1 differ both from one another and from that of genital HPVs, the existence of a similar regulatory element in genital HPVs cannot be predicted.

1.1.9 Replication

The replication of papillomavirus DNA has been reviewed (Lambert, 1991). After initiation at a single site within the LCR, replication of papillomavirus DNA proceeds bi-directionally (Waldeck *et al.*, 1984). In-vitro studies have shown that the replication start is identified by a single E1 binding site, which is located in the 3′ segment of the LCR. In genital HPVs, it lies approximately half way between the two E2 binding sites at the promoter and the single E2 binding site on the 5′ side of this segment (Mohr *et al.*, 1990; Lu *et al.*, 1993). The E1 protein recognizes A/T-rich motifs with only low sequence conservation, which, in the E1 binding site in HPV-16, has the sequence TAATACTTAAACTACAATAA. E2 protein forms heteromers with E1 protein in solution. These heteromers stimulate replication initiation by modulating E1 binding site recognition through binding of E2 to either of two flanking sites (Sverdrup & Kahn, 1994). Due to the overlap of alternative *cis*-responsive elements, replication can repress transcription from the E6 promoter (Sandler *et al.*, 1993). The E1 protein/DNA complex initiates replication and requires additional cellular factors similar to those required for replication of SV40 (Seo *et al.*, 1993). Papillomaviruses are able to control the copy number of their genomes in infected cells, a necessary prerequisite for episomal maintenance during persistent infection, and which is best exemplified in tissue culture by the ability of the BPV-1 genome to maintain a constant copy number of about 100 genomes per infected cell during prolonged amplification in mouse C127 fibroblasts (Lambert *et al.*, 1988). The control mechanism is poorly understood, but probably involves control of the extension of the replication fork rather than control of initiation events (Roberts & Weintraub, 1986). Productive infection and replication is restricted to differentiating non-dividing cells.

1.2 Serological response

Further information on the mechanisms of the immune response can be found in section 3.2.

1.2.1 Antigenic properties of HPVs

Papillomavirus capsids contain both type-specific and group-specific antigens. The group-specific antigens appear to be hidden within the intact particle since they become recognized only after disruption of the virions (Jenson *et al.*, 1980). Papillomavirus productive infection can be detected *in vivo* by staining sections from different lesions with a genus-specific antiserum (Jenson *et al.*, 1980; Woodruff *et al.*, 1980; Braun *et al.*, 1983; Taxy *et al.*, 1989; Lim *et al.*, 1990).

Since papillomaviruses cannot be grown in routine experimental systems, information about the epitopes that are involved in the interaction between the virus and its host cell is limited. Studies on such epitopes have been restricted to those papillomaviruses for which biological assays exist, i.e. BPV-1 (transformation of rodent cells in culture and induction of fibropapillomas in bovine fetal skin xenografts), CRPV (induction of warts in cottontail rabbits) and HPV-11 (infection after xenografting of human tissue). Antisera and monoclonal antibodies tested against complete particles of either HPV-11, BPV-1 or CRPV proved to inhibit infection in a virus-specific manner (Christensen & Kreider, 1990; Christensen et al., 1990; Christensen & Kreider, 1991; Ghim et al., 1991; Jenson et al., 1991; Christensen & Kreider, 1993; Lin et al., 1993; Christensen et al., 1994a); neutralizing activity was found in L1-specific and L2-specific sera (Roden et al., 1994b). In sera of patients with genital warts or laryngeal papillomas, neutralizing antibodies to HPV-11 virions were detected (Christensen et al., 1992).

A variety of different seroreactive regions was identified within the L1 and L2 proteins of HPV-1, -6, -11, -16, -18 and -33 by using either experimentally produced antisera or human sera from individuals with or without clinical HPV-related disease (Table 2). Seroreactive regions within the HPV E4 and E7 proteins have recently been discussed by Viscidi and Shah (1992) and by Dillner (1994). The significance of such epitopes during HPV infection is unknown.

Table 2. Seroreactive regions in HPV L1 and L2 proteins

HPV type	Gene	aa^a position	Serum used for detection^b	Specificity	Reference
HPV-1	L1	127–133	Anti-HPV-1	Type specific	Yaegashi et al. (1991)
	L2	102–108			
HPV-6	L1	417–437	Human	Type specific	Jenison et al. (1989)
HPV-6	L2	152–173, 175–191, 187–199, 201–217, 351–367	Human	Type-specific	Yaegashi et al. (1992)
		106–128, 187–199		Cross-reacting	
HPV-6	L2	196–205	Anti-BPV-1	Cross-reacting	Lehtinen et al. (1990)
HPV-11	L2	49–84, 147–162, 179–188, 180–200, 355–367	Human	Type specific	Yaegashi et al. (1992)
		103–127, 180–200		Cross-reacting	
HPV-16	L1	171–235, 411–475	Anti-BPV-1, COPV, APV	Cross-reacting	Dillner et al. (1991)
HPV-16	L1	473–492	Human	Cross-reacting	Cason et al. (1992)
		279–293		Type specific	
HPV-16	L2	149–204 (three regions)	Human	Type specific	Jenison et al. (1991)
HPV-16	L2	197–216	Human	Cross-reacting	Dillner et al. (1990a)

Table 2 (contd)

HPV type	Gene	aa[a] position	Serum used for detection[b]	Specificity	Reference
HPV-18	L2	110–211 (three regions)	Human	Type specific	Jenison et al. (1991)
HPV-33	L2	98–112, 107–117 82–94, 117–130	Anti-L2 fusion protein	Cross-reacting Type specific	Volpers et al. (1993)

[a]aa, amino acid
[b]COPV, canine oral papillomavirus; APV, avian papillomavirus

T-cell epitopes in HPV late proteins have been barely studied. Four T-cell determinants in the HPV-16 L1 protein were defined using synthetic peptides to stimulate peripheral blood mononuclear cells from asymptomatic individuals (Strang et al., 1990). This protein was also shown to contain three murine major histocompatibility complex (MHC)-class II-restricted T-cell determinants (Davies et al., 1990). For discussion of T-cell epitopes in HPV early proteins see section 3.2.3.

1.2.2 Immune response to papillomavirus infections

(a) Initial studies

Until recently, only very limited information was available about the humoral immune response to papillomavirus infections. There is no convenient experimental system for the large-scale production of papillomaviruses. Initially, only the structural proteins of those viruses that could be obtained in sufficient amounts (those from warts) were used as antigens. They were used in a variety of serological assays, such as immunoaggregation, immunodiffusion and radio-immunoassay (RIA) (Almeida et al., 1969; Pfister & zur Hausen, 1978; Pyrhönen & Neuvonen, 1978; Viac et al., 1978; Pfister et al., 1979a, 1981a; Kienzler et al., 1983; Steele et al., 1988; Anisimová et al., 1990; Steele & Gallimore, 1990; for review see Spradbrow, 1987). In these studies, HPV-specific antibodies were found to be associated with the presence of warts.

Nevertheless, some important aspects of the biology of papillomaviruses were discovered with the aid of serology. Work by Almeida et al. (1969) was the first to suggest that the papillomaviruses infecting the skin and the papillomaviruses infecting the mucosa are different from one another. The existence of a high prevalence of subclinical papillomavirus infections was first demonstrated through the detection of antibodies to HPV-8 particles in 10% of sera of asymptomatic individuals, in spite of the fact that HPV-8-induced lesions are extremely rare (Pfister et al., 1981a).

(b) Use of genetically engineered or synthetic viral antigens in serological assays

With the expression of recombinant papillomavirus proteins, it became feasible to measure antibodies directed to structural proteins of those HPV types that cannot be prepared from clinical lesions (e.g. the mucosotropic virus types such as HPV-16). In particular, the analysis of the humoral immune response against early proteins was not possible until the development of these genetically engineered reagents. In vitro recombination of the respective genes to heterologous promoters able to drive their expression efficiently and the introduction of such recombinant molecules into appropriate hosts, such as *Escherichia coli*, yeast, insect cells or mammalian cells, facilitated the production of the individual papillomavirus early or late proteins as well as of virus-like particles (Komly *et al.*, 1986; Matlashewski *et al.*, 1986a; Banks *et al.*, 1987; Bernhard *et al.*, 1987; Seedorf *et al.*, 1987; Thompson & Roman, 1987; Tomita *et al.*, 1987a,b; Sekine *et al.*, 1988; Tada *et al.*, 1988; Sato *et al.*, 1989a; Strike *et al.*, 1989; Meneguzzi *et al.*, 1990; Rose *et al.*, 1990; Tommasino *et al.*, 1990; Carter *et al.*, 1991; Zhou *et al.*, 1991a; Ghim *et al.*, 1992; Kirnbauer *et al.*, 1992; Stacey *et al.*, 1992; Wilson & Ludes-Meyers, 1992; Bream *et al.*, 1993; Hagensee *et al.*, 1993; Kirnbauer *et al.*, 1993; Park *et al.*, 1993; Rose *et al.*, 1993; Stacey *et al.*, 1993; Hines *et al.*, 1994). HPV proteins produced in prokaryotic or eukaryotic vector–host systems and synthetic peptides have all been used as antigens in different test systems, such as Western blot analysis, enzyme-linked immunosorbent assay (ELISA) and radioimmunoprecipitation. The different methods have been reviewed by Galloway (1992) and Gissmann and Müller (1994).

Expression of parts of proteins has been taken as a tool to identify seroreactive regions (Müller *et al.*, 1990; Bleul *et al.*, 1991; Jenison *et al.*, 1991). Synthetic peptides also proved suitable for the definition of seroreactive regions (Dillner, 1990; Dillner *et al.*, 1990a; Krchnák *et al.*, 1990; Müller *et al.*, 1990; Suchánková *et al.*, 1992). A compilation of epitopes used by different investigators was published recently (Viscidi & Shah, 1992; Dillner, 1994).

(i) Individuals with unknown disease status

There is limited information about the development of antibodies following natural papillomavirus infection in humans. A few reports indicate the presence of Ig(immunoglobuline)G or IgM antibodies to HPV-16 E4, E7, L1 or L2 or HPV-6 L1 proteins in up to 33% of children one month to 10 years of age and 40% in children 10–20 years of age (Li *et al.*, 1987; Jochmus-Kudielka *et al.*, 1989; Jenison *et al.*, 1990; Cason *et al.*, 1992; Müller *et al.*, 1995b). In view of the rare occurrence of clinically apparent papillomavirus infections in children, the significance of these data in unclear. No cases of seroconversion have so far been published.

Cross-sectional studies on the sera of healthy people demonstrated that antibody prevalence to HPV-16 E7 protein rises with age, whereas the prevalence of antibodies specific to HPV-16 E4 decreases in individuals over 20 (Jochmus-Kudielka *et al.*, 1989; Müller *et al.*, 1995b). Reactivity to HPV-16 virus-like particles was found to decrease in older women without HPV-16-related diseases (Jochmus-Kudielka *et al.*, 1989). There is evidence that antibodies decline after disappearance of warts (Bonnez *et al.*, 1993; Carter *et al.*, 1994) and that antibodies develop more frequently in females than in males (Tachezy *et al.*, 1994; Carter *et al.*, 1995). Veress *et al.* (1994) reported a peak of seropositivity of anti-HPV (HPV-11 L2 or HPV-16 E2, E7, L1 or L2) secretory IgA antibodies among cytologically normal women aged 25–32.

Lewensohn-Fuchs *et al.* (1993) investigated the serological responses to HPV-16 E2, L1 and L2 antigens before and after renal transplantation. Antibodies to the late proteins were shown to decrease after transplantation but remained detectable throughout the study (up to three years) whereas the number of patients with E2-specific antibodies increased after transplantation. A significant difference was found between 120 renal transplant recipients and 215 controls in the prevalence of antibodies to HPV-16 E4 (32% versus 10%; odds ratio, 4.7;

$p < 0.00001$) and E7 (15% versus 4%; odds ratio, 6.4; $p < 0.00001$) (Jochmus-Kudielka et al., 1992).

(ii) HPV-associated benign diseases

Antibodies to viral proteins of HPV-1, -6, -8, -11 or -16 are found in patients with papillomavirus-related benign lesions such as hand warts, condylomata acuminata, recurrent respiratory papillomas as well as in controls (Li et al., 1987; Steele & Gallimore, 1990; Steger et al., 1990; Suchánková et al., 1990; Bonnez et al., 1991, 1992; Carter et al., 1994; Kirnbauer et al., 1994).

The most remarkable differences in detection of antibodies between patients with benign lesions and healthy controls were measured when complete HPV particles were used, although a significant proportion of patients failed to react. In contrast, with synthetic peptides, reactivity was also seen in a proportion of sera obtained from asymptomatic individuals. In some studies applying bacterial fusion proteins or synthetic peptides, no differences were found (Jenison et al., 1990; Tachezy et al., 1994; for review see Viscidi & Shah, 1992).

By Western blot analysis using a bacterial HPV-6b L1 fusion protein, Li et al. (1987) found IgG antibodies in 18/30 sera from patients attending a colposcopy clinic and in 2/20 children below five years of age. Suchánková et al. (1990) detected IgG antibodies to a 17mer peptide shared between the HPV-6 and HPV-11 L2 proteins in the majority of patients with condylomata acuminata but in less than 15% of asymptomatic individuals.

HPV-11 particles produced from the mouse xenograft system were used to detect IgG antibodies by ELISA. The median optical density in patients with genital warts (0.32) or recurrent laryngeal papillomatosis (0.23) was greater than in controls (0.12 and 0.08, respectively) (Bonnez et al., 1991, 1992). It was demonstrated that in condyloma patients who responded to treatment, the median optical density dropped by 0.05% per day; it increased by 0.07% per day in non-responders (Bonnez et al., 1993).

Wikström et al. (1992) reported increased prevalence of serum IgG and IgA antibodies to HPV-6 L1 and L2 peptides in men with a history of genital warts in comparison to controls ($p < 0.05$ for both L1 and L2). However, the antibody prevalence was similar to that of controls.

Using a carboxyl-terminal 19mer peptide of the HPV-16 E2 protein and an HPV-16 E7 derived 30mer peptide, IgA antibodies were found more frequently in cervical secretions of 29 patients with genital condylomata than in 28 controls ($p < 0.025$ and $p < 0.005$, respectively) (Dillner et al., 1993).

In recent studies, virus-like particles have also been used to detect, by ELISA, antibodies in sera of patients with HPV-related benign lesions. Carter et al. (1994) reported antibodies to HPV-1 capsids in 16 out of 18 women with current foot warts, compared to 38 out of 73 individuals without a history of foot warts (odds ratio, 7.2 (95% CI, 1.5–69.4); $p < 0.01$). There was a loss of seroreactivity with time since the last appearance of the warts.

Using an HPV-11 virus-like particle-specific ELISA, Rose et al. (1994a) tested sera that had been analysed previously by whole-virion ELISA; they found a significant correlation between the individual seroreactivities obtained in both assays ($p < 0.000001$).

Antibodies to HPV-6 capsids were found more frequently among women with recurrent genital warts than among female controls without history of genital warts (58% versus 19%, odds ratio, 6.5; 95% CI, 3.0–14.1). This association was even stronger in pregnant women (88% versus 30%; odds ratio, 15.5 (95% CI, 1.8–735.7)) but was essentially absent in males (31% versus 26%; odds ratio, 1.3 (95% CI, 0.6–2.6)) (Carter et al., 1995). These authors also reported a positive association between HPV-6 virus-like particle-specific antibodies and both HPV DNA positivity in cervical swabs and number of sexual partners.

Only a few studies addressing the cell-mediated immune response to HPV antigens have been reported. Lymphoproliferative responses to the HPV-1 E4 and HPV-16 E4, E6, E7 and L1 proteins were observed in human donors, and no differences were found between normal donors and patients with HPV-related diseases (Cubie et al., 1989; Strang et al., 1990; Altmann et al., 1992; Steele et al., 1993; Kadish et al., 1994). Kadish et al. (1994) reported that cell-mediated immune response to a carboxyl-terminal peptide of the HPV-16 E7 protein was significantly associated with infections by HPV-16, -31 or -33 as compared to infections by other HPV types. These authors suggest that cell-mediated immune response may be associated to regression of the disease.

(iii) HPV-associated precancer and cancer

A number of studies have compared the immune response to HPV-associated precancers and cancers. They are discussed in section 3.2.

1.3 Methods for detection of HPV infections

HPV infections are detected by demonstration of HPV genomic sequences in infected tissues and, to a lesser extent, by identification of HPV proteins in tissues. HPVs cannot be propagated or isolated in tissue culture and, therefore, one of the most common methods of virus detection is not available for HPVs. The presence of HPVs is also inferred from cytological, histological, serological and clinical findings.

HPV detection methods have been developed most extensively for genital tract HPVs, because these infections have been linked to cervical cancer. Of the numerous HPVs that infect the genital tract, some types (e.g. HPV-16, -18, -31 and -45) are frequently found in cervical cancers (high-risk HPVs) whereas others (e.g. HPV-6, -11, -42, -43 and -44) are rarely detected in cervical cancers (low-risk HPVs). Therefore, in clinical and epidemiological investigations, diagnosis of HPV aims at identification of specific types of HPVs, particularly those associated with cancer. In addition to the extensive studies on genital HPVs, recently developed polymerase chain reaction (PCR) assays designed to amplify EV-associated HPVs have detected large numbers of novel HPVs in skin lesions.

1.3.1 HPV diagnosis by morphology

The link between koilocytosis in cervical smears and HPV infection was established by cytological and histological investigations in the mid-1970s (Meisels & Fortin, 1976; Purola & Savia, 1977; Della Torre et al., 1978). The presence of unequivocal koilocytes indicates productive viral infection with high specificity. However, with the advent of techniques for detection of viral genomes, it became evident that cytological and histological features are not sensitive indicators of the presence of HPVs. In a majority of individuals who are positive for HPV DNA, no cytological or histological correlates of HPV infection can be detected (Bauer *et al.*, 1991). In contrast, colposcopic visualization of the cervix after application of acetic acid identifies cervical HPV infection frequently, but the specificity of the procedure is unknown. Therefore, indirect detection of HPV infection by cytology, histology and colposcopy is of limited diagnostic accuracy. Moreover, these methods fail to discriminate between lesions produced by different HPV types.

1.3.2 Detection of HPV proteins in infected tissues

Detection of HPV capsid antigen in affected tissue with a broadly cross-reactive antiserum raised against disrupted viral capsids (see section 1.3.3) identifies productive HPV infection with a high specificity. Detection of capsid antigen is highly correlated with the presence of koilocytes. However, this antigen is seldom detected in individuals who are infected with HPVs but have no cytological abnormalities or in individuals who have high-grade cervical neoplasia or invasive cancer (Jenson *et al.*, 1985; Shah & Gissmann, 1989).

1.3.3 Detection of HPV genomic sequences

HPV genomic sequences are detected either by DNA amplification-based methods, in which targeted viral sequences are first amplified by PCR (Saiki *et al.*, 1988) and then identified, or by direct hybridization of the genomes in the specimens, in which identification takes place without prior amplification. The limitations of the methods are related to their analytical sensitivity, clinical utility, complexity, reliability, ease of performance and commercial availability.

Differences in the methods of specimen collection (e.g. cervical scrapes versus cervicovaginal lavage; the device used to collect specimens; the composition of transport medium) influence the reliability and analytical sensitivity of HPV diagnosis (Guerrero *et al.*, 1992; Schiffman, 1992a). For adequate diagnosis, non-amplification-based assays require a larger amount of specimen than PCR methods.

(a) PCR-based methods

PCR-based methods are now the most commonly used in HPV investigations. They have the highest analytical sensitivity and can detect as few as 10–100 copies of HPV genomes in the tested portion of the clinical specimens. PCR assays require very small amounts of specimen, and a simple one-step treatment prior to amplification. Initially, HPV type-specific primers were designed with the use of computer-assisted matrix comparison analyses for different parts of the genome. Type-specific primer pairs are very efficient and highly specific for the amplification and identification of the chosen types. However, more than 40 genital HPVs were cloned and had differing oncogenic potential. Therefore, it was useful to devise a strategy to amplify a broad spectrum of HPV types in a single PCR reaction using primer pairs based on highly conserved sequences (consensus or general primers). A single amplification reaction with these primers generates PCR products that are then utilized for type-specific identification of HPVs. Several of the PCR methods in use are suitable for large-scale studies. Epidemiological investigations related to questions of disease etiology, prevalence, persistence and latency of HPVs rely heavily on PCR-based diagnoses. False positive results due to contamination, which were frequent in the early studies, appear to be rare in more recent investigations. Strong laboratory discipline is needed to avoid contamination. A proportion of clinical specimens may be unsatisfactory for PCR assays because the cellular DNA is not amplifiable.

The PCR methods for diagnosis of genital HPVs have been reviewed (Gravitt & Manos, 1992; van den Brule *et al.*, 1993; Walboomers *et al.*, 1994). The main features of the two most widely used methods, as currently used, are shown in Table 3. The modifications in these methods, since their original descriptions (Manos *et al.*, 1989; van den Brule *et al.*, 1990; Snijders *et al.*, 1990), are referenced in the footnotes of Table 3. Both methods target sequences in the *L1* gene and detect HPVs in over 90% of invasive cancers (Walboomers *et al.*, 1994; Bosch *et al.*, 1995).

Table 3. Comparisons of two widely used HPV-PCR methods

	MY09–MY11	GP5+/GP6+
Primers	Consensus; degenerate; amplify a large number of HPVs; an additional primer added to amplify HPV-51[a]	Consensus; not degenerate; amplify a large number of HPVs; original primers extended to improve performance[b]
Amplification target	450 bp region of *L1* gene	140 bp region of *L1* gene
Probe label	Biotin	Radioactive
Identification of PCR products	(i) Dot blot hybridization with type-specific and generic probes using enhanced chemiluminescence (ii) Also adapted to ELISA format	(i) Hybridization with type-specific and generic (cock tail) probes (ii) Identification into low-risk and high-risk types[c]

[a] Hildesheim *et al.* (1994)
[b] de Roda Husman *et al.* (1995)
[c] Jacobs *et al.* (1995)

Both of the above methods employ consensus (or general) primers, which amplify a broad spectrum of HPV types in a single reaction. The primers are complementary to conserved sequences in the *L1* gene of HPVs. However, the different HPVs do not have identical sequences, even in the most conserved regions, so the goal of amplification of many HPV types in a single reaction is met by the design of primers. The MY09–MY11 primers are degenerate, i.e. they are a mixture of many primers, with nucleotide differences at several positions that render them complementary to the target DNAs of different HPV types. The GP5+/GP6+ primers are non-degenerate, i.e. they are a single set of primers that accept nucleotide mismatches. In the amplification reaction with GP5+/GP6+ primers, the stringency of primer annealing is reduced, so as to allow the primers to anneal to the target DNA, despite the mismatches in nucleotide sequences. The GP5+/GP6+ primers are more efficient in amplification of sequences from archival material where DNA may be degraded, because they target a smaller fragment of the gene.

The HPV sequences in the PCR products are identified to specific types in a number of ways. In both the MY09–MY11 and GP5+/GP6+ systems, type-specific probes for over 20 HPVs are available. These probes are employed to identify specific types in dot blot or Southern blot formats, or in an ELISA format. Alternatively, probe pools can be designed to distinguish high-risk HPVs from low-risk HPVs (Jacobs et al., 1995). PCR products may also be identified by their restriction enzyme digest patterns or by nucleotide sequencing (Lungu et al., 1992; Smits et al., 1992a; Bernard et al., 1994a). The nucleotide sequence of the amplified product can then be matched to the HPV nucleotide sequence database (Myers et al., 1994) in order to make a type-specific identification or to identify new HPV types. For establishment of a novel HPV type, the whole HPV genome must be cloned and evaluated at the HPV reference centre at Heidelberg.

The above two methods, MY09–MY11 and GP5+/GP6+, both amplify a region of the *L1* gene of genital HPVs. Lungu et al. (1995) recently described a PCR method with amplification of *E6* sequences of genital HPVs. The primers are designed to amplify selectively 10 high-risk HPVs. PCR methods have also been devised for the detection of a broad spectrum of cutaneous HPVs (Tieben et al., 1993; Shamanin et al., 1994a). Use of these methods in the study of skin cancers in renal transplant recipients has revealed that many of these lesions contain novel HPV types related to the EV-associated HPVs (Shamanin et al., 1994a; Berkhout et al., 1995).

(b) ViraPap™ and Hybrid Capture™

ViraPap™ (Digene Laboratories, Silver Spring, MD, USA) was one of the first commercially available HPV diagnostic tests and is approved by the US Food and Drug Administration (FDA). In this test, radioactive RNA probes of seven HPV types (HPV-6, -11, -16, -18, -31, -33 and -35), available as a single pool or as three separate pools (ViraType™ — HPV-6 and -11; HPV-16 and -18; HPV-31, -33 and -35), are employed to hybridize cellular DNA of clinical specimens placed on filters that are autoradiographed to reveal the hybrids in a dot blot format. The sensitivity and specificity of ViraPap™ as compared to other assays are discussed below. This test has now been replaced by a second-generation assay, Hybrid Capture™.

Hybrid Capture™ does not employ radioactive reagents and screens for a total of 14 HPVs with two RNA probe pools; probe A for five low-risk HPVs (HPV-6, -11, -42, -43 and -44) and probe B for nine types of HPV that are found in cancer (HPV-16, -18, -31, -33, -35, -45, -51, -52 and -56). The single-strand DNA in denatured specimens is reacted with the A and B RNA probes. The DNA–RNA hybrids are captured and immobilized with a hybrid-specific antibody and the hybrids are detected in an ELISA-type format with the use of a chemiluminescent compound. The presence of the viral DNA in the specimens is expressed as relative light units (RLUs). Higher ratios of specimen RLUs to control RLUs are indicative of a greater amount of viral DNA in the specimens, and in this way the test results allow quantification of viral DNA in the specimens (Cox et al., 1995).

The Hybrid Capture™ assay is available commercially and is approved by FDA. The analytical sensitivity of this test is 10^5 copies of HPV-16 genome. The negative and positive controls in the kit provide uniform standards for the testing laboratories. In a study of inter-laboratory variation in Hybrid Capture™ results among three laboratories, specimens were tested with probe pools A and B. Kappa values in inter-laboratory pairwise comparisons for positivity to either group A or group B ranged from 0.61 to 0.83. Of specimens that were positive for group B by the reference standard, 74% were positive in all three laboratories. The interlaboratory correlations of HPV quantitative data for probe B types ranged from 0.60 to 0.90. Probable false positive results were occasionally encountered, in less than 3% of the tests (Schiffman et al., 1995).

(c) Southern blot hybridization

In contrast to the PCR-based methods and Hybrid Capture™, which employ crude extracts of the clinical specimens as a starting point, Southern blot hybridization requires the purification of cellular DNA with a series of phenol:chloroform extractions. The purified cellular DNA is digested with restriction enzymes, electrophoresed, denatured, transferred to filters and hybridized at different stringencies with radiolabelled HPV probes. The identification of HPV types is based on the sizes of the hybridizing fragment and the stringency of hybridization.

The analytical sensitivity of Southern blot hybridization is similar to that for Hybrid Capture™. The sizes of the hybridizing fragments provide an internal control of the specificity of the annealing reaction; therefore, faint signals in Southern blot hybridization, if they correspond to the expected positions of the bands, can confidently be interpreted as positive. The test allows identification of viral subtypes and can provide evidence of viral integration.

The technique is labour-intensive and complex and employs radioactive probes. It is therefore not commonly used in large-scale epidemiological investigations. There is a significant inter-laboratory variation in detection and typing of HPVs by Southern blot hybridization. In a study of 40 clinical samples, pairwise agreement between four laboratories ranged from 66% to 97% for HPV detection and from 77% to 96% for typing of positive specimens (Brandsma et al., 1989).

(d) In-situ hybridization

This is the only method in which the viral genome can be identified in topographical relation to the pathological lesion. Cells or tissue sections on slides are hybridized using radioactive or nonradioactive DNA or RNA probes. Tests can be devised to detect viral DNA or viral transcripts of individual viral genes (Dürst et al., 1992; Iftner et al., 1992; Stoler et al., 1992).

The lower limit of detection of in-situ hybridization is 20–25 copies of the viral genome in the cell (Schneider et al., 1991). This limit of detection can be reduced further to one copy per cell by the use of special procedures such as in-situ PCR (Nuovo et al., 1991a,b; Bernard et al., 1994c).

Although labour-intensive, in-situ hybridization is very well suited for studies of molecular pathogenesis of HPV-associated diseases. The method can locate the viral genome in the tumour cells themselves, and correlate expression of specific viral genes with the evolution of the lesion. However, the technique is not suitable for epidemiological investigations, not only because of its complexity, but also because tissue specimens are generally not available from controls.

(e) Filter in-situ hybridization

This was the first HPV test designed for epidemiological study and was employed in several large-scale investigations (Reeves et al., 1989; de Villiers et al., 1992). In this assay, cells are placed on a filter and lysed, and the DNA on the filter is hybridized with radiolabelled probes and autoradiographed (Wagner et al., 1984).

This test is now seldom employed in HPV investigations. The test had a high interlaboratory variability, and in one study there was no correlation between the results of filter in-situ hybridization and the results of Southern blot hybridization (Schiffman, 1992a).

(f) Comparison of HPV testing methods

Results of selected studies comparing HPV testing methods are summarized in Table 4. ViraPap™ is compared to two reference tests (Southern blot hybridization and PCR) for detection of the seven HPV types included in ViraPap™. Southern blot hybridization is compared to PCR as the reference test. The specificity of both ViraPap™ and Southern blot hybridization was high, but their sensitivities varied over a wide range. The results of these comparisons should be interpreted with caution because the technical details of the tests between laboratories performing the tests were not identical. Also, in some instances, the small amounts of specimens available may have contributed to lower sensitivities of non-amplification-based assays (Guerrero et al., 1992; Schiffman, 1992a).

Table 4. Comparison of sensitivity and specificity of ViraPap™ and Southern blot hybridization

Reference test	Southern blot hybridization		PCR			
Comparison test	ViraPap™		ViraPap™		Southern blot hybridization	
	Sensitivity	Specificity	Sensitivity	Specificity	Sensitivity	Specificity
Kiviat et al. (1990)	0.90	0.94				
Bauer et al. (1991)			[0.54]	1		
Gravitt et al. (1991)			[0.39]	[0.96]		
Guerrero et al. (1992)	0.68	0.89	0.45	0.94	0.35	0.94

[ ] calculated by the Working Group

1.3.4 Detection of HPV infections and HPV-associated cancers by serological assays

The immunological responses to HPV infections and to HPV-associated cancers have been discussed in section 1.2 and 3.2. Currently, the ELISA antibody assay using virus-like particles as the antigen is the most promising assay for the detection of virus-specific antibody. However, the antibody response is low-titred and not detectable in all patients with documented infections. Likewise, at present, antibodies to E6 and E7 proteins are the most promising markers of HPV-associated invasive cancer.

These assays are now widely employed in HPV investigations. The results of these studies will indicate the extent to which the assays are useful as markers of HPV infection and of HPV-associated neoplasia.

1.4 Epidemiology of infection

Many detailed reviews of the epidemiology of genital HPV infection have been published (Koutsky *et al.*, 1988; Beutner *et al.*, 1991; Moscicki, 1992; Morrison, 1994; Schiffman, 1994; Schneider, 1994). Less is known about the epidemiology of non-genital HPV infections. This section focuses on new information and consistent themes that have emerged from studies of the transmission, incidence, prevalence and natural history of HPV infection. Within each sub-section data on genital infections are presented before data on non-genital infections.

1.4.1 Transmission

Results from several observational studies indicate that genital HPVs are transmitted primarily through contact with infected cervical, vaginal, vulvar, penile or anal epithelium. Barrett *et al.* (1954) reported that genital warts developed in four to six weeks in wives of servicemen who had returned from overseas and who had had genital warts. Oriel (1971) reported that 64% of sexual partners of individuals with genital warts developed genital warts themselves after a mean interval of two to three months. Similar results have been reported by others (Teokharov, 1969; Barrasso *et al.*, 1987a).

In studies of sexually inexperienced young women, HPV DNA and antibodies to genital types of HPV are rarely detected (Fairley *et al.*, 1992; Andersson-Ellström *et al.*, 1994; Gutman *et al.*, 1994; Rylander *et al.*, 1994; Carter *et al.*, 1995; Critchlow & Koutsky, 1995). Additional studies among young women show a positive trend between increasing numbers of recent sexual partners and increasing prevalence of genital HPV infection (Rosenfeld *et al.*, 1989; Moscicki *et al.*, 1990; Ley *et al.*, 1991; Bauer *et al.*, 1993). In a cohort study of 18–20-year-old female university students with a low-risk profile for sexually transmitted diseases (STDs), the overall prevalence of genital HPV infection as determined by PCR-based analysis was 35%. The prevalence at enrolment among the 183 sexually experienced women ranged from 17% of those reporting only one partner to 83% of those reporting more than five partners (Critchlow & Koutsky, 1995).

The above results indicate that, among adolescents and young adults, risk of genital HPV infection with each new sexual contact is high. Unlike the transmission dynamics for certain bacterial STDs (Brunham & Plummer, 1990), core groups (that is, small segments of the sexually active proportion of the population with very high rates of partner change) do not appear to be necessary to sustain high rates of genital HPV infection in communities throughout the world (Yorke *et al.*, 1978). To what extent the high prevalence of genital HPV infection among populations with relatively low rates of partner change can be attributed to a high rate of infectivity, a long duration of infectivity or a combination of both of these is currently not known.

Statistical evidence of HPV type-specific concordance in couples has been reported in two studies. Among a consecutive series of 50 couples attending an STD clinic, 63% of men and

72% of women were found to have HPV infection, as determined by PCR-based testing of anogenital samples. Of the 50 couples, five were excluded because one or both partners had an inadequate HPV DNA sample. In 20 couples both partners were HPV positive, in 21 couples only one partner was positive, and in four couples both were negative. Thirteen couples had the same HPV type detected, whereas only 8 would have been expected by chance ($p = 0.009$) (Baken et al., 1995). Among 32 married couples, HPV-16 was detected in both the husband and wife in 8 couples, of whom four demonstrated identical HPV-16 variants (Ho et al., 1993a). Although findings from these two studies support the role of sexual transmission in the epidemiology of genital HPV infection, they also demonstrate that quite often the same HPV type or variant cannot be detected in genital samples from both members of a sexual partnership.

Papillomavirus concordance was also studied in a group of rhesus monkeys, the sexual mating and offspring histories of which were known (Ostrow et al., 1990). Rhesus papillomavirus type 1 (RhPV-1) DNA was detected in cervical specimens from 20 of 30 female monkeys that had mated with one of two male monkeys infected with RhPV-1. None of 11 female monkeys that had not mated with either of the infected males was positive. The 'index' male monkey developed a penile carcinoma that metastasized to the lymph node, and two of the female mating partners developed cervical carcinoma. Both tumours and metastatic tissue were positive for RhPV-1.

Infections in the oral cavity of genital types of HPVs and HPV-associated recurrent respiratory papillomatosis (rare conditions) may be related to oral–genital contact (Kashima et al., 1992a). The occurrence of juvenile-onset recurrent respiratory papillomatosis in infants and young children indicates that HPV infections may be transmitted from mother to infant, probably at the time of delivery. There have been reports of HPV DNA detected in amniotic fluid, although in these studies transmission of the virus to the infant was not demonstrated (Sedlacek et al., 1989; Armbruster-Moraes et al., 1993). Age of mother, birth order of the infant and mode of delivery are important determinants of transmission. Most infants who develop juvenile-onset recurrent respiratory papillomatosis are delivered vaginally rather than by caesarean section (Shah et al., 1986), and many are the first-born single or twin infant of women who tend to be younger than other mothers delivering at the same institutions (Kashima et al., 1992a). Rare cases of ano-genital warts in new-borns have been reported (Tang et al., 1978) and HPV DNA has been detected in mucosal scrapes and washes obtained from infants (Roman & Fife, 1986; Jenison et al., 1990; Fredericks et al., 1993; St Louis et al., 1993). However, results from transmission studies of infants are not consistent, and do not provide a clear indication of the rate of infection among neonates who are exposed perinatally. Also, HPV type-specific concordance between mother–infant pairs has been observed only rarely.

Case reports of HPV-16 periungual infections and carcinomas (Moy et al., 1989; Euvrard et al., 1993) and of ano-genital warts in toddlers and children in whom sexual abuse has been ruled out (Handley et al., 1993) indicate that HPV (both genital and non-genital types) may be transmitted digitally from one epithelial site to another. Blood-borne transmission of HPV has not been reported. Studies of children sharing glue pots show that common non-genital warts on fingers and hands may be transmitted by fomites (glue in this instance) (Rowson & Mahy, 1967). Although fomite transmission of genital types of HPV has not been demonstrated, HPV

DNA has been detected on medical instruments and in laser plumes (Garden et al., 1988; Ferenczy et al., 1990).

Genital HPV infection may involve large areas of uro-genital, perineal, perianal, anal and scrotal epithelium. In men, a common site of genital warts is the base of the shaft of the penis (Chuang et al., 1984; Cook et al., 1993), a site that is not easily covered by a condom. For this reason, consistent and correct use of condoms probably does not protect against transmission of genital HPV as well as it does against transmission of bacterial STDs and human immunodeficiency virus (HIV).

A study by Mandal et al. (1991) included 105 men (median age, 26 years) without clinical evidence of anogenital warts who were attending an STD clinic. Pooled specimens consisting of exfoliated cells from the distal urethra, penile shaft, glans penis and anorectal junction were used for detection of HPV DNA using dot blot hybridization techniques. HPV DNA was detected in 21 (20%) men. Fifteen men (14%) regularly used condoms and 17 (16%) were circumcized but neither circumstance was associated with the detection of HPV DNA.

As with genital types (Oriel, 1971), transmission of non-genital types of HPV is probably more efficient in the presence of a macerated or abraded epithelial surface. Studies of plantar warts suggest that the virus may be transmitted from the soles of the feet of one individual to a concrete surface (such as found surrounding a swimming pool) to the feet of an unsuspecting individual walking barefoot on this abrasive, HPV-1 laden surface (Rasmussen, 1958; Koutsky et al., 1988). Common warts (verruca vulgaris) are frequently detected on the fingers and hands of butchers and workers who handle fish and poultry (Rüdlinger et al., 1989a; Melchers et al., 1993; Stehr-Green et al., 1993; Keefe et al., 1994a). Transmission of HPV (particularly HPV-7) in these occupational settings may be facilitated by the occurrence of accidental epithelial wounding from sharp objects and by the sharing of equipment and protective gear (Melchers et al., 1993).

1.4.2 Incidence

Few studies have been designed to provide estimates of the incidence of genital HPV infection. In one investigation of the general population of Rochester, MN, USA, the annual age- and gender-adjusted incidence of genital warts increased between the early 1950s and the late 1970s from 13 per 100 000 to 106 per 100 000 (Chuang et al., 1984). This time period corresponds to the years when the rates of other STDs were increasing dramatically in Europe and North America (Aral & Holmes, 1995). Additional studies using data obtained from a sample of private physician offices throughout the USA showed a 4.5-fold increase in the number of first visits for condyloma between 1966 and 1984 (Becker et al., 1987). In the United Kingdom, national STD data suggested a 2.5-fold increase in the incidence of condyloma for males and females between 1971 and 1982 (Koutsky et al., 1988). Incidence data for subclinical genital HPV infections are currently not available.

The incidence of common and plantar warts in the general population has not been studied. It has been suggested, from the data available, that the incidence is higher among children living in institutions than among those living in houses, and higher in children than in adults (Rasmussen, 1958; Massing & Epstein, 1963).

In children between 0 and 14 years of age, recurrent respiratory papillomatosis has an incidence per 100 000 of 0.7 in Denmark, 0.6 in the USA, 0.1 in Japan and of 2.8 in Thailand (Christensen *et al.*, 1984; Ushikai *et al.*, 1994).

1.4.3 Prevalence

Unlike incidence, which measures the rate of new infection in a population during a given time interval, prevalence measures the percentage of a population that has new, persisting or recurring infection at a given point or period in time. For genital infections such as gonorrhoea which are often symptomatic and clear with appropriate therapy, estimates of prevalence and incidence may be comparable. For infections such as HPV, which persist with or without treatment, measures of prevalence and incidence will be different. Host characteristics and clinical manifestations of incident versus prevalent cases are also likely to be different. Prevalence is an important measure of the burden of disease in a population. Measures of incidence are used to identify characteristics of individuals that are at risk of developing disease.

Using PCR-based HPV DNA detection methods, several investigators throughout the world have determined the prevalence of genital HPV infection among populations of women with normal Pap (Papanicolaou) smears (Table 5). Data in Table 5 are presented in descending order of positivity of HPV. However, the results from the various studies are not strictly comparable because Pap smears were evaluated by different criteria, and different HPV DNA assays, primers and methods of epithelial sampling were used (see Table 5 for references). Despite these methodological differences, some important conclusions can be drawn from the presented data. First, younger rather than older women are more likely to have HPV DNA detected in genital tract specimens. Secondly, HPV DNA is rarely detected in genital tract specimens of women who report no previous sexual activity (Fairley *et al.*, 1992; Rylander *et al.*, 1994; Critchlow & Koutsky, 1995). Thirdly, geographical differences in the prevalence of HPV infection are not readily apparent.

Results from these studies also indicate that, as with women with cervical neoplasia (McCance *et al.*, 1985; Lörincz *et al.*, 1990; Bergeron *et al.*, 1992), women with normal Pap smears are more likely to have HPV-16 infection than infection by any of the other classified types of HPV.

Sampling techniques for detecting HPV DNA may be less sensitive when used in men than women. Penile scrapings may yield limited cellular material and, thus, are often negative for HPV DNA when analysed by molecular methods that do not include an amplification step (Grussendorf-Conen *et al.*, 1987; Barrasso, 1992).

In one study (Kataoka *et al.*, 1991), urethral smears were obtained from 105 male Swedish Army recruits between the ages of 18 and 23 years. Their reported mean lifetime number of sexual partners was 1.4. Eighteen (17%) had HPV DNA detected in the urethral specimen. In addition, all those with visible lesions provided penile biopsy specimens for the detection of HPV DNA by a PCR-based method. Of these 39 men undergoing penile biopsy, 17 (44%) had HPV DNA detected in the biopsy specimen. Urethral specimens obtained from these same men were positive for HPV DNA in only 10 (26%).

Table 5. HPV DNA detection rates by PCR amplification among women with cytologically negative Pap smears

Reference	Study population	No. of subjects	Sites tested	HPV types tested for	Age of subjects (range, mean or SD)	Percentage HPV positive	Percentage HPV-16/18 positive
ter Meulen et al. (1992)	Gynaecology clinic, Tanzania	[261]	Cervix	HPV-6, -11, -16, -18, -31, -33, -35, -39, -40, -45, -51, X	15–70; 30.9 years	[47.9]	[16.9]
Wheeler et al. (1993)	University Health Service, USA	357	Cervix	HPV-6, -11, -16, -18, -31, -33, -35, -39, -45, -51, -52, -54, -59, PAP 88, PAP 238A, PAP 238B, W 13B	18–47; 23 years	44.3	8 (HPV-16)
Kjaer et al. (1993)	Random sample, Greenland	129[a]	Cervix	HPV-11, -16, -18, -33	20–39 years	43.4	35
Pao et al. (1990)	Clinic, Taiwan	102	Cervico-vaginal	HPV-6, -11, -16, -18, -33	NA	42.2	9.8
Lambropoulos et al. (1994)	Gynaecology clinic, Greece	201	Cervix	HPV-16, -18, X	17–45 years	40.8[i]	7.5
Becker et al. (1994)	Gynaecology clinics, USA	309	Cervix	HPV-6, -11, -16, -18, -31, -33, -35, -39, -45, -51, -52, -53, -54, -56, -58, -59, PAP 88, W 13B, PAP 238A	18–40; 26 years	40.1	11.7
Kjaer et al. (1993)	Random sample, Denmark	126[a]	Cervix	HPV-11, -16, -18, -33	20–39 years	38.9	44.4
Critchlow & Koutsky (1995)	University, USA, sexually active	183	Cervix, vulvo-vaginal	HPV-6, -11, -16, -18, -31, -33, -35, -45, X	18–20 years	35	14
Bauer et al. (1991)	University Health Service, USA	442[b]	Cervix	HPV-6, -11, -16, -18, -31, -33, -35, -39, -45, -51, -52, W 13 B, PAP 88, PAP 155, PAP 251, PAP 238B, X	mean, 22.9 years; SD, 4.2	32.5[b]	NA
Seck et al. (1994)	Infectious Disease Service, Senegal	47[i]	Cervix	HPV-6, -11, -16, -18, -31, -33, -35, X	NA	24.5[i]	NA
Czeglédy et al. (1992a)	Family planning clinic, Kenya	77	Cervix	HPV-6, -11, -16, -18, -31, -33	mean, 25.8 years	19.5	10.4

Table 5 (contd)

Reference	Study population	No. of subjects	Sites tested	HPV type tested for	Age of subjects (range, mean or SD, standard deviation)	Percentage HPV positive	Percentage HPV 16/18 positive
Schiffman et al. (1993)	Health Maintenance Organization clinics, USA	453	Cervico-vaginal	HPV-6, -11, -16, -18, -26, -31, -33, -35, -39, -40, -42, -45, -51, -52, -53, -54, -55, -57, -59, PAP 38, PAP 155, PAP 238A, PAP 251, PAP 291, W 13B	mean, 34 years	17.7	2.9
Engels et al. (1992)	STD clinic, Kenya	97	Cervix	HPV-6, -11, -16, -18, -31, -33, X	mean, 28 years; SD, 9.7	16.5	NA
Melkert et al. (1993)	Screening, Netherlands	156	Cervix	HPV-6, -11, -16, -18, -31, -33, X	mean, 15–34 years	14.1	3.8
Melkert et al. (1993)	Hospital, Netherlands	2320	Cervix	HPV-6, -11, -16, -18, -31, -33, X	mean, 15–34 years	13.9	3.9
Muñoz et al. (1992)	Random sample, Colombia	98	Cervix	HPV-6, -11, -16, -18, -31, -33, -35, X	mean, 47.5 years	13.3	11.2
van Doornum et al. (1992)	STD clinic, Netherlands, ≥ 5 partners 6 months before entry	108[d]	Cervix	HPV-6, -11, -16, -18, -33	mean, 29 years	11.9[d]	10.2
Bosch et al. (1993)	Random sample, Colombia	181	Cervix	HPV-6, -11, -16, -18, -31, -33, -35, X	19–70; 39.2 years	10.5	3.3
Melkert et al. (1993)	Hospital, Netherlands	1826	Cervix	HPV-6, -11, -16, -18, -31, -33, X	35–55 years	6.6	1.5
Bosch et al. (1993)	Random sample, Spain	193	Cervix	HPV-6, -11, -16, -18, -31, -33, -35, X	18–68; 36.1 years	4.7	0.5
Muñoz et al. (1992)	Random sample, Spain	130	Cervix	HPV-6, -11, -16, -18, -31, -33, -35, X	mean, 52.3 years	4.6	3.1
Melkert et al. (1993)	Screening, Netherlands	1555	Cervix	HPV-6, -11, -16, -18, -31, -33, X	35–55 years	4.2	0.9

Table 5 (contd)

Reference	Study population	No. of subjects	Sites tested	HPV type tested for	Age of subjects (range, mean or SD, standard deviation)	Percentage HPV positive	Percentage HPV 16/18 positive
Nishikawa et al. (1991)	Gynaecology clinic, non-pregnant women, Japan	52	Cervix	HPV-16, -18, -33	18–73; 38.5 years	3.8 (HPV-16 only)	3.8 (HPV-16 only)
Engels et al. (1992)	Family planning clinic, Kenya	109	Cervix	HPV-6, -11, -16, -18, -31, -33, X	mean: 28 years; SD, 9.7	3.7	NA
Critchlow & Koutsky (1995)	University, USA, no reported coitus	56	Cervix, vulvo-vaginal	HPV-6, -11, -16, -18, -31, -33, -35, -45, X	18–20 years	3.6	0.0
Rylander et al. (1994)	Adolescent clinic, Sweden, no reported coitus	130	Cervix	HPV-6, -11, -16, -18, -31, -33, -39, -40, -45, -55, -56, X	10–25; 18 years	1.5 (HPV-6 only)	0.0
Fairley et al. (1992)	Clinic, Australia, no reported coitus	55	Vagina	HPV-6, -11, -16, -18, -31, -33, X	13–41; 18 years	0.0	0.0

NA, not available; SD, standard deviation; X, primers
[a] Each group contains three women with dysplasia
[b] Excludes cases with cervical dysplasia and condylomatous atypia
[c] Excludes cervical dysplasia in HIV (human immunodeficiency virus)-negative cases
[d] Excludes three cases with Pap IIIa smear
[ ], calculated by the Working Group

Genital HPV DNA prevalence was also measured by PCR among 168 men (mean age of 46 years) and 327 women (mean age of 44 years) residing in Spain and 128 men (mean age of 46 years) and 308 women (mean age of 42 years) residing in Colombia (Bosch et al., 1994a). In Spain, 3.6% of men and 4.9% of women were positive for HPV, and in Colombia, 19% of men and 13% of women were positive.

Among men attending STD clinics for various reasons, higher prevalence estimates of genital HPV infection detected by PCR-based methods have been reported (84%, Wikström et al. (1991); 63%, Baken et al. (1995)).

Studies of HIV (human immunodeficiency virus)-infected men and women suggest that the prevalence of HPV infection as determined by PCR-based methods is high (over 75% for cervical infection among women and 54–55% for anal infection among men) (Caussy et al., 1990a; ter Meulen et al., 1992; Kiviat et al., 1993; Seck et al., 1994). The HPV type distribution among HIV-infected populations is similar to the type distribution seen in uninfected populations (Palefsky et al., 1990; Kiviat et al., 1993).

Recent data suggest that there may be geographical or ethnic differences in the prevalence of different variants of HPV. By sequencing segments from isolates of HPV-16 and -18 obtained from various patient populations from five continents, Ho et al. (1993b) and Ong et al. (1993) suggest that the observed distribution of variants of HPV-16 and -18 indicates that, to establish each phylogenetic branch, both of these viruses evolved separately for a period in both Africa and Eurasia. In addition, the investigators speculate that because representatives from both HPV-16 branches are present in American countries, the variants were probably transferred via immigration from Europe and Africa. Whether variants of oncogenic types of HPV are important in predicting increased risk for invasive cancer of the genital tract or anus remains to be determined.

Among adults, the prevalence of common warts among office workers and engineering fitters declined with age (Keefe et al., 1994a). Currently, data concerning the prevalence of subclinical infection by non-genital HPV types are not available.

1.4.4 Natural history

Little is known about the natural history of genital HPV infections. Nevertheless, clinical findings from a variety of studies suggest the following observations: (i) Although most individuals with genital HPV infection do not develop signs or symptoms that are brought to the attention of a clinician (Bauer et al., 1991), it is likely that many infections cause microscopically visible intraepithelial lesions that are never detected. (ii) Within a few years of initial infection, most individuals are clear of the molecular, microscopic and clinical signs of the initial infection (Evander et al., 1995). (iii) Severely impaired cell-mediated immunity appears to enhance replication of the virus, thereby increasing the probability of an individual developing new or recurrent lesions (Frazer et al., 1986; Halpert et al., 1986; Palefsky et al., 1990; Vermund et al., 1991; Kiviat et al., 1993; Maiman et al., 1993). (iv) Only a small percentage of individuals infected with an oncogenic type of HPV develop cancer (zur Hausen, 1990). (v) Cervical cancer is a common HPV-associated malignancy (Krone et al., 1995), perhaps in part because cells capable of proliferation at the junction of columnar and squamous epithelium are exposed to the surface and, therefore, are most susceptible to infection and transformation by HPV.

Additional findings that suggest how different clinical courses have evolved for specific types of genital HPVs include the following: (i) Most macroscopically visible genital warts are caused by HPV-6 or -11; HPV-6 in approximately two-thirds of cases and HPV-11 in one-third (Gissmann et al., 1983). (ii) Virtually all cases of recurrent respiratory papillomatosis are associated with HPV-6 or -11; HPV-11 in approximately two-thirds of cases and HPV-6 in one-third (Abramson et al., 1987). (iii) DNA from HPV-16, rather than DNA from other types of HPV, has been detected in genital tract specimens over the longest period of time (Hildesheim et al., 1994; Shoultz et al., 1994). (iv) High-grade cervical intraepithelial lesions, which often involve HPV-16 or -18, may arise spontaneously without prior development of a low-grade lesion (Koutsky et al., 1992). (v) Most patients with cervical cancers are infected with HPV-16 or -18 (Low et al., 1990; Lörincz et al., 1992; Bosch et al., 1995). (vi) In patients with cervical cancer, HPV-18 DNA is detected more often in adenocarcinomas, adenosquamous-cell carcinomas and small-cell carcinomas than in squamous-cell carcinomas (Barnes et al., 1988; Tase et al., 1988a; Stoler et al., 1991).

Persistence of HPV-16 variants was studied in a cohort of young women. A total of 127 HPV-16 specimens obtained from 40 women were tested for sequence differences in the non-coding region of the genome using single stranded conformational polymorphism of PCR-amplified material. Using this technique, 16 different variants of HPV-16 were detected, but only two variants accounted for over 50% of the infections. All HPV-16 specimens from 24 women who were repeatedly positive over two to six visits showed the same single stranded conformational polymorphism pattern at every visit. Sequencing of clones from a subset of specimens indicated that many women were infected by more than one variant, but that one variant seemed to predominate over time, with other variants detected only intermittently (Xi et al., 1995).

A variety of viral, host and exogenous factors may influence the course of HPV infection. The type(s) or variants of virus, anatomic site of infection and host response define whether a given genital HPV infection will be self-limited and escape detection, produce a clinically evident benign proliferative lesion, or slowly, over the course of several years, on average, induce malignant transformation of infected cells.

1.5 Pathology of HPV genital tract infection and evidence from pathology for progression to malignancy

A number of reviews have been written describing the changes that are associated with HPV infection of the epithelium of the male and female lower anogenital tract (Barrasso et al., 1987a; Fu et al., 1988; Fu & Reagan, 1989; Richart et al., 1992; Wright & Richart, 1992; Richart & Wright, 1994; Wright et al., 1994a). Similar reviews have been written for the putative HPV-related lesions of the skin (Price et al., 1988; Blessing et al., 1989; Jablonska & Majewski, 1994). At other epithelial sites, HPV infection has been described infrequently and few reviews are available linking HPV infection to histological changes at these sites.

1.5.1 Terminology

(a) Dysplasia and carcinoma in situ

By the late 1800s, the histological changes that occurred at the margins of invasive squamous-cell cancers of the cervix had been recognized and described (Williams, 1888). Their significance was not appreciated at the time, but these changes later came to be called carcinoma *in situ* (CIS), a term first introduced by Schottlander and Kermauner (1912) to describe cervical cancer precursors and later reintroduced by Broders (1932). Cullen (1900) first noted that these changes resembled the cytological and pattern alterations that were present in the adjacent invasive squamous-cell cancer and suggested that they may be precursor lesions.

Originally, only epithelia that contained atypical cells throughout their full thickness were regarded as cervical cancer precursors. However, with the introduction of exfoliative cytology, it became apparent that many cytological atypias reflected histological changes that, although lacking the full thickness de-differentiation of classical CIS, nevertheless shared some of the cytological and histological changes associated with CIS, which was recognized as a cancer precursor. When it became recognized that there was a wide spectrum of changes associated with histological alterations thought potentially to be cervical cancer precursors, it became important to define these minor atypias better, to understand their biology more completely and to devise an expanded terminology with which to identify them. Reagan and Hamonic (1956) introduced the term 'dysplasia' to designate cervical epithelia that contained cytologically atypical cells but lacked full thickness de-differentiation. The dysplasias were further divided into mild, moderate and severe grades, depending upon their differentiation (see Table 6). It was implicit in this terminology that the higher the grade, the closer the lesion was in aggregate to invasion. This assumption was based upon the observation that higher-grade dysplasias resembled CIS and invasive cancer more closely than those of lower grade. CIS remained in the clinicians' minds, however, as the only true cancer precursor. Patients with CIS were generally treated by total abdominal hysterectomy, and patients with lesser degrees of epithelial change — the dysplasias — were either treated by cervical conization or followed prospectively without treatment.

(b) Cervical intraepithelial neoplasia (CIN)

With continuing clinical experience, it became obvious both to pathologists and clinicians that there was extremely poor inter- and intra-observer reproducibility in differentiating CIS from dysplasia. It was particularly difficult for pathologists to distinguish severe dysplasia and CIS, and clinicians became increasingly sceptical of the rationale for therapy dictated by the dysplasia–CIS classification system.

In view of this, and after the completion of a number of laboratory and clinical studies that were begun in the 1960s, it became apparent that severe dysplasia and CIS could not be distinguished reproducibly at any level and that the lesser degrees of atypia — particularly moderate and severe dysplasia — merged imperceptibly in objective measurements with the higher-grade lesions (Richart, 1973).

Table 6. Summary of terms used for HPV-related non-invasive cervical abnormalities

		HISTOLOGICAL TERMS						CYTOLOGICAL TERMS	
		Normal	Inflammatory/ reparative responses, HPV related?	Mild dysplasia (koilocytosis, koilocytotic atypia, flat condyloma)	Moderate dysplasia	Severe dysplasia	Carcinoma in situ	Invasive cancer	
		Normal	Inflammatory/ reparative responses, HPV related?	CIN grade I	CIN grade II	CIN grade III		Invasive cancer	
		Normal	Inflammatory/ reparative responses, HPV related?	Low-grade CIN		High-grade CIN		Invasive cancer	
The Bethesda System		Within normal limits	ASCUS	Low-grade SIL	High-grade SIL			Invasive cancer	
Papanicolaou classification		Class I	Class II	Class III	Class IV			Class V	

CIN, cervical intraepithelial neoplasia; ASCUS, atypical squamous cells of undetermined significance; SIL, squamous intraepithelial lesion

These observations led to the introduction of the term 'cervical intraepithelial neoplasia' (CIN) to designate the spectrum of cervical diseases thought to play a role in cervical carcinogenesis (Richart, 1973). The implication of the CIN terminology was that there was a continuum of change that began with mild dysplasia and ended with invasive cancer after passing progressively through the intermediate stages of intraepithelial disease. The clinical implications of this new terminology were that presumed precursor lesions should be treated based on their size and location — not simply on their histological grade. Although the CIN lesions were graded CIN I, CIN II and CIN III, the CIN III category now included severe dysplasia and CIS (see Table 6), and, in terms of treatment, there was a lower emphasis on hysterectomy in favour of out-patient-directed methods and conservation of the uterus (Richart, 1987).

As molecular data accumulated, it became apparent that the spectrum of atypical epithelial changes that occurred in the female lower genital tract and were etiologically related to HPV could best be described as a two-tiered, rather than a three-tiered, disease process, and the CIN classification was modified appropriately (see Table 6) (Richart, 1990). Those lesions commonly referred to as mild dysplasia, flat condyloma or CIN I, which were thought to be the result of an acute epithelial viral infection, were designated low-grade CIN. Those lesions that contained more severe cytological atypia, which were thought to be true potential cancer precursors and to require treatment, were designated high-grade CIN. The distinction between low-grade CIN and high-grade CIN was based upon an assessment of cytological atypia and the presence or absence of abnormal mitotic figures. However, it was emphasized that the diagnostic decision should be taken at an operational level as well as a morphological level so that the clinician could infer accurately from the diagnosis whether the pathologist believed that the lesion being diagnosed was a true cancer precursor or not.

In several recent publications (Koutsky *et al*, 1992; Kiviat & Koutsky, 1993; Wright & Riopelle, 1984), it has been reported that, in incident cases of CIN, the mean age of low-grade CIN and high-grade CIN may be more similar than for prevalent disease and that some high-grade CINs may be the immediate result of high-oncogenic-risk HPV infection. High-grade CINs may occur *de novo* and may not require a pre-existing productive infection (Kiviat *et al.*, 1992). More data are needed to clarify these observations.

(c) Squamous intraepithelial lesion (SIL)

At this stage, cytological nomenclature was highly disparate, owing to the difficulties in communication and comparison of quality-control procedures between laboratories. Recognizing this, and the problems caused by an extremely low degree of intra-observer and inter-observer reproducibility in cytological diagnoses, a group was convened in Bethesda, MD, USA, to devise a uniform cytological terminology (National Cancer Institute Workshop, 1989; Luff, 1992). This meeting further recognized that the molecular data are most consistent with a two-tiered, rather than a three-tiered, system. This new nomenclature, known as 'The Bethesda System' (TBS), introduced the terms 'low-grade squamous intraepithelial lesion' (LSIL) and 'high-grade squamous intraepithelial lesion' (HSIL) (see Table 6). Low-grade SIL includes CIN I or mild dysplasia, koilocytosis, koilocytotic atypia and flat condyloma. The high-grade SIL designation includes CIN II and CIN III or moderate and severe dysplasia and CIS.

(d) Other organs in the male and female anogenital tract

Intraepithelial lesions of the vagina, vulva, penis and anus are generally diagnosed using a modification of the CIN terminology system and are generally graded in three classifications as in the original CIN nomenclature. The presumed precursor lesions for these organs are referred to as vaginal intraepithelial neoplasia (VaIN), vulvar intraepithelial neoplasia (VIN), penile intraepithelial neoplasia (PIN) and anal intraepithelial neoplasia (AIN).

1.5.2 *Temporal and spatial relationships between cervical cancer precursors and invasive cancer*

(a) Histological observations

The original observations that suggested the concept of a cervical cancer precursor and that led to the term CIS were made by pathologists who noted that the epithelium overlying or adjacent to cervical cancers contained cytological and pattern alterations that were similar to those found in invasive cancers. This simple, but profound, observation led to the concept that cancers were preceded by a precursor state that could be recognized histologically. The invention of the colposcope by Hinselmann (1925) allowed gynaecologists to recognize clinically alterations in the cervical epithelium that could be diagnosed, by punch biopsy, as CIS. These alterations could then be treated to prevent the development of invasive cancer. However, it was not until Papanicolaou and Traut (1943) published their observations on exfoliated cells that the true implications of these early histological and colposcopical observations could be utilized as part of mass screening programmes and be translated into cancer-prevention schemes. Subsequent observers noted that the mean age of diagnosis of mild, moderate and severe dysplasia, carcinoma *in situ* and invasive cancer increased progressively and that this increase was accompanied by an increasingly large lesional size. Increasing lesional size was accompanied by an increase in gland and canal involvement, and that, further still, the larger the lesion, the more likely it was to contain areas of invasion. These were compelling observations in support of the progression of CIN to cancer (Koss, 1992).

(b) Microinvasive and early invasive cervical cancers

The most important direct pathological evidence that putative cancer precursors are, in fact, precancerous lesions was the histological observation of invasion arising from such lesions. Tongues of invasion ranging from only one or two cells to larger lesions can be observed to arise directly from surface CIN lesions or from intraepithelial lesions involving the endocervical glands. These tongues of microinvasive carcinoma (Wright *et al.*, 1994b) may be single or multiple and are generally accompanied by a local inflammatory infiltrate and a desmoplastic response. For the cervix, the risk of metastasis depends upon the degree of stromal penetration. Microinvasive cancer with stromal penetration of 3 mm or less rarely metastasizes and such lesions are commonly treated conservatively by cervical conization alone.

(c) Clinical observations

Smith and Pemberton (1934) drew attention to the fact that patients who had invasive cervical cancer were commonly found to have had CIS in their prior biopsies; indeed, when patients with CIS diagnosed by biopsy were followed without treatment, a significant number of them developed invasion. Similar observations were made by Kottmeier (1961) who followed 31 women with CIS prospectively for at least 12 years. Seventy-two percent of these women developed invasive cancer. In a similar study in New Zealand (McIndoe et al., 1984), 131 patients with persistently abnormal Pap smears were followed for 4–23 years. Twenty-nine percent developed invasive carcinoma of the cervix or vaginal vault and 69% had persistent CIS, which was treated subsequently. These observations of the natural history of CIS suggest that, in the majority of patients, once it is established, CIS rarely regresses spontaneously. It is not clear why there is a discrepancy between the direct clinical follow-up observations and the data obtained from the population-based screening programme in British Columbia, which suggested that a high proportion of CIS regress without treatment. The 'yawning gap' between the cumulative incidence of CIS and that of invasive cancer which is seen in that study (Miller, 1992) is not concordant with clinical observations. The natural history of precursors of a lesser histological grade than CIS has been studied extensively. These studies have been reviewed by Östör (1993).

1.5.3 Histological changes in HPV-related lesions of the lower female genital tract

(a) Non-productive (latent) HPV infection

HPV is thought to infect the basal or parabasal cells of the squamous epithelium and to give rise either to a non-productive (latent) or a productive infection. The non-productive HPV infection is defined as one in which the virus's replication is synchronized with the cell cycle but in which none of the cytopathogenic effects of HPV can be detected — the epithelium appears normal cytologically and histologically. Although there is no direct evidence for a solely non-productive HPV infection, there are a number of clinical observations that suggest that it occurs.

(i) HPV DNA can be detected in patients with what appears to be normal cervical epithelium. In HPV DNA-positive/Pap smear-negative patients, the risk of developing an abnormal Papanicolaou smear within two years is substantially greater than that of HPV DNA-negative controls (Koutsky et al., 1992).

(ii) It is a common and widely known clinical observation that patients who have no clinical or cytological evidence of HPV while in the interpartum state may develop HPV-related lesions during the relatively immunocompromised pregnant state, only for such lesions to remit without treatment post partum.

(iii) Patients who had organ transplants may develop HPV-related lesions of the genital tract (Penn, 1986).

(iv) Patients in whom HPV-related lesions have been treated may have detectable HPV DNA despite normal cytological, colposcopical and histological findings. Such patients are at increased risk of recurrence compared to HPV DNA-negative controls (Koutsky et al., 1992).

(b) Low-grade CIN

A number of authors reported that it was possible to distinguish between flat condyloma and a true CIN lesion (Meisels & Fortin, 1976). However, in subsequent studies it was reported that the distribution of HPV types in those lesions designated as flat condyloma and CIN are indistinguishable from one another (Kadish et al., 1986; Willet et al., 1989), and that due to this lack of consistent morphological features, the ability to make such distinctions has extremely low inter- and intra-observer reproducibility. In addition, there are no differences in nuclear DNA content, as both have diploid/polyploid DNA distribution patterns (Fu *et al.*, 1983; Fujii *et al.*, 1984). It is not thought to be possible to separate flat condylomas from low-grade CIN or SIL lesions.

Low-grade CIN (Figures 4 and 5) is, by definition, a lesion that is well differentiated and contains alterations that are characteristic of the cytopathogenic effects of a replicative HPV infection. Operationally, it is a lesion that is thought by the pathologist to be the result of an acute viral infection and not to represent a true cancer precursor. Low-grade CIN lesions can arise through infection by any of the anogenital HPV types and the cytopathogenic effects of one type compared to another are generally reported to be indistinguishable at the level of the light microscope; however, some investigators have reported that HPV-16-induced lesions are more pleomorphic than those induced by other HPV types (Crum & Levine, 1984; Crum *et al.*, 1991)

Figure 4. Pap smear: low-grade CIN (SIL)

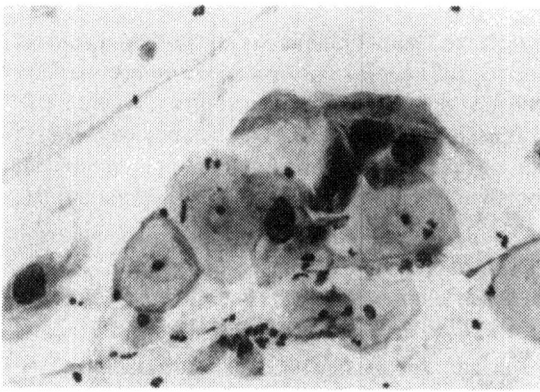

Normal superficial cells contain small, pyknotic regular nuclei. Abnormal cells are of superficial type but have irregular, hyperchromatic, large nuclei with a coarse, chromatin pattern.

Most low-grade CIN lesions contain a thickened epithelium due to the acanthosis that accompanies epithelial hyperplasia, and many also contain papillomatosis. The basal and lower parabasal layers characteristically have little cytological atypia, are arranged in a uniform fashion on the basal lamina and are not highly disorganized. As viral replication begins in the upper parabasal and lower intermediate layers of the epithelium, it is accompanied by the characteristic cytopathogenic effects of HPV infection and cytological and organizational alterations become evident. The effects that are most characteristic of an HPV infection include binucleation, perinuclear cytoplasmic cavitation with a thickened cytoplasmic membrane, and, most importantly, nuclear atypia. The expression of the E4-encoded proteins in squamous epithelial cells causes the cytokeratin matrix to collapse due to a specific binding to cytokeratin proteins (Doorbar, 1991; Doorbar *et al.*, 1991), possibly leading to the typical perinuclear cavitation, which is one feature of a productive HPV infection. The combination of nuclear atypia and perinuclear halo formation is referred to as koilocytosis or koilocytotic atypia (Koss & Durfee, 1955). These koilocytotic cells are the principal hallmark of a productive HPV infection of the cervical, vaginal or vulvar mucous membrane. It is important to emphasize that perinuclear halos may be produced as a result of vaginal infections or may accompany reparative or metaplastic processes.

Figure 5. Low-grade CIN

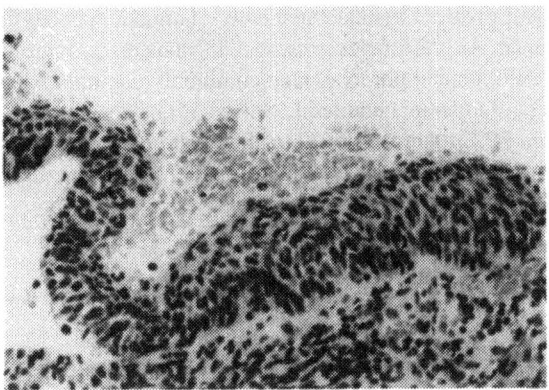

The epithelial cells are pleomorphic but differentiate as they reach the superficial layers. A tripolar mitosis is present consistent with the polyploidization that leads to cytological atypia.

The most characteristic histological feature of HPV infection, and the one that is most useful diagnostically, is nuclear atypia. HPV-related nuclear atypia is due to heteroploidy (Fu *et al.*, 1981), which appears to result from mitotic spindle abnormalities and leads to DNA replication without cytokinesis. The precise mechanism responsible for the abnormalities in mitosis and cytokinesis is not clear. The results of the interference with the mitotic process are the formation of bi- and multi-nucleated cells and enlarged atypical nuclei, accompanied by heteroploidization.

In the low-grade lesions, the nuclei are principally diploid and polyploid. Generally, mitotic figures are increased in low-grade lesions though this is generally confined to the lower third of the epithelium as are undifferentiated or basal-type cells. Mitotic figures are characteristically absent from the upper layers of the epithelium in low-grade CIN. Most of the mitotic figures have a normal appearance, but cells with tripolar mitoses or tetraploid-dispersed metaphases may also be seen (Winkler *et al.*, 1984). These two types of abnormal mitotic figures are also commonly found in polyploid lesions in other organs.

(c) High-grade CIN

High-grade CIN lesions (Figures 6–9) are substantially more atypical cytologically than low-grade CIN, have a higher degree of disorganization and have undifferentiated cells that extend past the lower third of the epithelium. This is reflected in the spectrum of HPV types found in low-grade CIN, which differs substantially from that found in high-grade CIN lesions (Matsukura & Sugase, 1995). In high-grade CIN, there is nuclear crowding, substantial pleomorphism, loss of both tissue organization and cellular polarity, and mitotic figures characteristically occur in the middle and upper third of the epithelium, in addition to the lower third. Cytological atypia that are found in high-grade CIN lesions differ substantially from those seen in the low-grade lesions. The nuclei in high-grade CIN are generally larger than those in low grade, their nuclear membranes are more prominent and tend to be convoluted and distorted, and the nuclear chromatin pattern is characteristically clumped, coarsely granular and contains prominent chromo-centers. As the nuclei enlarge, the nuclear:cytoplasmic ratio is altered in favour of the nucleus, and the cell borders, which commonly contain visible desmosomes in the low-grade lesions, become indistinct and hard to define. It has been reported that the E6 protein, particularly, and also the E7 protein of HPV-16 induce chromosomal aberrations (White *et al.*, 1994). The characteristic koilocyte of the low-grade CIN is generally absent or markedly attenuated in the high-grade lesions.

Figure 6. Pap smear: high-grade CIN (SIL)

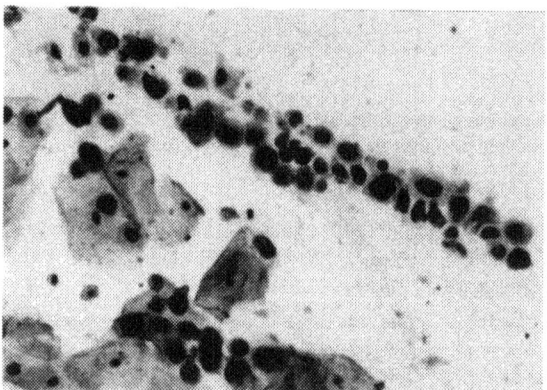

Normal superficial cells contain small, pyknotic, regular nuclei. Abnormal cells exfoliated from high-grade lesions are of the neoplastic basal and parabasal types, have an altered nuclear cytoplasmic ratio, and contain very hyperchromatic, irregularly shaped, pleomorphic nuclei with a dense, abnormal chromatin pattern.

One of the most important features distinguishing high-grade CIN from low-grade CIN is the presence of abnormal mitotic figures (AMFs) (Winkler *et al.*, 1984). Although many different types of AMFs are found in high-grade CINs, the most characteristic one is the three-group metaphase (i.e. chromosomal material on either side of the equatorial chromosomes in the metaphase) (Claas *et al.*, 1992). Other AMFs that are commonly seen include the two-group metaphase, multi-polar mitoses in excess of three, lagging metaphase chromosomes, coarsely clumped chromosomes and highly abnormal, bizarre mitotic figures. AMFs are found in aneuploid lesions (aneuploidy is a marker for cancer or precancer) and have been reported to be the histological marker that best predicts the biological behaviour of CIN (Fu *et al.*, 1981). As virtually all high-grade lesions and invasive squamous-cell cancers of the cervix are aneuploid, and as AMFs are an excellent surrogate marker for aneuploidy (Bergeron *et al.*, 1987a,b; Fu *et al.*, 1988), these mitotic abnormalities serve as a useful objective marker to distinguish between low-grade and high-grade CIN. In the presence of an AMF, a lesion will consistently be aneuploid and will be a true cancer precursor. In the absence of AMFs, the other histological features commonly used to classify these lesions should be taken into account.

Figure 7. High-grade CIN

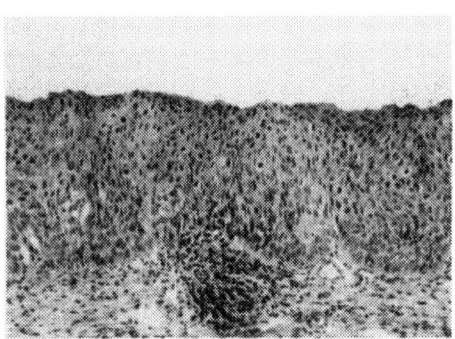

All the epithelial cells contain atypical nuclei with a pleomorphic, hyperchromatic pattern. The basal layer is disorganized, and basal-type cells extend through most of the thickness of the epithelium. Mitoses occur in all layers, and some contain coarsely clumped chromosomes.

(d) Microinvasive and invasive squamous-cell cancer of the cervix

Microinvasive squamous-cell cancer of the cervix (Figure 10) is a single or multiple irregular tongue of neoplastic squamous epithelium that breaks through the plane of the basal lamina and invades the cervical stroma or epithelial lamina propria. Characteristically, areas of microinvasion are better differentiated than the high-grade CIN from which they most commonly arise. They lack the smooth contour and crisp demarcation from the subjacent stroma that is found in both surface high-grade CIN and high-grade CIN with glandular involvement. Areas of microinvasion infiltrate in an irregular fashion, splitting collagen bundles. Microinvasive foci are commonly accompanied by an inflammatory and desmoplastic response. Microinvasion is defined as an invasive lesion that invades the cervical stroma to a depth of no more than 3 mm, and, frankly, invasive cancer (Figure 11) has a similar histological appearance to microinvasion but has invaded more than 3 mm into the cervical stroma. There is no convincing evidence that the histological appearance of invasive cancer or the patient's prognosis can be predicted from the HPV type that has produced the lesion.

Figure 8. High-grade CIN with glandular involvement

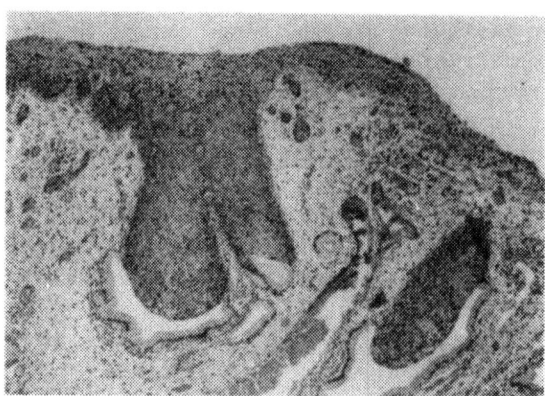

The epithelium is disorganized and has an irregular cytological appearance. The CIN extends into the endocervical glands but has a regular border and conforms to the shape of the gland. There is no stromal response. This lesion would be diagnosed as CIN grade II in a three-grade nomenclature system.

Figure 9. High-grade CIN

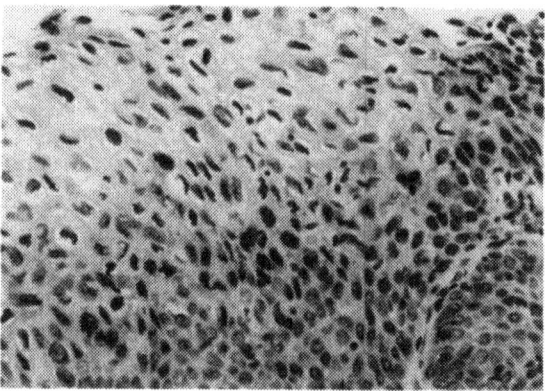

The full thickness of the epithelium is composed of highly pleomorphic, hyperchromatic cells that are disorganized and poorly attached to the basal lamina. Under a three-grade system of nomenclature, this would be diagnosed as CIN III and in current nomenclature as high-grade CIN.

(e) Vaginal intraepithelial neoplasia

The histological changes in the vaginal mucous membrane associated with HPV infection and HPV-induced neoplasia are similar to the changes that are seen in the cervical mucous membrane.

Figure 10. Microinvasive squamous-cell carcinoma

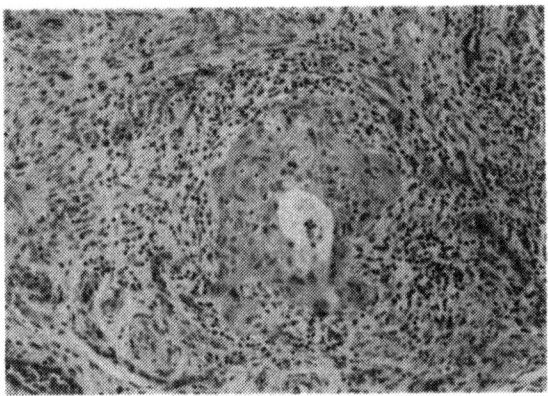

Multiple tongues of neoplastic squamous epithelium split collagen bundles in a focus of early invasion. The lesional tissue is more differentiated than in high-grade CIN, and the outline is irregular. The stromal invasion is accompanied by an inflammatory infiltrate and surrounded by a desmoplastic response.

Figure 11. Pap smear: invasive squamous-cell cancer

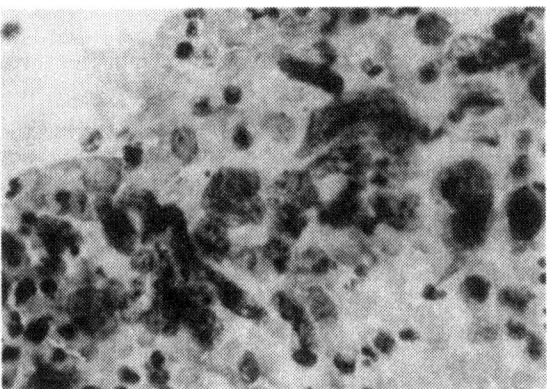

Highly atypical pleomorphic nuclei with an extremely irregular chromatin pattern and large irregular chromocenters in a background of necrotic cells.

(f) Vulva

The most characteristic HPV-related lesion found on the vulva is the acuminate wart. Condyloma acuminatum, which is almost always caused by HPV-6 or -11 (Gissmann & zur

Hausen, 1980; Gissmann *et al.*, 1982; Nuovo *et al.*, 1990; Matsukura & Sugase, 1995), is, by definition, an exophytic lesion. It has cytological and histological features and organizational alterations similar to those seen in the cervical and vaginal mucous membranes, except for the presence of substantial acanthosis and papillomatosis. Condylomata acuminata occurring on the mucous membranes characteristically have the full constellation of HPV-related cytopathogenic effects, including koilocytosis. Warts that occur in the keratinizing epithelium, however, commonly contain minimal cytological atypia, and koilocytes may be difficult to identify, particularly in clinically older lesions.

The intraepithelial lesions of the vulvar skin have a much more complicated histological pattern than those of the mucous membranes of the cervix and vagina (Wilkinson, 1994). It is common to distinguish three different VIN types histologically — basaloid, warty and well-differentiated. The basaloid type, as the name implies, is composed generally of small fairly uniform cells that are hyperchromatic and contain alterations in nuclear chromatin distribution patterns. They tend not to be highly active mitotically, and abnormal mitotic figures are seldom encountered. Warty type VIN is generally a highly pleomorphic lesion with multinucleated cells, cytological atypia, coarse chromatin clumping, large numbers of mitoses and AMFs. The warty type VIN is commonly associated with koilocytosis, and adjacent condylomatous-type changes are frequently seen. The well-differentiated type of VIN is characteristically composed of a complex, proliferative lesion, which is only minimally altered in pattern and contains minimal nuclear atypia. Dyskeratosis is a common feature. High-risk HPV types are found principally in the warty and basaloid types of VIN. They are uncommon in the well-differentiated type.

(g) Vagina, anus and penis

Squamous neoplasms of the vagina are similar in morphology to those of the cervix. Squamous neoplasms of the anus are similar morphologically to those arising in other keratinizing epithelia, including the HPV-related lesions of the vulva. The anus has a squamo-columnar junction and a transformation zone similar to that seen in the cervix. Squamous-cell cancers and their precursors develop at the squamo-columnar junction and in the transformation zone of the anus, as in the cervix.

(h) Adenocarcinoma in situ *and adenocarcinoma*

Just as the squamous intraepithelial lesions occur on the squamous side of the cervical squamo-columnar junction, so adenocarcinomas *in situ* and adenocarcinomas occur on the columnar side. They are commonly associated with CIN lesions, particularly those that are high grade (Luesley *et al.*, 1987). The endocervical epithelium appears not to support productive HPV infections, and low-risk HPV types have not been found in endocervical neoplasia (Higgins *et al.*, 1992a).

Adenocarcinoma *in situ* is characterized by complex gland formation in the distribution of the normal endocervical glands, cytological atypia (Figure 12), an increased mitotic rate and a gland-within-gland pattern. Cytological alterations similar to those seen in other aneuploid cellular populations are present and AMFs are common. Adenocarcinoma *in situ* is distinguished from invasive adenocarcinoma (Figure 13) by virtue of its pattern and lack of demonstrable invasion.

Figure 12. Pap smear: adenocarcinoma *in situ*

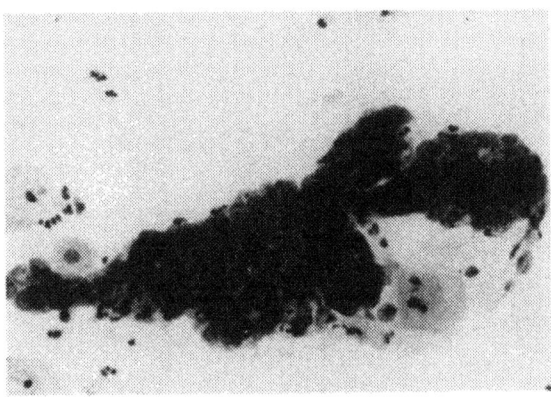

Endocervical cells appear in large, coarse aggregates. The nuclei are crowded and overlap, and the nuclear chromatin is irregular with coarsely clumped chromatin and large prominent chromocenters.

1.5.4 Pathology of non-melanoma skin cancer and cutaneous HPV infection

(a) Cutaneous HPV infection

In EV patients, skin wart infection takes the following three clinical forms, each with characteristic clinical and histopathological features: common and plane warts (verruca vulgaris and verruca planar), which are also seen in the general population, and EV-specific lesions, namely red plaque-like lesions and scaly pityriasis-like lesions (Orth *et al.*, 1979). In addition, seborrheic keratoses with typical EV-like histological changes have also been described in some patients (Jacyk *et al.*, 1993a; Tomasini *et al.*, 1993). The pathology of these lesions is reviewed by Jablonska & Majewski (1994).

(b) Non-melanoma skin cancer

Non-melanoma skin cancer refers to basal-cell and squamous-cell carcinoma and, conventionally, to the precancerous lesions actinic keratoses, Bowen's disease and intraepidermal carcinoma. This term also refers to keratoacanthoma, a common cutaneous lesion, which broadly resembles a squamous-cell carcinoma, but whose natural history is benign.

In immunosuppressed transplant patients, both the clinical and histopathological features of non-melanoma skin cancer differ. It is not possible to distinguish reliably keratoacanthoma and squamous-cell carcinoma in transplant recipients, for example, and for management and classification purposes they are referred to collectively as squamous-cell carcinoma. Similarly, in transplant recipients, actinic keratoses, intraepidermal carcinoma and Bowen's disease are not distinct entities. Since they are all thought to be dysplastic precancerous lesions, they are referred to collectively as verrucous keratoses (Blessing *et al.*, 1989). The pathology of non-melanoma skin cancer and the cytological evidence for a putative role for HPV in these lesions has been reviewed (Price *et al.*, 1988; Blessing *et al.*, 1989).

Figure 13. Pap smear: invasive endocervical adenocarcinoma

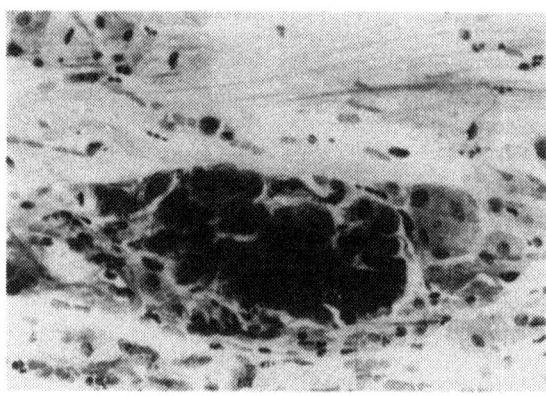

The abnormal glandular cells occur in clumps with irregularly shaped, pleomorphic nuclei with prominent large, highly irregular chromocenters.

1.5.5 Pathology of HPV-induced changes in the nude mouse system and tissue culture studies

When squamous epithelial cysts established beneath the renal capsule of nude mice are infected with HPV-11, changes occur similar to those seen in condylomata acuminata (Kreider *et al.*, 1986). When human-cultured epithelial cells are transfected with HPV-16 DNA and allowed to differentiate, the morphological changes resemble high-grade CIN (McCance *et al.*, 1988; McDougall, 1994).

1.6 Clinical disease of established HPV etiology (other than precancer and cancer)

Genital HPVs cause condylomata, laryngeal papillomas and some papillomas at other mucosal sites, e.g. the oral or sinonasal cavity and conjunctiva. Cutaneous HPV types and EV HPV types cause skin lesions. HPVs have been reported as being associated with many additional conditions, but the significance of these observations is as yet unclear (Shah & Howley, 1996). This section will only address benign conditions clearly associated with HPV.

1.6.1 Genital area

Condyloma acuminatum and genital wart are synonyms. The prevalence estimates of condyloma vary from 0.24 to 13%, depending mainly on the risk of sexually transmitted diseases (STD) and age distribution in the population examined (Kjaer & Lynge, 1989). The prevalence of condyloma in STD clinic patients was 11% compared with 2% in college students and was highest in the age group 16–24 years (Kiviat et al., 1989). Positivity for HPV DNA, which may reflect subclinical disease, was more than two-times higher than clinical disease in 377 first attendees of a STD clinic; 15% had genital warts, compared with 35% who were positive for HPV by ViraPap™/ViraType™ (Borg et al., 1993).

In women, the vulva, vestibule, vagina, perineum and perianal region are the most common sites for condylomata acuminata. HPV-6/11 was detected by Southern blot hybridization in up to 95% of condylomata acuminata (Gissmann et al., 1982; Johnson et al., 1991; Nuovo et al., 1991b).

Condylomata acuminata are rarely detected on the uterine cervix. HPV-6/11 was identified in 65% and HPV-16/18 in 8% of these lesions by Southern blot hybridization (Mitrani-Rosenbaum et al., 1988). Cervical condylomata may be hyperkeratotic and are sometimes confused with cancer owing to a bizarre pattern of vessels (Coppleson, 1991). The major capsid protein, L1, can be detected more often and in higher quantities in condylomata acuminata of the uterine cervix than in similar lesions of the penis or vulva (35% compared with 12% in a total of 95 cases) indicating a higher content of virus particles (Wools et al., 1994).

Genital warts are rarely observed in children. In a series of 25 children between seven months and 12 years in age, 74% of anogenital warts were HPV-6/11-positive and 17.4% were positive for HPV-2 by Southern blot hybridization. Clinical examination could not differentiate between HPV-2-positive and HPV-6/11-positive genital lesions. All children with HPV-2-positive condyloma also had cutaneous common warts which appeared to be due to auto-inoculation. One female newborn had anal warts one week after delivery and was probably infected in utero (Obalek et al., 1993). HPV-6-positive cutaneous lesions were found on an arm and a leg in a nine-year-old girl who was HPV DNA-negative in the genital tract and had no evidence of sexual abuse (Blauvelt et al., 1992).

In men, penile and urethral condylomata show a distribution of HPV types similar to that of genital warts in women. Lesions are condylomatous, macular, papular and may be keratotic (Barrasso et al., 1987a; Del Mistro et al., 1987; Zhu et al., 1993a; Labropoulou et al., 1994). Acuminate, papular and well-demarcated punctated lesions are most likely to contain HPV (Hippeläinen et al., 1993). In a series of 108 male patients, condylomata were located on the penile shaft in 51%, the shaft and perianal region in 14%, the shaft and scrotum in 2%, the shaft and urethral meatus in 15% and the urethral meatus alone in 18% (Rosemberg, 1991).

1.6.2 Upper respiratory and digestive tract and conjunctiva

HPV-11 is the most prevalent type (50–84%) found in laryngeal papillomas (Gissmann et al., 1983; Ushikai et al., 1994). When analysis is restricted to adult papillomas, HPV-6 is found most commonly (Corbitt et al., 1988). Recurrent respiratory papillomatosis originates in the upper respiratory tract where ciliated columnar and squamous epithelium are juxtaposed (Kashima et al., 1993). In adults with recurrent respiratory papillomatosis, biopsies of normal mucosa adjacent to papillomas were HPV DNA-positive in a majority of patients (Steinberg et al., 1983; Rihkanen et al., 1993, 1994), a finding that possibly explains frequent recurrences.

Oral verrucal-papillary lesions are clinically subdivided into verruca vulgaris, condyloma acuminatum, multiple and single papillomas, and focal epithelial hyperplasia (Scully *et al.*, 1985). All of 10 verrucae vulgares from the lip in one series were positive for HPV-2 DNA (Eversole *et al.*, 1987a), whereas the majority of oral lesions contained DNA from genital HPV types (Premoli-de-Percoco *et al.*, 1993). Oral condylomata acuminata resemble genital lesions with a 85% (17/20) positivity rate for HPV-6, -11 or related types (Eversole *et al.*, 1987b). HPV-13 and -32 are found almost exclusively in focal epithelial hyperplasia; 90% of these lesions are positive for one of these HPV types (Pfister *et al.*, 1983a; Beaudenon *et al.*, 1987). Of 202 cases of benign oral leukoplakia, 2.5% was positive for HPV-6/11 and 3.5% for HPV-16 by in-situ hybridization (Gassenmaier & Hornstein, 1988).

Conjunctival papillomas are positive for genital HPV types (Lass *et al.*, 1983). The prevalence of HPV-6 in conjunctival papillomas detected by in-situ hybridization decreases with age (McDonnell *et al.*, 1987). The authors suggested that HPV-6 infection of the conjunctiva is possibly acquired during passage through an infected birth canal.

1.6.3 Skin

Skin warts are classified according to macroscopic and microscopic morphological criteria. Infection with specific HPV types can be broadly correlated with these lesions (Gross *et al.*, 1982; Croissant et al., 1985; Jablonska *et al.*, 1985; Melton & Rasmussen, 1991).

(i) Typical common or mosaic warts, i.e. rough keratotic papules or nodules, on the hands, knuckles or periungual areas contain HPV-2, -4, -7, -26, -27, -28 or -29. Using PCR on specimens obtained from 111 immunocompetent patients, HPV-2a was found in 36% of the warts, HPV-2c in 23% (now known to be HPV-27; Chan *et al.*, 1994a), HPV-57 in 12%, a variant of HPV-57 in 14%, HPV-7 in 4% and HPV-4 in 1% (one endophytic common wart) (Rübben *et al.*, 1993). HPV-35 was found in a periungual wart of a patient with HPV-35-positive Bowenoid papulosis (Rüdlinger *et al.*, 1989b).

(ii) Butchers warts have the clinical appearance of common warts but occur on the hands of those who work with raw meat, fish, and poultry. Among 60 butchers, HPV-1 was found in 6.7% of warts examined by Southern blot hybridization, HPV-2 in 45%, HPV-3 in 15%, HPV-4 in 10% and HPV-7 in 23% (Orth *et al.*, 1981). A similar distribution of HPV types was seen with PCR analysis; 23/26 lesions were positive for HPV DNA: HPV-2 in 7.5%, HPV-4 in 11.5%, HPV-7 in 27% and unidentified HPV types (possibly containing HPV-1 or -3) in 42% (Melchers *et al.*, 1993). In another series, HPV-7 was found by PCR in 74/112 (66%) warts of men working in meat-processing plants (abattoir workers and butchers) (Keefe *et al.*, 1994b).

(iii) Filiform or papillomatous common warts found most frequently on the face, lips, eyelids or nares contain HPV-1, -2 or -7 (Jablonska *et al.*, 1985; Egawa *et al.*, 1993a). HPV-7 was found in two individuals with generalized or extensive facial warts with filiform appearance (de Villiers *et al.*, 1986a).

(iv) Flat or plane warts, which can appear at different locations on the body and can form a linear arrangement (i.e. Koebner warts), are associated with HPV-2, -3, -10, -26, -27, -28, -29 or -41 (Melton & Rasmussen, 1991).

(v) Deep plantar warts, i.e. hyperkeratotic plaques or nodules on the plantar surface of the foot, are usually positive for HPV-1 or -4 (Jablonska et al., 1985; Rübben et al., 1993). HPV-associated epidermal cysts of the sole of the feet of 33 Japanese patients contained HPV-60 (Kato & Ueno, 1992; Egawa et al., 1994). HPV-63 and -1 were present in the same nucleus of one plantar wart (Egawa et al., 1993b).

Morphological and virological findings of skin lesions found in immunocompromised patients after transplant or in patients with EV are discussed in section 2.5.

1.7 Therapy and vaccination

When treating patients with HPV infections and/or HPV associated neoplasia, the sexual partner may also be infected and lesions may be multifocal or multicentric. Strict therapeutic guidelines have not been established for HPV-related lesions since no valid studies have addressed the issues of treatment of the sexual partner or multiple body sites.

1.7.1 Therapy of benign disease

The choice for treatment of genital warts is chemical or physical destruction. Chemodestruction of genital warts with 20% podophyllin resin extract results in cure rates of between 35% and 45% (van Krogh, 1981; Rosemberg, 1991). In recent years, podophyllotoxin, the active ingredient in podophyllin resin, has become available for treatment of genital warts (Baker et al., 1990). A 0.5% podophyllotoxin solution reduced the mean number of warts from 6.27 to 1.1, destroyed about 70% of all warts and totally cleared the warts in 29–50% of patients (Baker et al., 1990; Bonnez et al., 1994b). In a randomized trial with 138 men and 67 women, 0.5% podophyllotoxin lotion was compared with 25% podophyllin solution. The former totally cleared 81% of warts compared with 61% by podophyllin ($p < 0.001$) (Kinghorn et al., 1993). In addition, podophyllotoxin solution is more efficacious than podophyllotoxin cream (Syed & Lundin, 1993). Podophyllin and its compounds should not be used in pregnant patients as it is a teratogen.

Topical trichloroacetic acid (TCA) is the alternative to podophyllin. It is applied topically to warts as a 50–85% solution and can be self-administered. A 85% solution gave a 60–80% eradication rate (Malviya et al., 1987; Menendiz Velazquez et al., 1993). The advantage of TCA is that it can be used in pregnancy. The clinical cure rate of TCA in pregnant patients with cervical condylomata was 83% with a 85% solution (Menendez Velasquez et al., 1993).

Five percent 5-fluorouracil (5-FU) ointment is recommended only for treating extensive and recalcitrant HPV-related vaginal lesions (Krebs, 1991). However, care must be taken not to overtreat — chronic vaginal ulcerations have been reported in some patients (Krebs & Helmkamp, 1991). Vaginal stenosis, burning vulva syndrome or dyspareunia may also occur in some women after 5-FU treatment. 5-FU is contraindicated in pregnant women. The neoadjuvant effect of 5-FU after CO_2 laser surgery is controversial (Reid et al., 1990) and may result in vaginal adenosis.

Excision, electrosurgical removal or cryotherapy are most frequently used for the treatment of HPV-related cutaneous lesions. After several sessions, cryotherapy or CO_2 laser therapy lead to the complete cure of genital warts in the majority of patients (Bergman et al., 1984; Reid *et al.*, 1985; Rosemberg, 1991). Similar success (78/91, i.e. 86% free of disease) is reported with the argon laser after one or two treatment sessions (Rotteleur *et al.*, 1986). The Nd:YAG (neodium:yttrium aluminium garnet) laser cured only 30% of 20 men with urethral condylomata after one course of treatment; to attain successful treatment, 40% received up to five courses (Volz *et al.*, 1994).

The antiviral, immunomodulating and antiproliferative action of interferon appeared to be promising for the treatment of genital warts. Although initial studies with recombinant α-interferon applied systemically or intra-lesionally resulted in significantly higher complete response rates in interferon-treated patients compared with placebo, i.e. 36% versus 17% (Eron *et al.*, 1986) and 62% versus 21% (Friedman-Kien *et al.*, 1988), two recent studies using various recombinant α-interferons found no significant effect (Reichman *et al.*, 1990; Condylomata International Collaborative Study Group, 1993a). After initial promising results on the effect of interferon in an adjuvant setting after laser therapy (Reid *et al.*, 1992), two recent studies showed no advantage when interferon was used after laser or cryotherapy compared with observation alone (Eron *et al.*, 1993; Condylomata International Collaborative Study Group, 1993b).

Similar data have been reported for the adjuvant treatment of recurrent respiratory papillomatosis. A study with 66 patients used α-n1-interferon in a randomized crossover trial as an adjuvant to surgery; it was reported that the papilloma growth rate was slowed by interferon treatment (Kashima *et al.*, 1985; Leventhal *et al.*, 1988). In a study of 123 patients randomly assigned to surgery plus interferon versus surgery alone there was no adjuvant effect of interferon (Healy *et al.*, 1988).

Since recurrent respiratory papillomatosis is a serious, recalcitrant disease that is difficult to treat, several drugs have been tested for their therapeutic efficacy in various small case series: 13-*cis*-retinoic acid showed some effect in combination with α-interferon in three recurrent respiratory papillomatosis patients, increasing surgical treatment intervals by a factor of two (Lippman *et al.*, 1994). Ribavirin showed a promising effect in the CRPV model (Ostrow *et al.*, 1992). It was used in four patients with recurrent respiratory papillomatosis. Complete remission was seen in two adults and partial remissions in another adult and one child resulting in a prolonged interval between required surgeries (McGlennen *et al.*, 1993). Photodynamic therapy was used in 33 patients who had moderate to severe recurrent respiratory papillomatosis. These patients were treated with dihaematoporphyrin ether intravenously 48–72 h prior to photo-activation with an argon pump dye laser system; a 50% decrease in papilloma growth rate was seen on average, with three patients remaining free of disease but continuing to be infected latently (Abramson *et al.*, 1992).

1.7.2 *Therapy of precancers*

Cervical intraepithelial neoplasia (CIN) is the most commonly detected genital precancer in humans. The following section will refer mainly to data regarding cervical disease but the principles apply generally to treatment of HPV-associated precancerous lesions of other body sites.

There are no strict clinical guidelines for the therapy of CIN; interim therapeutic guidelines were established at a recent consensus conference in the USA (Kurman *et al.*, 1994). However, there is general agreement that, prior to treatment, histological verification is mandatory in order to classify the lesion and to exclude invasive cancer. Overdiagnosis and overtreatment of lesions that are not CIN should be avoided. Ideally, therapy should be undertaken by a physician who understands the cytological, colposcopical, virological and histological aspects of cervical neoplasia and who takes into account the patient's physical and mental status as well. Treatment of CIN may be excisional or destructive. The main disadvantage of the destructive methods is that invasive cancer may be missed. The incidental finding of invasive cancer was reported in conization specimens in 0.8% patients in whom invasive cancer was missed by colposcopically directed biopsy preoperatively (Prendiville et al., 1989; Bigrigg et al., 1990; Luesley et al., 1990; Whiteley & Oláh, 1990). If invasive cancer is not detected in the triage procedure prior to destructive therapy, this diagnostic error may lead to recurrence and death (Sevin et al., 1979; Townsend et al., 1981). Destructive therapeutic techniques, such as CO_2 laser vaporization or cryotherapy, should be confined to the management of purely ectocervical low-grade lesions confirmed by colposcopy, cytology and histology (Sevin et al., 1979; Baggish, 1982; Andersen & Husth, 1992).

Cold knife conization has been used for decades to treat CIN but is increasingly being replaced by the CO_2 laser (Dorsey & Diggs, 1979) or high-frequency electrosurgical excision (large loop excision of the transformation zone, i.e. LLETZ, or loop electrosurgical excision procedure, i.e. LEEP) preoperatively (Prendiville et al., 1989; Bigrigg et al., 1990; Luesley et al., 1990; Whiteley & Oláh, 1990; Wright et al., 1992). Compared to LEEP excision, more tissue is removed by cold knife conization (15.8 mm versus 9.2 mm depth and 5.6 g versus 2.6 g of weight; $p < 0.01$) (Girardi et al., 1994). This is of special importance in young women since conization has a negative effect on fertility; in a case–control study following 56 patients and 112 controls, the duration of pregnancy was shorter ($p < 0.001$) and the incidence of premature delivery was higher ($p < 0.0001$) in women with a history of laser conization (Hagen & Skjeldestad, 1993). Similar data are reported for LEEP, after which 24% of women had babies with a birthweight of less than 2500 g as compared with 7% in controls ($p = 0.03$) (Blomfield et al., 1993). Other studies found no adverse effects of LEEP on fertility or pregnancy outcome (Cruickshank et al., 1995; Ferenczy et al., 1995). In a comparison of LEEP and cold knife conization patients in a case–control study with 43 women in each group, there was a mean operating time of 2.8 min versus 14 min ($p < 0.01$), blood loss of 3.3 ml versus 79 ml ($p < 0.01$) and postoperative complications such as haemorrhage in 4.7% versus 20.9% ($p < 0.05$) (Oyesana et al., 1993a). The same authors compared LEEP with CO_2 laser conization in a randomized trial with 150 patients in each group; significant differences were detected in operating time (2.5 min versus 24.2 min; $p < 0.001$), pain under local anaesthesia (7% versus 45%; $p < 0.001$), blood loss (2.77 ml versus 27.15 ml; $p < 0.001$) and thermal artifact on histological evaluation of the cone margins (5 versus 25 specimens; $p < 0.01$) (Oyesana et al., 1993b). Persistence rates for CIN after excisional treatment is about 4% (Prendiville et al., 1989; Bigrigg et al., 1990; Luesley et al., 1990). Persistence is more likely when the CIN involves the margins of excised tissue (Paterson-Brown et al., 1992; Lopes et al., 1993). The 'see and treat' approach using the LEEP technique (Keijser et al., 1992) eliminating histological evaluation prior to treatment should only be performed by experienced specialists who can ascertain whether or not invasive cancer is present. Many physicians prefer to obtain a histological diagnosis prior to treatment. Irrespective of the surgical technique, an endocervical curretage is usually performed following the treatment to verify that residual CIN is not present (Hatch et al., 1985).

Natural and recombinant interferon has been used as mono- and adjuvant therapy for treatment of CIN in a number of studies (Choo et al., 1986; Schneider et al., 1987a; Yliskoski et al., 1990, 1991; Schneider et al., 1995). A comparison of the therapeutic results is difficult since the studies vary in design, dosage, mode and duration of application and measurement of study outcome. Interferon is currently used principally for specific indications such as recurrent or extensive disease. Its therapeutic efficacy in the management of HPV-associated lesions remains controversial.

1.7.3 Vaccination

Therapeutic vaccination may potentially be used to treat patients with established HPV infections or HPV-associated precancer or cancer; prophylactic vaccination may potentially protect against HPV infection. Theoretically, protection can be achieved by induction of virus-neutralizing antibodies prior to exposure, and successful therapeutic vaccination will depend on stimulation of cellular immune response.

In animal models (BPV, CRPV and COPV), neutralizing antibodies produced after either natural infection or immunization with recombinant capsid proteins protect against subsequent viral challenge (Campo, 1991; Christensen & Kreider, 1991; Christensen et al., 1991; Jarrett et al., 1991; Lin et al., 1992; Campo et al., 1993; Chandrachud et al., 1995; Ghim et al., 1995). Antibodies often recognize conformation-dependent epitopes and are specific for individual papillomavirus types. Neutralizing antibodies are found in sera of HPV-positive patients (Christensen & Kreider, 1993; Kirnbauer et al., 1994), but regression or recurrence of HPV-induced lesions have not yet been correlated with previous antibody status. Recently, synthetic virus-like particles have been developed after expression of papillomavirus structural proteins *in vitro* (Zhou et al., 1991a; Hagensee et al., 1993; Kirnbauer et al., 1994). Studies using such particles in prophylactic vaccines will show whether anti-HPV neutralizing antibodies are able to protect against HPV infection.

Vaccination with non-structural papillomavirus proteins can generate a cellular immune response that may be effective in the treatment of papillomavirus-induced lesions. Regression of papillomas has been achieved in cattle by vaccination with BPV-4 E7 protein (Campo et al., 1993) and in rabbits by vaccination with CRPV E1 and E2 proteins (Selvakumar et al., 1995). In mice, the transforming proteins E6 and E7 of HPV-16 induce specific cytotoxic T cells (Chen et al., 1991, 1992a) or $CD4^+$ delayed type hypersensitivity T cells (McLean et al., 1993), which both mediate rejection of transplanted E6 or E7 expressing cells. Elimination of virus-infected cells by cytotoxic T cells depends on proper MHC (major histocompatibility complex) class I-restricted presentation of virus-derived peptides by the target cell. However, HPV-infected cells may escape immune surveillance since MHC (major histocompatibility complex) class I expression is downregulated in CIN or cervical cancer (Connor & Stern, 1990; Cromme et al., 1993a). Several potential cytotoxic T-cell epitopes of HPV-16 E6 and E7 have already been identified (Kast et al., 1993). Such epitopes as well as the proteins themselves are candidates for therapeutic anti-HPV vaccines. Several first phase trials are already in progress (Muñoz et al., 1995).

2. Studies of Cancer in Humans

In the following discussion of HPV infection as an exposure posing a risk of cancer, the importance of distinguishing 'transient' from 'persistent' infection is emphasized. Several lines of epidemiological evidence suggest that many incident HPV infections are transient, especially at younger ages, whereas less-common, persistent infections pose a higher risk for the development of subsequent cancer. These terms are admittedly ill-defined, as it is unclear whether persistent infection can include an undetectable 'latent' phase. Nevertheless, persistent cytological evidence of low-grade CIN has been shown to pose a higher risk of progression than the first occurrence of (incident) low-grade CIN (Richart & Barron, 1969; Nasiell et al., 1986). Also, persistent HPV DNA detection accompanying cytological/histological diagnosis of CIN has been associated with a high absolute and attributable risk of progression (Remmink et al., 1995).

In the absence of cytological evidence of CIN, 'high-risk' types of HPV (type 16 in particular) tend to persist longer than low-risk types (Hildesheim et al., 1994), and continued viral DNA detection is associated cross-sectionally with greater risk of incident CIN (Wideroff et al., 1995).

Persistence cannot be determined reliably by a single measurement of HPV infection. Moreover, it is not correct to assume that odds ratios or attributable proportion estimates from studies using cross-sectional assessment of past HPV infection are equivalent to prospective risk estimates. Typically, prospective risk estimates are lower than those from cross-sectional studies, because HPV infections appear to be lost more often in eventual 'controls' than in eventual 'cases', so that HPV positive cases in case–control studies are more likely to be persistent infections.

It is also worth noting here that there are too many anogenital HPV types to study each individually. For this reason, types are often grouped into putative 'high-risk' and 'low-risk' groups. These working definitions tend to be variable, as there are several possible sets of grouping criteria, based on either (i) biological behaviour in vitro, (ii) phylogeny imputed from DNA sequence homologies, or (iii) epidemiology. In epidemiological studies, the definition of 'high-risk' anogenital types can be based most liberally on finding type-specific HPV DNA (in the absence of other types) in cases of anogenital cancer. More strictly, 'high-risk' types have been defined as those associated with elevated relative risks of cancer in analytical studies.

Some authors have used the terms 'cancer-associated types' or 'oncogenic' types as synonyms for 'high-risk' types; all of these terms should be considered preliminary, given that the studies are designed to establish oncogenicity.

2.1 Descriptive studies of anogenital cancer

This section is limited to the descriptive epidemiological data addressing geographical and temporal correlations at the population level between cancer incidence and HPV prevalence at anogenital sites. To ensure comparability, the section includes only those studies in which the same HPV-testing methods were used for the populations being compared. There appear to be no relevant descriptive data relating rates of HPV infection to rates of cancer at non-anogenital sites.

Finally, because of the variability in exposure measurements of HPV and disease measurements of CIN, the results from different studies are only grossly comparable. Relative risks can be compared for general consistency and strength, but comparisons of absolute risk estimates are not reliable.

2.1.1 Cancer of the uterine cervix

Few studies have attempted to correlate rates (or time trends) of cervix cancer with rates (or time trends) of HPV infection in different parts of the world, but several studies have examined them separately.

Cervical cancer mortality trends in a number of countries have been surveyed by Cuzick and Boyle (1988), Beral *et al.* (1994) and others. Incidence and mortality trends are reported in a recent monograph (Coleman *et al.*, 1993a). The highest rates are found in South America, Asia and Africa, although there are few good data for the last. Very low rates are seen in Israel and the Middle East. The rates appear to be fairly stable in these areas and this is also true for southern and eastern Europe. However, marked declines have been observed in both incidence and mortality of cervical cancer in North America, western Europe and Japan. Much of the reduction has been attributed to an effect of screening (Hakama *et al.*, 1991; Aareleid *et al.*, 1993). An exception to the overall long-term decrease in these countries is a recent increase in rates among young women in the United Kingdom, Australia and New Zealand (Cuzick & Boyle, 1988). Even more recently, increases in cervical cancer rates among young women have been reported in Scandinavia and eastern Europe (Beral *et al.*, 1994). In the USA, blacks have approximately twice the cervical cancer rate of whites, but a study in Detroit of women aged 15–39 (Weiss *et al.*, 1994) found that the rates were decreasing more rapidly in blacks and were nearly equal to those of whites by 1991. The most recent incidence data from the USA suggest a stabilization or a slight increase in the rate of cervical cancer among white women under the age of 50 (Ries *et al.*, 1994). [Some of the international variation in rates of invasive cancer is likely to be due to the marked differences in the availability of screening and diagnosis and treatment of preinvasive lesions.]

No time-related trends in HPV DNA positivity have been identified in studies of archival CIN and cervical cancer specimens obtained from women residing in the USA and the United Kingdom (Collins *et al.*, 1988; Anderson *et al.*, 1993). Findings from these studies indicate that the association between specific types of HPV and cervical neoplasia has been consistent over the past 25–50 years. In each time period, high-risk types of HPV (HPV-16 and -18) were most frequently detected. Also, the more recently discovered HPV types (HPV-42, -45, -51, -52 and -56) were found in archival specimens, some of which were obtained 25 years earlier.

The early studies of the rates of HPV infection in normal women in high-risk and low-risk areas for cervical cancer yielded apparently paradoxical results (Table 7). Comparisons between Denmark and Greenland, the latter of which has a fivefold to sixfold higher cancer rate, did not show higher HPV rates in Greenland. In a population-based study of 1247 randomly selected women aged 20–39, cervical scrapes were analysed for HPV by filter in-situ hybridization (Kjaer et al., 1988). The positivity rate for HPV-16/18 was higher in Denmark (13%) than in Greenland (8.8%). Rates for HPV-6/11 were also slightly higher (7.5% versus 6.7%). In a second study of 255 women (Kjaer et al., 1993), similar prevalences were found in the two countries by dot blot (3.9% in Greenland versus 6.3% in Denmark) and PCR (43% versus 39%, respectively). [The Working Group noted that the apparent lower prevalence of HPV infection in the high-risk area may be explained by the earlier age at first intercourse among Greenlandic women causing an earlier peak and subsequent decline in the HPV–age curve. Consequently, studies covering only the age group 20–39 years may not be fully informative in this respect.]

In a study of 2330 women attending routine family planning and maternal and child health care clinics in Recife (high incidence) and São Paulo (lower incidence), Brazil, Villa and Franco (1989) found a threefold higher prevalence of HPV-16/18 by filter in-situ hybridization in women from the high-incidence area (5.9% versus 2.0% in the low-incidence area) and a 2.4-fold higher prevalence in women from the high-incidence area (5.1% versus 2.1%).

Muñoz et al. (1992) studied 228 population-based controls from a case–control study of invasive cancer and found a higher rate of HPV-positivity by PCR in Colombia compared to Spain (13.3% versus 4.6%), although the positivity rates were similar by Southern blot (4.2% versus 5.7%, respectively). In a comparison study in the same area (Bosch et al., 1993), controls to CIN III cases had twice the positivity rate for any HPV by PCR in Colombia compared to Spain (10.5% versus 4.7%). Rates for HPV-16 were also much higher (3.3% versus 0.5%). Cervical cancer incidence rates are about eight times higher in Colombia.

Hildesheim and colleagues (Hildesheim et al., 1993; Bauer et al., 1993) compared HPV DNA prevalences in two populations of cytologically normal women in the USA, presumed to vary substantially in their risk of cervical neoplasia. Specifically, 404 poor, white, black and Hispanic women in Washington, DC (high prevalence of cervical neoplasia) were compared with 483 middle class, predominantly white women attending a pre-paid health plan in Portland, Oregon (low prevalence of cervical neoplasia) using the same $L1$ consensus primer PCR test method. The prevalence of HPV DNA was 33.7% in the Washington population, compared to 17.7% among the Portland women.

2.1.2 Other anogenital cancers

Other anogenital cancers have been associated with HPV, notably vulvar, penile and anal cancer. Trends in the incidence of anal cancer have been studied in Denmark by Frisch et al. (1993) who found that they were stable between 1943 and 1957, but increased by 50% in men and tripled in women between 1957 and 1987. A similar pattern was observed in Connecticut, USA, where, on the basis of tumour registry data, the incidence of anal cancer increased 2.3-fold among women and 1.9-fold among men between 1960–88. An increase has also been observed in other parts of the USA, and anal cancer is now more frequent in women than men, in blacks than whites, and in residents of metropolitan rather than rural areas (Melbye et al., 1994a).

Table 7. Comparison of HPV detection rates in populations at different risk of cervical cancer

Reference	Location	Cervical cancer incidence per 10⁵ population	Source of study population	No. of participants	HPV type-specific detection rate (%)					HPV-positive	Detection method (types included)
					6/11	16/18	16	18	6/11 + 16/18 + 31/33/35		
Kjaer et al. (1988)	Greenland Denmark	1.98[a] 0.35[a]	Random samples of the general female population (1986)	586 661	6.7 7.5	8.8 13.0					Filter in-situ hybridization
Kjaer et al. (1993)	Greenland Denmark	1.98[a] 0.35[a]	Random samples of the general female population (1988)	129 126					3.9 6.3		ViraPap™/ViraType™
	Greenland Denmark						20.2 24.6	14.7 19.8		43.4 38.9	PCR (11,16,18,33)
Villa & Franco (1989)	Recife São Paulo	96.5 35.1	Random samples of women attending 3 family-planning and maternal and child health clinics	Total: 2330	5.2 2.4	5.9 2.0					Filter in-situ hybridization
Muñoz et al. (1992)	Colombia Spain	48.2 5.7–6.1	Random samples of women in participating areas	98 130			9.2 3.1			13.3 4.6	PCR (6,11,16,18, 31,33,35)
Bosch et al. (1993)	Colombia Spain	48.2 5.7–6.1	Women attending screening programmes and family-planning clinics	181 193			3.3 0.5			10.5 4.7	PCR (6,11,16,18, 31,33,35)
Hildesheim et al. (1993); Bauer et al. (1993)	Washington, DC, USA Portland, OR, USA	High risk Low risk	Women attending screening programmes	404 483						33.7 17.7	PCR (L1 consensus primers)

[a] Cumulative incidence per 100 women (20–39 years)

In contrast, the incidence of penile cancer was observed to decline during 1943–90 in uncircumsized populations despite the lack of screening procedures and changes in diagnostic criteria (Frisch et al., 1995).

Correlation analyses based on data from 136 cancer registries around the world revealed statistically significant correlations between the rates of cervical cancer and cancers of the mouth and oesophagus and between cancer of the penis and cancers of the mouth and hypopharynx (Muñoz et al., 1990). Bosch and Cardis (1990) used a similar approach to show a correlation between the incidence of cervical cancer and that of cancer of the penis, vagina and vulva. These reports are in line with previous studies in England and Wales (Smith et al., 1980), China (Li et al., 1982) and Brazil (Franco et al., 1988).

Further support for an etiological parallel between anal and cervical intraepithelial neoplasia (Scholefield et al., 1989, 1992) and between anal and cervical cancer has been substantiated in recent linkage studies of multiple primary cancers undertaken in Denmark and the USA (Melbye & Sprøgel, 1991; Rabkin et al., 1992).

2.2 Case reports and case series

Nearly 20 years ago H. zur Hausen suggested that human papillomavirus (HPV) could be causally involved in cervical carcinogenesis (zur Hausen, 1976). Subsequently, HPV DNA has been found repeatedly in cervical cancers and has also been implicated in the genesis of several other human cancer types, particularly neoplasms of the anogenital area, as well as of the skin and the respiratory and digestive tracts.

2.2.1 Cancer of the uterine cervix

(a) Pre-invasive cervical lesions

Table 8 gives a summary of case series of cervical intraepithelial neoplasia (CIN) that included more than 70 cases and gave the HPV results by cytological/histological category. The range of HPV results is broad, but in general the HPV detection rate increased with the severity of the lesion independent of the detection method used. [Cytological/histological misclassification of less-severe diagnoses may explain much of this trend.] The prevalence of HPV in CIN III was reported to be more than 70% in 13 out of the 21 studies. The variation in detection rate between studies was lowest for the PCR method for all cytological/histological groups. The variety of HPV types found in less-severe lesions is greater than that in more-severe lesions, in which the cancer-associated types are typically found.

In the six case series including more than 10 patients with adenocarcinoma *in situ* (Table 9), HPV DNA was found in 25–97% of cases. [The diagnosis of glandular intraepithelial lesions is more problematic than squamous intraepithelial diagnoses.]

(b) Squamous-cell carcinoma

Microscopic evidence of HPV infection has been linked to adjacent cervical cancer for decades. Table 10 summarizes the prevalence of HPV DNA in series ($\geq$ 40 cases) of patients with cervical squamous-cell carcinoma recorded in studies published from 1988 to date. In studies using PCR-based tests designed to detect more than a single HPV type, the HPV

Table 8. Prevalence of HPV DNA in cervical intraepithelial neoplasia (CIN) case series[a] (≥ 70 cases)

Reference	Study area	Detection method (types included)	No. of cases	Overall HPV positivity (%)[b]	HPV type-specific positivity (%)						Comments
					6	11	16	18	Others		
Fuchs et al. (1988)	Austria	Southern blot (6, 10, 11, 16, 18, 31, 33)	33 CIN I 43 CIN II 140 CIN III	36 40 56		27 9 6	9 35 48	3 2 7			Frozen tissue
Kurman et al. (1988)	USA/Brazil	Southern blot (6, 11, 16, 18, 31)	63 CIN I 61 CIN II 32 CIN III	71 87 97	11 15 3	5	19 41 66	2 2 6	35 30 22	Frozen tissue. 'Others' = HPV-31 and uncharacterized types
Lim-Tan et al. (1988)	Singapore	Southern blot (11, 16, 18)	37 CIN I 11 CIN II 41 CIN III	22 55 61		7	3 9 27	3 2	16 45 24	Frozen tissue
McNicol et al. (1989)	Canada	Filter in-situ hybridization (6/11, 16/18)	44 CIN I 18 CIN II 36 CIN III	84 72 81	64 67 56		27 56 33		14 19	Cervical swabs
Amortegui et al. (1990)	USA	In-situ hybridization (6/11, 16, 18, 31)	312 CIN I 114 CIN II 46 CIN III	50 54 43	17 5		12 25 24	7 7 9	15 17 11	Fixed tissue. 'Others' = HPV-31 and -16/18/31 unspecified
Billaudel et al. (1991)	France	Southern blot (6, 16, 18)	41 CIN I 20 CIN II 32 CIN III	27 50 63	9 5		9 15 28	3	22 30 31	Frozen tissue
Cooper et al. (1991a)	South Africa	In-situ hybridization (6, 11, 16, 18, 31, 33, 35)	17 CIN II 55 CIN III 24 CIN II 49 CIN III	53 49 58 73			6 27 42 49	6 11 4 14	41 11 13 10	Fixed tissue. 'Others' = HPV-31 and -33
	United Kingdom										
Nuovo et al. (1991b)	USA	In-situ hybridization (6/11, 16/18, 31/33/35, 42/43/44, 51/52, 45/56)	174 LSIL 70 HSIL	89 71	18		29 49		41 23	Fixed tissue. 'Others' predominantly HPV-31, -33, -35
Cornelissen et al. (1992)	Netherlands	PCR (LI) consensus primers and 6/11, 16, 18, 31, 33)	19 CIN I 16 CIN II 73 CIN III	68 81 90	5		21 50 53	5 6 7	37 25 33	Fixed tissue. 'Others' = HPV-31, -33 and unidentified
Meguenni et al. (1992)	Algeria	Southern blot (6/11, 16)	83 CIN I/II 92 CIN III	42 54	7 3		35 51			Frozen tissue
Saragoni et al. (1992)	Italy	In-situ hybridization (6/11, 16/18, 31/35/51)	26 LSIL 45 HSIL	38 36			19 24		19 16	Fixed tissue

Table 8 (contd)

Reference	Study area	Detection method (types included)	No. of cases	Overall HPV positivity (%)[a]	HPV type-specific positivity (%)					Comments
					6	11	16	18	Others	
Anderson et al. (1993)	USA	In-situ hybridization (6/11, 16/18, 31/33/35, 42/43/44, 45/56, 51/52)	159 HPV/CIN I 136 CIN II/III	43 55	9 4			14 27	23 27	Fixed tissue. 'Others' predominantly HPV-31/33/35
Cromme et al. (1993a)	Netherlands	PCR:GP 5/6, TS (6, 11, 16, 18, 31, 33)	34 CIN I 32 CIN II 28 CIN III	68 91 100				53* 75* 96*		Fixed tissue. *HPV types 16, 18, 31
Hellberg et al. (1993)	Sweden	In-situ hybridization (6, 11, 16, 18, 31, 33)	50 CIN I 54 CIN II 23 CIN III	60 81 100	2	24 2	12 54 70	4 9 9	18 17 22	Fixed tissue. HPV-positive cases younger than HPV-negative cases
Cuzick et al. (1994)	United Kingdom	PCR (semi quantitative) (6/11, 16, 18, 31, 33, 35)	13 CIN I 12 CIN II 61 CIN III	77 75 95			23 42 67	23 25 20		Cervical swabs
Delvenne et al. (1994)	Belgium	In-situ hybridization, immunohistochemistry, PCR (L1 consensus primers)	90 LSIL 50 HSIL	64 86	24 10		16 50		36 36	Fixed tissue. 'Others' include HPV-31, -33, -35 (21% in LSIL, 20% in HSIL) plus cases positive only by immunohistochemistry or PCR.
Hippeläinen et al. (1994)	Finland	In-situ hybridization (6/11, 16/18, 31/33, 42)	127 CIN I/II 25 CIN III	69 96	20 4		30 80		19 12	Fixed tissue
de Roda Husman et al. (1994)	Netherlands	PCR GP-5/6 and TS-PCR (6, 11, 16, 18, 31, 33) Southern blot of GP-PCR products (21 types)	971 Pap IIIa 295 Pap IIIb 107 Pap IV	72 85 100	2 1 1	1 1	25 50 51	5 8 12	35 23 31	Cervical swabs. 'Others' primarily HPV-31 and -33 or unknown

Table 8 (contd)

Reference	Study area	Detection method (types included)	No. of cases	Overall HPV positivity (%)[a]	HPV type-specific positivity (%)					Comments
					6	11	16	18	Others	
Sebbelov et al. (1994)	Denmark	In-situ hybridization (16)	52 CIN I/II	21			31			Fixed tissue
			53 CIN III	25			25			
		PCR (in β-globin positive) (16, 18, 31, 33, 35, 45)	40 CIN I/II				53		15	
			34 CIN III				85		29	
	Greenland	In-situ hybridization (16)	49 CIN I/II	14			14			Fixed tissue
			46 CIN III	20			20			
		PCR (in β-globin positive) (16, 18, 31, 33, 35, 45)	24 CIN I/II				54		13	
			30 CIN III				70	3	17	
Burger et al. (1995)	Netherlands	PCR (6/11, 16, 18, 31, 33)	32 CIN I	44	3		16	19	16	Cervical scrapes. Multiple types found in many samples
			39 CIN II	69	3		31	8	36	
			49 CIN III	86	2		59	8	27	
Matsukura & Sugase (1995)	Japan	Dot blot (27 HPV types)	71 CIN I	94			10	3	82	Frozen tissue. 'Others' predominantly HPV-52, -58 (CIN I, II, III), -56 (CIN I), -31 (CIN III)
			56 CIN II	100			23	1	75	
			93 CIN III	95			45		49	

PCR, polymerase chain reaction; GP, general probe; TS, type-specific; Pap, Papanicolaou smear test result; LSIL, low-grade squamous intraepithelial lesions; HSIL, high-grade squamous intraepithelial lesions

[a] Including studies that used hybridization methods
[b] Of those types tested

Table 9. Prevalence of HPV DNA in cervical adenocarcinoma *in situ* case series (≥ 10 cases)

Reference	Study area	Detection method (types included)	No. of cases	Overall HPV positivity (%)[a]	HPV type-specific positivity (%)					Comments
					6	11	16	18	Others	
Farnsworth et al. (1989)	Australia	In-situ hybridization (6, 11, 16, 18, 31)	17	88			29	59		Fixed tissue
Okagaki et al. (1989)	USA	In-situ hybridization (6, 16, 18)	21	67			24	48		Fixed tissue
Nicklin et al. (1991)	Australia	ViraType™ *in-situ* (6/11, 16/18, 31/33/35)	28	25			25		4	Fixed tissue. HPV status and smoking had no significant effect on behaviour of the lesions.
Higgins et al. (1992a)	Australia	In-situ hybridization (6, 11, 16, 18, 31, 33)	37[b]	97			32	65		Fixed tissue
Duggan et al. (1993)	Canada	Dot blot (6, 11, 16, 18, 31, 33, 35)	37	27			14	14		Fixed tissue. HPV positive cases tended to be older than HPV negative cases.
Lee et al. (1993)	USA	PCR (16, 18)	36	42			22	22		Fixed tissue. No association between HPV status and age

[a]Of those types tested
[b]Cervical intraepithelial glandular neoplasia (CIGN) grade III. CIGN I/II also present in 27 of the women

Table 10. Prevalence of HPV DNA in squamous-cell cervical cancer case series (≥ 40 cases)

Reference	Study area	Detection method (types included)	No. of cases	Overall HPV positivity (%)	HPV type-specific positivity (%)					Comments
					6	11	16	18	Others	
Fuchs et al. (1988)	Austria	Southern blot (6, 10, 11, 16, 18, 31, 33)	44	68			57	9	7	Frozen tissue. All lymph node metastases had HPV DNA of the same type as the primary tumour. 'Others' = HPV-10
Kurman et al. (1988)	USA/Brazil	Southern blot (6, 11, 16, 18, 31)	58	86			41	22	22	Frozen tissue. 'Others' = HPV-31 and uncharacterized types
Meng et al. (1989)	China	Dot blot (11, 16, 18)	46	48		2	39	7		Frozen tissue
Walker et al. (1989)	USA	Southern blot (6, 11, 16, 18, 31)	62	71			63	6	2	Frozen tissue. HPV-18-positive cases had a worse prognosis than HPV-16-positive and HPV-negative cases.
Ji et al. (1990)	China	In-situ hybridization (6, 11, 16, 18, 31, 33)	43	44			44			Fixed tissue. No information on histological group
Low et al. (1990)	Singapore	Dot blot (16, 18)	75	72			63	16		Frozen tissue
		Southern blot (16, 18)	58	78			66	21		
Riou et al. (1990)	France (~50%) Africa (~50%)	Southern blot/PCR (6, 11, 16, 18, 31, 33, 35, 39, 42)	89	83			61	8	18	HPV-negative women had a worse prognosis than HPV-positive women. No association between HPV status and age
van den Brule et al. (1991a)	Netherlands	PCR:GP 5/6, TS PCR (6/11, 16, 18, 31, 33)	50	100			84	26	6	Frozen/fixed tissue. 'Others' = HPV-31 and -33
Cooper et al. (1991b)	South Africa	In-situ hybridization (6, 11, 16, 18, 31, 33, 35)	69	64			42	22		Fixed tissue. No association between HPV status and age
Higgins et al. (1991a)	Australia	In-situ hybridization (6/11, 16, 18, 31/33)	171	83			63	11	9	Fixed tissue. HPV-negative cases were older and had a worse prognosis than HPV-positive cases. Survival was not related to HPV type. 'Others' = HPV-31/33

STUDIES OF CANCER IN HUMANS

Table 10 (contd)

Reference	Study area	Detection method (types included)	No. of cases	Overall HPV positivity (%)[b]	HPV type-specific positivity (%) 6	11	16	18	Others	Comments
Sebbelov et al. (1991)	Norway	Southern blot (11, 16, 18)	50	62			54	8		Frozen tissue. No association between HPV status and age, stage or survival
Hørding et al. (1992)	Denmark	PCR (16, 18)	50	72			60	12		Fixed tissue. No association between HPV status and tumour grade
Czeglédy et al. (1992b)	Hungary	PCR (16)	75	48			48			No information on histology. Presence of HPV-16 DNA in the majority of metastasizing lymph nodes of HPV-16-positive cases
Meguenni et al. (1992)	Algeria	Southern blot (6/11, 16)	78	76	3		73			Frozen tissue. No information on histological groups
Sarkar et al. (1992a)	India	In-situ hybridization (16, 18)	49	86			86	6		Fixed tissue
Chen et al. (1993a)	Taiwan, China	PCR (6, 11, 16, 18, 31, 33, 42, 52, 58)	40	78		3	50	5	20	Frozen tissue. No association between HPV status and stage or differentiation
Falcinelli et al. (1993)	Italy	PCR (6/11, 16, 18)	42	69			64			Fixed tissue. No mutation of Ki-*ras* gene was found.
Kenter et al. (1993)	Netherlands	PCR (16)	69	49			49			Fixed tissue. HPV-positive cases older than HPV-negative cases. No association between HPV status and prognosis
Kristiansen et al. (1994a)	Norway	PCR/Southern blot (6, 11, 16, 18, 33)	105	69			53	11		Frozen tissue. No association between overall HPV and age or differentiation. HPV-18 positivity was associated with younger age and poorly differentiated tumours.
Matulic & Saric (1994)	Croatia	Southern blot (6, 16/18)	44	61			61			Frozen tissue
Ngan et al. (1994)	Hong Kong	PCR/Southern blot (*L1* consensus primers and 16, 18)	64	73			67	39		Frozen tissue
Pao et al. (1994a)	Taiwan, China	PCR (*L1* consensus primers)	61	89			75			Frozen or fixed tissue. No information on histological groups
			49	57			43			

Table 10 (contd)

Reference	Study area	Detection method (types included)	No. of cases	Overall HPV positivity (%)[a]	HPV type-specific positivity (%)					Comments
					6	11	16	18	Others	
Williamson et al. (1994)	South Africa	PCR (L1 consensus primers and 6, 11, 16, 18, 31, 33, 45)	59	78			44	2	34	Frozen tissue. 'Others' predominantly unclassified types
Bosch et al. (1995)	22 countries[c]	PCR (L1 consensus primers and type specific, 26 types)	881	93			51	12	33	Frozen tissue. β-globin-positive (see also Table 12) 'Others' predominantly types related to HPV-16 and -18

PCR, polymerase chain reaction; GP, general probe; TS, type-specific

[a]Including studies published ≥ 1988 having used hybridization methods
[b]Of those types tested
[c]Africa (Algeria, Benin, Guinea, Mali, Tanzania, Uganda), Central and South America (Argentina, Bolivia, Brazil, Chile, Colombia, Cuba, Panama, Paraguay), Southeast Asia (Indonesia, Philippines, Thailand), North America (Canada, USA) and Europe (Germany, Poland, Spain)

prevalence is in the range of 57–100% with most studies detecting HPV in more than 75% of cases. The prevalence from the largest study was 93% (Bosch et al., 1995). In studies using Southern blot or in-situ hybridization, the ranges are 61–86% and 44–86%, respectively. HPV-16 is by far the most prevalent type. The data currently available do not support a relationship between HPV detection in cervical cancers and the age of the patients.

Figures 14 and 15 show the percentage positivity in squamous-cell cervical cancer case series of HPV and HPV-16, respectively.

(c) Adenocarcinoma and adenosquamous carcinoma

Table 11 summarizes cervical adenocarcinoma case series published since 1988 that included more than 15 cases and used hybridization methods for HPV detection. The prevalence of HPV ranged from 15 to 88% in nine studies using PCR or Southern blot. In six studies using in-situ hybridization, HPV was detected in 0–69% of cases. In the majority of investigations, HPV-18 was the predominant type; however in some studies, HPV-16 was as prevalent as HPV-18. HPV-positive cases tended to be younger than HPV-negative cases for unknown reasons.

A few studies of HPV in adenosquamous carcinomas have been conducted. The detection rate in series with more than 10 cases ranged from 18 to 94%. In the most recent study, HPV-16 and -18 were detected with about the same frequency (Tase et al., 1988; Walker et al., 1989; Leminen et al., 1991; Duggan et al., 1993; Bosch et al., 1995).

(d) Geographical and temporal variation

Little geographical variation is seen in the overall prevalence of HPV invasive cancers but there is some difference in the distribution of types. The best data come from a study by Bosch et al. (1995) in which nearly 1000 invasive cancer specimens, from 22 countries covering most parts of the world, were analysed in a single laboratory. The assay was based on PCR amplification using *L1* consensus primers, and samples were probed with different oligonucleotides capable of detecting and discriminating between 26 different anogenital HPV types. HPV DNA was detected in 93% of the tumours, with no significant geographic variation in overall positivity. HPV-16 was present in 50% of the specimens, HPV-18 in 14%, HPV-45 in 8% and HPV-31 in 5%. HPV-16 was the predominant type in all countries except Indonesia and Algeria, where HPV-18 was more common. There was significant geographical variation in the prevalence of some of the less-common virus types. A clustering of HPV-45 was apparent in western Africa, while HPV-39 and -59 were virtually confined to cancer cases from Latin America. In squamous-cell tumours, HPV-16 predominated, but HPV-18 predominated in adenocarcinomas and adenosquamous tumours. Further details on type-specific positivity by area are shown in Table 12.

In a series of smaller studies, Sebbelov et al. (1994) found similar rates of HPV-16 positivity by PCR in archival specimens from two additional countries, Greenland and Denmark (pre-invasive lesions, 63% and 68%, respectively; invasive cancers, 82% and 70%, respectively). Acs et al. (1989) found a slightly higher rate of HPV-16 positivity by Southern blot in 82 cancers in eastern Panama (43%) than in 69 from central Panama (29%). In a small study of 37 invasive cancers in two Mexican cities with high cervical cancer rates (Mexico City and Monterrey),

González-Garay et al. (1992) found similar positivity rates for HPV-16 (29% and 26%, respectively) and HPV-18 (7% and 10%, respectively) by Southern blot.

Figure 14. Detection of HPV DNA in sqamous-cell cervical cancer case series

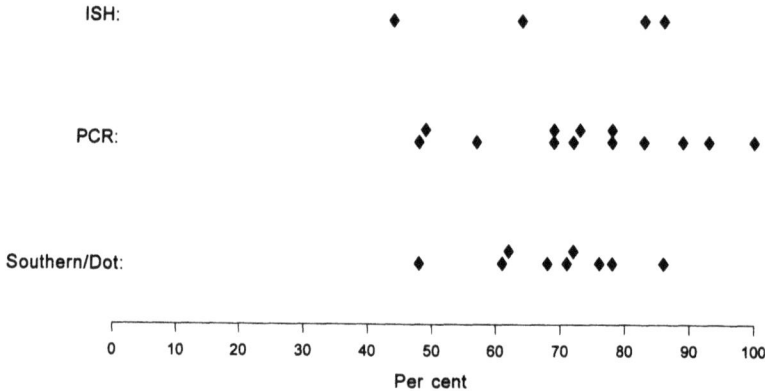

ISH, in situ hybridization; PCR, polymerase chain reaction
Data are taken from Table 10.

Figure 15. Detection of HP-16 in squamous-cell cervical cancer case series

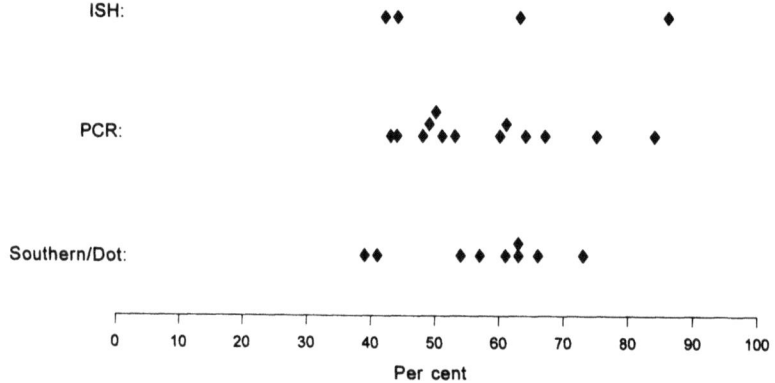

ISH, in situ hybridization; PCR, polymerase chain reaction
Data are taken from Table 10.

Two historical studies of biopsy material have yielded possibly conflicting data regarding changes in HPV positivity in neoplastic specimens over time. Anderson et al. (1993) compared 176 cervical tissues showing cervical intraepithelial neoplasia from 1964 to 1965 with 165 cases from 1988 to 1989 in Richmond, VA, USA, and found virtually the same positivity rate (43%

STUDIES OF CANCER IN HUMANS

Table 11. Prevalence of HPV DNA in cervical adenocarcinoma case series[a] (≥ 15 cases)

Reference	Study area	Detection method (types included)	No. of cases	Overall HPV positivity (%)[b]	HPV type-specific positivity (%)					Comments
					6	11	16	18	Others	
Tase et al. (1988)	USA	In-situ hybridization (2, 6, 16, 18)	40	43			3	40		Fixed tissue. No association between HPV and histological differentiation
Walker et al. (1989)	USA	Southern blot (6, 11, 16, 18, 31)	25	52			20	32		Frozen tissue. HPV-18-positive cases had a worse prognosis than HPV-16-positive and HPV-negative cases.
Riou et al. (1990)	France & Africa	Southern blot/PCR (6, 11, 16, 18, 31, 33, 35, 39, 42)	17	88			24	59	12	Fixed tissue
Bjersing et al. (1991)	Sweden	PCR (16, 18)	26	42			15	27		Fixed tissue. HPV-positive cases were younger than HPV-negative cases.
Griffin et al. (1991)	United Kingdom	In-situ hybridization (6, 11, 16, 18)	16	6				6		Fixed tissue
		PCR (11, 16, 18)	16	31			25	6		
Leminen et al. (1991)	Finland	In-situ hybridization (16, 18)	95	20			4*	16*		Fixed tissue. No correlation between HPV status and age, ploidy or survival, but correlation with both stage and tumour size. *Including 11 adenosquamous cancers
Young et al. (1991)	United Kingdom	In-situ hybridization (6, 11, 16, 18)	21	0						Fixed tissue
Hørding et al. (1992)	Denmark	PCR (16, 18)	50	70			18	52		Fixed tissue. No association between HPV status and tumour grade. Higher rate of HPV-18-positive carcinoma among younger women
Cooper et al. (1992)	United Kingdom	In-situ hybridization (6, 11, 16, 18, 31, 33, 35)	16	69			25	44		Fixed tissue. No association between HPV status and tumour differentiation
	South Africa		22	41				41		

Table 11 (contd)

Reference	Study area	Detection method (types included)	No. of cases	Overall HPV positivity (%)[b]	HPV type-specific positivity (%)					Comments
					6	11	16	18	Others	
Johnson et al. (1992a)	USA	PCR (16, 18)	19	79			21	58		Fixed tissue. HPV-positive cases were younger than HPV-negative cases.
Duggan et al. (1993)	Canada	Dot blot (6, 11, 16, 18, 31, 33, 35)	60	42			15	25	2	Fixed tissue. HPV-positive cases tended to be younger than HPV-negative cases.
Fulcheri et al. (1993)	Italy	In-situ hybridization (6/11, 16/18, 31/35/51)	18	6			6			Fixed tissue
Lee et al. (1993)	USA	PCR (16, 18)	20	15			10	5		Fixed tissue
Matsuo et al. (1993)	Japan	PCR (L1 consensus primers and 16, 18)	24	25			17	13		Fixed tissue. HPV-positive cases were younger than HPV-negative cases.
Milde-Langosch et al. (1993)	Germany	PCR (consensus primers) (6/11, 16, 31)	24	63			38	29		Fixed tissue. HPV-positive cases were younger than HPV-negative cases.
Bosch et al. (1995)	22 countries[c]	PCR (L1 consensus primers and type specific, 26 types)	25	96			28	56	12	Frozen tissue. 'Others' related to HPV-18

PCR, polymerase chain reaction
[a] Including studies published ≥ 1988 having used hybridization methods
[b] Of those types tested
[c] Africa (Algeria, Benin, Guinea, Mali, Tanzania, Uganda), Central and South America (Argentina, Bolivia, Brazil, Chile, Colombia, Cuba, Panama, Paraguay), Southeast Asia (Indonesia, Philippines, Thailand), North America (Canada, USA) and Europe (Germany, Poland, Spain)

versus 47%) by in-situ hybridization. However, Kock and Johansen (1987) compared 208 biopsy specimens from 1972 and 225 from 1983 in Denmark and found a large increase in the proportions showing condylomatous atypia (12% versus 50%, respectively). Within this group, immunoperoxidase staining for the HPV antigen was performed and an increase in positivity in the more recent samples was also found (12% versus 21%, respectively).

Table 12. Prevalence of individual HPV types by geographical region

HPV type	Region					
	Africa	Central and South America	Southeast Asia	Europe	North America	Total
	No. (%)	No. (%)	No. (%)	No. (%)	No. (%)	No. (%)
HPV-16 and related						
HPV-16	79 (42.5)	255 (50.5)	42 (42.9)	56 (65.1)	33 (57.9)	465 (49.9)
HPV-31	5 (2.7)	35 (6.9)	1 (1.0)	5 (5.8)	3 (5.3)	49 (5.3)
HPV-33	5 (2.7)	18 (3.6)	2 (2.0)	1 (1.2)	0	26 (2.8)
HPV-35	4 (2.2)	10 (2.0)	1 (1.0)	1 (1.2)	0	16 (1.7)
HPV-52	4 (2.2)	16 (3.2)	2 (2.0)	3 (3.5)	0	25 (2.7)
HPV-58	5 (2.7)	11 (2.2)	2 (2.0)	1 (1.2)	0	19 (2.0)
HPV-18 and related						
HPV-18	33 (17.7)	48 (9.5)	31 (31.6)	7 (8.1)	9 (15.8)	128 (13.7)
HPV-39	0	13 (2.6)	1 (1.0)	0	0	14 (1.5)
HPV-45	23 (12.4)	37 (7.3)	8 (8.2)	2 (2.3)	8 (14.0)	78 (8.4)
HPV-59	0	14 (2.8)	1 (1.0)	0	0	15 (1.6)
HPV-68	4 (2.2)	2 (0.4)	1 (1.0)	3 (3.5)	1 (1.8)	11 (1.2)
Other						
HPV-6	0	1 (0.2)	0	0	0	1 (0.1)
HPV-11	0	1 (0.2)	0	0	0	1 (0.1)
HPV-56	6 (3.2)	3 (0.6)	3 (3.1)	2 (2.3)	2 (3.5)	16 (1.7)
Miscellaneous	5 (2.7)	16 (3.2)	4 (4.1)	1 (1.2)	0	26 (2.8)
Undetermined	2 (1.1)	8 (1.6)	0	1 (1.2)	1 (1.8)	12 (1.3)
HPV negatives	19 (10.2)	36 (7.1)	3 (3.1)	4 (4.7)	4 (7.0)	66 (7.1)
Total specimens	186	505	98	86	57	932

Adapted from Bosch et al. (1995)

2.2.2 Anogenital cancers

(a) Cancer of the vulva and vagina

In Table 13, results from vulvar cancer case series ($\geq$ 10 cases) are summarized. The HPV prevalence ranged from 0% to 100%. No HPV DNA was seen in 29 tumours with substantial keratinization and adjacent lichen sclerosus, but without adjacent vulvar intraepithelial neoplasia

Table 13. Prevalence of HPV DNA in vulvar cancer case series' (≥ 10 cases)

Reference	Study area	Detection method (types included)	No. of cases	Overall HPV positivity (%)[b]	HPV type-specific positivity (%)					Comments
					6	11	16	18	Others	
Di Luca et al. (1986)	Italy	Southern blot (16)	10 SCC	20			20			Frozen tissue
Macnab et al. (1986)	United Kingdom	In-situ hybridization (16, 18)	10 SCC	80			80			Frozen tissue
Gupta et al. (1987)	Italy	In-situ hybridization (6/11, 16, 18)	10 early SCC 6 verrucous carcinomas	50 0		10	40			Fixed tissue. Among cases with histological evidence of viral infection, 78% were HPV positive. In those without signs of viral infection 33% were HPV positive.
Bender et al. (1988)	Germany	In-situ hybridization (6/11, 16/18)	27	59		19	41			No information on histological group
Carson et al. (1988)	USA	Southern blot/in-situ hybridization (1–6, 16, 18)	16 ASCC 26 SCC	6 19	4		12		6 4	Fixed tissue. The prognosis was worse for ASCC than for SCC.
Ikenberg et al. (1988)	Germany	Southern blot (16)	18	33			33			Frozen tissue. No correlation between HPV status and grade or stage of tumours
Venuti & Marcante (1989)	Italy	Dot blot/Southern blot (16, 18)	15 SCC	87			20	80		Frozen tissue
Neill et al. (1990)	United Kingdom	Southern blot (16, 18, 31, 33)	10 SCC with lichen sclerosus 10 SCC with VIN III	0 64*			55*			*11 lesions tested
Pilotti et al. (1990)	Italy	In-situ hybridization/Southern blot (6, 11, 16, 18, 31) PCR	10 SCC	10 75			10 75			Fixed/frozen tissue. Data only given for HPV-16

Table 13 (contd)

Reference	Study area	Detection method (types included)	No. of cases	Overall HPV positivity (%)[a]	HPV type-specific positivity (%)					Comments
					6	11	16	18	Others	
Andersen et al. (1991)	USA	In-situ hybridization (Vira type) (6/11, 16/18, 31/33/35)	30 SCC 12 intraepithelial like SCC	13 67						Fixed tissue. Cases with intraepithelial-like SCC were younger and more often smokers than cases with ordinary SCC.
Bloss et al. (1991)	USA	Southern blot/PCR (6, 11, 16, 18, 31)	21 SCC	48	10		48			Frozen tissue. No association between HPV and stage or prognosis. HPV-positive cases were younger than HPV-negative cases.
Hørding et al. (1991a)	Denmark	PCR (16)	24 SCC	58			58			Frozen tissue
Marcante & Venuti (1991)	Italy	PCR (11, 16, 18)	10	90			80	10		Fixed tissue. In all screened metastases, the same HPV type was found as in the primary tumour.
Nuovo et al. (1991c)	USA	PCR (E6 and L1 consensus primers and 6, 11, 16, 18, 31, 33, 35)	10 SCC (minimal keratinization) 13 SCC (substantial keratinization)	70 0			40		30	Fixed tissue. Adjacent VIN in 86% of HPV-positive cases compared to 6% of HPV-negative cases
Rusk et al. (1991)	USA	Dot blot/Southern blot (6/11, 16, 18)	31 SCC	23	6	6	10		6	Frozen tissue. No association between HPV and age or tumour grade
Toki et al. (1991)	USA	In-situ hybridization (6/11, 16, 18) PCR (6/11, 16, 18)	19 SCC 8 basaloid carcinomas 3 warty carcinomas	21 75 100			16 75 67	5 13 33		Fixed tissue. HPV-positive cases younger than HPV-negative cases
Brandenberger et al. (1992)	Switzerland	In-situ hybridization (6/11, 16, 18)	38 SCC	11	3		8			Fixed tissue. No association between HPV status and survival

Table 13 (contd)

Reference	Study area	Detection method (types included)	No. of cases	Overall HPV positivity (%)[a]	HPV type-specific positivity (%)					Comments
					6	11	16	18	Others	
Felix et al. (1993)	USA	PCR (6, 11, 16, 18, 33)	(Bartholin's gland) 7 SCC	86			86			Fixed tissue
			2 adenoid cystic carcinomas 1 AC	0						

SCC, squamous-cell carcinoma; ASCC, adenosquamous-cell carcinoma; VIN, vulvar intraepithelial neoplasia; PCR polymerase chain reaction; AC, adenocarcinoma
[a] Including studies having used hybridization methods
[b] Of those types tested

(VIN); however, HPV DNA was detected in 41% of tumours with minimal keratinization and/or adjacent VIN. HPV-16 was the predominant type detected, but cases containing HPV-6/11 have also been reported.

The prevalence of HPV in VIN III ($\geq$ 20 cases) ranges from 30 to 95% with four of seven studies finding HPV in more than 80% of cases (Table 14). The prevalence tends to be consistently higher than in series of vulvar cancer.

In vaginal cancer case series (3–18 cases), the range of positivity was 21–67%, with HPV detected in 48% of cancers overall (see Table 15). HPV-6 and -18 were the predominant types.

(b) Cancer of the penis

Table 16 summarizes the prevalence studies of penile cancer that included more than five cases. Studies in which in-situ hybridization was used detected HPV in 5–40% of squamous-cell carcinoma, whereas Southern blot and PCR studies found HPV in 44–100% and 18–82%, respectively. It seems that HPV (predominantly HPV-16) is found in penile squamous-cell carcinomas in some regions of the world, but, curiously, HPV has not been found in the five small studies of 'verrucous' carcinomas conducted to date.

(c) Cancer of the anus

In Table 17 results from anal cancer case series ($\geq$ 5 cases) are shown. In-situ hybridization studies found 24–73% of cases (squamous-cell carcinomas) to be HPV positive. The corresponding figures for Southern blot and PCR studies are 63–85% and 24–100%, respectively, and HPV-16 is the type most commonly observed. Scholefield *et al.* (1991) examined 173 anal squamous-cell cancers from fixed sections in six countries and found HPV-16 DNA in 29% of those using DNA-hybridization. Much lower positivity rates were found in India (3%) and South Africa (11%) than in Poland, Switzerland, Brazil and the United Kingdom, where the rates were similar (approximately 40%).

2.2.3 Other cancers

The presence of HPV at other cancer sites has been studied considerably less often and in far fewer patients compared to cancer of the cervix and anogenital areas. Some positive findings reported below may have been inflated by publication bias, as suggested by some especially high HPV prevalences in early reports that are refuted in more recent studies (e.g. prostatic cancer). From an interpretative viewpoint, it is also important to bear in mind that the presence of HPV according to any technique does not constitute a proof of causality *per se*, and the finding of HPV in cancer tissues frequently goes along with detection of several other viruses (e.g. Epstein–Barr virus, hepatitis C virus (see IARC, 1994a), etc.). Conversely, negative results also cannot be used confidently, since the type-specific methods developed for search of the genital tract (e.g. to detect HPV-6, -11, -16 and -18) may not be informative in cancers at different sites where other, perhaps not yet identified, site-specific types may play a role.

Table 14. Prevalence of HPV DNA in high-grade vulvar intraepithelial neoplasia (VIN III) case series (≥ 20 cases)

Reference	Study area	Detection method (types included)	No. of cases	Overall HPV positivity (%)[a]	6	11	16	18	Others	Comments
Bornstein et al. (1988)	USA	In-situ hybridization (6/11, 16/18/31)	46	83		37	48		9	Frozen tissue. No difference in HPV status between cases with multicentric and unicentric disease
Buscema et al. (1988)	USA	Southern blot (6, 11, 16, 18, 31)	22 (37 lesions)	84			68	5	11	Frozen tissue
Kaufman et al. (1988)	USA	In-situ hybridization (6, 11, 16, 18, 31)	46	83	20	24	17	24	9	Frozen tissue. HPV DNA more often present in older cases. Prevalence of HPV DNA similar in multifocal and unifocal lesions
Jones et al. (1990a)	New Zealand	In-situ hybridization (6, 11, 16, 18)	29	52			52			Fixed tissue. HPV positive cases were younger than HPV negative cases. Five cases progressed to cancer. All five had multifocal anogenital neoplasia. In four cases, HPV-16 was found in both VIN III and cancer tissue.
Beckmann et al. (1991a)	USA	In-situ hybridization, PCR (6, 16)	21	95	29		76		14	Fixed tissue. All women had multicentric squamous-cell neoplasia of the anogenital region.
Park et al. (1991)	USA	PCR, in-situ hybridization (6, 11, 16, 18)	20 warty 10 basal	65 30			65 30			Fixed tissue. HPV positive cases were younger than HPV negative cases.
Nuovo et al. (1991c)	USA	PCR (E6, L1 consensus primers and 6, 11, 16, 18, 31, 33, 35)	22	59			41		18	Fixed tissue

PCR, polymerase chain reaction
[a] Of those types tested

Table 15. Prevalence of HPV DNA in vaginal cancer case series[a] (≥ 3 cases)

Reference	Study area	Detection method (types included)	No. of cases	Overall HPV positivity (%)[b]	HPV type-specific positivity (%)					Comments
					6	11	16	18	Others	
Mitrani-Rosenbaum et al. (1988)	Israel	Southern blot (6/11, 16/18)	3	33				33		Frozen tissue
Ostrow et al. (1988)	USA	In-situ hybridization/filter in-situ hybridization (2, 6, 16, 18)	14	21			14			Fixed tissue
Kiyabu et al. (1989)	USA	PCR (16, 18)	14	64			57	7		Fixed tissue
Ikenberg et al. (1990)	Germany	Southern blot (6/11, 16, 18)	18	56			44		11	Frozen tissue
Kulski et al. (1990)	Australia	Histological filter in-situ hybridization (6, 11, 16, 18)	3	67						Fixed tissue

PCR, polymerase chain reaction
[a]Including studies having used hybridization methods
[b]Of those types tested

Table 16. Prevalence of HPV DNA in penile cancer case series[a] (≥ 5 cases)

Reference	Study area	Detection method (types included)	No. of cases	Overall HPV positivity (%)[b]	HPV type-specific positivity					Comments
					6	11	16	18	Others	
McCance et al. (1986)	Brazil	Southern blot (16, 18)	53	51			49	9		Frozen tissue
Villa & Lopes (1986)	Brazil	Southern blot (6, 11, 16, 18)	18 SCC	44		6		39		Frozen tissue. Presence of HPV DNA was not related to age, extent of disease or prognosis.
Kiyabu et al. (1989)	USA	PCR (16, 18)	5	40			40			Fixed tissue
Weaver et al. (1989)	USA	In-situ hybridization (6, 11, 16, 18, 31, 33)	9 SCC	11			11			Fixed tissue. HPV-6/11 was found in 25/30 penile condylomas.
Higgins et al. (1992b)	Australia Brazil	In-situ hybridization (6, 11, 16, 18, 31, 33)	20 SCC 6 SCC 5 verrucous carcinomas	35 33 0			35 33			Fixed tissue. Verrucous carcinomas from Australia (2) and Brazil (3)
Kulski et al. (1990)	Australia	Histochemical filter in-situ hybridization (6, 11, 16, 18)	10 SCC	20						Fixed tissue
Moriyama et al. (1990)	Japan	In-situ hybridization (6/11, 16/18, 31/33/35)	19	5				5		Fixed tissue. HPV-6/11 was found in 11/12 penile condylomas.
Varma et al. (1991)	USA	PCR (6/11, 16) In-situ hybridization (6, 11, 16, 18, 31, 33, 35)	16 SCC 2 verrucous carcinomas	81 0	6*		56		19*	Fixed tissue. *Only positive by in-situ hybridization
Sarkar et al. (1992b)	USA	PCR (6/11, 16, 18)	11 SCC 1 verrucous carcinoma	82 0			82			Fixed tissue. Bowenoid CIS: 7/7 HPV-16 positive; non-Bowenoid CIS: 0/8 HPV positive
Tornesello et al. (1992)	Uganda	Dot blot/Southern blot (6, 11, 16, 18, 31, 33)	13 SCC	100			100			Frozen tissue. Samples contained DNA with low homology to HPV-16/18.

Table 16 (contd)

Reference	Study area	Detection method (types included)	No. of cases	Overall HPV positivity (%)[a]	HPV type-specific positivity					Comments
					6	11	16	18	Others	
Wiener et al. (1992a)	USA	PCR (16, 18)	29 SCC	31			28	3		Fixed tissue. No association between HPV status and age, grade or survival
Iwasawa et al. (1993)	Japan	PCR (16, 18, 33)	111 SCC (untreated)	63			61	2		Fixed tissue. HPV-positive cases younger than HPV-negative cases; lymph node metastases from HPV-16-positive cases were also HPV-16 positive. Lymph nodes from HPV-negative cases were HPV negative.
			12 SCC (treated)	17			17			
Malek et al. (1993)	USA	PCR (L1 consensus primers)	7 SCC	71						Fixed tissue; 75% of cases were heavy smokers.
Masih et al. (1993)	USA	In-situ hybridization (6, 11, 16, 18, 31)	10 SCC	40			40			Fixed tissue
			10 verrucous carcinomas	0						
Chan et al. (1994b)	Hong Kong	PCR (16, 18)	34 SCC	18			12	12		Fixed tissue. HPV positive cases older than negative cases
			7 verrucous carcinomas	0						
Suzuki et al. (1994)	Japan	PCR (L1, E6 consensus primers)	13 SCC	54			31		23	Frozen/fixed tissue. 'Others' = HPV-31 and -33. No p53 mutation was found among HPV-positive or -negative cases.

SCC, squamous-cell carcinoma; PCR, polymerase chain reaction; CIS, carcinoma in situ
[a] Including studies having used hybridization methods
[b] Of those types tested

Table 17. Prevalence of HPV DNA in anal cancer case series* (≥ 5 cases)

Reference	Study area	Detection method (types included)	No. of cases	Overall HPV positivity (%)[b]	HPV type-specific positivity (%)					Comments
					6	11	16	18	Others	
Löning et al. (1988)	Germany	In-situ hybridization (6, 11, 16, 18)	8 SCC 2 verrucous carcinomas	25 100	100		25	13		Fixed tissue
Taxy et al. (1989)	USA	In-situ hybridization (6/11, 16, 18, 31)	12 SCC (9 F, 3 M)	25		8	17			Fixed tissue
Kulski et al. (1990)	Australia	Histochemical filter in-situ hybridization (6, 11, 16, 18)	18 SCC	39						Fixed tissue
Scholefield et al. (1990a)	United Kingdom	In-situ hybridization (16)	207 SCC	24			24			Fixed tissue. 1948–77: 15% HPV-16-positive cases; 1978–82: 33% HPV-16-positive cases; 1983–87: 50% HPV-16-positive cases
Scholefield et al. (1990b)	United Kingdom	Southern blot (6/11, 16, 18)	67 SCC (37 F, 30 M)	63			60	3		Frozen tissue. HPV status not related to any of the clinico-pathological variables examined
Wolber et al. (1990)	Canada	In-situ hybridization (6/11, 16/18)	9 CIS 12 SCC (F:M = 0.9) 14 cloacogenic carcinomas (F:M = 1.3)	78 58 0		22	56 58			Fixed tissue
Aparicio-Duque et al. (1991)	USA/Spain	In-situ hybridization (6/11, 16/18, 31/35/51)	5 cloacogenic carcinomas (3 M, 2 F)	80			80			Fixed tissue
Crook et al. (1991a)	United Kingdom	PCR/Southern blot (16, 18)	50 SCC	NA			76	8		Amplification of c-myc was demonstrated in 15/50 cancers, of which 13 were HPV-16-positive and one also HPV-18-positive.
		Southern blot (16, 18)		NA			58	6		

Table 17 (contd)

Reference	Study area	Detection method (types included)	No. of cases	Overall HPV positivity (%)[b]	HPV type-specific positivity (%)						Comments
					6	11	16	18	Others		
Duggan et al. (1991)	Canada	In-situ hybridization with: Horseradish peroxidase Alkine phosphatase Dot blot (6, 11, 16, 18, 33)	13 SCC (9 F, 4 M)	0 62 85	8 23	8	54 70				Fixed tissue
Higgins et al. (1991b)	Australia	In-situ hybridization (6, 11, 16, 18, 31, 33)	41 SCC 6 AC	73 0			68	2	2		Fixed tissue. HPV-positive cases were younger than HPV-negative cases.
Koulos et al. (1991)	USA	PCR (16, 18, 31, 35)	6 AC 2 SCC	33 100			100	33 50			Fixed tissue
Palefsky et al. (1991)	USA	PCR (6/11, 16, 18, 31, 33)	13	85	15		77		31		Fixed tissue
Scholefield et al. (1991)	India, South Africa, Switzerland, Poland, Brazil, United Kingdom	In-situ hybridization (16)	173 SCC	29			29				Fixed tissue. HPV prevalence significantly lower in samples from India and South Africa compared to the samples from Switzerland, Poland, Brazil and United Kingdom
Zaki et al. (1992)	USA	PCR (L1 consensus primers)	7 CIS 11 SCC (7 F, 4 M)	86 73	9	9	29 18	14	43 36		Fixed tissue

SCC, squamous-cell carcinoma; F, females; M, males; CIS, carcinoma in situ; PCR, polymerase chain reaction; AC, adenocarcinoma; NA, not available
[a]Including studies having used hybridization methods
[b]Of those types tested

(a) Oral cancer

In Table 18, results from case series of oral cancer (≥ 15 cases) are presented. Studies using in-situ hybridization detected HPV in 0–24% of squamous-cell carcinomas while HPV was detected by Southern blot in 12–70% and by PCR in 0–100%. In verrucous carcinomas, HPV was detected in 0–48% of cases. Generally, HPV-16 was the most frequent type observed, although HPV-18 and other types have been observed with equal frequency in some studies (e.g., Kashima *et al.*, 1990; Yeudall & Campo, 1991; Woods *et al.*, 1993). This area has recently been reviewed by Snijders *et al.* (1994a).

(b) Cancer of the pharynx and tonsil

Among patients with cancer of the pharynx, four studies found HPV DNA, of types 16 and 18, in 13–67% of cases (Brandsma & Abramson, 1989; Watts *et al.*, 1991; Arndt *et al.*, 1992; Ogura *et al.*, 1993), whereas Dickens *et al.* (1992) found no HPV in 16 cases using PCR to test for HPV-16/18. In two studies of tonsillar carcinoma, HPV-16 was detected by Southern blot in two of three cases (Brachman *et al.*, 1992) while in the other study, using general primer mediated PCR, HPV DNA was detected in 12 of 14 (86%) cases (Snijders *et al.*, 1994a). In this latter study, HPV-16 and -33 were detected most frequently (in eight and four carcinomas, respectively)

(c) Oesophageal cancer

Table 19 gives a summary of oesophageal cancer case series of more than 10 cases. The HPV prevalences found in studies using in-situ hybridization range between 0% and 43%. One study detected HPV in 45% using Southern blot. Four PCR studies found that 0–10% of cases were positive while another study detected HPV in 49% of oesophageal cancer patients. HPV-16 and -18 have been observed with similar frequency.

(d) Cancer of the colon and rectum

One study found one HPV-positive case of caecum cancer out of 27 malignant colon cancers (Ostrow *et al.*, 1987a). Several other studies detected no HPV in this type of neoplasia (Grimmel *et al.*, 1988; Kulski *et al.*, 1990; Higgins *et al.*, 1991b; Koulos *et al.*, 1991; Nuovo, 1991; Shah *et al.*, 1992; Shroyer *et al.*, 1992).

(e) Nasal/sinonasal cancer

In invasive nasal/sinonasal cancer series (≥ 5 cases), HPV has been detected in 0–25% of cases, with HPV-16 being the most common type (Klemi *et al.*, 1989; Ishibashi *et al.*, 1990; Furuta *et al.*, 1991; Judd *et al.*, 1991; Furuta *et al.*, 1992; Kashima *et al.*, 1992b; Ogura *et al.*, 1993).

(f) Laryngeal cancer

Table 20 summarizes laryngeal cancer series (≥ 25 squamous-cell carcinoma cases, ≥ 3 verrucous carcinoma cases). Among squamous-cell carcinomas and carcinomas of unknown

Table 18. Prevalence of HPV DNA in oral cancer case series[a] (≥ 15 cases)

Reference	Study area	Detection method (types included)	No. of cases	Overall HPV positivity (%)[b]	HPV type-specific positivity (%)				Comments
					6	11	16	18	Others	
Maitland et al. (1987)	United Kingdom	Southern blot (16)	15 SCC	47			40		7	Frozen tissue
Gassenmaier & Hornstein (1988)	Germany	In-situ hybridization (2, 6, 11, 16)	68 SCC	24 9	HPV-11 and -16 (relaxed conditions) HPV-6, -11, -16 (stringent conditions)					Fixed tissue
Syrjänen et al. (1988)	Finland	In-situ hybridization (6, 11, 13, 16, 18, 30)	51 SCC	12			6	8		Fixed tissue
Chang et al. (1990a)	Finland	In-situ hybridization (6/11/16/18) PCR (6, 11, 16, 18)	40 SCC	3 28	3		23	3		Fixed tissue
Greer et al. (1990)	USA	In-situ hybridization (6, 11, 16, 18, 31, 33, 35)	50 SCC 20 verrucous carcinomas	6 20	5		2 15	2	2	Fixed tissue
Kashima et al. (1990)	USA	Southern blot/reverse blot (6, 11, 16, 18, 31)	29	17	3		3		10	Frozen tissue. 'Others' = HPV-3, -13 and -57 related types
Tsuchiya et al. (1991)	Japan	Southern blot (6/11, 16/18, 31/33/35)	25 SCC	12						Frozen tissue
Watts et al. (1991)	USA	Southern blot (2, 6/11, 13, 16/18, 32) PCR (6, 11, 16, 18)	23 SCC 14 SCC	70 100	7	35 50	48 79	14		Frozen tissue
Yeudall & Campo (1991)	United Kingdom	Southern blot/PCR (4, 16, 18)	39 SCC	46			26	21		Frozen tissue
Young & Min (1991)	USA	In-situ hybridization (6/11, 16/18, 31/33/35)	17 SCC 10 verrucous carcinomas	0 0						Fixed tissue

Table 18 (contd)

Reference	Study area	Detection method (types included)	No. of cases	Overall HPV positivity (%)[b]	HPV type-specific positivity (%)					Comments
					6	11	16	18	Others	
Zeuss et al. (1991)	Spain	In-situ hybridization (6/11, 16/18, 31/33/35)	15 SCC 5 CIS	0 0						Fixed tissue
Shindoh et al. (1992)	Japan	PCR (16, 18, 33)	24 SCC (tongue only)	33			33	4		Fixed tissue. HPV-positive cases tended to be older than HPV-negative cases.
Holladay & Gerald (1993)	USA	PCR (L1 consensus primers)	37 SCC 2 verrucous carcinomas	19 0			19	3		Fixed tissue
Noble-Topham et al. (1993)	Canada	PCR (6/11, 16, 18)	25 verrucous carcinomas	48	4		8	40		Fixed tissue
Ogura et al. (1993)	Japan	PCR (16, 18)	15 SCC	0						Frozen tissue
Shroyer et al. (1993)	USA	PCR (generic), in-situ hybridization (6/11, 16/18, 31/33/35)	17 verrucous carcinomas	41	18	29				Fixed tissue
Woods et al. (1993)	USA	PCR (L1 consensus primers)	18 SCC	78	28		61	61		Fixed tissue. No association between HPV status and age, gender, tobacco usage or alcohol consumption

SCC, squamous-cell carcinoma; PCR, polymerase chain reaction; CIS, carcinoma *in situ*
[a] Including studies having used hybridization methods
[b] Of those types tested

Table 19. Prevalence of HPV DNA in oesophageal cancer case series[a] (≥ 10 cases)

Reference	Study area	Detection method (types included)	No. of cases	Overall HPV positivity (%)[b]	HPV type-specific positivity (%)				Comments
					6	11	16	18	Others	
Kiyabu et al. (1989)	USA	PCR (16, 18)	13 SCC	0						Fixed tissue
Chang et al. (1990b)	China	In-situ hybridization (6, 11, 16, 18)	51 SCC (25 F, 26 M)	43	6	8	18	16		Fixed tissue. Koilocytosis present in 55% of cases
Kulski et al. (1990)	Australia	Histochemical filter in-situ hybridization (6/11/16/18)	39	23						Fixed tissue
Loke et al. (1990)	Hong Kong	In-situ hybridization Slot blot (6, 11, 16, 18)	37 SCC	0						Fixed tissue Frozen tissue
Chang et al. (1992)	China	Southern blot (11, 16, 18, 30)	20 SCC	45						Frozen tissue
		PCR (6, 11, 16, 18)	51 SCC* (25 F, 26 M)	49	6	14	18	14		Fixed tissue. Koilocytosis present in 49% of cases *Same material as Chang et al. (1990b)
Toh et al. (1992)	Japan	PCR (L1 consensus primers) (16, 18, 31, 33, 52, 58)	45 SCC	7			2	4		Fixed tissue
Chang et al. (1993)	China	In-situ hybridization (6/11, 16, 18, 30, 53)	363 SCC (148 F, 215 M)	23	2		4	2	16	Fixed tissue. HPV DNA was found in 7/57 of the lymph node metastases. 'Other': unidentified types
Furihata et al. (1993a)	Japan	In-situ hybridization (16, 18, 31, 33)	71 SCC (9 F, 62 M)	34			14	20		Fixed tissue. HPV positivity and especially high-level expression of p53 were both markers of poor prognosis.

Table 19 (contd)

Reference	Study area	Detection method (types included)	No. of cases	Overall HPV positivity (%)[b]	HPV type-specific positivity (%)[a]					Comments
					6	11	16	18	Others	
Ogura et al. (1993)	Japan	PCR (16, 18)	14 SCC	7			7			Frozen tissue
Poljak & Cerar (1993)	Slovenia	In-situ hybridization (6/11, 16/18, 31/33/51) PCR	20 SCC (M)	0 10			10			Fixed tissue
Togawa et al. (1994)	International	PCR (consensus primer) and RFLP (6, 11, 16, 18)	72	24	0	0	13	1	10	Fixed or frozen tissue. HPV-16, -18 not detected in adjacent normal tissue

SCC, squamous-cell carcinoma; PCR, polymerase chain reaction; M, males; F, females; RFLP, restriction fragment length polymorphism
[a] Including studies having used hybridization methods
[b] Of those types tested

Table 20. Prevalence of HPV DNA in laryngeal cancer case series[a] (SCC, ≥ 25 cases; verrucous carcinomas, ≥ 3 cases)

Reference	Study area	Detection method (types included)	No. of cases	Overall HPV positivity (%)[b]	HPV type-specific positivity (%)					Comments
					6	11	16	18	Others	
Abramson et al. (1985)	USA	Southern blot (11, 16, 18)	5 verrucous carcinomas	100			100			Frozen tissue
Brandsma et al. (1986)	USA	Southern blot (6, 11, 16, 18)	6 verrucous carcinomas	100			100			Frozen tissue
Kahn et al. (1986)	Germany	Southern blot (30)	41	0						Frozen tissue
Scheurlen et al. (1986a)	Germany	Southern blot (16)	36	3			3			Frozen tissue
Syrjänen et al. (1987a)	Finland	In-situ hybridization (6, 11, 16, 30)	116 SCC	13	4	8	5			Fixed tissue
Hoshikawa et al. (1990)	Japan	PCR (6, 16)	34 SCC	21	3		18			Fixed tissue
Perez-Ayala et al. (1990)	Spain	PCR (11, 16)	48 SCC 3 verrucous carcinomas	54 100			54 100			Frozen tissue. HPV-16 prevalence increases with decreasing differentiation.
Somers et al. (1990)	USA	Southern blot (2, 6, 11, 16, 18, 30, 31, 33, 35)	25 SCC	4					4	Frozen tissue. 'Others' = HPV-35
Arndt et al. (1992)	Germany	In-situ hybridization (6/11, 16/18)	27 SCC	63		37		71		Fixed tissue. Most cases were heavy smokers.
Brandwein et al. (1993)	USA	PCR (L1 consensus primers)	40 SCC	8			3		5	Fixed tissue. All but one HPV-negative cases were smokers.

Table 20 (contd)

Reference	Study area	Detection method (types included)	No. of cases	Overall HPV positivity (%)[b]	HPV type-specific positivity (%)					Comments
					6	11	16	18	Others	
Kasperbauer et al. (1993)	USA	PCR (L1 consensus primers)	20 verrucous carcinomas	85						Fixed tissue
		In-situ hybridization (6/11, 16/18, 31/33/35)		0						
Ogura et al. (1993)	Japan	PCR (16, 18)	31	20			16	3		Frozen tissue

SCC, squamous-cell carcinoma; PCR, polymerase chain reaction
[a]Including studies having used hybridization methods
[b]Of those types tested

histology, two studies using in-situ hybridization found 13% and 63% of cases to contain HPV, respectively. Southern blot studies found 0–4% HPV-positive patients and studies that used PCR detected HPV in 8–54% of the cases. In contrast, in four studies of laryngeal verrucous carcinoma, which is a variant of well-differentiated squamous-cell carcinoma that clinically resembles laryngeal papilloma, HPV DNA was detected in 85–100% of cases (a total of 31 cases out of 34 were positive). HPV-16 was by far the most frequent type detected in these tumours.

(g) Lung cancer

Development of HPV-11-positive lung cancer subsequent to (juvenile) recurrent laryngo-tracheo-bronchial papillomatosis has been reported (Byrne *et al.*, 1987; Bejui-Thivolet *et al.*, 1990a; Guillou *et al.*, 1991). In one report of a single patient, respiratory papillomatosis was associated with HPV-6/11 infection but HPV-16 was detected with increasing frequency as the atypia progressed to carcinoma over a period of nine years (Doyle *et al.*, 1994).

Four case series have reported HPV in primary lung cancers. Stremlau *et al.* (1985) found HPV-16 in one of 24 (4%) cases of various histologies; Ostrow *et al.* (1987a) found HPV-16 in one of 20 (5%) cases; Bejui-Thivolet *et al.* (1990b) found predominantly HPV-16 and -18 in six of 33 (18%) cases of squamous-cell cancer and Yousem *et al.* (1992) found HPV (predominantly HPV-16/18, -31/33 and -35) in six of 20 (30%) squamous-cell cancers. In other case series, no HPV DNA was detected (Carey *et al.*, 1990; Shamanin *et al.*, 1994b; Szabó *et al.*, 1994). In 131 bronchial squamous-cell carcinomas, Syrjänen *et al.* (1989) found 12 HPV-positive cases (9%) using in-situ hybridization.

In a series of 31 bronchial squamous-cell papillomas, Popper *et al.* (1994) found that HPV-11, detected by in-situ hybridization, was frequently associated with benign papillomas (9 of 16, 56%) while HPV-16 and -18 were found in 11 of 12 (92%) papillomas associated with squamous-cell carcinomas.

(h) Cancer of the skin

The evidence available to date suggests a very low prevalence of mucosal-associated HPV types in all non-genital skin cancers other than those occurring at periungual and palmoplantar sites. In these rare tumours [sometimes found in patients who also have HPV-16/18-positive cervical disease], the high prevalence of HPV-16/18 DNA suggests possible genital transmission of HPV infection from genital sites.

It should be noted that many studies employ methods suitable for the detection of mucosal-associated HPV types only. This may not be informative in determining the true prevalence of HPV in non-genital skin cancers. Recent studies, employing degenerate and nested primers designed to detect EV-related HPV types, have found a higher prevalence of HPV DNA in skin cancer, both in immunosuppressed patients and (in preliminary studies) in skin cancers in the general population (Berkhout *et al.*, 1995). These early data need further evaluation.

Squamous-cell carcinoma and keratoacanthoma

A very low prevalence of HPV (0–20%) is found in squamous-cell carcinoma and keratoacanthoma in most studies where tumour site is not specified (Table 21). However, HPV-9 and -37 were found in a single keratoacanthoma in one case series of seven tumours and

Table 21. Prevalence of HPV DNA in skin cancer case series — Squamous-cell carcinoma and keratoacanthoma

Reference	Study area	Detection method (types included)	Number and type of lesions	Overall HPV positivity (%)[a]	HPV type-specific positivity (%)				Comments
					6/11	16/18		Other types detected	
Scheurlen et al. (1986b)	Germany	Blot hybridization and cloning/recombination	7 KA	14				9, 37*	Frozen tissue. *In a single KA. Present at ~10 copies/cell. HPV-37 not found in any of 35 malignant melanomas or 190 other skin tumours
Grimmel et al. (1988)	Germany	Southern blot (41)	6 KA 10 SCC	0 20				41	Frozen tissue. HPV-41 not found in any of 44 melanomas or 47 non-malignant skin lesions
Eliezri et al. (1990)	USA	In-situ hybridization (NA)	16 SCC	0					Fixed tissue
Kawashima et al. (1990)	Poland	Southern blot/PCR (5/8/14, 17/20/23/24, 6/11, 16/18/33, 1–4/7, 10/28)	33 KA 51 SCC (location NA) 25 SCC (lip)	0 2 4		4*		untyped	Frozen tissue. *HPV-16. No HPV DNA found in any of 14 cutaneous horns
Pierceall et al. (1991)	USA	PCR (6/11, 16, 18)	21 SCC	19		19*			Frozen tissue. *All HPV-16. 0/7 normal biopsies contained HPV.

KA, keratoacanthoma; SCC, squamous-cell carcinoma; NA, not available; PCR, polymerase chain reaction
[a] Percentage of those types tested

HPV-41 was found in two (of 10) squamous-cell carcinomas in another. HPV-16, although not found in most studies other than those examining periungual tumours, was found in four (of 21) squamous-cell carcinomas in one case series and in one (of 25) in another.

HPV-16/18 was found in 60% of 21 periungual squamous-cell carcinomas (based on two case series). Individual case reports also document the presence of HPV-16/18 in periungual squamous-cell carcinoma (Table 22). It should be emphasized that tumours at this site are extremely rare.

Verrucous carcinoma (epithelioma cuniculatum)

Individual reports document HPV-1, -6/11 and -16/18 in single cases of verrucous carcinoma, a rare, indolent (typically non-metastasizing) tumour occurring at acral sites. However, HPV was not identified in any of 11 tumours in one case series (Table 23).

Premalignant cutaneous disease (Bowen's disease and actinic keratoses)

There is a very low prevalence of HPV in Bowen's disease and actinic keratoses where the tumour site is not specified. HPV-1 and -2 have been reported in single cases and HPV-2, -34, -36 and -41 have been found in occasional lesions in larger case series. HPV-16 was found in one (of three) Bowen's tumours in one study and in one (of 18) cases in another (Table 24). These data contrast with the high prevalence of HPV found in periungual and palmoplantar Bowen's disease, where HPV-16/18 is found in 57–70% of lesions in several case series (Table 25). Again, it should be emphasized that disease at this site is very rare.

Basal-cell carcinoma

There is a very low prevalence of HPV in basal-cell carcinoma in most case series (0–2%), but in one study HPV-16 was found in three (of 16) cases (Table 26).

Other skin lesions

HPV has not been identified in other benign skin lesions at non-genital sites, including seborrheic keratoses (Zhu *et al.*, 1991), trichilemmomas (Leonardi *et al.*, 1991a) or acanthomas (Leonardi *et al.*, 1991b) in single case series. HPV-38 has been found in a single malignant melanoma (out of 36) in one study (Scheurlen *et al.*, 1986b).

(i) Breast cancer

HPV DNA was not detected in one series of 25 breast cancer cases where low-stringency Southern blot was used (Ostrow *et al.*, 1987a) and in a study of 80 breast cancers (consensus PCR) (Wrede *et al.*, 1992). In contrast, one other PCR study found HPV-16 in 30% of 17 cases (Di Lonardo *et al.*, 1992).

(j) Ovarian cancer

Among ovarian cancer cases, HPV was not detected in five studies (≥ 5 cases). However, in one study HPV-6 was detected in 10/12 cases using in-situ hybridization, and in another HPV-16 DNA was found in nine (50%) and HPV-18 DNA in three (17%) cases (of 18) using PCR (Table 27). One case contained both HPV-16 and -18.

Table 22. Prevalence of HPV DNA in skin cancer case series — Periungual/palmar squamous-cell carcinoma

Reference	Study area	Detection method (types included)	Number and type of lesions	Overall HPV positivity (no. or %)[a]	HPV type-specific positivity (no. or %)			Comments
					6/11	16/18	Other types detected	
Moy et al. (1989)	USA	Dot blot (6/11, 16/18)	10 periungual SCC	60		60		Fixed tissue. Episomal HPV-16 found in 4/6 HPV-16-positive specimens
Ostrow et al. (1989a)	USA	Southern blot and two-dimensional gel electrophoresis (2, 6, 16, 18, 31)	1 SCC, finger	1/1		1/1		Episomal and integrated HPV-16 demonstrated in tumour tissue
Eliezri et al. (1990)	USA	In-situ hybridization (NA)	11 periungual SCC	81		63*	2 untyped	Fixed tissue. *HPV-16 also found in 25/40 anogenital SCC
Guitart et al. (1990)	USA	In-situ hybridization (6/11, 16/18)	1 SCC, nail bed	1/1		1/1		Clinicopathological study of 12 cases. Only one examined for HPV patient also had HPV-16 in cervical tissue.
Ashinoff et al. (1991)	USA	PCR (16/18) In-situ hybridization (6/11, 16/18, 31/35/51)	2 SCC, finger	2/2		2/2		Fixed tissue
Moy & Quan (1991)	USA	Dot blot (6/11, 16/18)	1 SCC, finger	1/1		1/1		Frozen tissue

SCC, squamous-cell carcinoma; NA, not available; PCR, polymerase chain reaction
[a] Percentage of those types tested

Table 23. Prevalence of HPV DNA in skin cancer case series — Verrucous carcinoma/epithelioma cuniculatum

Reference	Study area	Detection method (types included)	Number and type of lesions	Overall HPV positivity	HPV type-specific positivity			Comments
					6/11	16/18	Other types detected	
Knobler et al. (1989)	Austria	Dot blot (6, 11, 16/18)	1 EC, lower leg	1/1	1/1			Frozen tissue
Garven et al. (1991)	USA	In-situ hybridization (11, 16, 18)	1 VC, leg	1/1	1/1	1/1		Fixed tissue. A single tumour contained HPV-11 and -18.
Noel et al. (1993)	Belgium	In-situ hybridization (1–5, 11, 16, 18)	1 VC, leg	1/1			1	Frozen tissue. Tumour contained HPV-1.
Petersen et al. (1994)	Denmark	PCR (consensus primer)	13 CC*, site not specified	0/11				Fixed tissue. *2 of 13 specimens did not amplify β-globin.

PCR, polymerase chain reaction; EC, epithelioma cuniculatum; VC, verrucous carcinoma; CC, carcinoma cuniculatum belonging to the group of VC

Table 24. Prevalence of HPV DNA in skin cancer case series — Bowen's disease and actinic keratoses

Reference	Study area	Detection method (types included)	Number and type of lesions	Overall HPV positivity (no. or %)[a]	HPV type-specific positivity (%)			Comments
					6/11	16/18	Other types detected	
Ikenberg et al. (1983)	Germany	Southern blot (16)	3 BD	33*		33		Frozen tissue. *HPV containing BD at unspecified site. HPV-16 in 12/15 genital BD
Pfister & Haneke (1984)	Germany	Southern blot (1, 3, 6, 8, 11, 13)	1 non-genital BD	1/1			2	
Grimmel et al. (1988)	Germany	Southern blot (41)	6 AK	17			41	Frozen tissue
Guerin-Reverchon et al. (1990)	France	In-situ hybridization (1, 2, 5, 6/11, 16/18)	11 non-genital BD	45		18	2 and untyped	Fixed tissue. HPV-16/18 found in 1/6 bowenoid papulosis and in 0/10 control skin samples
Kawashima et al. (1990)	Poland	Southern blot/PCR (5/8/14, 17/20/23/24, 6/11, 16/18/33, 1–4/7, 10/28)	83 non-genital BD 55 AK	2.4 5.5			34 36	Frozen tissue. HPV-16 found in 9/23 genital BD and HPV-33 in a further 4/23 cases
Kettler et al. (1990)	USA	In-situ hybridization (1, 6/11, 16/18)	18 non-genital BD	6		6		Fixed tissue
Inaba et al. (1993)	Japan	In-situ hybridization (NA)	1 BD forearm (6-year-old boy)	1/1			1	Frozen tissue

BD, Bowen's disease; AK, actinic keratoses; PCR, polymerase chain reaction; NA, not available
[a] Percentage of those types tested

Table 25. Prevalence of HPV DNA in skin cancer case series — Periungual and palmoplantar Bowen's disease

Reference	Study area	Detection method (types included)	Number and type of lesions	Overall HPV positivity (no. or %)	HPV type-specific positivity (no. or %)[a]			Comments
					6/11	16/18	Other types detected	
Ikenberg et al. (1983)	Germany	Southern blot (16)	1 periungual BD	1/1		1/1		Frozen tissue
Kawashima et al. (1986)	Poland	In-situ hybridization (16 followed by cloning and recombination)	1 periungual BD	1/1			34*	Frozen tissue. *HPV-34 also found in 1/36 genital bowenoid papulosis but in 0/13 non-genital SCC and 0/12 non-genital BD
Stone et al. (1987)	USA	In-situ hybridization (1, 4, 6/11, 16/18)	1 plantar BD	1/1		1/1		
Rüdlinger et al. (1989b)	USA	In-situ hybridization (NA)	1 periungual BD	1/1			35	
Ketler et al. (1990)	USA	In-situ hybridization (1, 6/11, 16/18)	7 palmoplantar BD	70		70		Fixed tissue
Ashinoff et al. (1991)	USA	PCR (16/18) In-situ hybridization (6/8, 16/18, 31/35/51)	5 periungual BD	60		60		Fixed tissue
McGrae et al. (1993)	USA	Dot blot hybridization and PCR (NA)	3 BD finger (1 patient)	100		100		
Nordin et al. (1994)	Netherlands	NA	1 BD finger	1/1		1/1		HPV-16 also found in vulvar and cervical dysplastic tissue from this patient
Sau et al. (1994)	USA	In-situ hybridization (6/11, 16/18, 31/33/51)	7 BD nail bed	57		57		Fixed tissue

BD, Bowen's disease; SCC, squamous-cell carcinoma; NA, not available; PCR, polymerase chain reaction
[a] Percentage of those types tested

Table 26. Prevalence of HPV DNA in skin cancer case series — Basal-cell carcinoma

Reference	Study area	Detection method (types included)	Number and type of lesions	Overall HPV positivity (%)[a]	HPV type-specific positivity (%)			Comments
					6/11	16/18	Other types detected	
Grimmel et al. (1988)	Germany	Southern blot (41)	13 BCC	0				Frozen tissue
Eliezri et al. (1990)	USA	In-situ hybridization (NA)	26 BCC	0				Fixed tissue
Kawashima et al. (1990)	Poland	Southern blot/PCR (5/8/14, 17/20/23/24, 6/11, 16/18/33, 1-4/7, 10/28)	53 BCC	2			20	Frozen tissue
Pierceall et al. (1991)	USA	PCR (6/11, 16,18)	16 BCC	19		19*		Frozen tissue. *All HPV-16. 0/7 normal skin biopsies contained HPV.
Nahass et al. (1992)	USA	PCR (*L1* consensus primers)	3 scrotal BCC	0				Fixed tissue
Zhu et al. (1993b)	USA	PCR and Southern blot	13 BCC	0				

BCC, basal-cell carcinoma; NA, not available; PCR, polymerase chain reaction
[a] Percentage of those types tested

Table 27. Prevalence of HPV DNA in ovarian cancer case series (≥ 5 cases)

Reference	Study area	Detection method (types included)	No. of cases	Overall HPV positivity (%)[a]	HPV type-specific positivity (%)					Comments
					6	11	16	18	Others	
de Villiers et al. (1986b)	Germany	Reverse Southern blot	7 malignant cancers	0						Frozen tissue. No information on histology
Kaufman et al. (1987)	USA	In-situ hybridization (6, 11, 16, 18)	12 adenocarcinomas	83			83			Frozen tissue
Ostrow et al. (1987a)	USA	Filter in-situ hybridization (low stringency)	10 malignant cancers 4 metastatic cancers	0 0						Frozen tissue
Leake et al. (1989)	USA	Southern blot (6, 16, 18, 31, 35) PCR (6/11)	12 adenocarcinomas 3 tumours of low malignant potential	0 0						Frozen tissue. Histopathological changes suggestive of HPV infection (koilocytosis) in 5/15 tumours
McLellan et al. (1990)	USA	PCR (6, 11, 16, 18)	24 tumours of low malignant potential	0						Fixed tissue
Beckmann et al. (1991b)	USA	PCR (L1 consensus primers)	18 malignant cancers 11 'borderline'	0 0						Fixed tissue. β-Globin was successfully amplified in each tissue sample.
Lai et al. (1994)	Taiwan, China	PCR (16, 18)	18 cases	61			50	17		Frozen tissue

PCR, polymerase chain reaction
[a] Of those types tested

(k) Cancer of the bladder and urethra

For these tumours, contamination during tissue acquisition is a particular concern. The range in prevalence of HPV detected in bladder cancer cases is wide. In six studies, HPV was detected in 0% (0/5), 2% (1/44), 5% (1/22), 16% (12/76), 20% (4/20) and 29% (26/90) of cases, respectively, with HPV-16 being the most common type (Ostrow et al., 1987a; Bryant et al., 1991; Kerley et al., 1991; Chetsanga et al., 1992; Shibutani et al., 1992; Furihata et al., 1993b). No HPV DNA was found in a total of 150 bladder cancers from three further studies using PCR (Knowles, 1992; Saltzstein et al., 1993; Sinclair et al., 1993).

In urethral carcinomas, HPV has been detected in 29–100% of the cases based on four case series including one, four, 14 and 18 cases, respectively (Grussendorf-Conen et al., 1987; Mevorach et al., 1990; Wiener et al., 1992b; Wiener & Walther, 1994).

(l) Prostate cancer

Concerning HPV in prostatic cancer tissue (Table 28), four studies found HPV in 41–75% of cases using Southern blot or PCR. HPV-16 was the type most frequently detected. In contrast, three studies found no HPV DNA and two studies found 3/23 cases (13%) and 6/34 (25%) to be positive for HPV-16. Cuzick (1995) has recently reviewed the data on HPV and prostate cancer. He noted that the positivity rates were as high in benign prostatic hypertrophy as in invasive cancer, raising doubt about any direct role of HPV in prostatic cancer.

(m) Cancer of the eye

HPV has been found in both intraepithelial neoplasia of the conjunctiva (0–80%) and in 62–100% of invasive carcinomas of the conjunctiva, eyelid and lacrimal sac (Table 29).

2.3 Cohort studies

Virtually all prospective studies of HPV infection and cancer have focused on the cervix. The pathogenesis of HPV-related cervical cancer is usually pictured as a multistage process with at least three pathological stages: (i) HPV infection, (ii) increasingly severe grades of intraepithelial neoplasia (CIN I–III) and (iii) invasive cancer. In practice, these postulated stages cannot be distinguished perfectly. The cytological/histological signs of HPV infection and CIN I in particular tend to be overlapping and transient. Despite the resultant methodological difficulties, prospective epidemiological studies have adopted this useful three-stage model.

Accordingly, two different types of cohort studies of cervical HPV infection have been conducted. The first type examines the postulated transition from HPV infection to development of CIN. The second focuses on the apparent 'progression' of CIN (including the cytological diagnosis of HPV) to cancer or, more commonly, to high-grade CIN as a surrogate or intermediate endpoint for cancer. These two complementary types of cohort studies will be discussed in turn.

Table 28. Prevalence of HPV DNA in prostatic cancer case series[a]

Reference	Study area	Detection method (types included)	No. of cases	Overall HPV positivity (%)[b]	HPV type-specific positivity (%)					Comments
					6	11	16	18	Others	
McNicol & Dodd (1990)	Canada	Southern blot (16, 18)	4	75						Frozen tissue
Masood et al. (1991)	USA	In-situ hybridization (6, 11, 16, 18, 31, 33, 35)	20	0						Fixed tissue
McNicol & Dodd (1991)	Canada	PCR (16, 18)	27	52			52	4		Frozen tissue. Specimens obtained by transuretheral resection and suprapubic prostatectomy
Anwar et al. (1992a)	Japan	PCR (16, 18, 33)	68	41			16	25	7	Fixed tissue
Effert et al. (1992)	USA	PCR (16, 18)	30	0						Fixed tissue. Specimens obtained by radical prostatectomy
Ibrahim et al. (1992)	USA	PCR/in situ hybridization	24	25			25			Frozen and fixed tissue
Rotola et al. (1992)	Italy	PCR (6/11, 16)	8	NA	50		75			Frozen tissue
Serfling et al. (1992)	USA	PCR (6, 11, 16, 18, 33)	30	0						Frozen tissue
Sarkar et al. (1993)	USA	PCR (6/11, 16, 18)	23	13			13			Fixed tissue
Moyret-Lalle et al. (1995)		PCR (16, 18)	17	53			53			

PCR, polymerase chain reaction; NA, not available
[a] Including studies having used hybridization methods
[b] Of those types tested

Table 29. Prevalence of HPV DNA in eye lesion case series[a] (≥ 2 cases)

Reference	Study area	Detection method (types included)	No. of cases	Overall HPV positivity (no. or %)[b]	HPV type-specific positivity (no. or %)					Comments
					6	11	16	18	Others	
Conjunctiva										
Lass et al. (1983)	USA	Southern blot (11)	2 papillomas	50		50				Frozen tissue
McDonnell et al. (1987)	USA	In-situ hybridization (2, 6, 16, 18)	28 dysplasias 23 papillomas	0 65	65					Fixed tissue. Of papilloma cases, 14 contained koilocytosis.
McDonnell et al. (1989a)	USA	PCR (16, 18)	5 dysplasias 1 carcinoma 1 melanoma	100 1/1 0			100 1/1			Fixed tissue
Lauer et al. (1990)	USA	PCR (16, 18)	5 intraepithelial neoplasias	80			80	20		Fixed tissue
Odrich et al. (1991)	USA	PCR (E1 consensus primers and 6, 11, 16, 18, 33)	3 SCC (bilateral)	100			100			Frozen tissue
McDonnell et al. (1992)	USA	PCR (16, 18)	42 neoplasias	88			88			Fixed tissue. 11 invasive carcinomas, 12 severe dysplasias/CIS and 19 mild/moderate dysplasias
Eyelid										
McDonnell et al. (1989b)	USA	PCR (16/18)	1 SCC	1/1			1/1			Fixed tissue
Hayashi et al. (1994)	Japan	In-situ hybridization (6, 11, 16, 18, 31, 33)	21 sebaceous carcinomas (14 F, 7 M)	62	19	24	52	33	48	Fixed tissue. 12 cases had antibodies to p53. The presence of antibodies was more frequent in advanced cases.
Lacrimal sac										
Madreperla et al. (1993)	USA	PCR/in-situ hybridization (6, 11, 16, 18, 31, 33, 35)	3 carcinomas 3 papillomas	100 100		100		33	67	Fixed tissue

SCC, squamous-cell carcinoma; CIS, carcinoma in situ; PCR, polymerase chain reaction; F, female; M, male
[a] Including studies having used hybridization methods
[b] Percentage of those types tested

2.3.1 Following HPV DNA detection in normal women to cytological diagnosis of CIN

Cohort studies of HPV infection as a risk factor for incident CIN have enrolled apparently normal women, using DNA diagnostic assays to test for HPV infection. However, no examination of the cervix *in vivo* can rule out the presence of CIN in its most subtle form, when only a few cell clusters might be affected. Thus, no prospective study of HPV infection and 'incident' CIN can claim truly to have started with a completely CIN-free cohort. As a result, the strong cross-sectional association between HPV DNA detection and prevalent CIN unavoidably biases (upwards) estimates of absolute and relative risk for newly developed CIN, especially in the early months of follow-up.

At the practical (e.g. clinical) level, the importance of this bias is unclear. In effect, the cohort studies are determining whether the detection of HPV DNA precedes the diagnosis of CIN. In the published prospective studies, the diagnosis of the initial absence of CIN in the cervix has been based upon two common clinical techniques, exfoliative cytology and colposcopy. Most cohorts have been composed of women who are normal at enrollment and report no medical histories of abnormal cervical cytological (Papanicolaou smear) diagnoses except for benign inflammatory or reactive changes. For greater certainty of lack of disease, some groups have also subjected the key enrollment slides to review, or have examined all women colposcopically to rule out prevalent cervical lesions missed by cytology. The development of CIN within the cohorts has been diagnosed either by cytological or colposcopic screening at regular intervals, with the endpoint defined either as first cytological appearance of CIN, or more accurately a colposcopically directed biopsy diagnosed as CIN.

Using these available diagnostic techniques, the microscopic diagnoses of HPV infection and CIN overlap. Recognition by pathologists that the cytological diagnosis of HPV infection (koilocytotic atypia) is practically indistinguishable morphologically from the mildest grade of CIN (CIN I) has introduced logical circularity into the prospective studies of HPV infection and incident CIN I. If the diagnosis of CIN I includes the cytological evidence of HPV infection, then, of course, the relative risk of CIN I will be elevated following detection of HPV DNA. Some investigators have attempted to address this issue by presenting relative risks following HPV infection for koilocytotic atypia and various grades of CIN separately, even if the pathological distinctions are unreliable.

In addition, the Working Group was aware of several large unpublished studies of HPV infection in women with normal cytological diagnoses. The major (> 1000 women) ongoing cohorts include, at minimum, the work of the groups of R. Burk in the USA, J. Cuzick in the United Kingdom, E. Franco in Brazil, R. Herrero in Costa Rica, S. Kjaer in Denmark, L. Koutsky in the USA, C. Meijer in the Netherlands, A.B. Moscicki in the USA, J. Peto in the United Kingdom and India, M. Ronderos in Colombia and M. Schiffman in the USA.

Lörincz *et al.* (1990) followed a cohort of 215 cytologically normal women from a single gynaecologist's practice in Washington DC, USA, testing them for over 15 types of HPV DNA using low-stringency Southern blot. Mean follow-up was about two years, during which time three (15%) of the 20 women initially HPV-positive were diagnosed with cervical or vaginal intraepithelial neoplasia, compared to only nine (5%) of the 195 women who were initially HPV-negative. However, medical abstracting revealed that 10 of the 12 women developing neoplasia had already had CIN prior to their cytological normalcy at enrollment. In other words, HPV positivity was, at least in part, predicting recurrent rather than incident disease.

Badaracco et al. (1992) followed 82 cytologically normal women with HPV-16 or -18 (by dot blot) for approximately 18 months. They observed 22 new cytological diagnoses of 'HPV effect' [koilocytotic atypia] and three new diagnoses of CIN among the initially infected women. However, they also observed seven new cytological diagnoses of 'HPV effect' among 20 women without HPV-16 or -18 at enrolment. Thus, the relative risk of cytological abnormality following detection of HPV DNA was not elevated. [The study population was not well described and no types other than HPV-16 or -18 were assayed.]

Koutsky et al. (1992) studied a cohort of 241 cytologically normal women who had no past medical history of CIN and had been recruited in a sexually transmitted disease clinic in Seattle, USA. HPV-6, -11, -16, -18, -31, -33 and -35 were assayed using dot blot or Southern blot hybridization. The population was followed every four months by repeated HPV testing and cytological and colposcopic examinations for an average of 25 months. Twenty-eight women developed histologically confirmed high-grade CIN. CIN I was not an endpoint. A Cox regression analysis, treating the repeated HPV test results as a time-dependent covariate, indicated that HPV DNA positivity was associated with an adjusted relative risk (RR) for high-grade CIN of 11 (95% CI, 3.7–31). The RR was highest for women with HPV-16 and -18 (RR, 11 (95% CI, 4.6–26)) and for those with repeated positive tests (for ≥ 3 tests: RR, 26 (95% CI, 6.5–112)). On the basis of survival analysis, the cumulative incidence of biopsy-confirmed high-grade CIN among HPV-positive women was 28% at two years, compared with 3% among HPV-negative women. Most of the incident high-grade CIN occurred within the first two years of follow-up.

In Helsinki, Finland, Stellato et al. (1992) followed a cohort of 214 cytologically normal women of whom 145 were HPV DNA positive and the remainder were age-matched HPV-DNA-negative patients from the same clinical setting. The commercial dot-blot system, ViraPap™/ViraType™, was used for HPV testing. The subjects were followed actively every four months for a mean of about one year, with cytological evidence of CIN triggering a colposcopically directed biopsy. During follow-up, cytological evidence of CIN was seen in 25 (17%) HPV-positive women compared with only one (1%) HPV-negative woman ($p = 0.005$ by χ^2 test). Of these 25 women, histological confirmation of CIN was reported for 10. The increased risk of incident CIN was restricted to women with the 'cancer-associated' or 'high-risk' types of HPV (HPV-16, -18, -31, -33 and -35).

de Villiers et al. (1992) used filter in-situ hybridization to assay for HPV-6/11 and -16/18 in a large cohort of cytologically normal women in south-western Germany. Two out of 13 women (15.4%) who developed carcinoma in situ or invasive cancer during five years of passive cytological follow-up were HPV-positive at enrolment, compared to 8.8% of all women who were cytologically normal at enrolment. [The study cohort was not well defined.]

Prospective data from a cohort study of HPV infection and incident CIN among 11 200 cytologically normal women with no past history of CIN, recruited in 1989–90 from cytological screening clinics at the Portland, Oregon, USA, Kaiser-Permanente prepaid health plan, have been reviewed by Shah and Howley (1996). The length of follow-up extended to four years. Incident cases of CIN were mainly low-grade or koilocytotic atypia, HPV DNA positivity at enrolment (defined by Hybrid Capture™) was associated with an elevated risk of subsequent CIN. The risk peaked in the first two years following enrolment. Using life-table methods, the cumulative risk of new CIN following HPV DNA detection using Hybrid Capture™ approached 60% by four years of follow-up.

2.3.2 *Following mild dysplasia/koilocytotic atypia to CIN III/invasive cancer*

Prospective studies of the progression of HPV-associated mild dysplasia are designed to begin where the incidence studies end. In other words, they follow prospectively women with cytological or histological diagnoses of CIN to an endpoint of progression to more severe cervical neoplasia. The startpoint is usually mild dysplasia, and, for obvious ethical reasons, the endpoint in truly prospective (not historical cohort) studies is high-grade CIN and not invasive cancer, unless cases develop inadvertently despite surveillance.

Accurate assessment of disease states is difficult without interfering with the natural history of the disease. Cytological, histological and colposcopic assessments may all be inaccurate and, moreover, biopsy may lead to regression.

In the USA, CIN I and the cytological evidence of HPV are now formally combined as 'low-grade squamous intraepithelial lesions' (LSIL) (Solomon, 1989). Similarly in the forthcoming World Health Organization histopathology classification, changes associated with HPV infection are included under CIN I. There is a large literature dating back two decades regarding the natural history of mild dysplasia, which has also been called 'minimal dysplasia', 'slight dysplasia', 'mild dyskaryosis' or 'CIN I'. Correspondingly, previous terms for the cytological evidence of HPV infection in the absence of dysplasia were 'koilocytotic atypia', 'condylomatous atypia' or 'flat condyloma'. Prospective studies with any of these terms as an enrolment diagnosis were considered relevant for the evaluation of carcinogenicity of HPVs.

(a) Prospective studies of mild dysplasia/koilocytotic atypia without HPV DNA testing

The cytological/histological diagnosis of cervical HPV infection is neither sensitive nor specific (Sherman *et al.*, 1994; Kato *et al.*, 1995). Moreover, 'HPV effect' cannot reproducibly be distinguished from CIN I, which is associated with the same spectrum of HPV types. As mentioned above, the two diagnoses are combined as 'LSIL' in both the Bethesda system and the forthcoming WHO classification.

Nevertheless, it is useful to summarize briefly the many important studies that preceded the advent of HPV DNA testing, but which demonstrated the prospective risk of high-grade cervical cancer precursor lesions following the diagnosis of low-grade lesions now thought to be HPV-induced. Representative prospective studies of cohorts thought to have specifically cytologically or clinically defined HPV infections of women (koilocytotic atypia, condylomatous atypia, flat condyloma or venereal warts) will be reviewed individually. The many similar prospective studies of cohorts diagnosed with CIN I (mild, minimal or slight dysplasia or dyskaryosis) will be summarized in aggregate, because some groups continue to view CIN I as more severe (e.g. more of a cancer precursor) than the cytologic evidence of HPV infection alone.

(i) Follow-up of cohorts with HPV infection diagnosed microscopically or clinically

Meisels and Morin (1981) analysed the cytological records of 234 715 women participating in a mass screening programme in Quebec, Canada, from 1975 to 1979. Of these women, 3977 were diagnosed with 'flat condyloma'. Within the five-year study period, 4.7% of the 3670 patients with condyloma and 10% of the 307 patients with condyloma with nuclear atypia were subsequently diagnosed with dysplasia, carcinoma *in situ* or cancer.

Using a historical cohort approach, Franceschi *et al.* (1983) in Oxford, United Kingdom, compared the risk of diagnosis of CIN following an initial clinical diagnosis of genital warts with the risk following diagnosis of other sexually transmitted diseases. Genital warts are now known to be associated with HPV-6, -11 and related types (see section 1.6). Among the cohort of 489 women who had a smear three to four years after first attendance, the risk of CIN III or microinvasive carcinoma in women diagnosed with genital warts (7/206) appeared to be higher than among the women with other diseases (2/283), although the numbers of events were quite small.

Chuang *et al.* (1984) conducted a historical cohort study of cervical cancer risk in Minnesota, USA, following the diagnosis of genital warts. Among the 500 women, 11 cases of cervical carcinoma *in situ* were diagnosed after an average of four years giving a RR of 3.8 (95% CI, 1.9–6.8) compared to historical rates from the local area.

In the United Kingdom, Evans and Monaghan (1985) observed that, in a group of 51 patients with histological diagnoses of HPV infection, 16% progressed to high-grade cervical neoplasia within 12 months. This included one case of microinvasive carcinoma.

In Melbourne, Australia, Mitchell *et al.* (1986) followed 846 women, diagnosed in 1979 as having cytological evidence of HPV, and carried out repeated cervical examinations during 1980–85. Women with previous or concurrent diagnoses of dysplasia were excluded. Over these six years, carcinoma *in situ* developed in 30 women, compared to 1.9 cases expected from general population incidence rates, yielding an RR of 16 (95% CI, 11–22).

Pagano *et al.* (1987) followed 251 patients referred to a colposcopy clinic in Melbourne, Australia, for cytological diagnoses of HPV infection without CIN. Over up to three years of follow-up, 10% of women developed histologically confirmed CIN. Nearly all progressions occurred within the first 12 months following initial assessment.

To examine whether HPV predicted an increased risk of subsequent cytological or histological diagnosis of CIN, Boyle *et al.* (1989) established a historical cohort of women diagnosed in Connecticut, USA, in 1973–81, 631 with cytological evidence of HPV and 410 with *Trichomonas* infections. Average follow-up time was about two years. Thirteen women with HPV and two with *Trichomonas* had CIN diagnosed within six months of the identifying smear and were excluded from the analyses. The absolute risk of CIN following HPV infection was 8.7%, yielding an RR of 2.7 (95% CI, 1.4–4.9) when compared to the *Trichomonas*-infected cohort, after adjustment for age, nulliparity and frequency of cytological examination. The RR for CIN II–III was 3.2 (95% CI, 1.3–7.8).

Kataja *et al.* (1989) presented a life-table analysis of the best-known cohort study of cervical HPV infection defined cytologically (Syrjänen *et al.*, 1987b). A cohort composed of

256 women with cytological evidence of HPV infection without CIN and 106 women with HPV and CIN was established in Finland beginning in 1981. They were examined by colposcopy, cytology and/or punch biopsy every six months. From life-table analyses, the cumulative risk of progression to carcinoma *in situ* was estimated to be about 15% at 78 months for the group with HPV infection alone. The cumulative risk of progression among women with HPV/CIN I was 20–25% at 78 months. The two risk curves were not significantly different in the earlier years of follow-up when the person-years were greatest. However, longer follow-up of the group with HPV and CIN I indicated a continued substantial risk of progression up through the longest observation period of 96 months.

Sigurgeirsson *et al.* (1991) estimated the relative risks of cervical cancer and carcinoma *in situ* associated with a diagnosis of venereal warts by constructing a historical cohort from patients' records. They compared the incidence of cervical cancer among 711 Swedish women with venereal warts diagnosed during 1969–84 to national registry data. With a mean follow-up of eight years, the RR for cervical cancer was 1.8 (95% CI, 0–10; one case); that for carcinoma *in situ* was 1.5 (95% CI, 0.9–2.5; 17 cases). However, among a corresponding group of 2549 men with venereal warts, the RR of anogenital malignancy was 2.6 (95% CI, 1.2–5.0; nine cases).

Gram *et al.* (1992) linked hospital records to Norwegian cancer registry data to examine the temporal relationship between the cytological diagnosis of HPV or *Trichomonas* infection and subsequent risk of CIN III in northern Norway. From 1980 to 1989, HPV infection was noted in 678 of 43 016 women with negative Pap-smears, while *Trichomonas* was diagnosed in 988. The age-adjusted incidence rates of CIN III were as follows: 225 per 10^5 person-years follow-up among women with neither infection, 459 per 10^5 person-years among women with *Trichomonas* and 729 per 10^5 person-years among women with HPV. The RR for the development of CIN III among women with HPV, adjusted for several possible confounding variables, was 3.5 (95% CI, 1.9–6.6) compared to uninfected women.

Montz *et al.* (1992) followed 203 women in Los Angeles, USA, with cytological diagnoses of low-grade SIL. The presence of occult high-grade CIN missed by cytology was minimized by enrollment colposcopy. Seven women (3.4%) progressed to high-grade SIL: one at three months, one at six months and five at nine months.

(ii) Follow-up of cohorts with mild dysplasia

The many cohort studies of women diagnosed with CIN I were comprehensively reviewed recently by Östör (1993) who provided useful aggregate estimates by pooling the data from over 15 studies. In total, he reviewed the follow-up of about 4500 women with CIN I from published studies. The observed risk of progression to CIN III in the studies was 11%, with 1% observed progression to invasive cancer during follow-up (which was often short and truncated by treatment). The remaining cases persisted (32%) or regressed (57%).

Soutter and Fletcher (1994) reanalysed five studies (Robertson *et al.*, 1988; Fletcher *et al.*, 1990; Cooper *et al.*, 1992b; Hirschowitz *et al.*, 1992; Kirby *et al.*, 1992) of cytological follow-up of women with mildly abnormal cervical smears. The four latter studies were too recent to be included in Östör's pooled estimates (Östör, 1993). Soutter and Fletcher estimated that the annual incidence of invasive cancer among women with mild cytological abnormalities was between 143 and 420 per 10^5 person-years, which is comparable to Östör's cumulative incidence of 1%. The magnitude of risk of cervical cancer following diagnosis of CIN I was calculated to be 16–47 times greater than the incidence of cervical cancer in women of similar age in the general population of England and Wales.

(b) Prospective studies of mild dysplasia/koilocytotic atypia with HPV DNA testing

In recent prospective studies of CIN I/koilocytotic atypia, HPV DNA typing has sometimes been included as an independent covariate. The aim of including HPV typing in progression studies has been to determine whether HPV type predicts the risk of progression independently of microscopic diagnosis.

Campion *et al.* (1986) in London, United Kingdom, used filter in-situ hybridization to test for HPV-6 and -16 among 100 women aged < 30 years with persistent CIN I (mild dyskaryosis on three consecutive smears taken within 16 weeks). No biopsies were taken at enrolment. The cohort was examined every four months by colposcopy and cytology for a range of 19 to 30 months. Of the 26 women who progressed to histologically confirmed CIN III, 22 (85%) had tested positive for HPV-16 DNA at enrolment; only 17 of the 74 women (23%) who did not progress to CIN III had tested positive for HPV-16 DNA. Thus, the presence of HPV-16 was significantly associated with risk of (and time to) progression; presence of HPV- 6 was not. [The HPV test method used in this study is now obsolete and possibly inaccurate with regard to typing. For example, the possibility of cross-reactivity between HPV-16 and related types not known at the time of the investigation should be considered.]

Schneider *et al.* (1987b) monitored 48 HPV-positive West German women cytologically over a period of three to 24 months. Filter in-situ hybridization had been used to detect HPV-6/11 and -16/18. Of the 17 women with an initial cytological diagnosis of 'condyloma', two progressed to histologically confirmed CIN III. Both were HPV-16/18-positive at enrolment (one was also positive for HPV-6/11), whereas there were no instances of progression among the seven women positive for HPV-6/11 only. The same association of risk of progression with HPV-16/18 positivity was seen among the six women who progressed to CIN III among the 26 who were initially diagnosed as 'CIN I/II'.

Caussy *et al.* (1990b) studied 47 cases of invasive cancer and 94 matched controls in British Columbia, Canada, using archival pathology specimens. The cases were women treated for invasive cancer from 1960 to 1986, and archival biopsies showing CIN, taken at least two years before the diagnosis of cancer, used to test for HPV DNA at the pre-invasive stage using tissue in-situ hybridization. HPV-6/11, -16/33 and -18 were assayed. The controls were women with previous, available CIN biopsies who had not progressed to invasive cancer. [An appreciably larger percentage of controls than cases had been treated at the CIN stage.] The controls were matched to cases on a variety of factors, including date of the biopsy showing CIN. The investigators observed non-significantly elevated HPV prevalence for all three type groups among the case group (6.4% for HPV-18; 8.5% for HPV-6/11; 19% for HPV-16/33) compared with their matched controls (2.1%, 3.2% and 11%, respectively).

Kataja *et al.* (1990) performed a survival analysis of enrolment HPV typing data from the long-term Finnish prospective study of women with cytological evidence of HPV infection (Syrjänen *et al.*, 1987b). Starting in 1981, the cohort was followed every six months by cytology and colposcopy (with or without biopsy, depending on the study subgroup) for a mean of 50 months. For 458 women in the cohort, archival enrolment specimens were assayed for HPV-6, -11, -16, -18, -31 and -33 using in-situ hybridization. Clinical progression was defined as a change from no CIN to CIN or from lower to higher grade CIN. The overall rate of progression was 16.4%. The risk of progression was highest in 91 women positive for HPV-16 (35.2%) or 14 having multiple infections (28.6%), intermediate for 205 women with other HPV types (15%), and lowest in 48 HPV-negative women (6.1%). These differences were statistically significant in both contingency-table and survival-curve analyses. [The inconsistency of finding HPV DNA negativity in women diagnosed with cytological changes supposedly indicating HPV infection raises the possibility of either false positive cytological diagnoses or false negative DNA hybridization.]

Using a retrospective cohort design, Weaver *et al.* (1990) studied 32 patients in Ohio, USA, with histological diagnoses of CIN I 'with koilocytosis', testing archival paraffin-embedded specimens with in-situ hybridization for HPV-6/11, -16, -18, -31 and -33. The cytological follow-up, a minimum of two examinations over at least 1 year, ranged from 12 to 80 months with a mean of 27 months. The cumulative rate of progression to CIN II or greater was 9% (3 cases), with no apparent difference in rates of progression between the HPV-positive (7%) and HPV-negative (12%) subcohorts. [The Working Group noted the small sample size of this study.]

Byrne *et al.* (1990) followed 42 women in the United Kingdom with cytological evidence of CIN I or II at four-monthly intervals, using cytology and colposcopy, with an endpoint of histologically confirmed CIN III. Enrolment and follow-up specimens were tested for HPV-6, -11, -16 and -18 using a slot blot DNA hybridization method. The women were seen from three to 11 times over the 45-month follow-up period. Thirty of the 42 women (71%) were positive for HPV-16 or -18 DNA at some time during the study. In this subgroup, five of 30 (16.7%) progressed, compared to one of the 12 women (8.3%) who were HPV-16/18-negative throughout. [The HPV exposure measurement mixes enrolment and follow-up positivity into a cumulative positivity measurement that is not strictly prospective.]

Parry *et al.* (1990) reported on 44 women with CIN I–II, whom they followed by quarterly cytological and colposcopic examination over a two- to three-year period. The women were tested by dot blot at each visit for HPV-6, -11, -16 and -18. The detection of HPV-16 or -18 at any time during follow-up was associated with a significantly increased risk of progression to CIN III. [The enrolment DNA data are not reported separately to permit a strictly prospective analysis.]

Using cytology and colposcopy quarterly for up to 36 months, Hørding *et al.* (1991b) monitored 15 women in Copenhagen, Denmark, diagnosed histologically with mild dysplasia. Filter in-situ hybridization was used to test enrolment and follow-up specimens for HPV-11, -16 and -18. HPV positivity at any time was found in seven of the women, all of whom had progressive or persistent lesions. In comparison, only four of the eight persistently HPV-11/16/18-negative patients had persistent or progressive CIN. [When combined with similar results for women found initially to have CIN II, the differences by HPV positivity/negativity were statistically significant. However, this study mixes enrolment and follow-up HPV positivity into a cumulative HPV positivity measurement that is not strictly prospective. The HPV test used is obsolete.]

Pich et al. (1992) followed 24 women in Italy, with CIN I or CIN II lesions immunohistochemically positive for HPV antigens. The biopsies were further analysed for HPV-6/11 and -16/18 DNA. Follow-up included quarterly cytological, colposcopic and histological examinations over a two-month to 65-month period. Four of 10 women with HPV-16/18 progressed to histologically diagnosed CIN III, compared with none of 14 HPV-16/18-negative women. [This investigation combines CIN I and II, and does not separate clearly enrolment versus follow-up HPV positivity.]

Hellberg et al. (1993) conducted a historical cohort study of 201 women with CIN lesions tested for HPV-6, -11, -16, -18, -31 and -33 by in-situ hybridization. The mean follow-up time was 17.3 years. In a multivariate analysis, HPV type was significantly associated with risk of progression, independent of grade of CIN. [Crude data permitting analyses specific for HPV type among women with low-grade CIN were not presented].

Downey et al. (1994) followed 92 women in the United Kingdom with cytologically/histologically diagnosed CIN I or 'wart virus infection' for up to 70 months of passive surveillance (medical record review and quarterly cytology with colposcopy following any abnormal cytological diagnoses). The endpoint, reached by 25 patients, was the histological diagnosis of CIN II or more-severe disease. Cervical DNA from samples taken at enrolment was tested for HPV-16 using 'semiquantitative' PCR only. The presence of HPV-16 DNA was non-significantly (but negatively) associated with risk of progression. Also, counter to the expectations raised by cross-sectional data from the same population (Bavin et al., 1993), greater viral burden was not predictive of progression. [The Working Group noted that HPV testing was conducted for HPV-16 only, and that other high-risk types could be present in the 'HPV-negative' group. Also HPV-16 positivity was unusually prevalent among the low-grade cases (51/92), raising a concern about the accuracy of the viral typing.]

Gaarenstroom et al. (1994) performed a retrospective cohort study of HPV testing by general primer PCR among 227 patients with frozen cervical swabs taken at the time of first abnormal cervical cytological diagnosis. All women had colposcopically directed biopsies at entry. Cohort members were followed subsequently by colposcopy and cytology at 3-month intervals, without therapeutic interventions for at least 6 months. The presence of HPV-16 DNA at enrolment predicted the following: a significantly elevated 29% risk of progression to higher-grade neoplasia (defined histologically); a 10% risk of progression for HPV-18, -31, -33 and unknown types; and a 0% risk of progression among women positive only for HPV-6 or -11 or negative for HPV. [The cohort included 100 women with underlying CIN II–III at enrolment, as well as 101 with underlying CIN I and 26 with no CIN demonstrated histologically. Excluding the 24 women with CIN III did not alter the conclusions but further recalculations are not possible from the data presented.]

Remmink et al. (1995) prospectively followed a cohort of 342 women in Amsterdam, with a new cytological diagnosis of 'Pap IIIb' or lower, suggestive of mild, moderate or severe dysplasia. Surveillance every three to four months included cytology, colposcopy without biopsy and HPV DNA testing for 27 types by a well-validated PCR technique. The mean follow-up of the entire cohort was about 16 months. At the start of follow-up, 62% of women were HPV-positive. Nineteen women (5.6%) progressed, defined as developing a lesion with a colposcopic impression of CIN III over more than two quadrants of the cervix or a Pap smear of class V (highly suggestive of malignancy). All 19 women subsequently had histologically confirmed CIN III and all were HPV-positive both at enrolment and continuously during follow-up.

2.3.3 Prospective studies of HPV infection at body sites other than the cervix

In Australia, Planner and Hobbs (1988) followed, without treatment, 103 women with colposcopic and histological evidence of HPV infection of the vulva, with no associated VIN. One patient experienced progression to a VIN III lesion after two years.

Arndt et al. (1993) studied the prospective risk of carcinoma of the larynx related to laryngeal infection with HPV-16 or -18 among 150 patients with chronic laryngeal inflammation, followed for up to 3.5 years. PCR was used to test for HPV-16 and -18 DNA in laryngeal biopsies. Fifteen (16.5%) of the 91 patients positive for HPV-16 or -18 developed laryngeal cancer, compared to only one patient (1.7%) among the 59 in the HPV-negative group.

2.4 Case–control studies

To date, case–control studies contribute the bulk of the epidemiological evidence linking HPV to cervical cancer and to CIN III. The initial studies were severely hampered by test validity and study design (for reviews see Koutsky et al., 1988; Muñoz et al., 1988; Bosch & Muñoz, 1989; zur Hausen, 1989; Franco, 1992; Bosch et al., 1994b; Schiffman & Schatzkin, 1994). In addition to the general concern on the comparison of studies based on HPV DNA assays of different sensitivity and specificity, the interpretation of case–control studies is difficult because, in many cases, the published investigations were not based on cases and controls drawn from defined and comparable populations; rather, they consisted of a series of cases collected in a medical facility and compared to an undefined group of women without cervical abnormalities. In addition, many studies were based on small numbers of cases and controls, and potential confounders, such as age, were not controlled for.

This monograph includes a comprehensive compendium of published reports of different quality. The data on cervical cancer and CIN lesions are presented in an ordered fashion by stage of disease and by HPV detection method employed. Tables 30, 31 and 36 include studies of CIN lesions in which HPV was detected by non–hybridization methods (Table 30), hybridization methods not including amplification (Table 31) and PCR based methods (Table 36). In a similar manner, Tables 38, 39 and 40 summarize studies on invasive cervical cancer. Table 37 and 41 summarize studies of CIN and invasive cancer in which serological assays were used to assess HPV exposure.

Of the studies included, only a limited number fulfil the epidemiological requirements of a case–control study. These are the studies in which the following criteria are met:

(i) There is a recognizable study design aiming at avoiding bias in the recruitment of cases and the selection of controls.

(ii) The study subjects are representative of the general population.

(iii) There is a comprehensive effort to evaluate all known or suspected risk factors for cervical cancer.

(iv) The size of the study is sufficiently large to allow precise estimates of risk.

(v) The estimates of HPV exposure are based on state-of-the-art PCR methods.

(vi) The statistical analysis includes multivariate techniques.

The few studies that fulfilled these criteria were highly influencial in the Working Group's final evaluation and they are placed as first entries in Tables 36 and 40.

Of all the variables that may affect the results, test validity seems to be the main one. In this light, it is remarkable that hospital-based studies (Eluf-Neto *et al.*, 1994) produce similar risk estimates to population-based studies (Muñoz *et al.*, 1992). The increased detection level afforded by PCR-based methods over previous assays provided more accurate estimates of the HPV prevalence in cases and controls, but in many studies, quantitative information on the level of HPV DNA is not available, so the importance of high-level positivity cannot be investigated.

2.4.1 Cervical cancer

Reviews of the case–control studies relating HPV DNA detection and cervical neoplasia are largely consistent in showing that the association is strong with odds ratios greater than 10 in the majority of studies. The association is specific to a limited number of HPV types. HPV-16, -18, -31, -33 and -45 account for perhaps 80% of the types found in biopsies of invasive cervical cancer worldwide (Bosch *et al.*, 1995). The association is also consistent geographically in all countries in which studies have been conducted. The increased detection level afforded by PCR-based methods over previous assays has provided more-accurate estimates of the HPV prevalence in cases and controls. In general, odds ratios and attributable risks (ARs) are higher in PCR-based studies (although the association is consistently present and statistically significant irrespective of the HPV detection method used) (for reviews, see Bosch *et al.*, 1992; Muñoz & Bosch, 1992; Schiffman, 1992a,b).

(a) HPV and CIN III

Table 30 summarizes case–control studies in which exposure to HPV was assessed using morphological criteria of diagnosis in cells or biopsies or using immunoperoxidase staining to detect HPV capsid antigen in biopsies. It is known that the sensitivity of morphological changes such as koilocytosis is low and that the presence of markers associated with a productive HPV infection decreases as the severity of the intraepithelial process advances (see section 1.5). Many of these studies are crude by current standards but were of importance at the time when the association between HPV and cervical neoplasms was unknown. However, it soon became clear that DNA-based studies were capable of detecting HPV DNA in a large fraction of cervical cancer. The studies listed in Table 30 are therefore of limited value concerning the association between HPV and cervical cancer.

Reid *et al.* (1982) examined the margins of neoplastic lesions in women undergoing hysterectomy for cervical cancer, CIS or for reasons not related to cervical neoplasia. A semi-objective rating system of HPV-related morphological changes was used to evaluate specimens. Cases and controls were classified according to a wart score and a categorical division into

Table 30. Case–control studies of CIN I–III using HPV non-hybridization methods

Reference and study area	Cases (number and type)	Controls (number and type)	HPV prevalence (%)	Odds ratio (95% CI)	HPV test/comments/adjustments
Reid et al. (1982) Detroit, MI, USA	All women with hysterectomy 20 CIN I 20 CIN III	40 age-, race- and SES-matched women with hysterectomy and no cervical pathology	Cases Controls Negative 0 80.0 Suspect 12.5 10.0 Infected 87.5 10.0	Definite HPV versus negative or suspect [CIN I–III, 63 (13.4–345.5)]	Criteria for seven histological parameters scored in 3 levels: negative; suspect; infected
Grunebaum et al. (1983) New York, USA	251 patients referred to colposcopy with CIN I–III	90 normal cervices from same clinic	Control, 24.4 Mild dysplasia, 62.5 Moderate dysplasia, 59.8 Severe dysplasia, 22.9 CIS, 14.3	[CIN I–III, 2.5 (1.9–4.4)]	Koilocytosis, multinucleation, parakeratosis, dyskeratosis
Syrjänen (1983) Finland	345 dysplasias, CIS, invasive condylomatous lesions	275 dysplasias, CIS, invasive non-condylomatous lesions	Control, 0 (0/129) All, 56.2 (122/217) Papillomatous, 100 Inverted, 69.7 Flat, 52.5	[∞ (115–∞)] [∞ (187–∞)] [∞ (159–∞)] [∞ (98–∞)]	Staining, immunoperoxidase-PAP (paraffin sections), HPV Ag in cells
Syrjänen et al. (1983) Finland	79 dysplastic and/or CIS with condylomatous lesions	31 dysplastic and/or CIS without-condylomatous lesions	Control, 0 All cases, 70.8 Papillomatous, 100 Inverted, 83.3 Flat, 66.7	[∞ (44–∞)] [∞ (32–∞)] [∞ (43–∞)] [∞ (36–∞)]	Staining, immunoperoxidase-PAP (paraffin sections), HPV Ag in cells
Adam et al. (1985) Houston, USA	23 CIN	23 matched, no CIN	Control, 0 (0/10) CIN I–II, 27 (3/11) CIN III, 0 (0/2) All, 22.2 (4/18)	[∞ (0.4–∞)] Not computable Any lesion, [∞ (0.4–∞)]	Presence of structural antigen in biopsy specimens. Prospective cohort study of women exposed to diethylstilboestrol
Guijon et al. (1985) Manitoba, Canada	33 CIN I–III referred to colposcopy	54 women with no CIN attending family-planning clinic	Case, 45 Control, 3.7	[21.7 (4.1–152.8)]	Koilocytosis

Table 30 (contd)

Reference and study area	Cases (number and type)	Controls (number and type)	HPV prevalence (%)	Odds ratio (95% CI)	HPV test/comments/adjustments
Zaninetti et al. (1986) Italy	126 abnormal Pap smears in women less than 20 years of age	1914 normal cervices, same age and clinic		Ever having genital warts 9.15 (5.1–16.3)	History of genital warts. OR adjusted for number of sexual partners
Höckenström et al. (1987) Gothenburg, Sweden	49 women with a consort with genital warts	124 women age, parity, OC use and date-of-examination matched to the case attending family-planning clinics	Dysplasia or HPV infection: Case, 37 Control, 6	[8.4 (3.1–23.5)]	Koilocytosis, atypia, dysplasia
Alberico et al. (1988) Trieste, Italy	533 cases attending colposcopy with dyskaryosis to CIN III and CIS. Of these, 299 CIN I–III	533, age matched to the cases, with no CIN	Dyskeratosis, 26 CIN I, 39 CIN II, 51 CIN III–CIS, 25 Normal, 0.19	Any CIN versus normal [333 (45–6460)]	Detection of condylomatous cytohistological features
Cuzick et al. (1990) United Kingdom	110 CIN I 103 CIN II 284 CIN III	833 family-planning clinic and local GPs	Control, 5 CIN I, 33 CIN II, 28 CIN III, 16	CIN I, 8.4 CIN II, 7.1 CIN III, 3.4	History of genital warts. $p < 0.05$
Seshadri (1991) India	16 CIN I 29 CIN II 25 CIN III	50 controls	Control, 28.9 CIN I, 62.5 CIN II, 75.9 CIN III, 60.0	[4.2 (1.1–16.9)] [7.8 (2.6–27.0)] [3.8 (0.4–49.4)]	Histopathological evidence of HPV infection
Kjaer et al. (1992) Denmark	586 CIS 59 invasive cancers	614 population based		Ever genital warts 1.7 (1.2–2.5)	History of genital warts. OR increased with early age at first episode of genital warts. OR adjusted for age, smoking, number of partners, oral contraception, and parity
Thanapatra et al. (1992) Thailand	970 specimens with CIN I–III	22691 specimens with no CIN or carcinoma from screening programme	CIN I–III, 26 Control, 1.2	[28.8 (23.8–34.9)]	Koilocytosis, atypia

[ ] Calculated by the Working Group
CIN, cervical intraepithelial neoplasia; SES, socio-economic status; CIS, carcinoma *in situ*; OC, oral contraceptive; Ag, antigen; Pap, Papanicolaou; PAP, peroxidase-antiperoxidase; GP, general practitioner; OR, odds ratio
^{a} ∞, zero cases in control group

definite HPV changes, suspected HPV changes and no HPV changes. Using as cases those that had definite HPV changes and comparing these to those that were negative or suspected, the odds ratios were [107 (95% CI, 17.6–877)] for invasive cervical cancer (see also Table 38) and [63 (95% CI, 13.4–345.5)] for CIN lesions.

Grunebaum et al. (1983) evaluated HPV signs in 348 patients referred to a colposcopy clinic. Of these, 251 women had histologically confirmed CIN I–III and they were compared to 90 women with normal cervices. The presence of HPV signs was 44.6% among cases and 24.4% among controls [OR, 2.5 (95% CI, 1.9–4.4)]. Of seven cases of invasive cancer diagnosed in this series, none had HPV signs.

In two studies, Syrjänen (1983) and Syrjänen et al. (1983) compared the presence of HPV signs in cervical lesions ranging from dysplasia to CIS in 79 and 345 patients with 31 and 275 patients without concomitant condylomatous lesions. HPV antigens were investigated using the immunoperoxidase–peroxidase–antiperoxidase method. Cases without associated condyloma (controls) were consistently negative and cases with associated condyloma were HPV antigen-positive in 70.8% and 56.2% of patients, respectively.

Adam et al. (1985) studied 23 cases of CIN lesions arising in a cohort of women exposed *in utero* to diethylstilboestrol. A control group of 23 cohort members without CIN were identified. The peroxidase–antiperoxidase method was used to detect HPV structural antigen and part of the biopsies were also reviewed for the presence of HPV signs. Of CIN I–II cases, 27% were immunoperoxidase-positive compared to none of the controls. None of the differences was statistically significant [$p > 0.05$]. Of 18 cases investigated (CIN I–III, HPV and squamous metaplasia), 15 had HPV-related changes histologically and four had HPV structural antigen reactivity.

Guijon et al. (1985) compared the presence of HPV signs in 33 women with colposcopically detected and biopsy-proven CIN I–III and 54 women with normal cervices; 45% of cases and 3.7% of the controls had HPV signs [OR, 21.7 (95% CI, 4.1–152.8)].

Zaninetti et al. (1986) conducted a similar study in Italy including 126 women below 20 years with abnormal Pap smears and 1914 women of the same age with a normal Pap smear. A history of warts was reported by 15 cases (11.9%) and 22 controls (1.1%). The estimated relative risk, adjusted for number of sexual partners, was 9.15 (95% CI, 5.1–16.3).

Höckenström et al. (1987) investigated the presence of dysplasia or HPV signs in 49 female consorts of men with condylomata acuminata and compared them to a group of 124 women from family-planning clinics matched to cases on age, oral contraceptive use, parity and date of examination. Thirty-seven percent of cases had HPV-related signs compared to 6% of controls [OR, 8.4 (95% CI, 3.1–23.5)].

Alberico et al. (1988) evaluated condylomatous signs in 533 women attending a colposcopy clinic with diagnoses ranging from dyskaryosis to carcinoma *in situ*. A control group of 533 women with normal cervices were also evaluated. The prevalence of HPV colposcopic signs in the 299 CIN I–III lesions was 38.5% compared with 0.19% in controls [OR, 333 (95% CI, 45–6460)].

Cuzick et al. (1990) investigated 497 women under the age of 40 with CIN I–III and 833 controls from general practitioners' files or family-planning clinics. A history of genital warts was reported by 5% of the controls, 33% of the CIN I cases, 28% of the CIN II cases and 16% of the CIN III cases ($p < 0.05$ for each CIN stage as compared to controls).

Seshadri et al. (1991) compared 70 women with CIN I–III to 50 controls with normal cervices. HPV exposure was assessed using the standard histopathological criteria. The presence of HPV changes was reported in 28.9% of the controls, 62.5% of CIN I cases, 75.9% of CIN II cases and 60.0% of CIN III cases. The estimated odds ratio for the group of CIN I–III was [OR, 5.9 (95% CI, 2.3–15.4)].

Kjaer et al. (1992) compared the history of genital warts in 586 cases of carcinoma *in situ* of the cervix, 59 cases of invasive carcinoma and 614 controls drawn from the general population that generated the cases. One-hundred-and-two cases reported having had episodes of warts (17.9%) as well as 62 controls (10.3%). The odds ratio adjusted for age, smoking, number of partners, oral contraception and parity was 1.7 (95% CI, 1.2–2.5). The risk increased with earlier age at first episode of genital warts.

Thanapatra et al. (1992) compared the presence of HPV signs and a cytological diagnosis of CIN in women participating in a national screening programme in Thailand. Of 970 women diagnosed as CIN I–III, 26.0% had HPV signs compared to 1.2% of the controls [OR, 28.8 (95% CI, 23.8–34.9)].

Evans et al. (1992) investigated the history of anogenital warts in relation to the presence of CIN I–III in the United Kingdom. The reported odds ratio for a history of vulvar warts was 0.34 (95% CI, 0.13–0.84).

In China, Su (1987) used the peroxidase stain to explore HPV genus specific antigen in 244 cervical tissue specimens. Six of 52 cases of carcinoma (12%) were HPV positive as compared to none of the 20 controls tested.

In the USA, Amburgey et al. (1993) conducted a case–control study of 102 cases of CIN I–III matched to an equal number of controls. No HPV detection method was used but cases reported genital warts more often than controls (OR, 2.5 (95% CI, 1.0–6.4)).

In Durban, Kharsany et al. (1993) examined a series of patients attending an STD clinic. HPV exposure was found cytologically in 22/48 (46.0%) cases, colposcopically in 28/48 (58.3%) and histologically in 26/45 (57.8%). Women with CIN had clinical HPV signs in 13/28 (46.4%).

Kjaer et al. (1991) investigated the history of genital warts in husbands of monogamous women with CIN and in the husbands of a control group in Denmark. The study group included 41 case couples and 90 control couples. Genital warts were reported in 9/41 (22.0%) husbands of cases and in 2/90 (2.2%) husbands of controls. The odds ratio, adjusted for age and use of a condom with the partner, was 17.9 (95% CI, 3.3–98.3). Cell specimens from the male genital warts were analysed using ViraPap™ and ViraType™ and only two husbands of cases were found to be HPV-positive (one had HPV-6/11 and the other HPV-16/18). [The Working Group noted that ViraPap™ assays in specimens from the male genitalia may be inaccurate in detecting HPV DNA prevalence.]

Table 31 contains a summary of case–control studies investigating preinvasive lesions (CIN I–III) using hybridization assays without amplification techniques, including Southern blot, dot blot, filter in-situ hybridization (FISH) and variants of these methods.

Table 31. Case–control studies of CIN I–III lesions using HPV hybridization assays without amplification

Reference and study area	Cases (number and type)	Controls (number and type)	HPV prevalence (%)	Odds ratio (95 % CI)	HPV test	Comments/adjustments
McCance et al. (1985) London, United Kingdom	Colposcopy clinic 20 CIN I 30 CIN II 28 CIN III	17 without cervical abnormality	HPV-16 CIN I, 55 CIN II, 66 CIN III, 71 Control, 18	HPV-16 [5.7 (1.1–35.6)] [9.3 (1.8–53.6)] [11.7 (2.2–70.5)]	DNA hybridization Probes: 6, 16 and low stringency	
Demeter et al. (1987) Australia	6 minor cell atypias 29 CIN I 35 CIN II 62 CIN III	23 normal	Any HPV Minor cell atypia, 33.3 CIN I, 72.4 CIN II, 77.1 CIN III, 71.0 Normal, 30.4 HPV-16/18 Minor cell atypia, 16.6 CIN I, 51.7 CIN II, 51.4 CIN III, 53.2	Any HPV [1.1 (0.1–10.5)] [6.0 (1.5–24.4)] [7.7 (2.0–30.8)] [5.6 (1.8–18.2)] HPV-16/18 [0.7 (0.03–9.9)] [3.9 (1.0–16.0)] [3.8 (1.0–15.0)] [4.1 (1.2–14.5)]	Filter in-situ hybridization Probes: 6/11 and/or 16/18	Colposcopy clinic attendees
Pao et al. (1989) Taipei, Taiwan, China	276 urogenital condylomata, 47 cervical dysplasias	39 symptom free	Symptom free, 15.4 Urogenic condylomata, 84.4 CIN or CIS, 72.3	Any HPV [29.8 (11.0–84.8)] [14.4 (4.4–49.7)]	In-situ DNA hybridization 6/11, 16, 18, 31, 33	Detection in exfoliated cervicovaginal cells
Duggan et al. (1990) Canada	300 CIN/condylomata	90 normal	CIN/condylomata, 60 Normal, 26.6	Any HPV [4.1 (2.4–7.2)] High-risk HPVs [18.8 (7.6–49.4)]		
Kataoka & Yakushiji (1990) Japan	37 clinical findings	71 symptom free	Case, 32.4 Control, 5.6	Any HPV [8.0 (2.1–33.0)]	Non-isotopic subgenomic probes on Southern blot hybridization	Young women (14–27)
Becker et al. (1991) New Mexico, USA	52 atypias 77 slight dysplasias 27 moderate–severe dysplasias	1447 Pap negative	Pap negative, 5.6 Atypia, 21.2 Slight dysplasia, 45.5 Moderate–severe dysplasia, 66.7%	HPV [4.5 (2.1–9.5)] [14.0 (8.3–23.9)] [33.7 (13.8–84.1)] Any Pap abnormalities, [11.7 (7.8–17.6)]	Dot-blot hybridization assay (ViraPap™)	Random sample of patients undergoing a pelvic examination. Prevalence varies with ethnicity.

Table 31 (contd)

Reference and study area	Cases (type and number)	Controls (type and number)	HPV prevalence (%)	Odds ratio (95 % CI)	HPV test	Comments/adjustments
Lindh et al. (1992) Sweden	52 CIN I 23 CIN II–III	416 with no CIN	No CIN, 14 CIN I, 50 CIN II–III, 39	*HPV* [6.3 (3.3–12.1)] [4.8 (1.9–12.5)] All CIN, [5.5 (3.1–9.7)] *HPV-16* All CIN, [3.4 (1.1–9.8)] *HPV-18* All CIN, [12.3 (4.3–36.1)]	Southern blot, probes 6, 11, 16, 18, 31, 33, 35	Women attending outpatient clinics
Lörincz et al. (1992) USA	270 borderline atypias 638 definite cervical diseases: LSIL & HSIL	1566 normal cervices	Normal, 6.4 Borderline atypia, 23.7 Cervical disease, 79.3 LSIL, 69.5 HSIL, 87.4	*HPV* Any cervical disease, 27.1 ($p < 0.0001$) Definite cervical disease, [55.4] *LSIL* HPV-16, 36.9 (25.0–54.5) HPV-18, -45, -56, 32.7 (19.2–55.8) *HSIL* HPV-16, 235.7 (198.5–279.5) HPV-18, -45, -56, 65.1 (50.2–84.5)	Southern hybridization	Pooled analysis and HPV testing of subjects from 8 studies. No adjustments, crude odds ratios
Manavi et al. (1992) Austria	411 dysplasias	240 normal cytologies	Prevalence given by Pap grade	*HPV* II, [27.9 (11.2–73.5)] III, [52.9 (20.3–146.4)] IV, [136.5 (44.3–447.7)] V, [468.0 (130.9–1852.7)]	In-situ nucleic acid hybridization	
Meekin et al. (1992) New Zealand	87 dysplasias 84 atypias 495 infections/benign atypias	1347 normal cytologies	Control, 8.3 Dysplasia, 48.3 Atypia, 20.2 Infection/benign atypia, 10.1	Odds ratio for atypia or dysplasia: HPV, 5.8 (4.0–8.6) HPV-16/18, 6.4 (3.3–5.9)	Dot-blot DNA hybridization	Attendees of family planning clinics
Tanaka et al. (1992) Japan	145 abnormal cytologies	100 normal cytologies	Normal, 2 Benign, 2 Condyloma, 100 Mild–moderate dysplasia, 39 Severe dysplasia/CIS, 44 Invasive, 70 Any abnormal, 30	*HPV* [$p < 0.001$] [31.8 (6.8–204.1)] [38.1 (5.8–318.5)] [114.3 (12.9–1463.2)] [20.7 (4.7–126.8)]	Southern blot, probes 6, 11, 16, 18, 31, 33, 35	HPV and HPV type specific prevalence. No multivariate analysis. HPV prevalence by age and type of lesion

Table 31 (contd)

Reference and study area	Cases (type and number)	Controls (type and number)	HPV prevalence (%)	Odds ratio (95 % CI)	HPV test	Comments/adjustments
Levine et al. (1993) USA	34 cytological SIL 25 equivocal atypias 19 histological HSIL	147 cytological controls 150 histological controls	Cytological control, 16 Histological control, 19 Cytological SIL, 58 Equivocal atypia, 40 Histological HSIL, 68	7.3 (3.3–17.0) 3.4 (1.4–8.5) 10.3 (3.3–32.0)	ViraPap™	Population-based case–control study of college students. Age: 18–35. Covariates: age, multiple lifetime sexual partners, oral contraceptive use
Meyer et al. (1993) USA	61 LSIL 16 HSIL	72 cytologically normal women	Normal, 6.9 LSIL, 29.5 HSIL, 68.7	HPV [5.6 (1.8–18.8)] [29.5 (6.2–158.1)]	ViraPap™ combined with ViraType™ in-situ hybridization	Patients: high risk for HPV infection. Type-specific information also available. No odds ratios, no multivariate analysis
Becker et al. (1994) New Mexico, USA	201 H dysplasias	337 hospital controls	Case, 66.5 Control, 13.9	12.8 (8.2–20.0)	ViraPap™	
Brisson et al. (1994) Canada	548 H CIN 338 L CIN	612 hospital controls	H CIN, 42.5 L CIN, 12.0 Control, 6.02	8.7 (5.1–15.0) 1.6 (0.9–3.0)	Southern blot for HPV-16	
Davidson et al. (1994) Alaska, USA	74 atypias 68 LSIL 96 HSIL	723 normal cervices	Normal, 14.1 Atypia, 29.7 LSIL, 64.7 HSIL, 89.6	1.0 2.7 (0.8–9.5) 10.4 (6.1–17.8) 14.4 (9.6–21.8)	ViraPap™, ViraType™	Alaska native women. 3 groups: routine care clinics (n = 492), referral colposcopy clinic (n = 385) and population-based (n = 249). Odds ratio combined for HPV-16/18 and -31/33/35
Marin et al. (1994) Slovenia	109 abnormal smears 22 LSIL 7 CIN I 14 CIN II–III	42 normal smears	HPV-16 / HPV-18 Normal, 11.9/4.8 LSIL, 13.6/13.6 CIN I, 14.3/0.0 CIN II–III, 21.4/14.3	HPV-16 [1.2 (0.2–6.5)] [1.2 (0.0–15.0)] [2.0 (0.3–12.2)] Any CIN/HPV-16/18 [1.9 (0.6–6.3)]	In-situ hybridization	Age: 17–51

[ ] Calculated by the Working Group
CIN, cervical intraepithelial neoplasia; CIS, carcinoma in situ; HSIL, high-grade squamous intraepithelial lesion; LSIL, low-grade squamous intraepithelial lesion; H, high grade; Pap, Papanicolaou smear

McCance et al. (1985) investigated 78 cases of CIN I–III with FISH using probes for HPV-6 and -16. The CIN cases were compared to 17 controls. HPV-16 positivity was found in 18% of the controls and 55%, 66% and 71% of CIN I–III, respectively [ORs, 5.7 (95% CI, 1.1–35.6); 9.3 (95% CI, 1.8–53.6); 11.7 (95% CI, 2.2–70.5)].

Demeter et al. (1987) conducted a FISH-based study of 132 cases of CIN I–III using probes for HPV-6/11 and -16/18. The CIN cases were compared to 23 controls. HPV-16/18 positivity was 21.8% among controls and 51.7%, 51.4% and 53.2% for CIN I–III respectively [ORs, 3.9 (95% CI, 1.0–16.0); 3.8 (95% CI, 1.0–15.0); 4.1 (95% CI, 1.2–14.5)].

Pao et al. (1989), using in-situ hybridization, investigated 47 cases of dysplasia and 39 controls. Prevalence rates of HPV DNA positivity were 15.4% among controls and 72.3% among cases [estimated OR, 14.4 (95% CI, 4.4–49.7)].

In Venezuela, Azocar et al. (1990) investigated 119 non-monogamous women using ViraPap™ and cytological criteria (normal/abnormal). HPV DNA positivity rates among cases with abnormal cytology were 88% (16/18) and 26% (26/101) among women with normal cytology [OR, 23 (95% CI, 4.6–157)].

In Canada, Duggan et al. (1990) used the dot blot system to investigate a series of 401 patients attending a colposcopy clinic in which a cytological/histological diagnosis was available. Of the 300 subjects classified as CIN/condyloma, 60% were HPV DNA positive. In the group with normal cytology, 26.6% had evidence of HPV DNA [OR, 4.1 (95% CI, 2.4–7.2)]. The HPV types identified were largely high-risk types (HPV-16/18/33) or HPV-6/11. HPV-16 was the predominant virus detected [OR for high-risk types, 18.8 (95% CI, 7.6–49.4)]. There was a strong trend of increasing prevalence of high-risk types in relation to the severity of the CIN lesion ($p < 0.001$).

Kataoka and Yakushiji (1990) used Southern blot hybridization to investigate 37 cases of dysplasia and 71 controls. HPV prevalence rates were 5.6% among controls and 32.4% among cases [estimated OR, 8.0 (95% CI, 2.1–33.0)].

In the USA, Becker et al. (1991) studied 1603 randomly selected Hispanic, native American and non-Hispanic white women to determine the prevalence of cervical HPV infection according to Pap smear results. These results included atypia (52 cases), slight dysplasia (77 cases) and moderate to severe dysplasia (27 cases). Women with normal Pap smears (1447 cases) served as controls. The method used to detect HPV was dot-blot hybridization (ViraPap™). The HPV DNA prevalence in the group with negative Pap smears was 5.6%, 21.2% for atypia, 45.5% for slight dysplasia and 66.7% for moderate–severe dysplasia [estimated crude ORs, 4.5 (95% CI, 2.1–9.5) for atypia; 14.0 (95% CI, 8.3–23.9) for slight dysplasia; and 33.7 (95% CI, 13.8–84.1) for moderate–severe dysplasia; 11.7 (95% CI, 7.8–17.6) for any Pap abnormality].

In northern Italy, Garuti et al. (1991) investigated HPV DNA prevalence in 276 biopsies using Southern blot hybridization. They reported an increased trend in the prevalence of HPV-16 from specimens with normal cytology to invasive carcinoma. The opposite trend was observed for HPV-6 and -11.

In Sweden, Lindh et al. (1992) compared the HPV DNA prevalence using Southern blot in 416 women with no clinical signs of HPV-related disease with that of 75 women with CIN (52 with CIN I and 23 with CIN II–III). A mixture of subgenomic probes were targeted at HPV-6, -11, -16, -18, -31, -33 and -35. HPV prevalences were 14% for asymptomatic women, 50% for women with CIN I lesions, and 39% for women with CIN II–III lesions [estimated crude ORs for any HPV: 6.3 (95% CI, 3.3–12.1) for CIN I; 4.8 (95% CI, 1.9–12.5) for CIN II–III; and 5.5 (95% CI, 3.1–9.7) for all CIN]. The type-specific prevalences for cases (all CIN) and controls were, respectively: 8% versus 3% for HPV-6, 4% versus 1% for HPV-11, 8% versus 4% for HPV-16, 15% versus 2% for HPV-18, 12% versus 4% for HPV-31, 8% versus 3% for HPV-33, 1% versus 1% for HPV-35, and 1% versus 0.5% for undetermined HPV [ORs for CIN: 3.4 (95% CI, 1.1–9.8) for HPV-16, and 12.3 (95% CI, 4.3–36.1) for HPV-18].

In the USA, Lörincz et al. (1992), in a pooled analysis of eight studies of the relationship between HPV infection and cervical neoplasia, compared 1061 cases of cervical disease (atypia (270), LSIL (377), HSIL (261) and carcinoma (153)) with 1566 women with a normal cervix. The method used to detect HPV was low-stringency and high-stringency Southern blot hybridization with specific probes for HPV-6/11, -16, -18, -31, -33, -35, -42, -43, -44, -45, -51, -52, -56 and -58. The overall HPV DNA prevalence among cases was 23.7% for borderline atypia and 79.3% for cervical disease. The HPV DNA prevalence for controls was 6.4%. Risk estimates (not adjusted for other risk factors) were 27.1 for any cervical disease and [55.4] for definite cervical disease. Type specific HPV prevalences are shown in Table 32.

Table 32. Distribution of HPV types by diagnosis

HPV type	Normal (%) (n = 1566)	Atypia (%) (n = 270)	LSIL (%) (n = 377)	HSIL (%) (n = 261)
Negative	93.6	76.3	30.5	12.6
6/11	0.5	2.2	16.7	3.1
16	1.0	4.4	16.2	47.1
18	0.3	1.9	4.0	5.0
31/33/35	0.8	3.0	11.1	19.2
42/43/44/45	0.5	2.6	4.5	1.5
51/52/56/58	1.2	2.2	7.7	5.7
Unclassified	2.1	7.4	9.3	5.7

From Lörincz et al. (1992)

The crude odds ratios (95% CI) for type-specific HPVs are shown in Table 33.

In Austria, Manavi et al. (1992) compared the HPV DNA prevalence using in-situ hybridization in 411 patients with cytological dysplasia with that of 240 cytologically normal women. HPV prevalences according to the Papanicolaou classification were: 2.5% for Pap grade I, 41.7% for Pap grade II, 57.6% for Pap grade III, 77.8% for Pap grade IV and 92.3% for Pap grade V. The corresponding crude ORs as compared to women with a Pap grade I were: [27.9 (95% CI, 11.2–73.5)] for Pap grade II, [52.9 (95% CI, 20.3–146.4)] for Pap grade III, [136.5 (95% CI, 44.3–447.7)] for Pap grade IV and [468.0 (130.9–1852.7)] for Pap grade V.

Table 33. Crude odds ratios for HPV types in relation to atypia, LSIL and HSIL

HPV type	Atypia	LSIL	HSIL
6/11, 42, 43, 44	6.1 (3.1–12.1)	52.6 (36.0–76.9)	24.1 (13.4–43.4)
31,33,35,51,52	2.6 (1.2–5.2)	21.6 (17.9–26.1)	71.9 (51.0–101.6)
16	5.0 (2.5–9.9)	36.9 (25.0–54.5)	235.7 (198.5–279.5)
18,45,56	6.6 (2.8–15.7)	32.7 (19.2–55.8)	65.1 (50.2–84.5)

From Lörincz et al. (1992)

In New Zealand, Meekin et al. (1992) compared the HPV DNA prevalence using dot blot in 1347 cytologically normal women with that of 666 women with dysplasia (n = 87), atypia (n = 84) or a cytology showing the presence of infection or benign atypia (n = 495). HPV prevalences were as follows: 8.3% for control women, 48.3% for dysplasia, 20.3% for atypia and 10.1% for infection or benign atypia. The OR associated with any HPV was 5.8 (95% CI, 4.0–8.6) for atypia or dysplasia. The corresponding OR for HPV-16/18 was 6.4 (95% CI, 3.3–5.9).

In Japan, Tanaka et al. (1992) compared the HPV DNA prevalence using Southern blot in 100 women with normal cytology with that in 145 women with an abnormal cytology. Probes for HPV-6, -11, -16, -18, -31, -33 and -35 were used. The HPV DNA prevalence in the group with normal cytology was 2%. The overall HPV prevalence in women with abnormal cytology was 30% — 2% for benign lesions, 100% for condylomas, 39% for mild–moderate dysplasia, 44% for severe dysplasia/CIS and 70% for invasive cancer. [Estimated crude ORs were 31.8 (95% CI, 6.8–204.1) for mild–moderate dysplasia, 38.1 (95% CI, 5.8–318.5) for severe dysplasia/CIS, 114.3 (95% CI, 12.9–1463.2) for invasive carcinoma and 20.7 (95% CI, 4.7–126.8) for any abnormality.]

In the USA, Goff et al. (1993) examined 360 biopsies of attendees of a colposcopy clinic with ViraPap™. Of 71 CIN I–III cases, 35 (49.3%) were HPV positive as were 31 of 225 controls (13.8%) [OR, 6.1 (95% CI, 3.2–11.6)].

Levine et al. (1993) conducted a population-based case–control study of US college students aged 18–35 years to estimate the effect of HPV infection on SIL of the uterine cervix. Cases included 34 cytological SIL and 25 equivocal atypia as well as 19 histologically confirmed HSIL. The control group consisted of 147 subjects with a normal cervical cytology. The method used to detect HPV was ViraPap™. The HPV prevalence among cases was 58% among cytological SIL, 40% among cases of equivocal atypia and 68% among histological HSIL. The HPV prevalence among cytological controls was 16% and among histological controls 19%. Risk estimates were adjusted for age, multiple lifetime sexual partners and oral contraceptive use. The adjusted odds ratios for HPV DNA presence were as follows: for cytological SIL, 7.3 (95% CI, 3.3–17.0); for equivocal atypia, 3.4 (95% CI, 1.4–8.5); and for histological HSIL, 10.3 (95% CI, 3.3–32.0). The distribution of HPV types among cases and controls are shown in Table 34.

Table 34. Distribution of HPV types by diagnosis

HPV type	Cytological diagnosis			Histological diagnosis	
	Control (%)	Equivocal (%)	SIL (%)	Control (%)	HSIL (%)
Negative	85.4	60.0	42.4	82.4	33.3
6/11	0.0	16.0	6.1	0.7	5.6
16/18	1.4	8.0	18.2	2.7	33.3
31/33/35	4.2	0.0	12.1	4.7	5.6
6/11 + 31/33/35	0.0	0.0	3.0	0.0	5.6
16/18 + 31/33/35	0.0	8.0	0.0	0.0	0.0
Indeterminate	9.0	8.0	18.2	9.4	16.7

From Levine et al. (1993)

The type-specific crude odds ratios (95% CI) for a larger sample selected subsequently from the same population are shown in Table 35.

Table 35. Odds ratios for HPV-types in relation to LSIL and HSIL

HPV type	Cytological LSIL	Cytological HSIL
6/11	6.9 (1.6–29.0)	–
16/18	12.9 (4.7–35.0)	12.4 (3.3–46.0)
31/33/35	5.2 (1.7–16.0)	10.8 (3.0–39.0)

From Levine et al. (1993)

In the USA, Meyer et al. (1993) estimated the HPV DNA prevalence in 61 patients with LSIL, 16 patients with HSIL and 72 cytologically normal women. The method used to detect HPV was ViraPap™ combined with ViraType™ in-situ hybridization. HPV prevalences were: 6.9% for cytologically normal women, 29.5% for LSIL and 68.7% for HSIL. Crude ORs were [5.6 (95% CI, 1.8–18.8)] for LSIL and [29.5 (95% CI, 6.2–158.1)] for HSIL.

In a young population in the USA, Moscicki et al. (1993) compared HPV-positive and HPV-negative women who were also studied with colposcopy. Detailed criteria to evaluate colposcopy findings were used. Women who were HPV-16/18-positive by ViraPap™ had a higher mean number of lesions (1.7 versus 0.7; $p < 0.001$) and higher lesional scores (3.4 versus 1.0; $p < 0.001$) than women who were HPV-negative or HPV-positive for HPV-6, -11, -31, -33 or -35.

Becker et al. (1994) conducted a case–control study in New Mexico, USA, including 201 cases of high-grade dysplasia and 337 hospital controls. Scraped specimens from the cervix were investigated using ViraPap™ and ViraType™ and PCR. The corresponding HPV DNA prevalences for ViraPap™ were as follows: cases 66.5%, controls 13.9% (OR, 12.8 (95% CI, 8.2–20.0)).

In Canada, Brisson *et al.* (1994) investigated the presence of HPV DNA using Southern blot in 548 cases of high-grade CIN, 338 cases of low-grade CIN and 612 hospital controls. The corresponding HPV DNA prevalences were 42.5%, 12.0% and 6.0%, respectively, and the ORs adjusted for age, number of sexual partners, age at first intercourse, smoking, oral contraceptive use, DNA source and DNA load were 1.6 (95% CI, 0.9–3.0) for low-grade CIN and 8.7 (95% CI, 5.1–15.0) for high-grade CIN. A dose-response was observed with increasing load of HPV-16 DNA. The association with low-grade CIN was not statistically significant.

In the USA, Davidson *et al.* (1994) estimated HPV prevalences in 961 Alaska native women, of which 723 had a normal cytology, 74 had atypia, 68 LSIL and 96 HSIL. ViraPap™ and ViraType™ were used to detect HPV DNA. The HPV prevalences were 14.1% for normal women, 29.7% for atypia, 64.7% for LSIL and 89.6% for HSIL. As compared to normalcy, the crude ORs were: 2.7 (95% CI, 0.8–9.5) for atypia, 10.4 (95% CI, 6.1–17.8) for LSIL and 14.4 (95% CI, 9.6–21.8) for HSIL. The corresponding odds ratios for HPV types 16/18 were 1.5 (95% CI, 0.7–3.4) for atypia, 2.6 (95% CI, 1.2–5.6) for LSIL and 7.1 (95% CI, 4.5–11.3) for HSIL. Odds ratios for HPV-31/33/35 were: 2.4 (95% CI, 1.3–4.5) for atypia, 3.9 (95% CI, 2.1–7.4) for LSIL and 6.3 (95% CI, 3.7–10.5) for HSIL.

In Slovenia, Marin *et al.* (1994), using in-situ hybridization, investigated 109 cases of abnormal smears, 22 with LSIL, 7 with CIN I and 14 with CIN II and 42 controls. Among controls, the prevalence rate of HPV-16 was 11.9% and of HPV-18 4.8%. Among cases the prevalence was 32.1% for HPV-16 and 10.4% for HPV-18. The estimated OR for any CIN and HPV-16/18 combined was [1.9 (95% CI, 0.6–6.3)].

Table 36 summarizes the results of case–control studies that investigated preinvasive lesions (CIN I–III) using hybridization assays with amplification techniques. There are two PCR techniques that were used by most of the studies. One uses consensus primers based on approximately 450 bp of the *L1* region of HPV-16/18, and utilizes type-specific and generic probes. The other amplifies a smaller region of *L1*, detects a broader range of types, and is often followed by a separate type-specific PCR (see section 1.3.3). The two tests have not been formally validated against each other. During the period in which they have been used, the number of HPV-specific probes has increased and the strategies to collect, store and analyse specimens have improved considerably. Therefore, any variation in the prevalences observed may be an artefact, partially due to differences in the methodology employed.

In Spain, Bosch *et al.* (1993) compared 157 cases of severe dysplasia, carcinoma *in situ* or CIN III with 193 controls having normal cytology, nonspecific inflammatory changes or Pap grades I and II. The method used to detect HPV was PCR based on consensus primers of the *L1* region with probes for HPV-6, -11, -16, -18, -31, -33 and -35. The HPV DNA prevalence was 70.7% among cases and 4.7% among controls. Risk estimates were adjusted for age, geographical area, number of sexual partners, age at first sexual intercourse, *Chlamydia trachomatis* and husband's sexual partners. The adjusted OR for HPV DNA presence was 56.9 (95% CI, 24.8–130.6; attributable fraction, 72.4%). The distribution of HPV types in cases was HPV-16 (69.4%), HPV-18 (0.9%), HPV-31 (1.8%), HPV-33 (8.1%), HPV-35 (0.9%) and HPV unknown (18.9%). The distribution of HPV types in controls was as follows: HPV-16 (11.1%), HPV-18 (0.0%), HPV-31 (11.1%), HPV-33 (11.1%), HPV-35 (0.0%) and HPV unknown (66.7%). The adjusted

Table 36. Case-control studies of CIN I–III lesions using HPV hybridization assays, including amplification (PCR) methods

Reference and study area	Cases (number and type)	Controls (number and type)	HPV prevalence (%) Type	Cases	Controls	Odds ratios (95% CI)	HPV test	Comments/adjustments
Bosch et al. (1993) Spain	157 severe dysplasias, carcinomas in situ, CIN III	193 normal cytology, nonspecific inflammatory changes or Pap I and II	HPV 16 18 31 33 35	70.7 69.4 0.9 1.8 8.1 0.9	4.7 11.1 0 11.1 11.1 0	56.9 (24.8–130.6) 295.5 (44.8–1946.4) 28.9 (5.5–152.8)	PCR 6, 11, 16, 18, 31, 33, 35	Attributable fraction, 72.4%. Age, geographical area, number of sexual partners, age at first intercourse, *Chlamydia trachomatis*, husband's sexual partners
Colombia	125 severe dysplasias, carcinomas in situ, CIN III	181 normal cytology, nonspecific inflammatory changes or Pap I and II	HPV 16 18 31 33 35	63.2 51.9 0 3.8 3.8 2.5	10.5 31.6 0 0 5.3 0	15.5 (8.2–29.4) 27.1 (10.6–69.5) 23.4 (2.8–190.6)	PCR 6, 11, 16, 18, 31, 33, 35	Attributable fraction, 60.3%
Coker et al. (1993) South Carolina	114 CIN I 28 CIN II/III 115 atypias 140 inflammatory	223 normal cytology	HPV-16/18/33 CIN II/III CIN I Atypia Inflammatory Normal	35.7 24.5 6.1 10.7 2.7		21.9 (6.4–74.5) 11.7 (4.3–32) 3.0 (0.9–9.8) 2.6 (0.8–8.4) 1	PCR 6b, 11, 16, 18, 33	Age, race, smoking, sexual behaviour, use of oral contraceptives. 60% were black and of low socioeconomic level.
Schiffman et al. (1993) Portland, OR, USA	319 condylomatous atypias 131 CIN I 50 CIN II/III	453 randomly selected from 17 654 women with normal cytology and no known history of CIN	*CIN I* HPV-16/18 31, 33, 35, 39, 45, 51, 52 6/11, 42, other or unknown *CIN II–III* HPV-16/18 31, 33, 35, 39, 45, 51, 52 6/11, 42, other or unknown	36.0 34.4 21.6 62 10 18	2.9 3.3 11.5 2.9 3.3 11.5	200 (68.0–570.0) 130 (47.0–370.0) 24 (9.3–60.0) 180 (49.0–630.0) 22 (4.8–97) 10 (3–36)	PCR 6/11, 16, 18, 26, 31, 33, 35, 39, 40, 42, 45, 51, 52, 53, 54, 55, 57, 59	Age, HPV test results and lifetime numbers of sex partners

Table 36 (contd)

Reference and study area	Cases (number and type)	Controls (number and type)	HPV prevalence (%) Type	Cases	Controls	Odds ratios (95% CI)	HPV test	Comments/adjustments
Van der Brule et al. (1991a) Amsterdam, Netherlands	124 Pap IIIa 31 Pap IIIb 22 Pap IV	(a) 1346 symptom-free population (b) 239 gynaecological outpatient population without history of cervical pathology, (c) 177 gynaecological outpatient population having history of cervical pathology	HPV overall Pap IIIa Pap IIIb Pap IV (a) (b) (c) HPV-16/18 Pap IIIa Pap IIIb Pap IV (a) (b) (c)	70 84 100 41 58 70	3.5 9.2 21.5 0.9 2.5 12	HPV overall [68.1 (45.4–102.4)] HPV-16/18 [135.8 (82.5–225.9)]	PCR 6/11, 16, 18, 31, 33	No adjustments. Cases: Pap IIIa + Pap IIIb + Pap IV Controls: (a) + (b) + (c)
Morrison et al. (1991) Bronx, NY, USA	Hospital 65 non-pregnant with histopathological documentation of SIL	Family-planning clinic 59 women with normal cytology	HPV One HPV type > one HPV type	84.6 53.8 30.8	39.0 35.6 3.4	10.4 (3.6–30.4) 7.2 (2.4–21.9) 43 (6.9–266.6)	PCR 16, 18, 33	Age, ethnicity, education, number of cigarettes daily, current use of oral contraceptives, age at first coitus, HPV infection determined by PCR. SIL: including atypia, CIN I, CIN II and CIN III
Pasetto et al. (1992) Urbino, Italy	Hospital 23 CIN II–III cytology specimens	Hospital 148 normal cytology specimens	HPV-16	32.4	8.9	[12.8 (4.4–38.8)]	PCR 16	
Nakazawa et al. (1992) Osaka, Japan	Hospital 37 CIN III	Hospital 69 normal	HPV-16 HPV-18 HPV-16 and -18	24.3 2.7 0	8.7 5.8 1.4	[2.8 (0.8–9.4)] [0.4 (0.02–4.1)]	PCR 16, 18	No odds ratios given in the paper. No adjustments
Bavin et al. (1993) London, United Kingdom	Hospital 35 CIN III	Hospital 54 normal	HPV HPV-16	27 74.3	16 63	[1.95 (0.67–5.73)] [1.7 (0.61–4.84)]	PCR 16	Use of semiquantitative PCR for HPV-16

Table 36 (contd)

Reference and study area	Cases (number and type)	Controls (number and type)	HPV prevalence (%)				Odds ratios (95% CI)	HPV test	Comments/adjustments
			Type	Cases		Controls			
Margall et al. (1993) Barcelona, Spain	Hospital 66 biopsies/cervical scrapes of patients with cervical lesions:	Hospital: 64 women with normal Papanicolaou test	*16 and/or 18*	Biopsy (cases)	Scrape (cases)	Scrape (cases)	HPV-16 and/or -18 Odds ratios for CIN using cervical scrapes [1.7 (0.5–5.8)]	PCR 16, 18	The prevalence of HPV-16 in controls was 11%.
	14 chronic inflammations (ChI)		ChI	43	0				
	5 cervical condylomas (CC)		CC	80	20				
	24 CIN I		CIN I	50	17				
	12 CIN II		CIN II	50	17				
	10 CIN III		CIN III	70	20				
	1 invasive carcinoma (IC)		IC	0	0				
Becker et al. (1994) New Mexico	201 H dysplasias	337 hospital controls		93.8		42.1	20.8 (10.8–40.2)	PCR *L1* consensus primers	
Cuzick et al. (1995) London, United Kingdom	81 CIN II–III	1904 negative cytology or CIN I	HPV					Type-specific PCR (16, 18, 31, 33)	Cases and controls from women undergoing routine screening
			16	75		4.5	[65 (33–113)]		
			18	44		1.6	[50 (28–88)]		
				6		0.8	[13 (5.4–31)]		
			31	25		1.4	[24 (13–45)]		
			33	9		0.8	[12 (4.7–30)]		
Liaw et al. (1995) Taiwan	40 CIN I 48 CIN II–III, invasive cervical cancers	261 normal cytology		92		9	CIN I, 14.0 (6.1–32) CIN II–III, invasive, 122.3 (38.5–388.9)	PCR	HPV-16 predominant in CIN II–III and invasive cancers; HPV-52 and -58 predominant in CIN I and controls
Strickler et al. (1995) Jamaica	49 CIN III, cervical cancers	40 women with normal cervix or CIN I		92.1		25.7	[2.7 (1.1–7.0)] *p* for trend with HPV grade < 0.001	PCR *L1* consensus primers	HTLV-1 was also identified as a risk factor for CIN III/cervical cancer.

[ ] Calculated by the Working Group
Pap, Papanicolaou smear test result; CIN, cervical intraepithelial neoplasia; H, high-grade; PCR, polymerase chain reaction; HTLV-1, human T-lymphotropic virus; SIL, squamous intra-epithelial lesion

ORs for specific HPV types were: for HPV-16, 295.5 (95% CI, 44.8–1946.4); for HPV-31, -33 and -35, 28.9 (95% CI, 5.5–152.8); and HPV unknown, 18.7 (95% CI, 6.6– 54.8).

In Colombia, Bosch et al. (1993) compared 125 cases of severe dysplasia, carcinoma in situ or CIN III with 181 controls having normal cytology, nonspecific inflammatory changes or Pap grades I and II. The method used to detect HPV was PCR with probes for HPV-6, -11, -16, -18, -31, -33 and -35. The HPV DNA prevalence was 63.2% among cases and 10.5% among controls. Risk estimates were adjusted for age, geographical area, number of sexual partners, age at first sexual intercourse, C. trachomatis and smoking. The adjusted OR for HPV DNA presence was 15.5 (95% CI, 8.2–29.4; attributable fraction, 60.3%). The distribution of HPV types in cases was HPV-16 (51.9%), HPV-18 (0.0%), HPV-31 (3.8%), HPV-33 (3.8%), HPV-35 (2.5%) and HPV of unknown type (38%). The distribution of HPV types in controls was HPV-16 (31.6%), HPV-18 (0.0%), HPV-31 (0.0%), HPV-33 (5.3%), HPV-35 (0.0%) and HPV of unknown type (47.4%). The adjusted ORs for HPV type specific were as follows: HPV-16, 27.1 (95% CI, 10.6–69.5); HPV-31, -33 or -35, 23.4 (95% CI, 2.8–190.6); HPV of unknown type, 12 (95% CI, 5.1–28.6).

In the same study (Bosch et al., 1993), 852 specimens were tested using the commercial dot blot system, ViraPap™. The results were as follows: in Spain the study included 207 CIN III cases and 209 controls, and HPV DNA prevalences were 33.8% and 3.8% and the OR was 13.4 (95% CI, 5.9–30.6); in Colombia, the subjects included were 187 cases and 249 controls and HPV DNA prevalences were 28.9% and 10.0% and the OR was 8.7 (95% CI, 4.9–15.3). These risk estimates were adjusted for all variables that showed an association with cervical cancer in the study.

The comparison of results when testing the same specimens with ViraPap™, Southern hybridization and PCR showed concordant results for the presence or absence of HPV DNA in 65% of the cases. PCR and Southern blot hybridization were concordant in the type specific result in 86% of the specimens (see also section 1.3; Guerrero et al. 1992).

In South Carolina, USA, Coker et al. (1993) compared 114 cases of CIN I, 28 cases of CIN II–III, 115 cases of atypia and 140 cases of infection or inflammatory changes with 223 controls selected from normal cytology. The method used to detect HPV DNA was PCR and specific probes were used for HPV-6b, -11, -16, -18 and -33. The HPV DNA (HPV-16, -18 or -33) prevalence was 35.7% among cases with CIN II or III and 2.7% among controls. Risk estimates were adjusted for age, race, smoking, number of sexual partners and current use of oral contraceptives. The adjusted OR for HPV DNA (type HPV-16, -18 or -33) was 21.9 (95% CI, 6.4–74.5) for CIN II/III.

In Portland, Oregon, USA, Schiffman et al. (1993) compared 50 cases of CIN II–III with 453 controls selected randomly from 17 654 women with normal cytology and no known history of CIN (not matched). Cervico-vaginal lavages were used to collect cytological specimens. The method used to detect HPV was PCR and specific probes were used for HPV-6/11, -16, -18, -26, -31, -33, -35, -39, -40, -42, -45, -51, -52, -53, -54, -55, -57 and -59. Risk estimates were adjusted for age, HPV test results, and lifetime numbers of sexual partners. The distribution of HPV types in cases of CIN II-III was as follows: HPV-16 or -18: 62%; HPV-6, -11, -42, other or unknown: 18%; and HPV-31, -33, -35, -39, -45, -51 or -52: 10%. The distribution of HPV types in controls was: HPV-16 or -18: 2.9%; HPV-6, -11, -42, other or unknown: 11.5%; and HPV-31, -33, -35, -39, -45, -51 or -52: 3.3%. The adjusted ORs for type-specific HPV in CIN II–III were: HPV-16 or -18, 180 (95% CI, 49-630); HPV-6, -11, -42, other or unknown, 10 (95% CI, 3–36);

HPV-31, -33, -35, -39, -45, -51 or -52, 22 (95% CI, 4.8–97). The study also included 319 women with condylomatous atypia, randomly chosen among the 492 women diagnosed in the screening programme. Taken together, the 492 cases with lesions classified as condylomatous atypia or above and the 453 controls, the odds ratios were: HPV-6, -11, -42, other or unknown, 8.7 (95% CI, 5.8–13.0); HPV-31, -33, -35, -39, -45, -51 or -52, 33.0 (95% CI, 18.0–59.0); HPV-16 or -18, 51.0 (95% CI, 28.0–94.0).

Further analyses of this study were reported following correspondence by Luthi and Burk (1993). This association of CIN I and CIN II–III was not modified by age.

In Amsterdam (Netherlands), van den Brule *et al.* (1991a) compared 124 cases of Pap IIIa (mild and moderate dysplasia), 31 cases of Pap IIIb (severe dysplasia) and 22 cases of Pap IV (carcinoma *in situ*) with 1346 controls selected from a symptom-free population of women, 239 female gynaecological outpatients without a history of cervical pathology and 177 gynaecological outpatients having a history of cervical pathology. The method used to detect HPV was PCR testing for HPV-6/11, -16, -18, -31 and -33. The HPV DNA prevalence among cases was 70% in Pap IIIa, 84% in Pap IIIb, 100% in Pap IV, 3.5% among symptom-free controls, 9.2% in women without a history of cervical pathology and 21.5% in women having a history of cervical pathology. The distribution of HPV-16 and -18 in cases was: Pap IIIa, 41%; Pap IIIb, 58%; and Pap IV, 70%. The distribution of HPV types 16 and 18 in controls was 0.9% in the symptom-free population, 2.5% in the gynaecological outpatient population without a history of cervical pathology and 12% in the gynaecological outpatients having a history of cervical pathology.

In New York (USA), Morrison *et al.* (1991) compared 65 nonpregnant woman who had histopathological documentation of a cervical SIL (including atypia, CIN I, II, III), with 59 controls selected from family-planning or other gynaecology clinics in order to obtain cytologically normal specimens. The method used to detect HPV was PCR for HPV-16, -18 and -33. The HPV DNA prevalence was 84.6% among cases and 39% among controls. Risk estimates were adjusted for age, ethnicity, education, number of cigarettes smoked daily, current use of oral contraceptives, age at first coitus and HPV infection determined by PCR. The adjusted ORs for HPV DNA presence was 10.4 (95% CI, 3.6–30.4). One HPV-type was found in 53.8% of cases, and more than one type was found in 30.8%. One HPV type was found in 35.6% of controls, and more than one type in only 3.4%. The adjusted ORs for HPV type specific were: one HPV type, 7.2 (95% CI, 2.4–21.9); more than one HPV type, 43 (95% CI, 6.9–266.6). In this study there was an attempt to quantify the intensity of the HPV viral load by visual inspection of the signal and the size of the band. The dose–response relationship was then assessed by stratifying the results of the Southern blot and the PCR assays into three categories (negative, weak, strong). The ORs were as follows: Southern blot — weak signal, 15.7 (95% CI, 4.4–56.3); strong signal, 21.1 (95% CI, 4.9–91.0; p for trend < 0.01); PCR — weak signal, 8.0 (95% CI, 2.3–27.5); strong signal, 12.7 (95% CI, 3.8–42.4; p for trend < 0.01).

In Urbino (Italy), Pasetto *et al.* (1992) compared 23 cases of CIN II and CIN III with 148 controls selected from women with a normal colposcopic examination, i.e. the absence of vaginal or vulvar lesions. The method used to detect HPV was PCR, HPV-16. The HPV DNA prevalence was 32.4% among cases and 8.9% among controls. [The crude OR for HPV-16 DNA was 12.8 (95% CI, 4.4–38.8).]

In Japan, Nakazawa et al. (1992) compared 37 cases of CIN III with 69 controls from the outpatient clinic of the department of obstetrics and gynaecology of Osaka University Medical School. The method used to detect HPV was PCR, for types 16 and 18. The HPV DNA prevalence was 27% among cases and 16% among controls. [The crude OR for HPV DNA presence was 1.95 (95% CI, 0.67–5.73)]. The distribution of HPV types in cases was: HPV-16, 24.3%; HPV-18, 2.7%; HPV-16 and -18, 0.0%. The distribution of HPV types in controls was: HPV-16, 8.7%; HPV-18, 5.8%; HPV-16 and -18, 1.4%. [Crude odds ratios for HPV-16, 2.8 (95% CI, 0.8–9.4); for HPV-18, 0.4 (95% CI, 0.02–4.1).]

In London, Bavin et al. (1993) studied 179 women sequentially referred to the Royal Free Hospital Colposcopy Clinic because of a smear suggesting mild dyskaryosis. The method used to detect HPV was PCR and the probe used was type 16. All women were explored with colposcopy and, when required, with biopsy, and a final diagnosis was reached. Of 179 women investigated, 35 were considered CIN III and 54 were considered normal. The HPV-16 DNA prevalence was 74.3% among cases and 63% among controls. [The crude OR for HPV-16 DNA presence was 1.7 (95% CI, 0.61–4.84)].

In Barcelona (Spain), Margall et al. (1993) compared 66 women who had had either abnormal Papanicolaou smears or abnormal biopsies (14 chronic inflammatory lesions, 5 cervical condylomata, 24 CIN I, 12 CIN II, 10 CIN III and 1 invasive carcinoma) with 64 controls with normal Papanicolaou tests. The method used to detect HPV was PCR, testing HPV-16 and -18 in the biopsies and cervical scrapes. The HPV-16 and/or -18 DNA prevalence in biopsies among cases was: chronic inflammatory lesions, 43%; cervical condyloma, 80%; CIN I, 50%; CIN II, 50%; CIN III, 70%; and invasive carcinoma, 0%; that in cervical scrapes was: chronic inflammatory lesions, 0%; cervical condyloma, 20%; CIN I, 16.6%; CIN II, 16.6%; CIN III, 20%; and invasive carcinoma, 0%. The HPV-16 prevalence in cervical scrapes among controls was 11%. The crude OR for HPV DNA presence in cervical scrapes for CIN I–III was [1.7 (95% CI, 0.5–5.8)]. This study showed that among cases, the observed HPV DNA prevalence varies according to the sampling method. PCR performed on biopsies yielded systematically higher positivity rates than PCR performed on cytological specimens (see Table 36). Comparing the HPV DNA prevalence rates in cytological specimens from cases and controls, there is no significant association between HPV and CIN. [Using the HPV results obtained using the biopsies in cases and the cytology among controls, the estimated OR for CIN I–III was [9.7 (95% CI, 3.3–29.2)].]

Becker et al. (1994), in a study described on p. 153, analysed 201 high-grade dysplasia patients and 337 controls. Using PCR and common primers, HPV prevalences were 93.8% in cases and 42.1% in controls (OR, 20.8 (95% CI, 10.8–40.2)).

In the United Kingdom, Cuzick et al. (1995) compared the use of cytology and HPV testing for the detection of cervical abnormalities in 1985 women undergoing routine screening. Semiquantitative PCR was used to detect HPV-16, -18, -31 and -33 and only 'high-level' infections were called positive. Women who were either HPV-positive or who had some degree of dyskaryosis on cytology were referred for colposcopy. Of 81 women found to have CIN II–III on colposcopy, 61 (75%) were HPV-positive in comparison with 85 of 1904 (4.5%) women with negative cytology or biopsies showing CIN I or less (control group) [OR, 65 (95% CI, 38–113)]. HPV-16, -18, -31 and -33 were found in 44%, 6%, 25% and 9%, respectively, of women with CIN

II–III and in 1.6%, 0.8%, 1.4% and 0.8%, respectively, of control women. Some women were infected with more than one HPV type. In comparison with HPV-negative women, the OR associated with infection with different HPV types were [50 (95% CI, 28–88)] for HPV-16, [13 (95% CI, 5.4–31)] for HPV-18, [24 (95% CI, 13–45)] for HPV-31 and [12 (95% CI, 4.7–30)] for HPV-33.

In Taiwan, Liaw et al. (1995) conducted a study including 88 patients with biopsy-confirmed CIN I–III and invasive cervical cancer (three cases). PCR was used to detect HPV DNA. The prevalence of HPV DNA was 92% among high-grade cases (CIN II–III, invasive cervical cancer) and 9% among controls (OR, 122.3 (95% CI, 38.5–388.9)). The viral types identified differed between high-grade cases (HPV-16 was predominant) and low-grade CIN and controls (HPV-52 and -58 were predominant).

Strickler et al. (1995) investigated a series of cases in Kingston, Jamaica, an area where human T-cell lymphotropic virus type 1 (HTLV-1) is prevalent. The HPV DNA prevalence, as assessed by PCR was as follows: benign (n = 40), 25.7%; ASCUS (atypical squamous cells of unknown significance) (n = 11), 50.0%; koilocytosis atypia/CIN I (n = 60), 49.2%; CIN II (n = 29), 63.0%; and CIN III/carcinoma (n = 49), 92.1%. The trend in HPV prevalence increased significantly with severity of the lesion ($p < 0.001$). The study also identified HTLV-1 seroprevalence as an independent risk factor for cervical cancer (OR, 3.82 (95% CI, 1.03–14.2)).

In Belgium, Vandenvelde and Van Beers (1993) used a PCR system to screen 71 dysplastic or neoplastic specimens and 323 normal specimens. HPV-33 was found to be highly prevalent in this population and HPV-16 and -18 were the types more strongly related to advanced CIN.

Table 37 summarizes the results of case–control studies that investigated preinvasive lesions (CIN I–III) using serological assays. In aggregate, the studies demonstrate that even relatively minor cervical abnormalities elicit a systemic immune response. Antigen choice was observed to influence greatly the epidemiological associations, suggesting that various stages of HPV natural history may be marked by different immune responses.

Serum IgA antibodies to a carboxyl-terminal 19mer peptide of the HPV-16 E2 protein was present in 20/30 CIN patients but only in 6/27 controls without CIN (Dillner et al., 1989a).

Local IgA antibodies to BPV virions were detected more frequently in cervical secretions of 18 women presenting with an abnormal smear (with or without CIN) than in 24 controls ($p < 0.005$) (Dillner et al., 1989b). Baird (1983) described an increased prevalence of serum IgG antibodies to disrupted BPV virions in sera of patients with CIN and cervical cancer (included in Table 37). This result was not confirmed in a subsequent study (Dillner et al., 1990b), but an increase in serum IgA antibodies to disrupted BPV virions was found by these investigators.

Cason et al. (1992) investigated sera of 52 patients with CIN and of 21 children by ELISA using an HPV-16 L1-specific peptide (aa 473–492). Ninety-one percent of the 23 patients with HPV-16 DNA-positive CIN compared to only 66% of 29 HPV-16 DNA-negative patients ($p < 0.05$) and only 24% of the 21 children ($p < 0.001$) had measurable IgG antibodies.

Strickler et al. (1994) compared 21 women with incident SIL (16 koilocytotic atypia, 3 CIN I and 2 CIN III) to 56 matched controls with regard to HPV seropositivity using a panel of synthetic peptides. Many of the cases had only very slight cytological abnormalities (koilocytotic atypia), yet an elevated percentage (86%) of case sera was seroreactive to HPV-16 for IgG and/or IgA

Table 37. Case–control studies of preinvasive CIN lesions using serological assays for HPV antigens

Reference and country	Cases (number and type)	Controls (number and type)	HPV serological prevalence (%)	Odds ratio (95 % CI)	Serological tests/comments/adjustments
Dillner et al. (1989a) USA	30 CIN	27 without CIN	Case, 66.7 Control, 22.2	[6.7 (1.9–27.5)]	Serum IgA antibodies to a HPV-16 E2 peptide
Dillner et al. (1989b) Sweden	18 abnormal smears, with or without CIN	24 normal smears	Case, 61 Control, 25	[4.5 (1.1–21.9)]	Local IgA antibodies to BPV virions
Cason et al. (1992) United Kingdom	23 HPV-16 DNA positive CIN	29 HPV-16 DNA negative CIN	Case, 91 Control: Adult, 66 Child, 24	[5.4 (1.0–56.5)]	ELISA, using HPV-16 L1-special peptide
Stricker et al. (1994) USA	21 SIL	56 matched	Case, 86 Control, 54	HPV-16 5.76 (1.24–26.8)	
Wideroff et al. (1995) USA	152 pathologically confirmed squamous intraepithelial lesions: 76 low-grade 21 high-grade 55 ASCUS	688 normal cytology	Case: Low-grade, 34.2 High-grade, 52.4 ASCUS, 14.5 Control, 16.1	[2.7 (1.5–4.6)] [5.7 (2.1–15.4)] [0.9 (0.4–2.0)]	Serum IgG antibodies to HPV-16 virus-like particles

[ ] Calculated by the Working Group
CIN, cervical intraepithelial neoplasia; ASCUS, atypical squamous cells of undetermined significance; SIL, squamous intraepithelial lesion

(adjusted OR, 5.76 (95% CI, 1.24–26.8)). In contrast, seroreactivity to HPV-6 was negatively associated with risk of incident SIL (OR, 0.13 (95% CI, 0.02–0.77)) for IgG.

Wideroff et al. (1995) used an enzyme-linked immunosorbent assay to detect serum IgG antibody response to HPV-16 virus-like particles in a nested case–control study of cervical neoplasia. One hundred-and-fifty-two cases with pathologically confirmed squamous intra-epithelial lesions and 688 controls with normal cytology were tested. Of cases with low-grade and high-grade lesions, 34.2% and 52.4% were seropositive, respectively, compared to 16.1% of the controls. However, in multivariate analyses, seropositivity was associated more with HPV-16 DNA status (especially HPV-16 DNA persistence) than with pathology grade *per se*.

(b) HPV and invasive cancer of the uterine cervix

Table 38 summarizes the findings of five studies that investigated the association of HPV infections with invasive cervical cancer using non-hybridization methods.

A study from Detroit, MI, USA, described in detail on p. 142, used morphology to assess HPV exposure and included women undergoing hysterectomy for cervical cancer (40 cases) or for other reasons and who showed a normal cervix (40 controls). Using the women who clearly presented HPV signs as exposed and comparing them to women who were negative or suspect, [the OR was 107 (95% CI, 17.6–877)] (Reid et al., 1982).

One study used history of genital warts and number of episodes of genital warts as a surrogate measure of exposure to HPV. The study found an excess risk for two or more episodes of warts and a trend with increasing number of episodes (Peters et al., 1986). [The Working Group noted that genital warts is likely to be a surrogate of HPV-6/11 infection.]

Su (1987) used peroxidase–antiperoxidase staining and found no association of HPV signs with invasive cancer.

In a study from Thailand, described p. 146, 417 cases of cervical carcinoma were identified of which 19 showed HPV signs (4.6%). Among 22 691 controls, the prevalence was 1.2% [OR, 3.9 (95% CI, 2.3–6.4)] (Thanapatra et al., 1992).

In a study from India (Thankamani et al. (1992a), using indirect immunofluorescence staining, HPV DNA was found in 41% of invasive cervical carcinomas compared to none in oral cancers.

Table 39 summarizes studies that used hybridization methods without amplification procedures to assess exposure to HPV. Most are listed below.

McCance et al. (1985) investigated, in London, UK, the prevalence of HPV-16 among 13 cases of invasive carcinoma with DNA hybridization with HPV probes 6 and 16. These were compared to 17 controls. HPV-16 positivity was 18% among controls and 92% among cases [OR, 45.2 (95% CI, 4.3–2555.9)].

Lörincz et al. (1987) examined 190 biopsies with southern hybridization for HPV-6/11, -18, -31 and others. Cases of CIN I–III were HPV positive in 77% of instances, invasive cervical cancer biopsies in 89% and controls in 9% [OR for CIN I–III, 35.0 (95% CI, 6.9–239.9); OR for invasive cervical cancer, ∞ (95% CI, 5.9–∞)]. The study noted the predominance of HPV-18 in cervical adenocarcinomas and suggested that HPV-16 was more common in specimens from Brazil and Peru than in specimens from the USA.

Table 38. Case–control studies of invasive cervical cancer using HPV non-hybridization assays

Reference and study area	Cases (number and type)	Controls (number and type)	HPV prevalence (%)	Odds ratio (95 % CI)	HPV test/comments/adjustments.
Reid et al. (1982) Detroit, MI, USA	40 ICC All women with hysterectomy	40 age-, race- and SES-matched women with hysterectomy and no cervical pathology	*Negative* Case, 0 Control, 70.0 *Suspect* Case, 5.0 Control, 15.0 *Infected* Case, 95.0 Control, 15.0	[107 (17.6–877)]	Criteria for seven histological parameters scored in 3 levels: negative, suspect and infected
Peters et al. (1986) USA	200 population-based registry ICC	200 matched neighbourhood controls	*One episode* Case, 5.5 Control, 2.5 *More than one episode* Case, 4.5 Control, 1.0	2.5 (0.8–7.3) 5.0 (1.1–23.5)	Self-reported genital warts. Adjusted odds ratios (genital warts)
Su (1987) China	30 ICC 22 ICC with condyloma	20 of unknown origin	ICC, 0 ICC + condyloma, 27 Control, 0		Peroxidase. Paraffin blocks (n = 244) classified by diagnosis
Thanapatra et al. (1992) Thailand	417 ICC	22 691 specimens with no CIN or carcinoma	Case, 4.6 Control, 1.2	[3.9 (2.3–6.4)]	Koilocytosis, atypia. Description of HPV signs in all smears (first visit and follow-up) attending a national screening program for a period of 1 year
Thankamani et al. (1992a) India	64 ICC 10 oral cancers	5 normal cervices	Normal, 0 ICC, 41 Oral cancer, 0	[∞ (0.6–∞)]	Indirect immunofluorescence staining and peroxide antiperoxidase

[ ] Calculated by the Working Group
ICC, invasive cervical cancer; SES, socioeconomic status

Table 39. Case–control studies of invasive cervical cancer using HPV hybridization assays without amplification

Reference and study area	Cases (number and type)	Controls (number and type)	HPV prevalence (%)	Odds ratio (95 % CI)	HPV test	Comments/adjustments
McCance et al. (1985) London, United Kingdom	13 ICC	17 with no cervical abnormality	HPV-16 ICC, 92 Control, 18	[45.2 (4.3–2555.9)]	DNA hybridization Probes: 6, 16 and low stringency	
Kulski et al. (1987) Australia	54 ICC (45 SCC) 11 CIN I–II CIN III	5 biopsies from healthy women	CIN, 74 ICC, 73 HPV-16, 65 HPV-18, 7 Control, 0	[∞ (1.9–∞)] [∞ (3.0–∞)] [∞ (1.5–∞)] [∞ (0.1–∞)]	Southern blot 11, 16, 18	Cross-sectional; 82 biopsies classified by diagnosis
Lörincz et al. (1987) USA, Brazil, Peru	78 CIN I–III 64 SCC	23 biopsies	CIN I–III, 77 SCC, 89 Control, 9	[35.0 (6.9–239.9)] [∞ (5.9–∞)]	Southern hybridization 6/11, 18, 31, others	Study in biopsies for the USA, Peru and Brazil
Meanwell et al. (1987) United Kingdom	47 ICC	26 benign gynaecologically	ICC, 66 Control, 35	HPV-16 [3.7 (1.3–10.0)]	Southern hybridization	Also risk factors but no adjustment
Schneider et al. (1987b) Germany	73 ICC 47 CIN	442 hysterectomies	ICC, 26 CIN, 45 Control, 14	HPV, [2.2 (1.2–3.9)] HPV-16/18, [2.8 (1.4–5.5)]	Filter in-situ hybridization 16, 18, 6/11	Hysterectomy cases classified by reason: cancer/benign
Zhang et al. (1987) China	29 ICC 2 dysplasias	9	Cases HPV-16, 52 HPV-18, 9 Controls HPV-16, 11	HPV, [13.1 (1.4–119)] HPV-16, [8.2 (0.9–405.3)]	Hybridization 16, 18	Cross-sectional; biopsy specimens
Choo et al., 1988 Taiwan, China	31 ICC (biopsy) 7 ICC (cytology)	190 (cytology)	ICC (biopsy) HPV-16, 51 HPV-18, 5 HPV-31, 0 HPV-33, 3 ICC (cytology) HPV-16, 43 Controls HPV-16, 2.6	HPV, [28 (5–158)] HPV-16, [39 (13–123)]	Southern blot 16, 18, 31, 33	Controls not comparable to cases. Different series with only 7 ICC cases. No real case–control
Fuchs et al. (1988) Austria	216 CIN I–III 44 ICC	31 hospital controls	CIN I–III, 50.0 ICC, 68.2 Control, 3.2	[30.0 (4.3–601.9)] [37.7 (5.3–1673.1)]	Southern hybridization	
Hsieh et al. (1988) China	77 ICC	16 other tissues, including normal cervix	ICC, 63.6 Control, 6.3	HPV, [∞ (2.9–∞)]	Southern hybridization	

Table 39 (contd)

Reference and study area	Cases (number and type)	Controls (number and type)	HPV prevalence (%)	Odds ratio (95 % CI)	HPV test	Comments/adjustments
Wilczynski et al. (1988a) USA	11 adenocarcinomas	11 other cancers 6 hysterectomies	ICC HPV-16, 18.2 HPV-18, 45.5 Control, 0	[∞ (0.3–∞)] [∞ (1.9–∞)]	Southern blot 16, 18, 31, 6/11	Adenocarcinomas only
Zhang et al. (1988) Australia	24 ICC 15 CIN III 20 CIN I–II	33 with non-cancer gynaecological problems	ICC, 96 CIN III, 80 CIN I–II, 65 Control, 9	HPV. [230 (22–2359)]	Dot hybridization/ Southern blot 6/11, 16/18	Cross-sectional study in gynaecologic clinic. Data from biopsy tabulated. Also good correlation with scrapes
Colgan et al. (1989) Canada	7 ICC 30 CIN/condylomata	12 hysterectomies	CIN, 60 ICC, 57 Control, 0	[∞ (1.5–∞)]	Southern blot HPV-16 /31	Cross-sectional; only biopsy
Czeglédy et al. (1989) Hungary	41 ICC 12 CIN III 7 CIN I–II 3 vaginal cancers 18 condylomata	22 scrapes	ICC, 60 HPV-16, 46 HPV-18, 15 CIN III, 66 CIN I–II, 43 Control, 14	[9.9 (2.5–39.0)] [40.1 (4.3–937)] [∞ (0.7–∞)] [12.7(2.3–70)] [11.1 (2.0–6.2)]	Southern blot/dot blot/filter in-situ hybridization 4, 11, 16, 18	Cross-sectional: 336 samples tested, 22 of them were normal
Donnan et al. (1989) China	68 ICC 48 dysplasias HPV: subsample of 58	116 hospital: surgical and gynaecological outpatient controls matched by age. 17 controls for HPV, different from previous ones	ICC, 11/30, 37 Dysplasia, 5/28, 18 Controls, 1/17, 6	HPV-16 ICC: 9.3 (1.0–84.1) Dysplasia: 3.5 (0.3–118)	Filter in-situ hybridization	HPV determined only in subsample
Reeves et al. (1989) Panama, Costa Rica, Colombia, and Mexico	759 hospital-based cases	1467 (age-matched) community and hospital controls	HPV Case, 67.1 Control, 35.4 HPV-16/18 Case, 62 Control, 32 HPV-6/11 Case, 17 Control, 7	HPV [3.7 (3.0–4.5)] HPV-16/18 signal +/–: 2.1 (1.6–2.8) 1+: 4.1 (3.2–5.4) 2–4+: 9.1 (6.1–13.6) HPV-6/11 signal +/–: 2.2 (1.5–3.1) 1+: 4.6 (2.6–8.2) 2–4+: 3.9 (0.8–17.9)	Filter in-situ hybridization, 6/11, 16/18	Adjusted for age, number of sexual partners, age at first sexual intercourse, number of live births, interval since last Pap, years of education
Chang et al. (1990c) China	5 condylomata acuminata 21 SCC	11 normal	Normal, 0 Condylomata acuminata, 100 SCC, 57.1	[∞ (5.6–∞)] [∞ (2.4–∞)]	DNA in-situ hybridization, 6, 11, 16 and 18	Series of genital biopsies from pathology departments

Table 39 (contd)

Reference and study area	Cases (number and type)	Controls (number and type)	HPV prevalence (%)	Odds ratio (95 % CI)	HPV test	Comments/adjustments
Yokota et al. (1990) Japan	31 ICC	666 with normal cervices from outpatient clinics and screening centers	*Cases* HPV-16, 39 HPV-18, 10 HPV-6/11, 3 *Controls* HPV-16, 2 HPV-18, 1 HPV-6/11, 1	HPV, [31.2 (13.7–71.1)] HPV-16, [34.4 (13.7–86.4)] HPV-18, [32.2 (5.2–193.6)]	Filter in-situ hybridization 6/11, 16, 18	Outpatients
Zhang (1990) China	116 ICC	36	ICC, 51 Control, 6	HPV, [17.6 (5.2–53.7)] HPV-16, [∞ (5.1–∞)]	Southern blot 16, 33, 31	Cross-sectional
Hildesheim et al. (1991) Latin-America	766 ICC	1532 hospital and community controls		HPV-16/18, 4.3 (3.0–6.0) HPV-16/18+HSV, 8.8 (5.9–13.0)	Filter in-situ hybridization 6/11, 16/18	Same study as Reeves et al. (1989). This analysis focuses on the interaction HSV/HPV.
Ohta et al. (1991) Japan	24 ICC 62 Pap IIIa 56 Pap III 29 Pap IIIb 8 CIS	124 (Pap I–II)	ICC, 65 Pap II, 50 Pap I–II, 6	HPV, [72.1 (14–361)]	ViraPap™ ViraType™	
Si et al. (1991) China	318 ICC 14 CIN 48 condylomata 34 cervicitis	24 normal biopsies	ICC, 60 CIN, 50 Condylomata, 28 Cervicitis, 20 Control, 8.3	HPV, [22 (5.0–95.4)] HPV-16, [16.1 (3.9–149.8)] HPV-18, [∞ (0.2–∞)]	Dot blot/Southern blot 16, 11	Cross-sectional
Wei et al. (1991) China	169 for HPV 34 CIS 10 ICC 8 CIN I 6 CIN II 5 CIN III	77 cervicitis 2 cervical polyps	ICC, 40 CIS, 71 CIN III, 40 CIN II, 33 CIN I, 25 Control, 36.7	[1.23 (0.3–4.8)] [4.44 (1.9–10.7)]	Dot blot 6b, 11, 16, 18	Survey of 6710 women. Biopsy of those with abnormalities. HPV in biopsies
Kadish et al. (1992) USA	63 LSIL 126 HSIL/ICC	122 controls	LSIL, 92.1 HSIL/ICC, 66.7 Control, 40	[17.3 (6.1–52.9)] [3.0 (1.7–5.2)]	Southern	
Kanetsky et al. (1992) New York, USA	4 ICC 1 CIS 1 CIN I	272 (226 tested for HPV)	Case, 33 Control, 2.7	HPV, 18.3 (1.9–121)	ViraPap™ 6/11, 16/18, 31/33/35	278 black/elderly women attending screening program. Also questionnaire for risk factors

Table 39 (contd)

Reference and study area	Cases (number and type)	Controls (number and type)	HPV prevalence (%)	Odds ratio (95 % CI)	HPV test	Comments/adjustments
Lörincz et al. (1992) USA	153 ICC	1566 normal cervices	Control, 6.4 Case, 89.5 HPV-16, 52.6 HPV-18, 26.3	HPV-16, 260.0 (216.9–311.9) HPV-18, –45, –56, 296.1 (198.9–441.1)	Southern hybridization	Pooled analysis and HPV testing of subjects from 8 studies. No adjustments, crude odds ratios
Mandelblatt et al. (1992) New York, USA	6 (4 ICC, 2 CIN)	226	Case, 33.3 Control, 2.7	[12.2 (1.2–122.9)]	Dot blot	Women aged 65 or more
Saito et al. (1992) Japan	20 CIN I–III 22 ICC	599 hospital	CIN I–III, 45 ICC, 68.2 Control, 4.2	[180 (6.2–52.3)] [47.2 (16.3–141.7)]	Dot blot	
Thankamani et al. (1992b) India	102 ICC	12 hysterectomies	HPV-11, 36 Control, 0 HSV, 53	[10 000 (1.5–10 000)]	Hybridization 11, (HSV-2)	HPV-11 only. Also HSV-2
Marin et al. (1994) Slovenia	60 SCC 6 adenocarcinomas	42 normal	Adenocarcinoma HPV-16, –18 33.3 33.3 SCC 43.3 7.0 Control 11.9 4.8	HPV-16 [3.7 (0.4–36.0)] [5.7 (1.8–19.1)]	In-situ hybridization	

[ ] Calculated by the Working Group
SCC, squamous-cell carcinoma; ICC, invasive cervical carcinoma; CIN, cervical intraepithelial neoplasia; LSIL, low grade squamous intraepithelial lesion; HSIL, high grade squamous intraepithelial lesion; Pap, Papanicolaou smear; HSV, herpes simplex virus

Schneider *et al.* (1987b) studied HPV in Germany by filter in-situ hybridization methods with probes for HPV-6/11, -16 and -18 in 616 women with a history of hysterectomy. HPV was present in 33% of 120 women with cervical neoplasia and in 14% of 442 women with benign disease. [The OR was 2.2 (95% CI, 1.2–3.9) for any HPV and 2.8 (95% CI, 1.4–5.5) for HPV-16/18.]

Choo *et al.* (1988), in Taiwan, used dot blot and Southern blot hybridization to search for HPV-16, -18, -31 and -33 in 31 cases of invasive cervical carcinoma and 190 cytologically healthy women (viral DNA was studied in cervical swabs). The prevalences of HPV-16 were 51% among carcinoma cases and 2.6% among controls [OR, 39 (95% CI, 13–123)].

In Austria, Czerwenka *et al.* (1989) examined a series of cytology specimens with southern blot, dot blot and in-situ hybridization. Specimens classified as normal or Pap II were HPV positive by Southern blot in 27/166 (16.3%) whereas smears that were Pap III-IV were HPV positive in 55/77 (74%) [OR, 14.7 (95% CI, 7.3–29.9)].

In a study from Hong Kong, Donnan *et al.* (1989) assessed prevalence of HPV-16 by Southern blot in 30 invasive cervical cancer cases and 17 gynaecological controls. A total of 11 cases and one control were positive (OR, 9.3 (95% CI, 1.0–84.1)).

Reeves *et al.* (1989) conducted a population-based case–control study in Panama, Costa Rica, Colombia and Mexico including 759 cases and 1467 age-matched, randomly selected controls. HPV DNA was determined by filter in-situ hybridization with probes for HPV-16/18 and -6/11. Known and suspected risk factors for cervical cancer were assessed via direct interview. Prevalences for any HPV were 67.1% for cases and 35.4% for controls; those for HPV-16/18 were 62% for cases and 32% for controls; and those for HPV-6/11 were 17% for cases and 7% for controls. Relative risks for cancer, adjusted for age, number of sexual partners, age at first sexual intercourse, number of live births, interval since last Pap smear and years of education were: for any HPV, [3.7 (95% CI, 3.0–4.5)]; for HPV-16/18 signal +/–, 2.1 (95% CI, 1.6–2.8); signal 1+, 4.1 (95% CI, 3.2–5.4); signal 2–4+, 9.1 (95% CI, 6.1–13.6); for HPV-6/11 signal +/–, 2.2 (95% CI, 1.5–3.1); signal 1+, 4.6 (95% CI, 2.6–8.2); signal 2–4+, 3.9 (95% CI, 0.8–17.9). [Several publications based on the same study provided slightly different risk estimates (Reeves *et al.*, 1987; Brenes *et al.*, 1987; Reeves *et al.*, 1989; Herrero *et al.*, 1990; Hildesheim *et al.*, 1991; Herrero *et al.*, 1992)].

Yokota *et al.* (1990) studied HPV infection in women from Tokyo, Japan, attending out-patient gynaecology clinics and screening centres. Filter in-situ hybridization methods were employed with probes for HPV-6/11, -16 and -18. In 31 invasive cervical cancer cases, the prevalences were 3%, 39% and 10% and in 666 control women without cervical pathology were 1%, 2% and 1%. For invasive cervical cancer cases, the ORs were [31.2 (95% CI, 13.7–71.1)] for any type of HPV, [3.7 (95% CI, 0.4–31)] for HPV-6/11, [34.4 (13.7–86.4)] for HPV-16, and [32.2 (95% CI, 5.2–193.6)] for HPV-18.

Kadish *et al.* (1992) in the USA used cervicovaginal lavage and Southern hybridization to investigate 329 women attending a colposcopy clinic. The HPV DNA prevalence was 49/122 (40.2%) among controls and 142/189 (75.1%) of patients with SIL or cancer [OR, 4.5 (95% CI, 2.7–7.6)]. Among patients with LSIL, 58/63 (92.1%) were HPV positive [OR, 17.3 (95% CI, 6.1–52.9)]. Of the patients with HSIL or cancer, 84/126 (66.7%) were HPV positive [OR, 3.0 (95% CI, 1.7–5.2)].

Lörincz et al. (1992) reported on a pooled analysis of subjects included in eight studies that were investigated using Southern blot, including the aforementioned Lörincz et al. (1987). A total of 153 cases of invasive carcinoma were compared to 1566 controls with normal cervices. The prevalence of HPV in controls was 6.4%. The prevalence among cases was 89.5%, of which 52.6% was HPV-16 and 26.3% HPV-18. The type specific ORs were 260.0 (95% CI, 216.9–311.9) for HPV-16, 296.1 (95% CI, 198.9–441.1) for HPV-18, -45 or -56, and 31.1 (95% CI, 18.7–51.8) for HPV-31, -33, -35, -51 and -52.

Mandelblatt et al. (1992) investigated HPV DNA by dot blot in six cases of cervical neoplasia and 226 controls aged 65–96 years from New York, USA. HPV DNA was detected in two cases and six controls [OR, 17.6 (95% CI, 1.4–155.0)].

Saito et al. (1992) assessed HPV DNA by dot blot in 22 invasive cervical cancer cases and 599 cytologically normal women from Osaka, Japan. The prevalence of infection was 68.2% in cases and 4.2% in controls [odds ratio, 47.3 (95% CI, 16.3–142)].

Monsonego et al. (1993) studied a series of patients from Paris, France, with squamous genital cancer of the cervix (15), vagina (3), vulva (3) and anus (2). The study also included 48 specimens from the same locations without abnormal cytological features that served as controls. Blot hybridization was used to detect and type HPV DNA. The prevalence of all types of HPV among controls was 26/48 (54.2%). Among squamous genital cancer cases the HPV DNA prevalence was 19/23 (82.6%) [OR, 4.0 (95% CI, 1.1–16.5)]. The study also included the male partners of cases and controls. The HPV DNA prevalences in the lesions sampled were 6/16 (37%) in spouses of squamous cancer patients and 18/43 (42%) in spouses of negative controls.

Marin et al. (1994) investigated 66 invasive cancers and 42 hospital controls from Ljubljana, Slovenia, using in-situ hybridization. Among controls, the prevalence rate of HPV-16 was 11.9% and that of HPV-18 was 4.8%. The HPV prevalence in 60 squamous-cell carcinomas was 43.3% for HPV-16 and 7.0% for HPV-18. In six cases of adenocarcinoma the prevalence of HPV-16 was equal to the prevalence of HPV-18 (33.3%). The estimated odds ratios for HPV-16 were [3.7 (95% CI, 0.4–36.0)] for adenocarcinoma and [5.7 (95% CI, 1.8–19.1)] for squamous-cell carcinoma (see also Table 31).

Table 40 includes the case–control studies that used PCR amplification methods to assess exposure to HPV.

In Spain and Colombia, Muñoz et al. (1992) conducted a population-based case–control study including 436 incident cases of squamous-cell invasive cervical cancer and 387 population controls. Specimens tested with PCR were 229/436 (53%) of the cases and 228/387 (60%) of the controls. HPV detection was carried out using PCR methods based on the $L1$ region consensus primers. Hybridization was performed sequentially with probes to HPV-6, -11, -16, -18, -31, -33, -35 under high-stringency conditions. Subsequently, the filters were screened with a generic probe containing a mixture of amplifiers of HPV-16 and -18 (Bauer et al., 1991). The ORs for HPV DNA were 46.2 (95% CI, 18.5–115.1) in Spain and 15.6 (95% CI, 6.9–34.7) in Colombia. The attributable fraction derived from this study indicated that 67.5% of cases in Spain and 66.0% in Colombia could be attributed to HPV. Odds ratios were also calculated by type specific HPVs for Spain and Colombia combined, as follows: HPV-16 (29.7 (95% CI, 14.5–57.4)), HPV-18 (19.4 (95% CI, 4.0–93.7)), HPV-31, -33, -35 [21.4 (95% CI, 6.1–75.6)] and

Table 40. Case–control studies of invasive cervical cancer using HPV hybridization assays including amplification (PCR) methods

Reference and country	Cases (number and type)	Controls (number and type)	HPV prevalence (%) Type	Cases	Controls	Odds ratio (95 % CI)	HPV test/comments/adjustments
Muñoz et al. (1992) Spain	250 incident cases	238 population-based controls	All	69.0	4.6	46.2 (18.5–115.1)	PCR. Adjusted for age, study area, number of sexual partners, education, age at first birth and history of a prior Pap smear
Cali, Colombia	186 incident cases	149 population-based controls	All	72.4	73.3	15.6 (6.9–34.7) Spain and Colombia, combined HPV-16, 29.7 (14.5–57.4) HPV-18, 19.4 (4.0–93.7) HPV-31, -33, -35, 21.4 (6.1–75.6) HPV unidentified, 79.6 (11.1–572.4)	
Eluf-Neto (1994) Brazil	199 hospital-based cases	225 hospital-based controls	Any 16 18 31/33 16/18/31/33 Undefined	84 54 9 3 66 19	17 5 1 0 6 10	37.1 (19.6–70.4) 74.9 (32.5–173) 56.9 (11.7–276) 75.1 (34.2–165) 13.8 (6.4–29.6)	PCR. Odds ratios adjusted for age, socioeconomic status, number of Pap smears, parity, number of sexual partners, age at first sexual intercourse and duration of oral contraceptive use
Peng et al. (1991) China	101 hospital-based cases	146 gynaecological clinic-based controls	16 33 16/33	31.7 3.0 34.7	1.4 0 1.4	32.9 (7.7–141.1)	PCR. Adjusted for age, income, residence, age at first marriage and cigarette smoking
ter Meulen et al. (1992) Tanzania	50 cervical carcinomas (hospital-based) 3 vaginal carcinomas	359 non-cancer gynaecological patients	Any 16 18 45 Other	89 38 32 6 13	59	[1.6 (0.8–3.2)] [6.6 (2.9–15.4)] [4.2 (1.8–9.9)]	Southern blot and/or PCR

Table 40 (contd)

Reference and country	Cases (number and type)	Controls (number and type)	HPV prevalence (%) Type	HPV prevalence (%) Cases	HPV prevalence (%) Controls	Odds ratio (95 % CI)	HPV test/comments/adjustments
Das et al. (1992a) India	96 hospital-based cases	22 asymptomatic normal women	Any 16 18	98 64 3	18 18 0	[211.5 (30.1–2048)]	Southern blot and/or PCR
Shen et al. (1993) Taiwan, China	78 cervical cancers	55 uterine leiomyomas		66.7	5.5	HPV, [33.6 (9.5–184.2)] HPV + CMV, [∞ (13.6–∞)]	PCR. Results show a strong interaction between HPV and CMV.
Asato et al. (1994) Japan	52 cervical cancers	2873 Pap I–II		88.5	9.5	[72.5 (30.5–209.6)]	PCR, $L1$ consensus primers
Griffin et al. (1990) United Kingdom	19 squamous-cell carcinomas	10 normal	Any	84.2	60	[3.6 (0.5–31.0)]	PCR. HPV tested in paraffin wax-embedded material
Arends et al. (1993) United Kingdom	47 cervical cancers	24 normal	16/18	79	0	[∞ (17.2–∞)]	PCR

[ ] Calculated by the Working Group
CMV, cytomegalovirus; PCR, polymerase chain reaction; Pap, Papanicolaou smear

unidentified HPV-types [79.6 (95% CI, 11.1–572.4)]. An additional analysis stratified by HPV status was performed. This analysis showed that, among HPV-negative cases, the risk factors identified were related to sexual behaviour. However, among HPV-positive cases and controls, the only significant differences were the use and the duration of use of oral contraceptives (Bosch et al., 1992).

Of the subjects included in these studies, 823 cervical specimens were also tested by ViraPap™. In Spain, 250 cases and 238 controls were investigated. The HPV DNA prevalence was 41% among cases and 2.5% among controls (OR, 29.1 (95% CI, 10.3–81.9)). In Colombia, 186 cases and 149 controls were investigated. The HPV DNA prevalence was 30.4% for cases and 0.7% among controls (OR, 93.2 (95% CI, 12.6–687.3)). The intensity of the hybridization signal in the ViraPap™ system was quantified into five categories. The corresponding odds ratios were: very weak positive, 1.0; positive (2–3), 8.6 (95% CI, 1.7–42.2); strong positive (4–5), 10.3 (95% CI, 1.7–64.2). Southern hybridization was also used in 617 specimens. In Spain, 184 cases and 158 controls were tested. The HPV DNA prevalence among cases was 36.4% and among controls 5.7% (OR, 8.8 (95% CI, 4.1–19.0)). In Colombia, 132 cases and 143 controls were tested. The HPV DNA prevalence was 25.0% for cases and 4.2% among controls (OR, 9.6 (95% CI, 3.7–25.1)). The results of this study have also been partially reported elsewhere (Muñoz et al., 1994).

Moreno et al. (1995) conducted a statistical analysis of the CIN III and cervical cancer studies in Spain and in Colombia. Risk factors were compared between the two types of cases and between cases and controls to ascertain factors that might favour the progression from CIN III to invasive cancer. Neither entity differed in exposure to HPV, HPV types or estimates of HPV viral load in any significant way.

In São Paulo, Brazil, Eluf-Neto et al. (1994) conducted a hospital-based case–control study including 199 histologically confirmed consecutive cases and 225 controls from a diversity of diagnoses. A PCR system was performed directly on crude cell suspensions by a combination of general primer-mediated and type-specific PCR (GP-PCR/T-PCR). The HPV attributable fraction calculated from this study was 86%. The ORs for type specific HPVs were 74.9 (95% CI, 32.5–173.0) for HPV-16, 56.9 (95% CI, 11.7–276.0) for HPV-18, 75.1 (95% CI, 34.2–165.0) for HPV-16, -18, -31 and -33 and 13.8 (95% CI, 6.4–9.6) for unidentified HPV types. After adjustment, a residual association was found for increasing parity (p for trend = 0.02). A non-statistically significant trend was observed for number of sexual partners and for duration of use of oral contraceptives (Eluf-Neto et al., 1994).

Peng et al. (1991) conducted a case–control study in Sichuan, China, with 101 cases and 146 hospital controls. HPV-16 and -33 were detected by PCR. Prevalences were 31.7% in cases and 1.4% in controls for HPV-16, 3.0% in cases and 0% in controls for HPV-33 and 34.7% in cases and 1.4% in controls for HPV-16/33 with an odds ratio of 32.9 (95% CI, 7.7–141.1) adjusted for age, income, residence, age at first marriage and cigarette smoking. In this study, no association was found between cervical cancer and herpes simplex virus type 2 (OR, 1.3; 95% CI, 0.7–2.3).

ter Meulen et al. (1992) determined HPV by PCR in 50 biopsies of invasive cervical cancer and 359 cervical swabs of noncancer gynaecological patients in Tanzania. Any HPV was found in 59% of controls and 89% of cases. Type-specific prevalences in cases were 38% for HPV-16,

32% for HPV-18, 6% for HPV-45 and 13% for other HPV type. Crude relative risks were: [1.6 (95% CI, 0.8–3.2)] for any HPV, [6.6 (95% CI, 2.9–15.4)] for HPV-16 and [4.2 (95% CI, 1.8–9.9)] for HPV-18. In this study, HIV seroprevalence was also investigated and found to be strongly correlated to HPV prevalence. The controls were HIV-positive in 12.8% of instances. In contrast, among 270 cases of cervical carcinoma, only 3% were HIV-positive. Among controls, the stronger risk factors for HPV positivity was young age and HIV seropositivity. [The Working Group noted the high prevalence of HIV among controls, the young age of controls as compared to cases and the fact that HPV was detected in biopsies among cases and in cervical swabs among controls.]

Das et al. (1992a) reported a series of biopsies from 96 consecutive cases of cervical cancer from India and compared them with 22 biopsies from normal controls attending the same clinic. All specimens were investigated with Southern hybridization, and 91.7% of the cases were found to be HPV-positive. The eight cases that tested HPV negative were further investigated using PCR and six were found to be HPV-positive. HPV-16 accounted for 64% of the HPV types. Four of the 22 controls were HPV-positive using PCR (18%) [OR, 211.5 (95% CI, 30.1–2048)]. [The Working Group noted the lack of systematic investigation of specimens using PCR.]

Shen et al. (1993) conducted a case–control study in Taiwan with 78 invasive cervical cancer cases and 55 controls with uterine leiomyoma. HPV and cytomegalovirus (CMV) infections were determined by PCR. Prevalence of HPV was 66.7% in cases and 5.5% in controls. The odds ratio for any HPV was [33.6 (95% CI, 9.5–184.2)] and a strong interaction with CMV was found giving an infinite odds ratio for HPV plus CMV, based on 40 cases and no controls positive for both.

In a short communication, Asato et al. (1994) reported PCR-*L1* consensus primer-based HPV prevalence rates in 52 cervical cancer cases and 2873 women with Pap I–II cervices from Ryukyus, Japan. A total of 46 cases (88.5%) and 274 (9.5%) controls were positive [crude OR, 72.5 (95% CI, 30.5–209.6)].

Griffin et al. (1990) assessed the prevalence of HPV-6, -11, -16 and -18 using PCR and Southern blot in paraffin-embedded blocks from 19 cases of squamous-cell carcinoma and 10 normal cervices from Leeds, UK. HPV-6/11 was detected in 10 cases and five controls [OR, 1.1 (95% CI, 0.2–5.1)]; HPV-16/18 was detected in 16 cases and five controls [OR, 5.3 (95% CI, 0.9–31)].

Arends et al. (1993) used a type-specific PCR-based assay for HPV-6, -11, -16, -18 and -33 on 47 cervical carcinomas and 24 samples of histologically normal cervices. The incidence of HPV-16 and -18 was 79% in carcinomas and 0% in the normal controls [OR, ∞ (95% CI, 17.2–∞)]. HPV-6 and -11 were not found in cancer cases or controls.

Figures 16 and 17 show the odds ratios and 95% confidence intervals for associations found in case–control studies between HPV-16 (or its nearest surrogate) and risk of invasive cervical cancer. Figures 16 and 17 show data obtained by methods other than PCR and by PCR, respectively.

Table 41 summarizes studies that used serological assays to detect antibodies against HPV proteins. The table includes mainly studies of anogenital cancer. Some published studies have also explored HPV seropositivity in cases of CIN (see above and Table 37) and in skin cancer (Steger *et al.*, 1990). Much additional work is currently underway in this active area.

Figure 16. Odds ratios and 95% confidence intervals for associations found in case–control studies using non-PCR methods between HPV-16 (or its nearest surrogate) and invasive cervical cancers

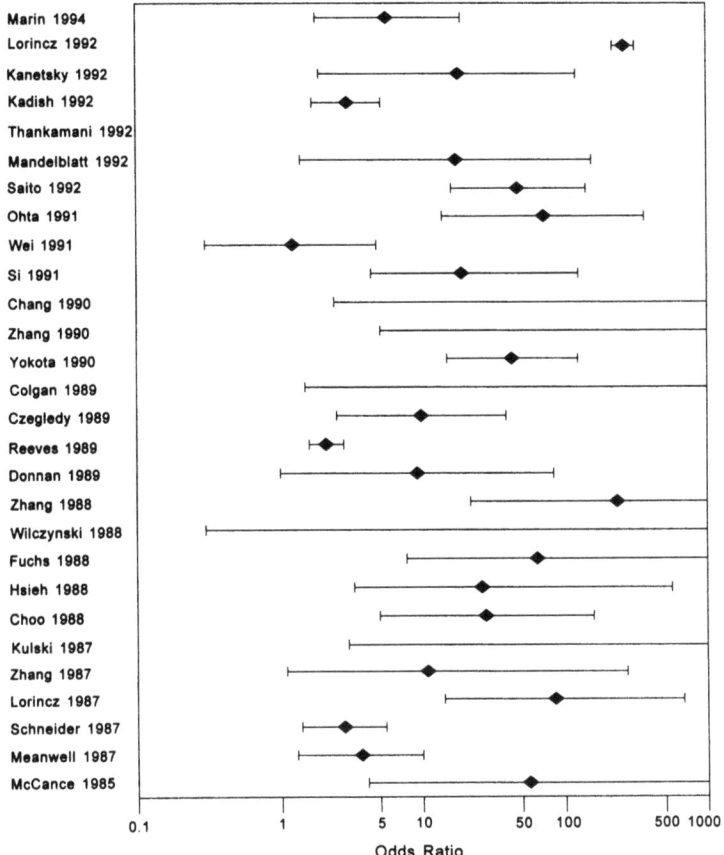

Data are taken from Table 39

Several antibody-detection systems have been used and the majority have been validated against cervical cytological/histological diagnoses and/or HPV DNA in cervical cells. The serological detection rate among HPV DNA-positive cases in the studies reported range between 50 and 70%. Moreover, some of the assays perform differently in cases of invasive cervical cancer (seropositivity rates are higher) than in cases of preinvasive lesions (see also section 1.3.4).

Figure 17. Odds ratios and 95% confidence intervals for associations found in case–control studies using PCR methods between HPV-16 (or its nearest surrogate) and invasive cervical cancers

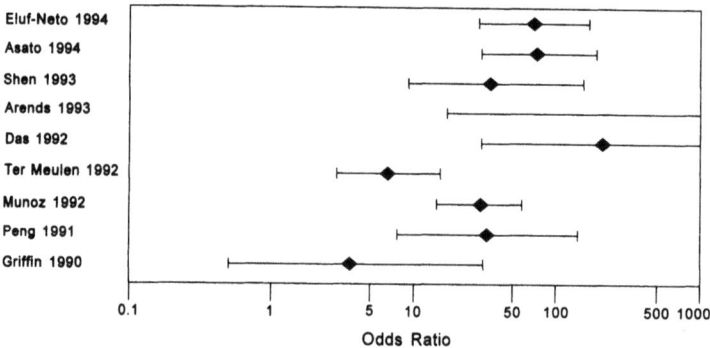

Data are taken from Table 40.

This section focuses on the studies that have reported antibody seroprevalence rates in cases and in a group of non-cervical cancer controls. However, with few exceptions these comparisons rarely comply with the requisites of design and analysis of rigorous epidemiological investigations.

In a study in Australia, Baird (1983) collected sera from 60 cases of anogenital warts, 92 cases of CIN and 46 cases of cervical cancer. The sera was examined for IgG antibodies to a group-specific BPV-2 antigen using a solid-phase enzyme-linked immunosorbent assay, and compared with sera collected from 256 controls (48 children, 108 adults, 60 attendees of STD clinics and 40 non-cervical cancer patients). Prevalences were 10% in controls, 95% in cases of anogenital warts, 60% in CIN cases and 93% in cervical cancer patients. Estimated crude odds ratios were [171 (95% CI, 40.6–845.3)] for anogenital warts, [13.4 (95% CI, 5.8–31.5)] for CIN and [129 (95% CI, 30.3–643.8)] for cervical cancer.

In Germany, Jochmus–Kudielka et al. (1989) collected sera from 46 patients with HPV-associated lesions, 88 patients with cervical cancer and from 385 controls (49 laboratory personnel and 336 patients, both men and women, with no HPV-related infections) and tested them by the Western blot technique for the presence of antibodies to HPV-16 proteins E4 and E7 that had been expressed in *Escherichia coli* as fusion proteins. Prevalences of E4 and E7 were 18% and 4% respectively for control patients with no HPV-related infections, 12% and 2% for control laboratory personnel, 23% and 0% for patients with condyloma acuminata, 43% and 0% for CIN I–II patients, 32% and 16% for CIN III patients and 16% and 20% for cervical cancer patients. Compared to an age-matched selection of controls, the crude ORs for cervical cancer were 2.3 [(95% CI, 0.9–5.6)] for E4 and 18.0 [(95% CI, 3.9–115.7)] for E7. The authors

STUDIES OF CANCER IN HUMANS

Table 41. Case–control studies of CIN, invasive cervical cancer and cancer at other sites using serological assays for HPV antigens

Reference and study	Cases (number and type)	Controls (number and type)	HPV prevalence (%)	Odds ratio (95 % CI)	HPV serology test	Comments/adjustments
Baird (1983) Australia	60 anogenital warts 92 CIN 46 cervical cancers	48 children 108 adults 60 STD clinic 40 non-cervical cancers	Anogenital wart, 95 CIN, 60 Cervical cancer, 93 Control, 10	[171 (40.6–845.3)] [13.4 (5.8–31.5)] [129 (30.3–643.8)]	Solid-phase enzyme-linked immunosorbent assay for an IgG antibody to a group-specific BPV-2 antigens	Odds ratios calculated using STD clinic patients and non-cervical cancer patient as controls
Jochmus-Kudielka et al. (1989) Germany	44 HPV-associated lesions 88 cervical cancers	336 patients with no HPV-related infections 49 laboratory personnel	E4/E7 Control, 18/4 Laboratory personnel, 12/2 Condyloma, 23/0 CIN I–II, 43/0 CIN III, 32/16 Cervical cancer, 16/20	Compared to age-matched controls: Cervical cancer for E4, 2.3 [(0.9–5.6)] ($p = 0.53$) Cervical cancer for E7, 18.0 [(3.9–115.7)]	Western blot HPV-16 ORFs E4 and E7 proteins	Anti-E7 antibodies may represent a marker for cervical development. Anti-E4 antibody may be correlated with virus replication.
Mann et al. (1990) Panama	186 invasive cervical cancers	172 age-matched controls	Cases/controls IgA to E7, 21/9 IgG to E7, 25/6 IgA to 245, 15/11 IgG to 245, 19/11	5.3 (2.4–11.6) 2.7 (1.3–5.3) 1.7 (1.2–3.3) 1.0 (0.4–1.6)	ELISA IgG and IgA antibodies to HPV-16 (E7 peptide and to peptide 245, epitope in E2)	Odds ratios adjusted for cigarette smoking, education, pregnancies, time since last Pap and age at first sexual intercourse. Conclusions: Antibodies to E7 are markers for invasive cervical cancer. Seropositivity correlated poorly with clinical stage, survival, or the presence of HPV-DNA in tumour.
Steger et al. (1990) Germany	54 malignant melanomas 60 basal-cell carcinomas 44 Hodgkin's diseases 11 squamous-cell skin carcinomas 32 cervical cancers	445 randomly selected controls	Malignant melanoma, 28 Basal-cell carcinoma, 40 Hodgkin's disease, 48 Squamous-cell skin carcinoma, 73 Cervical cancer, 37 Control, 20	[1.6 (0.8–3.1)] [2.7 (1.5–4.9)] [3.7 (1.9–7.3)] [10.8 (2.5–52.6)] [2.4 (1.1–5.5)]	HPV-8-specific IgG antibodies to L1 (Western blot analysis with the entire HPV-8 L1 as antigen)	
Bleul et al. (1991) Tanzania and Germany	Invasive squamous-cell cervical carcinomas Tanzania: 116 Germany: 94	Age-matched controls with other gynaecological problems Tanzania: 116 Germany: 94	Tanzania Control, 0; case, 8.6 Germany Control, 0; case, 3.2	[∞ (237–∞)] [∞ (0.4–∞)]	Anti HPV-18 E6 and E7 antibodies ELISA	Analysis with a synthetic 28-mer peptide comprising E7/1 region

Table 41 (contd)

Reference and study	Cases (number and type)	Controls (number and type)	HPV prevalence (%)	Odds ratio (95 % CI)	HPV serology test	Comments/adjustments
Köchel et al. (1991) Germany	46 cervical cancers	31 non-genital cancer patients 41 healthy women	HPV-16/18 E6 & E7 Case, 63 Cancer control, 6.5 Healthy control, 9.8 HPV-16/18 L1 & L2 Case, 54.3 Cancer control, 41.9 Healthy control, 43.9	As compared to healthy controls: HPV-16/18 E6 & E7 [15.8(4.3–63.3)] HPV-16/18 L1 & L2 [1.5 (0.6–3.9)]	Antibodies to HPV-6b, HPV-16 and HPV-18 L1, L2, E4 and E7 Western blot	
Kanda et al. (1992) Japan	12 CIN 108 cervical cancers	140 healthy women	Anti-HPV-16 E1/E4 cases/controls CIN, 0/0 Cancer, 10.2/0 Anti-HPV-16 E7 cases/controls CIN, 0/0 Cancer, 20.4/0	One-tailed p values [< 0.0001] [< 0.0001]	ELISA Western blot HPV-16 E1/E4 and E7	Prevalences available for other cancers: ovarian (n = 28), endometrial (n = 6), choriocarcinoma (n = 3), vulvar (n = 2), VIN (n = 3)
Lehtinen (1992) Finland	Newly diagnosed cervical carcinomas: 42 squamous-cell carcinomas 19 adenocarcinomas	61 age-matched controls	Squamous-cell carcinomas cases/controls HPV-6 E2, 17/5 HPV-16 E2, 43/13 Adenocarcinoma cases/controls HPV-6 E2, 11/11 HPV-16 E2, 42/16 Any cases/controls HPV-6 E2, 15/7 HPV-16 E2, 43/15	IgA HPV-16 E2 peptide 245 Squamous-cell, 13 (2.4–249) Adenocarcinoma, 9 (1.8–194) Any, 9.5 (2.8–57.2) No difference with HPV-6 No differences with IgG	ELISA HPV-16 E2 IgA and IgG antibody levels	Unadjusted odds ratios
Mandelson et al. (1992) USA	69 invasive cervical cancers	81 controls	HPV-16 E7 Level Cases/controls 0 66/71 +1 12/17 >+1 22/12	+1, 0.8 (0.4–1.8) >+1, 3.8 (1.7–8.5) Others (HPV-6, 16/18 L1 & L2 & other Es) were not associated)	IgG antibodies to HPV-6 (L1, L2) HPV-16/18 (E2, E4, E6, E7, L1 & L2) Western blot assay	Adjusted for age, cigarette smoking, age at first sexual intercourse, lifetime number of sexual partners, number of prior births, number of prior Pap smears in previous decade

Table 41 (contd)

Reference and study	Cases (number and type)	Controls (number and type)	HPV prevalence (%)	Odds ratio (95 % CI)	HPV serology test	Comments/adjustments
Müller et al. (1992) Colombia and Spain	100 HPV-16 invasive 15 HPV-other invasive 62 HPV-negative invasive cancers 49 HPV-16 CIN III	177 controls of invasive cases 49 controls of CIN cases	Any E6/any E7 Invasive control, 4/15 CIN-control, 6/20 HPV-16-invasive, 16/42 HPV-other-invasive, 0/27 HPV-negative-invasive, 2/23 HPV-16 CIN, 4/18 HPV-positive-invasive	Any E7 [4.0 (2.2–7.4)] [2.0 (0.5–7.6)] [1.6 (0.7–3.5)] [0.9 (0.3–2.7)] [3.7 (2.0–6.7)]	ELISA with 4 HPV-16 E6-E7 peptides	Results for E6 can be also computed but the prevalences are much smaller than E7. Cases were selected because of HPV DNA status and controls.
Sasagawa et al. (1992) Japan	30 invasive cervical cancers 26 CIN III	38 healthy women	E6/E7 CIN, 19/8 Invasive cancer, 27/33 Control, 0/0	One-tailed p-values E6/E7 [< 0.01/0.16] [< 0.001/0.0001]	HPV-16 E6 & E7 ELISA	
Ghosh et al. (1993) United Kingdom	92 cervical cancers 90 CIN	84 healthy women	L1/E4/E6/E7 Control, 4/24/5/10 CIN I/condyloma, 18/36/14/14 CIN II-III, 10/39/13/6 Cervical cancer, 5/43/35/25	Age-sex-matched (69 cases and 69 controls) Cervical cancer E4, [2.5 (1.1–5.5)] E6, [16.7 (3.5–108.3)] E7, [3.9 (1.2–13.0)]	E4, E6, E7, L1 Western blot analysis of recombinant HPV proteins	
Jha et al. (1993) United Kingdom	219 population-based cervical cancers	387 age-matched women	Cases/controls HPV-16 E7, 14/7 HPV-18 E7, 7/5 HPV-16/18 E7, 20/12	1.9 (1.1–3.5) 1.8 (0.8–3.9) 1.9 (1.2–3.2)	HPV-16 E7 and /or HPV-18 E7 ELISA	Adjusted for age, number of sexual partners, age at first sexual intercourse, years of oral contraceptive use, number of normal Pap smears in the past four years
Heino et al. (1993) Sweden	64 anal epidermoid carcinomas	79 healthy blood donors	Prevalence IgA E2:9 Case, 89; control, 24	IgA E2:9, [25.7 (9.3–74.3)] L1, L3, E7 not significantly associated	ELISA IgA and IgG antibodies to 5 HPV-16 peptide antigens	
Paez et al. (1993) Japan	51 squamous-cell carcinomas 4 adenosquamous-cell 2 adenocarcinomas	200 healthy blood donors	E7/L2 Squamous-cell, 20/29 Adenosquamous-cell, 0/75 Adenocarcinoma, 0/0 All cancer, 18/32 Control, 5/9	E7, [4.0 (1.4–11.3)] L2, [4.7 (2.1–10.4)]	Antibodies to HPV-16 E7 and L2 proteins Western blot assay	

Table 41 (contd)

Reference and study	Cases (number and type)	Controls (number and type)	HPV prevalence (%)	Odds ratio (95 % CI)	HPV serology test	Comments/adjustments
Stacey et al. (1993) Australia	Cervical cancers: 10 E7 seropositive 10 E7 seronegative	10 healthy controls	*Prevalence of bE7 RIPA* E7 seropositive, 100 E7 seronegative, 50 Any, 75 Control, 0	[$p = 0.0001$]	HPV-16 E7 protein by recombinant baculovirus (bE7 RIPA)	Authors conclude that the bE7 RIPA assay provides a more sensitive method for the detection of E7 antibodies in human sera than does the currently widely used Western blotting method.
Viscidi et al. (1993) Colombia and Spain	97 invasive cancers 49 CIN	121 controls of invasive cases 48 controls of CIN cases	*E6 or E7 cases/controls* CIN: 8 / 2 Invasive: 72 / 6	*E6 or E7 cases/controls* [4.2 (0.4–102.0)] [42.2 (16.4–113.7)]	HPV-16 E6 and E7 TT-RIPA	
Sun et al. (1994a) Colombia and Spain	97 population-based invasive cervical cancers	121 population-based controls	ELISA RIPA E6 15/5 56/2 E7 41/17 43/4 E6 or E7 46/21 72/6	E6 ELISA, 3.5 (2.1–5.8) E6 RIPA, 74.7 (25.2–219.5) E7 ELISA, 3.3 (2.7–4.0) E7 RIPA, 17.7 (11.1–29.7) E6 or E7 ELISA, 3.3 (2.8–3.9) E6 or E7 RIPA, 42.2 (28.3–62.7)	Radioimmunoprecipitation (in vitro-translated HPV-16 E6 & E7) versus ELISA (E6 and E7 synthetic peptides)	Comparison of peptide-ELISA versus TT-RIPA. Odds ratios not adjusted
Sun et al. (1994b) Brazil	194 hospital-based invasive cervical cancers	217 hospital-based controls	E6: 54/6 E7: 30/5 E6 or E7: 63/10 E6 and E7: 21/0.5 E6 or E7 high antibody titres: 41/0.5	35 (15–83) 10 (4–25) 28 (13–61) 87 (10–736) 239 (29–1946)	Radioimmunoprecipitation HPV-16 E6 and E7	Odds ratios adjusted for age, socioeconomic status, number of Paps, parity, NOSP, AFSI, duration and use of oral contraceptives sensitivity and specificity for invasive cancer: E6 or E7: 63 and 90; E6 or E7 (high titres): 41 and 99.7

[ ] Calculated by the Working Group

CIN, carcinoma *in situ*; TT-RIPA, radioimmunoprecipitation of the translated protein; NOSP, number of sexual partners; AFSI, age at first sexual intercourse; VIN, vulvar intraepithelial neoplasia; ORF, open reading frame; BPV, bovine papillomavirus; STD, sexually transmitted disease; ELISA, enzyme-linked immunosorbent assay; Pap, Papanicolaou smear conclude that the presence of anti-E7 antibodies may represent a marker for cervical cancer development and that the presence of anti-E4 antibodies may be correlated with virus replication.

In Panama, Mann et al. (1990), using an enzyme-linked immunosorbent assay, tested sera from 186 cases of invasive cervical cancer and from 172 age-matched controls for IgG and IgA antibodies to HPV-16 E7 peptide and to peptide 245, representing an epitope in E2. Prevalences (%) in cases and controls were 21 and 9 for IgA to E7, 25 and 6 for IgG to E7, 15 and 11 for IgA to peptide 245 and 19 and 11 for IgG to peptide 245, respectively. The ORs for cervical cancer, adjusted for cigarette smoking, education, number of pregnancies, age at first sexual intercourse and time since last Pap, were 5.3 (95% CI, 2.4–11.6) for IgG to E7, 2.7 (95% CI, 1.3–5.3) for IgA to E7, 1.7 (95% CI, 1.2–3.3) for IgG to peptide 245 and 1.0 (95% CI, 0.4–1.6) for IgA to peptide 245. Seropositivity correlated poorly with clinical stage, survival or the presence of HPV–DNA in tumour. The authors concluded that these data suggest that antibodies to E7 are markers for invasive cervical cancer.

In Germany, Steger et al. (1990), using Western blot analysis with the entire L1 as antigen to detect HPV-8-specific IgG antibodies, tested serum from 445 randomly selected controls and from 201 patients with various cancers (54 with malignant melanoma, 60 with basal-cell carcinomas, 44 with Hodgkin's disease, 11 with squamous-cell skin carcinoma and 32 with cervical cancer). Prevalences of HPV-8 L1 antibodies were 20% in the control group, 28% in patients with malignant melanoma, 40% in patients with basal-cell carcinomas, 48% in patients with Hodgkin's disease, 73% in patients with squamous-cell skin carcinoma and 37% in patients with cervical cancer. The corresponding estimated odds ratios were [1.6 (95% CI, 0.8–3.1)] for malignant melanoma, [2.7 (95% CI, 1.5–4.9)] for basal-cell carcinomas, [3.7 (95% CI, 1.9–7.3)] for Hodgkin's disease, [10.8 (95% CI, 2.5–52.6)] for squamous-cell skin cancer and [2.4 (95% CI, 1.1–5.5)] for cervical cancer.

Suchánková et al. (1991) tested a total of 140 sera from Czech women with either normal cervical diagnoses (n = 85), CIN (n = 21) or cervical cancer (n = 34) compared to 10 children's sera as controls. They assayed IgG antibody by ELISA against an HPV-16 E7 synthetic peptide (16/E7-2) and by Western blot against a genitally engineered HPV-16 E7 fusion protein. The two assay results were highly significantly correlated. Twelve of 34 cancer patients (35.2%) tested positive in one or both assays compared to six of 106 (5.7%) CIN and normal patients. None of the 10 children's sera was reactive.

In a study in USA, Mandelson et al. (1992) measured IgG antibodies to HPV-6-encoded L1 and L2 and to HPV-16- and HPV-18-encoded E2, E4, E6, E7, L1 and L2 bacterial fusion proteins in a Western immunoblot assay among 69 cases with invasive cervical cancer and 81 control women. The intensities of the Western blot bands were graded as 0 (negative), +1, +2 or +3. Prevalences (%) for anti HPV-16 E7 among cases and controls were 66 and 71 for grade 0, 12 and 17 for grade +1 and 22 and 12 for grade > +1. The OR (adjusted for age, cigarette smoking, age at first sexual intercourse, lifetime number of sexual partners, number of prior births, number of prior Pap smears in previous decade) for HPV-16 E7 was 3.8 (95% CI, 1.7–8.5) for grade > +1. Odds ratios for the other fusion proteins were not statistically significant. The authors conclude that these findings strongly support an association between antibodies to HPV-16 E7 and invasive cervical cancer.

Müller et al. (1992) collected sera from 177 cases of invasive cervical cancer and their 177 controls, and sera from 49 cases of CIN III and their 49 controls, all participating in a case–control study of cervical cancer and CIN III in Spain and Colombia, and examined them for antibodies to four HPV-16 E6 and E7 peptides. Cases of invasive cervical cancer were categorized, according to their PCR-based HPV DNA status, into HPV-16 DNA positive (n = 100), HPV DNA positive for other types (n = 15), and HPV DNA negative (n = 62). All CIN cases selected were positive for HPV-16 DNA. Prevalences (%) of antibodies to any of the four E6 peptides and to any of the four E7 peptides for each group were four and 15, respectively, for controls of invasive cases, 6 and 20 for controls of CIN cases, 16 and 42 for cases of HPV-16 positive invasive cancer, 0 and 27 for cases of invasive cancer positive for other HPV types, 2 and 23 for cases of invasive cancer HPV negative, and 4 and 18 for cases of HPV-16 positive CIN. Estimated crude ORs using positivity to any of the E7-related peptides were [3.7 (95% CI, 2.0–6.7)] for the HPV positive invasive group, [4.0 (95% CI, 2.2–7.4)] for the HPV-16 invasive group, [2.0 (95% CI, 0.5–7.6)] for the other HPV types group, [1.6 (95% CI, 0.7–3.5)] for the HPV-negative group and [0.9 (95% CI, 0.3–2.7)] for the HPV-16 CIN group. Thus, HPV-16 E6/E7 seropositivity was most associated with invasive cancer containing HPV-16.

In the United Kingdom, Ghosh et al. (1993) collected sera from 90 cases of CIN and 92 cases of cervical cancer and examined them in comparison with those of 84 healthy controls for antibodies to HPV early proteins E4, E6, E7 and the major capsid protein L1 using Western blot analysis of recombinant HPV proteins. Prevalences (%) for L1/E4/E6/E7 were 4/24/5/10 for controls, 18/36/14/14 for CIN I and condylomata, 10/39/13/6 for CIN II–III and 5/43/35/25 for cervical cancer. In an analysis of 69 cases and 69 controls matched by age, the estimated odds ratios for cervical cancer were [2.5 (95% CI, 1.1–5.5)] for E4, [16.7 (95% CI, 3.5–108.3)] for E6 and [3.9 (95% CI, 1.2–13.0)] for E7.

Jha et al. (1993) collected sera from 219 cases of cervical cancer and their 387 controls participating in a population-based case–control study in the United Kingdom and examined them for antibodies to HPV-16 E7 and/or HPV-18 E7 by ELISA. Prevalences (%) for cases and controls were 14 and 7 for HPV-16 E7, 7 and 5 for HPV-18 E7 and 20 and 12 for HPV-16/18 E7. The ORs adjusted for age, number of sexual partners, age at first sexual intercourse, years of oral contraceptive use and number of Pap smears in the past four years were 1.9 (95% CI, 1.1–3.5) for HPV-16 E7, 1.8 (95% CI, 0.8–3.9) for HPV-18 E7 and 1.9 (95% CI, 1.2–3.2) for HPV-16/18 E7. [The Working Group noted that blood collection followed case–control diagnosis by several years.]

Krchnák et al. (1993) studied seroreactivity to four HPV-18 E7 peptides in 65 invasive cancer patients and 65 controls matched on age and place of residence in the Czech Republic. Seroreactivity was extremely low in cases (< 5% to any peptide) and totally absent in controls.

Onda et al. (1993) in Japan tested seroreactivity to HPV-15 E4 and E7 ELISA antigens as well as HPV DNA type among 51 women with invasive cervical cancer compared to 22 women with CIN (10 with carcinoma *in situ*). The ELISA antigens were bacterially expressed. *L1* consensus primers were used for PCR. Ten out of 17 (58.8%) HPV-16 DNA-positive cancer cases were positive for either anti-E4 or anti-E7, compared to 24 women (12.5%) with cancer containing another HPV type and 0/10 women with HPV-negative carcinoma. The only other seropositive patient had HPV-negative carcinoma *in situ*.

Viscidi *et al.* (1993) collected sera from 97 cases of invasive cervical cancer and their 121 controls, and sera from 49 cases of CIN and their 48 controls, participating in a case–control study of cervical cancer and CIN in Spain and Cali, Colombia, and examined them for antibodies to HPV-16 E6 and E7 proteins by radioimmunoprecipitation of the in-vitro translated proteins (TT-RIPA). Prevalences (%) for invasive cases and controls were 56 and 2 for E6, 43 and 4 for E7, 72 and 6 for E6 or E7 and 26 and 0 for E6 and E7. Prevalences (%) for CIN cases and controls were 2 and 0 for E6, 6 and 2 for E7, 8 and 2 for E6 or E7 and 0 and 0 for E6 and E7. The estimated crude OR for E6 or E7 was [42.2 (95% CI, 16.4–113.7)] for invasive cervical cancer and [4.2 (95% CI, 0.4–102.0)] for CIN.

Dillner *et al.* (1994) conducted a seroepidemiological study of cervical cancer and HPV in northern Sweden. Sera from 94 cases of incident cervical cancer were compared to 188 age- and sex-matched controls. Twelve antigens from HPV-6, -11, -16 or -18 were tested as a panel for IgG and IgA reactivity. Significantly increased odds ratios of about 3 were found for multiple antigens with the highest OR (9.2 (95% CI, 4.4–19.4)) associated with IgG to an HPV-18 E2 antigen.

Nindl *et al.* (1994) analysed sera obtained from 137 Mexican cervical cancer patients using several different assays for HPV-16 proteins E6 and E7. Specifically, ELISA using as antigen either synthetic peptides or the complex E7 protein was compared to RIPA using viral protein made by in-vitro transcription/translation. As controls, sera from 163 healthy Mexican women and 35 healthy German men were tested. For all assays, cancer cases had higher seroreactivity (17–47%) than controls (who were rarely seropositive).

Sun *et al.* (1994a) extended the work of Viscidi *et al.* (1993) by testing sera further from 97 cases of invasive cervical cancer and 121 controls participating in a population-based case–control study of cervical cancer in Spain and Cali, Colombia. They examined them for antibodies to HPV-16 E6 and E7 by both the radioimmunoprecipitation assay with in-vitro-translated HPV-16 E6 and E7 proteins (TT-RIPA), and an enzyme-linked immunosorbent assay (ELISA). Prevalences (%) for cases and controls using peptide-ELISA were 15 and 5 for E6, 41 and 17 for E7, 46 and 21 for E6 or E7 and 8 and 2 for E6 and E7. Prevalences (%) for cases and controls using TT-RIPA were 56 and 2 for E6, 43 and 4 for E7, 72 and 6 for E6 or E7 and 27 and 0 for E6 and E7. The unadjusted ORs using peptide-ELISA were 3.5 (95% CI, 2.1–5.8) for E6, 3.3 (95% CI, 2.7–4.0) for E7, 3.3 (95% CI, 2.8–3.9) for E6 or E7 and 3.5 (95% CI, 1.4–8.9) for E6 and E7. In comparison, the unadjusted odds ratios using TT-RIPA were much larger: 74.7 (95% CI, 25.2–219.5) for E6, 17.7 (95% CI, 11.1–29.7) for E7, 42.2 (95% CI, 28.3–62.7) for E6 or E7 and [∞ (95% CI, 10.6–∞)] for E6 and E7.

Masked sera from 194 cases of invasive cervical cancer and 217 controls participating in a hospital-based case–control study of cervical cancer in Brazil were examined for antibodies to HPV-16 E6 and E7 by radioimmunoprecipitation assay (Sun *et al.*, 1994b). Prevalences (%) for cases and controls were 54 and 6 for E6, 30 and 5 for E7, 63 and 10 for E6 or E7, 21 and 0.5 for E6 and E7 and 41 and 0.5 for high antibody titres to E6 or E7. The ORs adjusted for age, socioeconomic status, number of Papanicolaou smears, parity, number of sexual partners, age at first sexual intercourse and duration of oral contraceptive use were 35 (95% CI, 15–83) for E6,

10 (95% CI, 4–25) for E7, 28 (95% CI, 13–61) for E6 or E7, 87 (95% CI, 10–736) for E6 and E7 and 83 (95% CI, 10–689) for high antibody titres (cpm > 6000) for E7 and 239 (95% CI, 29–1946) for high antibody titres (cpm > 6000) for E6 or E7. Antibody prevalences (%) for HPV-DNA 16 and HPV DNA-negative invasive cases were 61/41 for E6, 43/14 for E7, 73/41 for E6 or E7, and 31/14 for E6 and E7. The sensitivity and specificity for invasive cancer were 63% and 90% for E6 or E7 and 41% and 99.7% for high antibody titres (cpm > 6000) to E6 or E7.

Dillner et al. (1995) extended their previous seroepidemiological study of 94 Swedish cervical cancer cases and 184 matched controls by testing the sera for IgG and IgA to several promising new antigens. Seropositivity in the tests was, for most, significantly associated with risk of cervical cancer, with odds ratios ranging up to 15. The three serological assays showing the strongest associations with cervical cancer were E6 : 10 IgA (OR, 15 (95% CI, 6.0–49)), HPV-16 virus-like particle IgG (OR, 9.3 (95% CI, 3.8–27.5)) and E1: 19 IgG (OR, 7.8 (95% CI, 4.0–16)). Even higher odds ratios were observed when combinations of assays were used to discriminate cases from controls.

Nonnenmacher et al. (1995) tested the serological response to HPV-16 virus-like particles among 89 women with HPV-16 DNA-positive cervical cancer and 49 with CIN III compared to 162 controls in Colombia and Spain. Seropositivity was strongly associated with risk of cervical cancer [OR, 9.5 (95% CI, 4.9–19.3)] and CIN [OR, 22.6 (95% CI, 9.7–56.8)] in both countries. In contrast to E6 and E7 RIPA data from the same population (Müller et al., 1992), seropositivity to virus-like particles was significantly higher among CIN patients than among cancer patients.

From the studies in Table 41 the following conclusions seems to emerge:

(i)   The association of HPV derived antibodies with cervical cancer

Differences in HPV antibodies between cases of cervical cancer and controls have consistently been detected by serological assays. Studies based on HPV-derived antibodies are generally consistent with the findings of the studies based on HPV DNA detection, but with some exceptions, the magnitude of the risk estimates is lower than that obtained by recent HPV DNA-based comparisons.

(ii)   Titre of antibody

One study indicated that high antibody titres to E6 and E7 was a stronger discrimination between cases and controls than antibody positivity (Sun et al., 1994b).

(iii)   Clinical stage of cervical neoplasia

Although comparability of studies cannot be formally established, antibodies to HPV-derived proteins are more often found in cases of invasive cervical cancer than in cases of preinvasive lesions. One study suggested that seroprevalence of antibodies to E6 protein were directly related to clinical stage (Sun et al., 1994b). The finding is not replicated by other studies (Heino et al., 1993).

2.4.2 Other cancers

(a)   Anogenital cancers

There are few case–control studies of the association between HPV and cancers of the genital tract other than cervix (for review see Daling & Sherman, 1992; Holly & Palefsky,

1993). In this section, studies in which history of genital warts was analysed as a surrogate measurement of HPV infection are described.

(i) Cancer of the penis

Table 42 summarizes four studies. HPV-16 was the predominant HPV type (> 60%) in all the reports. One study using PCR reported HPV prevalences of 49% (Maden *et al.*, 1993) for penile cancer and another, using in-situ hybridization, found over 90% HPV positivity for penile intraepithelial neoplasia (PIN) II and III (Demeter *et al.*, 1993).

Maden *et al.* (1993) reported an odds ratio of 5.9 (95% CI, 2.1–17.6) for history of genital warts. A further study tested normal foreskin from adults and found strong associations between both overall HPV and HPV-16 and penile carcinoma (Varma *et al.*, 1991).

Brinton *et al.* (1991) conducted a case–control study of penile cancer in China involving 141 cases and 150 community controls. On examination, 13 cases and one control had genital warts at the time of the study [OR, 15.1 (95% CI, 2.2–647)].

(ii) Cancer of the anus

Six case–control studies have reported on HPV and anal cancer (Table 43). Control material included, variously, colon adenocarcinoma and anal tissue from the control patients. The HPV DNA prevalence observed in epidermoid anal cancer cases ranged from 21.3% (Beckmann *et al.*, 1989) to 80% (Ogunbiyi *et al.*, 1994a). The prevalence of HPV DNA in anal adenocarcinoma was zero in one study (Beckmann *et al.*, 1989). The prevalence among controls ranged from 0% to 14% and the odds ratio estimates were consistently greater than 20.

(iii) Cancers of the vulva

Three case–control studies have reported on cases of cancer of the vulva (see Table 44). In the USA, Brinton *et al.* (1990) compared the history of genital warts in a series of 209 cases of vulvar cancer and 348 community controls. Cases reported warts in 14.8% of instances and controls in 1.4%. The odds ratio was 15.2 (95% CI, 5.5–42.1). A possible interaction with smoking was suggested. Smokers with a history of warts had 35 times the risk of vulvar cancer over controls.

In Denmark, Hørding *et al.* (1993) tested 62 women with vulvar cancer and 110 specimens of vulvar tissue from women who died in accidents. Using PCR techniques, HPV (HPV-6/11, -16, -18, -33) DNA was detected in 30.6% of the cases and in none of the controls. HPV prevalence was more common if the cancer tissue had VIN III lesions in the adjacent region.

In Australia, Kulski *et al.* (1989) used filter in-situ hybridization to test for HPV DNA specimens from the cervix and the vulva of women referred because of clinical or morphological abnormalities or past HPV infection. Of the samples, 74% of the cervical scrapes and 68% of the vulvar scrapes were HPV positive. None of 35 women without signs of cervical abnormality tested positive for HPV DNA. [The difference in HPV prevalence between cases and controls may be overestimated due to the selection criteria of cases and controls.]

Table 42. Case–control studies of penile neoplasms

Reference and country	Cases (number and type)	Controls (number and type)	HPV prevalence (%)	Odds ratio (95% CI)	HPV test	Comments/adjustments
Brinton et al. (1991) China	141 cases of penile cancer	150 community controls	Case, 9 Control, 1 HPV prevalence assessed by genital warts	Genital warts: [15.1 (2.2–647)]	History of genital warts	
Varma et al. (1991) USA	23 cases (30 specimens) of penile carcinoma	20 foreskins from adults	Cases HPV, 87 HPV-16, 78 Controls, 0	[∞ (17.7–∞)] [∞ (11.3–∞)]	PCR In-situ hybridization	Cases and controls were tested on paraffin embedded specimens from archival material. Tests included HPV-6/11 and -16 probes. Prevalence reported includes the combined results of the PCR and in situ tests and refers to the 23 patients.
Demeter et al. (1993) USA	44 PIN	88 men with condyloma acuminatum (not tested for HPV)	PIN I, 62.5 (58% HPV-6/11) PIN II, 90 (60% HPV-16, -31) PIN III, 92.3 (92.3% HPV-16)		RNA–RNA in-situ hybridization Southern blot	Controls not tested for HPV. Concordance on HPV between in situ hybridization and Southern blot was 74%. Concordance on type among positive cases was 100%. No evidence of viral integration
Maden et al. (1993) USA	110 penile cancers (67 tested for HPV)	355 men from general population matched by age at date of diagnosis	Cases HPV, 49 HPV-16, 70 Controls, not tested HPV prevalence assessed by genital warts	History of genital warts: 5.9 (2.1–17.6)	PCR History of genital warts	Cases tested on paraffin-embedded specimens. Subjects interviewed were 50.2% of the cases and 70.3% of the controls.

[ ] Calculated by the Working Group
PIN, penile intraepithelial neoplasia; PCR, polymerase chain reaction

Table 43. Case–control studies of anorectal cancer

Reference and country	Cases (number and type)	Controls (number and type)	HPV prevalence (%)	Odds ratio (95% CI)	HPV test	Comments/adjustments
Daling et al. (1987) USA	148 anal cancers	166 colon cancers	*History of genital warts* Squamous-cell homosexual men, 47.1 heterosexual men, 28.3 women, 28.6 Transitional-cell, 0 Control, 1–2	26.9 (2.8–257.1)	History	No HPV tests performed
Palmer et al. (1989) United Kingdom	45 anal cancers	28 sex-matched patients undergoing rectal surgery	HPV, 61 HPV-16, 56 HPV-18, 5 Control, 0	[∞ (8.8–∞)] [∞ (7.4–∞)] [∞ (0.1–∞)]	Southern blot, dot blot In-situ hybridization	HPV-16 was predominantly integrated into cellular DNA
Beckmann et al. (1989) USA	23 anorectal carcinomas *in situ* 47 invasive carcinomas 42 transitional-cell carcinomas 14 adenocarcinomas	110 colon adenocarcinomas (fixed tissue)	*In situ*, 56.5 Invasive, 21.3 Transitional, 2.4 Adenocarcinoma, 0 Control, 0	[∞ (27–∞)] [∞ (6.2–∞)] [∞ (0.1–∞)]	In-situ hybridization	Type distribution was similar between in situ and invasive carcinomas. Of 23 HPV-positive cases, 8 were HPV-6, 10 were HPV-16, 1 was HPV-18, and 4 were HPV-X. Control tissue was a strip of anal epithelium extending from anorectal junction to the anal margin.
Scholefield et al. (1992) United Kingdom	152 women with CIN III investigated for AIN/anal cancer (n = 29)	50 women without CIN (2 with CIN I) (AIN, n = 0)	Case, 51 Control, 14	[6.5 (2.1–21.1)]	PCR	
Shroyer et al. (1992) USA	5 anorectal cancers	22 colon adenocarcinomas	Case, 100 Control, 0	[∞ (12.1–∞)]	PCR (100%) In-situ hybridization (80%)	
Ogunbiyi et al. (1994a) United Kingdom	40 invasive vulvar cancers investigated for HPV anal infection and anal cancers from biopsy material taken using a proctoscope in conjunction with a colposcope	80 hospital	Vulvar cancer, 75 Anal SIL, 76.9 Anal cancer, 80 Control, 13.7	Anal neoplasms: 22.0 (5.4–98.6)	PCR	Study of concurrent lesions in the vulva and the anal region. Controls were selected if they had no history of anogenital HPV infection or neoplasia. Cases were not excluded if history of HPV infection. Only HPV-16 investigated

[ ] Calculated by the Working Group
AIN, anal intraepithelial neoplasia (grades I, II, III); CIN, cervical intraepithelial neoplasia; PCR, polymerase chain reaction; SIL, squamous intraepithelial lesion; X, HPV type unknown

Table 44. Case–control studies of vulvar and ovarian cancers

Reference and country	Cases (Number and type)	Controls (Number and type)	HPV prevalence (%)	Odds ratio (95% CI)	HPV test	Comments/adjustments
Kaufman et al. (1987) USA	12 ovarian cancers	4 normal ovaries	Case, 83 Control, 0	HPV-6b, [∞ (1.1–∞)]	In-situ hybridization	Signal intensity specifically located in the nucleus using HPV-6b probe. Signal with HPV-11 very weak
Kulski et al. (1989) Australia	128 CIN or HPV signs	35 women free of cervical abnormalities	Cervical scrape, 74 Vulvar scrape, 68 Cervical + vulvar, 57 HPV-16/18, 61 HPV-6/11, 14 HPV-31, -33, 3 Control, 0	[∞ (23.6–∞)] [∞ (11.1–∞)]	DNA filter in-situ hybridization	Study of the coexistence of HPV infections in the vulva and the cervix. Cases included patients selected because of HPV clinical and/or morphological signs. HPV types investigated were 6/11, 16/18, 31/33.
Brinton et al. (1990) USA	209 vulvar cancers	348 community controls	History of genital warts Case, 14.8 Control, 1.4	15.2 (5.5–42.1)	History of warts	No HPV detection was performed. Interaction between genital warts and smoking is suggested.
Sherman et al. (1991) USA	53 vulvar cancers 180 VIN	466 population controls	Vulvar cancer, 41.7 VIN, 38.7 Control, 4.5	17.3 (6.3–47.2) 15.8 (8.4–29.8)	History of genital warts (condyloma)	
Hording et al. (1993) Denmark	79 vulvar cancers (62 tested)	110 normal vulvar tissues from accident casualties	Case, 30.6 (61% with associated VIN III and 13% without VIN III) HPV-16, 68.4 HPV-18, 15.8 HPV-33, 15.8 Control, 0	[∞ (40–∞)]	PCR	HPV-positive cases were younger and more frequently had multicentric neoplasms. HPV-6/11, -16, -18 or -33 were investigated. No cases of HPV-6/11 were found.

[ ] Calculated by the Working Group
VIN, vulvar intraepithelial neoplasia; PCR, polymerase chain reaction

(b) Other cancers

(i) Cancer of the mouth

Three studies have compared HPV DNA prevalence in cases of oral cancer and tissues from individuals without oral cancer (Table 45). In three of them the prevalence of HPV among cases was significantly higher than among controls.

In Taiwan, Chang *et al.* (1989) compared tissue specimens from 17 cases of oral cancer with specimens from normal gingival tissue from 17 patients using Southern blot techniques. Among cases, 13/17 (76.4%) were HPV-16 positive and, among controls, 1/16 (5.9%) was positive for an unknown type. The estimated OR was [52.0 (95% CI, 4.4–1454.0)]. Three oral papillomas were also studied and all were HPV-16 positive; the HPV-16 sequences detected in the oral cancers and papillomas were episomal. Twelve of the 17 cases were also betel chewers and/or smokers.

Brandsma and Abramson (1989) investigated 21 cases of cancer of the mouth (10) and tongue (11) using Southern blot and compared HPV detection with site-matched specimens from 18 controls. Two cases were HPV positive compared with none of the controls (see also Table 46).

Maden *et al.* (1992) investigated 131 male cases of oral cancer and 136 male population controls matched by age and date of diagnosis from Washington State, USA. Random digit dialling was used to identify eligible controls. Exfoliated cells from the mouth were used as primary material for HPV testing and PCR methods were used. The study included an extensive questionnaire on exposure to the key risk factors for oral cancer and the risk estimates were adjusted for age, smoking, alcohol consumption and lifetime number of sexual partners. The prevalence of HPV-6 DNA was 19% among cases and 9% among controls. The crude OR was 2.9 (95% CI, 1.1–7.3) and the adjusted OR was 2.8 (95% CI, 1.1–7.3). HPV-16 DNA was found in 6% of the cases and in 1% of the controls. The crude OR was 6.2 (95% CI, 0.7–52.2). In this study no association was found between oral cancer and history of the most common sexually transmitted diseases including herpes simplex virus (HSV)-1 or HSV-2. However, a non-significant increase in risk was associated with the presence of HSV-2 antibodies (adjusted OR, 1.8 (95% CI, 0.7–4.6)).

In Germany, Ostwald *et al.* (1994) used a PCR-based method to compare HPV DNA prevalence between 26 cases of oral carcinoma and 97 healthy volunteers. Cell scrapes from the buccal mucosa were collected from both cases and controls. From cases, additional specimens were taken from the normal mucosa distant from the cancer location. Among cases, 61% showed evidence of HPV DNA against 1% among controls [odds ratio, 153.6 (95% CI, 17.7–3449.4)] and 18 out of the 26 cases were smokers.

Table 46 summarizes studies that investigated cases of cancers from different sites in the upper digestive and respiratory tracts in relation to the presence of HPV DNA. Controls for these cases were normally obtained from normal patients undergoing scrapes or biopsies from matched sites for reasons other than cancer.

Table 45. Case–control studies of cancer of the oral cavity

Reference and country	Cases (number and type)	Controls (number and type)	HPV prevalence (%)	Odds ratio (95% CI)	HPV test	Comments/adjustments
Chang et al. (1989) Taiwan	17 oral carcinomas 3 oral papillomas	17 normal gingival tissues	*HPV-16* Carcinoma, 76.4 Papilloma, 100 *Any HPV* Control, 5.9	[52.0 (4.4– 1454.0)]	Southern blot	HPV-6/11, -16 and -18 investigated. Interaction between betel chewing and HPV is suggested.
Abdelsayed (1991) USA	18 dysplasias or carcinomas in non-alcohol/non-tobacco users	18 dysplasias or carcinomas in alcohol and/or tobacco users	Case, 0 Control, 11		In-situ hybridization	HPV-6/11, -16/18 and -31/33/35 investigated. One control was positive for HPV-6/11 and the other for HPV-16/18.
Maden et al. (1992) USA	131 oral cancers	136 population controls matched on age and date of diagnosis	*Case* HPV-6, 19 HPV-16, 6 *Control* HPV-6, 9 HPV-16, 1	2.8 (1.1–7.3) 6.2 (0.7–52.2)	PCR	Odds ratio for HPV-6 adjusted for age, smoking, alcohol consumption and lifetime number of partners
Müller et al. (1994) Germany	26 oral carcinomas	97 normal oral mucosae from volunteers	Case, 61 (HPV-16 and -18 predominant) Control, 1	[153.6 (17.7– 3449.4)]	PCR and Southern blot	HPV prevalence in the normal mucosa of cases decreased with distance from the cancer site.

[ ] Calculated by the Working Group
PCR, polymerase chain reaction

Table 46. Case–control studies of cancer of the upper digestive and respiratory tracts

Reference and country	Cases (Number and type)	Controls (Number and type)	HPV prevalence (%)	Odds ratio (95% CI)	HPV test	Comments/adjustments
Brandsma & Abramson (1989) USA	101 carcinomas Nose (2) Mouth (10) Tongue (11) Tonsil (7) Pharynx (8) Larynx (60) Oesophagus (3)	116 hospital controls matched by site	Nose, 0 Mouth, 0 Tongue, 18.2 Tonsil, 28.5 Pharynx, 12.5 Larynx, 5.0 Oesophagus, 0 Control, 1.7	All cases [4.90 (0.93–34.3)]	Southern blot	
Bryan et al. (1990) United Kingdom	13 pharynx and larynx carcinomas	14 with normal nasopharynx mucosa	Case, 84.6 HPV-11, 30.8 HPV-6/11, 53.8 Control, 64.3	[3.1 (0.37–30.26)]	PCR	Specimens tested for HPV-6 and -11 types
Niedobitek et al. (1990) Germany	28 carcinomas of the tonsil	30 chronic tonsilitis	Case, 21.4 Control, 0	[∞ (1.4–∞)]	In situ hybridization	
Williamson et al. (1991) South Africa	14 oesophageal carcinomas	41 hospital controls	Case, 43 Control, 15	[4.38 (0.92–21.5)]	PCR	Biopsies from normal mucosa of the cases showed 66.6% HPV positivity rate.
Benamouzig et al. (1992) France	12 oesophageal cancers	24 hospital controls	Case, 25 Control, 4.2 (dot blot results)	[7.67 (0.57–220.8)]	In-situ hybridization Dot blot	Dot blot hybridization gave higher positivity rates than in-situ hybridization. Normal mucosa of the cases showed HPV DNA in 41.6%.
Snijders et al. (1992b) The Netherlands	10 carcinomas of the tonsil	7 tonsilitis patients	Case, 100 HPV-16, 40 HPV-33, 40 HPV-16/33, 10 Control, 0	[∞ (7.5–∞)]	PCR Southern blot RNA-PCR In-situ hybridization	E7 transcripts of HPV-16 were exclusively located within carcinoma cells. Stroma was negative.
Tyan et al. (1993) Taiwan	30 carcinomas of the nasopharynx 44 other carcinomas of the head and neck	11 normal tissues from nasopharynx and oral cavity	Nasopharynx, 46.7 Other head and neck cancer, 29.5 Control, 9.1	[8.4 (1.0–406.3)] [4.1 (0.5–195.8)]	PCR and DNA sequencing	Coinfection of HPV with EBV occurred in 46.6% of nasopharingeal carcinomas and in 11.4% of the other head and neck cancers. HPV-16 accounted for 96% of the HPV DNA positive specimens. Only HPV-16 DNA was tested.

Table 46 (contd)

Country (Reference)	Cases (Number and type)	Controls (Number and type)	HPV prevalence (%)	Odds ratio (95% CI)	HPV test	Comments/adjustments
Watanabe et al. (1993) Japan	12 carcinomas of the tonsil and pharynx	28 tonsilitis	Case, 20 Control, 0 (PCR results)	[∞ (4.4–∞)]	Dot-filter Southern blot PCR	Study comparing primarily the results of the three detection methods

[ ] Calculated by the Working Group
PCR, polymerase chain reaction; EBV, Epstein-Barr virus

(ii) Cancer of the tonsil

Using in-situ hybridization with probes for HPV-6, -11 and -16 under high stringency, Niedobitek et al. (1990) tested 28 tonsillar carcinomas and 30 tonsils removed because of chronic inflammation. Six of the cases and none of the controls were HPV-16 positive [$p < 0.001$].

Snijders et al. (1992b) used PCR and Southern hybridization techniques to test 10 cases of carcinoma of the tonsil and seven cases of tonsillitis as controls. All cases tested positive for HPV against none of the controls [OR, ∞ (95% CI, 7.5–∞)]. The presence of HPV DNA in cancer cells was further tested with in-situ hybridization. In all instances, the stroma was HPV-negative and HPV DNA was detected in the cancer cells.

In Japan, Watanabe et al. (1993) tested 12 cases of carcinoma of the tonsil and pharynx and used 28 specimens from cases of acute tonsillitis as controls. Three methods for HPV testing were used, dot-filter, Southern hybridization and PCR. Using the PCR results, the HPV DNA prevalence was 20.0% among cases and zero in controls [OR, ∞ (95% CI, 4.4–∞)].

(iii) Cancer of the pharynx, larynx and oesophagus

Table 46 summarizes the results of studies that included short series of cases of cancers of the pharynx, larynx, oesophagus and a miscellaneous group of other cancer sites of the head and neck. HPV DNA was detected using a variety of hybridization methods. Brandsma and Abramson (1989) tested 101 cases of carcinomas of the upper respiratory and digestive tract against a site matched group of 116 of hospital controls. For all cancer sites combined, the OR was [4.9 (95% CI, 0.93–34.4)]. In most investigations, the HPV prevalence ratio among cases was higher than 1. However none of the studies showed statistically significant differences. [The number of specimens examined in each study was small (< 50). Lack of power may explain the lack of significance of the differences observed.]

(iv) Colon cancer

In the USA, three reports from the same research group explored the presence of HPV markers in specimens of colon cancer using different techniques. Kirgan et al. (1990a,b) compared 43 cases of colorectal cancer (30 invasive and 13 in situ), 30 adenomas of the colon and 30 specimens of normal colon. The methods used initially to detect HPV were immunohistochemistry on sections from paraffin-embedded blocks followed by in-situ hybridization of the specimens that tested positive. HPV antigen prevalence was 97% among cancers, 60% among adenomas and 23% among normal controls [$p < 0.001$ for comparisons of HPV antigen between each group of cases and controls]. HPV DNA was found by in-situ hybridization in 27% of adenomas, 43% of the carcinoma specimens tested and in none of the controls. [Differences in HPV DNA prevalence were significant only for the group of carcinoma in situ (69%) and controls (0%) ($p = 0.004$)]. In a third study, L1-PCR and Southern blot were used in specimens from 38 carcinomas, 21 adenomas and 24 normal mucosa. Prevalence rates were 32% in carcinomas, 38% in adenomas and 8% in normal mucosa [OR for carcinoma, 5.7 (95% CI, 1.0–41.4); OR for adenoma, 6.8 (95% CI, 1.1–55.0)] (McGregor et al., 1993). [These studies from one laboratory are not consistent with the case series reported in section 2.2.3.]

(v) Cancer of the ovary

One study (see Table 44) (Kaufman et al., 1987) compared HPV DNA prevalence in 12 ovarian cancers and from four ovaries of women with benign disease of the ovary or uterus. Ten of the cases of ovarian cancer (83%) were HPV positive against none in the control groups [$p < 0.001$]. HPV-6b was the only type identified.

(vi) Cancer of the urinary bladder

In Japan, Anwar et al. (1992b) compared 48 specimens from bladder cancer cases with 21 specimens from normal bladder. PCR methods were used in combination with dot and Southern blot hybridization. Prevalences of HPV DNA were 81% in cases and 33% in controls [OR, 8.67 (95% CI, 2.38–33.27)]. HPV-16, -18 and -33 accounted for 62% among cases and 14 % among controls [OR, 10.0 (95% CI, 2.3–50.0)]. [These data are not consistent with the case series reported in section 2.2.3.]

(vii) Cancer of the conjunctiva

In the USA, McDonnell et al. (1986) reported the prevalence of HPV capsid antigen using immunoperoxidase staining of 50 conjunctival papillomas and 61 dysplastic conjunctival lesions (24 mild to moderate dysplasia, 37 severe dysplasia to invasive cancer). Positive staining was seen in 23 papillomas (46%) and in five dysplastic lesions (8.2%) but in none (of 20) control conjunctival sarcoidosis biopsy specimens [OR, ∞ (95% CI, 3.6–∞) and OR, ∞ (95% CI, 0.3–∞), respectively].

(viii) Lung cancer

In France, Bejui-Thivolet et al. (1990b) reported on the prevalence of HPV DNA in 10 cases of squamous-cell metaplasia and 33 cases of squamous-cell carcinoma of the bronchus. In-situ hybridization with butinylated probes types 6, 11, 16 and 18 were used on paraffin-embedded tissue. HPV-6 DNA was identified in one bronchial metaplasia. HPV DNA was found in six carcinomas (18%). HPV-18 was found in three cases, HPV-16 in one case, HPV-11 in one case and HPV-6 in one case. Ten specimens from normal mucosa and alveolar tissues were used as controls and were all negative for HPV DNA [$p = 0.18$].

2.4.3 Cofactors

Given the high prevalence of anogenital HPV infections and the relative rarity of anogenital cancers, it is worth considering those additional carcinogenic cofactors that might cause a small proportion of infected persons to progress to malignancies. The discussion of HPV 'cofactors' refers, accordingly, to exposures that accelerate or otherwise increase the rate of transition to malignancy following HPV infection, including factors that increase the likelihood that infection will persist.

Possible HPV cofactors for cervical cancer will be mentioned briefly here for completeness, but a complete summary is not attempted. The magnitude of the association between HPV and cervical neoplasia is such that even if there is confounding or effect modification from other factors, this could not explain the large relative risks seen in the epidemiological studies. The separate topic of the identification of HPV-independent factors that might cause the small proportion of apparently HPV-negative cervical cancers will not be addressed and nor will HPV as a cofactor for other cancers be described, because of the scarcity of relevant data.

To study HPV cofactors for cervical cancer requires a study group known to be exposed to HPV. Thus, the review of studies of cofactors is restricted to recent projects with reliable HPV DNA typing data and odds ratios for other factors reported within a well-defined HPV-positive stratum (Bosch *et al.*, 1992; Koutsky & Kiviat, 1993; Muñoz *et al.*, 1993; Schiffman *et al.*, 1993; Eluf-Neto *et al.*, 1994; Muñoz *et al.*, 1994; de Sanjosé *et al.*, 1994; Strickler *et al.*, 1995).

The variable 'earlier age at first sexual intercourse' has been observed to be a risk factor among HPV-positive women for both invasive cancer (Bosch *et al.*, 1992) and CIN III (Muñoz *et al.*, 1993). This sexual behavioural variable is likely a proxy for age at first exposure to HPV infection and could be reflecting 'latency' (here meaning the long time from HPV exposure to cancer diagnosis) or a 'vulnerable period' in which infection at younger ages is more carcinogenic for some reason.

High parity (e.g. more than five live births) has been consistently observed to elevate the risk among HPV-positive women of both cervical cancer (Bosch *et al.*, 1992; Eluf-Neto *et al.*, 1994) and CIN III (Muñoz *et al.*, 1993; Schiffman *et al.*, 1993). However, interpretation is complicated by the finding of similar elevations of risk associated with multiparity among apparently HPV-negative women. In epidemiological terms, parity would therefore be considered to be an 'independent' risk factor if the HPV-negative women were truly negative (a questionable assumption). Hormonal, traumatic, immunological and nutritional hypotheses have been advanced to explain the risk associated with multiparity, but there are insufficient data to decide among them.

Also suggestive of hormonal influences, the use of oral contraceptives has been found to be a possible HPV cofactor in several studies of invasive cervical cancer (Bosch *et al.*, 1992; Eluf-Neto *et al.*, 1994) and CIN III (Negrini *et al.*, 1990; Muñoz *et al.*, 1993; Schiffman *et al.*, 1993). Because of the concordant findings regarding parity and oral contraceptive use, hormonal influences can be considered the most promising candidates in the search for HPV cofactors.

Two studies (Koutsky *et al.*, 1992; de Sanjosé *et al.*, 1994) have reported that seropositivity to *Chlamydia trachomatis* is associated with an elevated risk of CIN III among HPV-positive women. Another study (Strickler *et al.*, 1995) found HTLV-1 seropositivity to be a possible viral cofactor. However, no putative viral cofactor has been associated consistently with risk in the few studies presenting relevant data, with the obvious exception of HIV-associated immunosuppression leading to an increased risk of HPV infection and CIN (and anal neoplasia). A possible etiological role of HSV-2 in cervical carcinogenesis, suggested by a previous generation of seroepidemiological case–control studies, has not been consistently observed in more recent studies that take HPV infection properly into account (Hildesheim *et al.*, 1991; Bosch *et al.*, 1992; Jha *et al.*, 1993; Koutsky & Kiviat, 1993; de Sanjosé *et al.*, 1994).

Cigarette smoking has also not been observed to be a strong HPV cofactor for either cervical cancer, despite strong *a priori* suspicions (Bosch *et al.*, 1992; Eluf-Neto *et al.*, 1994) and consistently elevated risks in case–control studies (Winkelstein, 1990), or high-grade CIN (Koutsky *et al.*, 1992; Muñoz *et al.*, 1993; Schiffman *et al.*, 1993). However, no larger epidemiological study of smoking, HPV and invasive cervical cancer has yet been performed in a geographic region where intensive smoking among women is prevalent.

In addition to a possible genotoxic role, it is also possible that smoking plays a role in immunosuppression (Barton et al., 1988) permitting an incipient HPV infection to become persistent.

At least one group has presented case–control data suggesting that relative nutritional deficiencies of folate or other micronutrients (e.g. vitamin C, carotenoids) could be an HPV cofactor (Butterworth et al., 1992). The case–control and scant clinical trial evidence for nutritional cofactors are, overall, still weak.

Immunological variables are likely to be among the most important HPV cofactors, based on the HIV immunosuppression data and animal models. Ongoing case–control and cohort studies among HPV-infected women are considering, in particular, the roles of HLA genotypes, seroreactivity, and in-vitro measurements of cell-mediated immunity (e.g. lymphocyte IL-2 production following HPV antigen challenge).

Finally, it is interesting to consider that most HPV cofactors identified in epidemiological studies have tended to distinguish high-grade CIN and invasive cervical cancer on the one hand from low-grade CIN and HPV infection on the other. Few cofactors, if any, have been observed to distinguish invasive cancer from high-grade CIN, except for the substantially older age of invasive cases (Moreno et al.,1995). This observation, if confirmed, might suggest that the risk of progression of HPV infection/low-grade CIN to prevalent, chronic CIN III is more influenced (and modifiable) by external factors than the subsequent risk of invasion, which could be stochastic and primarily dependent on time spent with CIN III.

2.5 Special populations

2.5.1 Skin cancer in patients with epidermodysplasia verruciformis (EV)

Epidermodysplasia verruciformis (EV) is a very rare, inherited condition which was first described in 1922 (Lewandowsky & Lutz, 1922). During the subsequent 60 years, approximately 250 cases were reported worldwide (Lutzner & Blanchet-Bardon, 1985). The condition is usually recognized before puberty and is characterized by widespread HPV infection and the later development of multiple cutaneous squamous-cell carcinomas, predominantly on sun-exposed sites. Basal-cell carcinomas, although described, appear to be rare, and there are no reports of increased risk of malignant melanoma in EV patients. There are no published SMRs available for skin cancer in this population, but a squamous-cell carcinoma:basal-cell carcinoma ratio of 16:1 was reported in one study of 66 EV patients. A postal questionnaire sent to Japanese doctors found that most of these EV patients had developed virus warts by the age of 10 years, whilst squamous-cell carcinoma developed between the ages of 30–50 years. The average lag time between onset of EV-type skin wart infection and squamous-cell carcinoma was 24.5 years (Tanigaki et al., 1986).

Other virus-associated diseases, including hepatitis B infection (van Voorst Vader et al., 1986; see also IARC, 1994b), genital carcinoma and Burkitt's lymphoma have been described in EV patients (Lutzner & Blanchet-Bardon, 1985). The high level of consanguinity in EV families suggests an autosomal recessive mode of inheritance (Lutzner, 1978; Tanigaki et al., 1986), but in one family the inheritance appeared to be X-linked (Androphy et al., 1985). The genetic basis of this disease is not known.

The importance of sunlight (see also IARC, 1992) in the development of EV-associated squamous-cell carcinomas is suggested by the fact that, although skin warts are found on all body sites, the carcinomas occur almost exclusively on sun-exposed sites (Tanigaki et al., 1986). Furthermore, squamous-cell carcinomas appear to develop more frequently in Caucasian EV patients living in sub-tropical and tropical climates than in temperate climates, and are rare in black EV patients. Only two of 33 (6%) black South African EV patients developed squamous-cell carcinomas [van Voorst Vader et al., 1987] compared with 40–50% of Caucasian patients living in Europe (Orth et al., 1979), 58% in Japan (Tanigaki et al., 1986) and 100% of patients living in South America (Rueda & Rodriguez, 1976).

HPV types in warts and skin cancers in EV patients

(i) Skin warts

EV patients develop a variety of skin warts. Common and plane warts (verruca vulgaris (VV) and verruca planar (VP)) are also seen in the general population, but there are also EV-specific lesions, namely red plaque-like lesions (RP) and scaly, pityriasis versicolor-like lesions (PV) (Orth et al., 1979).

Table 47 summarizes studies of HPV typing of EV-associated skin warts. All studies used hybridization methods without amplification. Reports are based on a limited number of specimens, often from single patients, and only one study includes information on control material (Jacyk et al., 1993a). Some studies do not specify the type of skin wart examined and many do not specify the number of samples examined.

VP and VV lesions appear to be associated predominantly with HPV types 3 and 10. However, the large number of HPV types found in EV lesions where the clinical type of wart has not been specified (HPV-12, -15, -21, -22, -23, -25, -46 and -47; reviewed in de Villiers, 1989) suggests that this apparent association should be interpreted with caution. Kanda et al. (1989) found no relationship between HPV type and clinical lesion. HPV-5, -8, -9, -14, -17, -20 and -38 have been found in PV-like virus warts in EV-patients. Multiple HPV types were found in PV-like lesions.

(ii) Squamous-cell carcinoma

Table 48 summarizes data available on HPV types found in EV-associated skin cancer, including single case reports and case series. Reports are based on very limited numbers of tumours and no study includes information on control material. All studies were performed using hybridization methods without amplification.

HPV-5, -8, -14, -17 and -20 have been identified in EV-associated invasive squamous-cell carcinoma, although only in a small number of samples. HPV-16 was isolated from a case of Bowen's disease of the thumb in one patient (Ostrow et al., 1987b). HPV-5, -8 and -20 DNA has been found in squamous-cell carcinoma as oligomers and monomers, some in concatemeric form (approximately 100 copies/cell) (Pfister et al., 1983b; Deau et al., 1991; Yutsudo et al., 1994). HPV-20 transcripts in squamous-cell carcinomas were demonstrated in one study (Yutsudo et al., 1994).

Both wild-type HPV-5 genomes and deleted forms have been found in primary and metastatic tumour (Ostrow et al., 1982; Yabe et al., 1989). In addition, sequence variants of the

Table 47. HPV detected by Southern blot in skin warts in EV patients

Reference	Study area	No. of lesions (No. of patients)	Clinical description	Overall HPV positivity (%)	1-3 and 10	5	8	17	20	Others[a]
Orth et al. (1979)	Europe	Multiple lesions (14)	VP	NA	+					HPV-2
			RP	NA	+					
			PV	NA						
Ostrow et al. (1982)	USA	Multiple lesions (2)	NA	NA		+				
						+				
Pfister et al. (1983b)	Turkish patient	Multiple lesions (1)	NA	NA						4 others not identified
Kremsdorf et al. (1984)	France	Multiple lesions (8)	VV/VP	NA		+	+		+	HPV-14a, -14b, -15 and -21
			PV	NA				+		HPV-19, -21, -23 and -24
Lutzner et al. (1984)	France	Multiple lesions (11)	NA	NA	+	+	+	+	+	HPV-2, -14, -22, -9 and -9-related
van Voorst Vader et al. (1986)	Netherlands	Multiple lesions (1)	NA	NA		+	+	+		HPV-19 and -24
Ostrow et al. (1987b)	USA	6 (1)	VV/VP	83	4/6					One type not identified. HPV-16 in Bowen's disease
Kanda et al. (1989)	Japan	Multiple lesions (12)	VP, VV	NA	+					HPV-14 and -38
			PV	NA		+		+	+	HPV-12, -14 and -38 (multiple HPV types in some lesions)
			RP	NA						
			RP	NA						
Jacyk & de Villiers (1993)	South Africa	Multiple lesions (20)	VP	NA	+	+			+	HPV-14 and -21
			PV	NA		+		+		
Jacyk et al. (1993a)	South Africa	Multiple lesions (5)	Seborrheic keratoses	NA		+		+		No HPV found in 10 keratoses from non-EV patients
			PV	NA		+				
			VP	NA	+	+				
Jacyk et al. (1993b)	South Africa	Multiple lesions (1)	PV	NA						HPV-9
			VV	NA						HPV-4 and -9
Yutsudo et al. (1994)	Japan	Multiple lesions (1)	PV	NA				+		HPV-38
		Multiple lesions (1)	VV, VP	NA	+				+	

VV, verruca vulgaris; VP, verruca planar; PV, pityriasis versicolor-like lesions; NA, not available; RP, red plaque-like lesions
[a] Of those types tested

Table 48. HPV detected by Southern blot in skin cancer in EV patients

Reference	Study area	No. of tumours (No. of patients)	Overall HPV positivity (%)	HPV type-specific positivity number or (%)					Comments
				5	8	17	17	20	
Ostrow et al. (1982)	USA	2 (2)		(2/2)					HPV-5 found in PV lesions, primary SCC and metastatic SCC in same patient. Wild-type and sub-genomic HPV-5 found in primary and metastatic tumour
Pfister et al. (1983b)	Turkish patient	1 (1)		(1/1)					100 copies/cell. Oligomeric DNA, some persisting in concatemeric form
Lutzner et al. (1984)	France	7 (5)		57	29				HPV-14 found in one SCC. The seven skin cancers include three cases of Bowen's disease and four cases of SCC.
Orth (1986)	International	28* (14)	96	75	17				HPV-14b (1 tumour) (approximately 100–300 copies/cell). *Whether all of these are new cases that have not been reported previously is unclear.
van Voorst Vader et al. (1986)	Netherlands	1 (1)		(1/1)					HPV-17 and -24 found in peri-lesional tissue
Ostrow et al. (1987b)	USA	1 (1)							HPV-16 found in Bowen's disease of thumb
Kanda et al. (1989)	Japan	6 (NA)	33			17	17		
Yabe et al. (1989)	Japan	1 (1)		1/1					HPV-5 found in benign lesions. Deleted forms of HPV-5 found in both primary and metastatic tumour from same patient
Yutsudo et al. (1994)	Japan	1 (1)						(1/1)	100 copies/cell. Episomal DNA as oligomers and monomers. HPV transcripts in SCC suggests infection.

EV, epidermodysplasia verruciformis; NA, not available; SCC, squamous-cell carcinoma; PV, pityriasis versicolor-like lesion

HPV-5 and -8 *E6* gene have been demonstrated in some EV-associated cancers (Deau *et al.*, 1991). The significance of these findings and their role in transformation remains unclear.

2.5.2 Studies of cancer incidence in transplant patients

Tumours that may have a viral etiology may be those that occur at high frequency in transplant recipients. The most recent cohort study comparing cancer incidence in transplant recipients with that in the general population (Birkeland *et al.*, 1995), confirms the findings of many smaller studies (see, for example, Matas *et al.*, 1975; Kinlen *et al.*, 1979). In the study of Birkeland *et al.* (1995), 5692 transplant recipients (1964–82) were followed from 1968–86 using data from the Nordic cancer registries. The transplant recipients were found to have a twofold to fivefold increased risk of many common tumours, including those of the colon, rectum, larynx and lung. A very high, 10–30-fold increase was seen for non-Hodgkin's lymphoma, skin cancer and urogenital and anogenital carcinomas.

(a) HPV infection, CIN and invasive cervical and anogenital carcinoma in transplant recipients

A number of studies have been conducted to estimate the prevalence of cervical lesions and/or HPV infection among groups of women who are immunosuppressed following renal transplantation. Some have also included control groups of immunocompetent women. The results of these studies are summarized in Table 49.

(i) HPV infection and CIN

The prevalence of cervical HPV infection in transplant recipients has been estimated at between 20 and 45%, while condylomata have been reported in 8–30% of women (Table 49).

In one study (Alloub *et al.*, 1989) in the United Kingdom, there was no significant difference between the prevalence of HPV DNA in 49 renal transplant patients attending for routine follow-up and in 69 control women from a gynaecology ward who had no history of CIN and had had a negative smear within the last two years (45% and 38%, respectively). HPV-16/18 DNA was, however, more common in the transplant recipients than controls (27% and 6%, respectively; $p < 0.005$) but there was no significant difference in the prevalence of HPV-6/11 (24% and 32%, respectively).

Two other studies have reported significantly increased rates of HPV infection in transplant recipients. In the USA, Halpert *et al.* (1986) found cytological evidence of HPV in 18 of 81 women (22%) who had received a renal transplant more than one year previously, and in only two of 81 (2.5%; $p < 0.01$) hospitalized immunocompetent women, matched to the transplant patients by age, race and age at first coitus. Fairley *et al.* (1994a) used PCR to detect HPV in 15 of 69 (22% women who had received a renal transplant in Australia more than six months previously, compared with 18 of 89 (20%) of women on dialysis therapy and one of 22 (4.5%) 'normal' women with mild renal impairment. In this latter study, five (7%) transplant recipients, 4 (4%) women on dialysis and no 'normal women' had CIN.

Schneider *et al.* (1983) reviewed the histological reports and slides from a group of 132 women who received renal transplants in Virginia, USA, between 1962 and 1979. Eleven women (8%) developed koilocytotic atypia, which is considered diagnostic of condyloma, a

Table 49. Prevalence of cervical HPV infection, CIN and invasive carcinoma of the cervix in renal allograft recipients

Reference	Area	Detection method	Number and % with HPV or lesion				Relative risk and 95% CI	Comments
			Transplant patients		Controls			
			No.	%	No.	%		
HPV Infection								
Schneider et al. (1983)	USA	Cytology (koilocytotic atypia)	11/132	8	—			
Halpert et al. (1986)	USA	Cytology	18/81	22	2/81	2.5		$p < 0.01$
MacLean et al. (1986)	New Zealand	Cytology	5/24	21	—			
Alloub et al. (1989)	United Kingdom	DNA hybridization HPV-6/11 HPV-16/18	22/49 12/49 13/49	45 24 27	26/69 22/69 4/69	38 32 6		$p < 0.005$
Gentile et al. (1991)	Italy	Cytology/histology	12/39	31	—			
Gitsch et al. (1992)	Germany	Histology (condyloma)	7/23	30	—			
Fairley et al. (1994a)	Australia	PCR (*L1* consensus primers)	15/69	22	1/22	4.5		$p = 0.05$
Invasive carcinoma								
Schneider et al. (1983)	USA		1/132	0.8	—			
MacLean et al. (1986)	New Zealand		0/24	0	—			Mean time since transplant 61 months
Fairley et al. (1994b)	Australia & New Zealand		12 cases	NA	—		SIR, 3.3 (1.7–5.8)	Mean follow-up 5.8 years
Birkeland et al. (1995)	Denmark, Finland, Norway & Sweden		28 cases	NA	—		SIR, 8.6 (5.7–13)	Mean follow-up 4.8 years

Table 49 (contd)

Reference	Area	Detection method	Number and % with HPV or lesion				Relative risk and 95% CI	Comments
			Transplant patients		Controls			
			No.	%	No.	%		
CIN								
Porreco et al. (1975)	USA		3/131	2.3	–		SIR [14 (2.8–40)]	Mean follow-up 3.6 years
Cordiner et al. (1980)	United Kingdom	Cytology/histology	5/26	19	–			After a mean of 3.8 years immunosuppression
Ingoldby et al. (1980)	United Kingdom		0/50	0	–			Three years follow-up, 1–2 cases expected
Schneider et al. (1983)	USA		6/132	4.5	–			Mean time to CIN since transplant, 38 months
Halpert et al. (1986)	USA	Cytology	10/81	12	2/81	2.5	[5.6 (1.1–38)]	Mean time since transplant, 47 months
Alloub et al. (1989)	United Kingdom	Histology	24/49	49	7/69	10	[8.5 (3.0–25)]	
Gentile et al. (1991)	Italy	Cytology/histology	1/39	2.6	–			Mean time since transplant, 77 months
Gitsch et al. (1992)	Austria	Histology	2/23	8.7	–			
David et al. (1993)	Germany		5/58	8.6	–			
Fairley et al. (1994a)	Australia	Cytology	5/69	7.2	0/22	0		

[ ] Calculated by the Working Group
CIN, cervical intraepithelial neoplasia; SIR, standardized incidence ratio

mean of 22 months after transplantation. Of these eleven women, six also developed CIN a mean of 38 months after transplantation.

Gitsch *et al.* (1992) found cervical condyloma in seven of 23 renal transplant recipients (30%), six (86%) of whom were positive for HPV by in-situ hybridization (two each for HPV-6/11, -16/18 and -31/33). In comparison, eight of 14 (56%; $p > 0.1$) immunocompetent women with cervical condyloma, matched to the transplant patients by age and parity, were HPV positive (three each for HPV-6/11 and -16/18 and two for HPV-31/33).

CIN has been detected in up to 50% of women following renal transplantation (Table 49) and a number of case–control and cohort studies have suggested a higher incidence of CIN among transplant recipients than in the general population. These studies have not, in general, reported data for HPV infection.

Porreco *et al.* (1975) identified 131 women four months following renal transplantation in Colorado, USA. During an average of 3.6 years follow-up, three women developed intra-epithelial carcinoma of the cervix, compared with 0.22 expected on the basis of rates in Colorado, giving a standardized incidence ratio (SIR) of 14 [95% CI, 2.8–40].

Ingoldby *et al.* (1980) followed 50 women who had received renal transplants in the United Kingdom. There were no new cases of CIN during an average of three years of follow-up while one or two cases would have been expected.

In the study of Halpert *et al.* (1986) described above, 12% of renal transplant recipients had CIN compared with 2.5% of the matched control group [crude OR, 5.6 (95% CI, 1.1–38)]. In the study of Alloub *et al.* (1989) described above, 49% of transplant recipients had CIN, compared with 10% of the control group [OR, 8.5 (95% CI, 3.0–25)]. Blessing *et al.* (1990) used in-situ hybridization to test for HPV-4–6, -8, -11, -16 and -18 in 22 samples from seven women with cervical, vaginal and vulvar intraepithelial lesions. HPV-6 was identified in one sample, HPV-16 in 12 samples (from six patients) and HPV-18 in four samples (from three patients).

(ii) Invasive carcinoma

Two cohort studies have followed large groups of patients following renal transplantation. Fairley *et al.* (1994b) followed a cohort of 15 820 patients (8785 men and 7035 women) identified through the Australia and New Zealand Dialysis and Transplant Registry. A total of 8215 patients had received renal transplants and 7605 were on dialysis therapy between 1976 and 1992. The cohort was followed for cancer incidence until March 1992 and the expected numbers of cancers were calculated from national rates. Twelve women who had received renal transplants developed cervical cancer giving an SIR of 3.3 (95% CI, 1.7–5.8) compared with two women on dialysis therapy (SIR, 0.74 (95% CI, 0.1–1.2)).

Birkeland *et al.* (1995) identified 2369 women who had received renal transplants in Denmark, Finland, Norway and Sweden from 1964 to 1982. They were followed until 1986 and expected numbers of cancers were calculated based on the national rates. Twenty eight women developed cervical cancer, giving an SIR of 8.6 (95% CI, 5.7–13).

(iii) Other anogenital cancers

Few case series define and, therefore, reliably document the incidence of anogenital carcinoma in transplant recipients, but it does appear to be higher than that seen in the general population. In one series, Penn (1986) found that patients with anogenital carcinoma accounted for 2.8% (65/2150) of tumours in transplant recipients compared with 0.5% of tumours in the general population.

In two cohort studies (Fairley et al., 1994b; Birkeland et al., 1995), the incidence of anogenital cancer in renal transplant recipients has been reported to be between 2.1 and 56 times that expected from rates in the general population (Table 50). In one study (Fairley et al., 1994b), this excess was seen only in patients who had received renal transplants, and not in those on dialysis therapy; SIR for transplant and dialysis patients were as follows: vulvar cancer, 56 (95% CI, 36–83) and 4.2 (95% CI, 0.4–12), respectively; penile cancer, 24 (95% CI, 6.4–60) and no case observed but 0.23 expected; anal cancer, 40 (95% CI, 11–102) and no case observed but 0.13 expected.

Table 50. Incidence from cohort studies of anogenital carcinomas among renal transplant recipients

Reference	Country	Population (follow-up)	Cancer site	Sex	SIR	95% CI	Comments
Birkeland et al. (1995)	Denmark, Finland, Norway and Sweden	2369 women 3323 men (1964–86)	Vulva/vagina Rectum Rectum	F M F	31 4.5 2.6	15–55 2.3–7.9 0.7–6.6	11 observed 12 observed 4 observed
Fairley et al. (1994b)	Australia and New Zealand	7035 women 8785 men (1976–92)	Vulva Anus Penis	F M + F M	56 40 24	36–83 11–102 6.4–60	24 observed 4 observed 4 observed

The prevalence of anal HPV-16 infection has been determined in only one series of transplant patients using a PCR technique on anal biopsy material (Ogunbiyi et al., 1994b). HPV DNA was found in 36 of 76 biopsies from transplant patients (47%) compared with 18 of 145 biopsies from controls (12%; $p < 0.05$). Anogenital intraepithelial neoplasia was found in 26/133 patients compared with 1/145 control subjects ($p < 0.05$). Anogenital carcinoma was found in only one transplant patient and in no control in this series. HPV-6/11, -16/18 and -5 were found in one further giant anal condyloma using immunocytochemistry, in-situ hybridization, Southern blot and PCR (Soler et al., 1992). Only one report exists for HPV typing in anogenital carcinoma. This study, of a single case of a metastatic perianal squamous-cell carcinoma in a transplant recipient, documents integration of HPV-11 in both primary and metastatic tumour (Manias et al., 1989).

(b) HPV DNA in transplant-associated skin lesions

(i) Skin warts

Individual case reports document the presence of multiple HPV types, including EV-associated types, in skin warts of transplant recipients. These include HPV-2 (Euvrard et al., 1991; Purdie et al., 1993), HPV-5/8 (Lutzner et al., 1983; Purdie et al., 1993), HPV-27 (Ostrow et al., 1989b) and HPV-49 (Favre et al., 1989).

Table 51 summarizes the results of larger studies of transplant-associated virus warts (> 5 lesions). In studies using in-situ hybridization or Southern blot, the overall detection rate of HPV DNA where multiple probes were employed ranged from 20% to 82%, with most studies

Table 51. Prevalence of HPV DNA in skin warts of transplant recipients

Reference	Study area	Detection method (types included)	No. of cases	Overall HPV positivity (%)*	HPV type-specific positivity				Other HPV types (no. of lesions)	Comments
					1–4/10	5/8	6/11	16/18		
Gassenmaier et al. (1986)	Germany	Southern blot (1, 2, 3, 4, 5/8, 16/18)	16	8/16 (50)	6/16	1/16	1/16		–	Paraffin-embedded tissue
Rüdlinger et al. (1986)	United Kingdom	Southern blot (1–4, 10, 5, 6/11, 16)	54	39/54 (72)	39/54	0/54	0/54		–	Frozen tissue. Multiple HPV types found in single lesions. No control warts examined
Barr et al. (1989)	United Kingdom	Dot blot and Southern blot (1, 2, 4, 5/8)	77	NA	NA	12/77			–	Frozen tissue. No control virus warts examined
Wilson et al. (1989)	United Kingdom	Southern blot (1, 2, 3, 4, 5, 8)	18	13/18 (72)	9/18	0/18			4/18 not further characterized	Frozen tissue. Viral genome in HPV-2 warts showed polymorphism at PvuII and PstI sites.
Blessing et al. (1990)	United Kingdom	In-situ hybridization (4, 5, 8)	20	4/20 (20)	0/20	4/20			–	Frozen tissue. Simple warts, dysplastic warts and EV-like lesions (3) studied. No specimen contained > 1 HPV type. No control wart samples
Euvrard et al. (1993)	France	In-situ hybridization (1a, 2a, 5, 16/18)	17	14/17 (82)	9/17	0/17	10/17		–	Frozen and paraffin-embedded tissue. Multiple HPV types found in single lesions. No control warts examined
Soler et al. (1993)	France	Southern blot, in-situ hybridization and PCR (5, 6/11, 16/18, 1a, 2a)	18 (transplant) 3 (non-transplant)	11/18 (61) 0/3 (0)	1/18 0/3	1/18 0/3	4/18 0/3		–	Frozen tissue
Trenfield et al. (1993)	Australia	Southern blot (1, 2, 3, 4, 5/8, 10, 11, 16/18, 41)	18	5/18 (28)	5/18	0/18	0/18		–	Frozen tissue
Hepburn et al. (1994)	New Zealand	Dot blot (1–5, 6/11, 8, 41, 48, 49)	44 (36 patients)	19 (43)	26/44	4/44	5/44		41 (1)	Multiple types found in some lesions
Pélisson et al. (1994)	France	In-situ hybridization (1a, 2a, 5, 6a, 11a, 16 and 18)	8 (transplant) 7 (non-transplant controls) 7 (non-transplant normal skin)	5/8 (63) 4/7 (57) 0/7 (0)	4/8 4/7 0/7	1/8 0/7 0/7	4/8 0/7 0/7		– – –	Frozen tissue. Simple warts examined. Multiple HPV types found in single lesions

Table 51 (contd)

Reference	Study area	Detection method (types included)	No. of cases	Overall HPV positivity (%)	HPV type-specific positivity[a]			Other HPV types (no. of lesions)	Comments
					1–4/10	5/8	6/11 16/18		
Shamanin et al. (1994a)	United Kingdom	PCR and direct sequencing (1–4, 10, 5/8, 6/11, 16/18 and others)	50	28 (60)	2/50	0/50	1/50	27 (6), 28 (2), 57 (1), 12 (1), 15 (1), 17 (2), 25 (1), 29 (4), 49 (1), uncharacterized (14)	Frozen tissue. Benign warts and EV-like lesions (3) studied. No control warts examined
Stark et al. (1994)	United Kingdom	Southern blot and PCR (1, 2, 5/8, 6/11, 16/18 and others)	18 (transplant) 6 (non-transplant)	10/18 (55) 2/6 (33)	4/18 2/6	3/18 0/6	3/18 0/6	0/18 0/6	Frozen tissue

NA, not available; PCR, polymerase chain reaction; EV, epidermodysplasia verruciformis
[a] Of those types tested

identifying HPV DNA in over 60% of lesions. Three studies employed PCR amplification and, in these, the detection rate was between 55 and 61%. The failure to detect HPV DNA in a number of skin warts, even in studies employing PCR, suggests that the results should be interpreted with caution. Since control skin warts from immunocompetent patients were not employed in many studies, it is not known whether this reflects the limitations of the methods employed or a potential reservoir of currently unknown, and therefore undetectable, HPV types in transplant recipients.

Common skin-associated HPV types 1, 2, 3, 4 and 10 were by far the most common types to be identified in skin warts in studies where probes for these HPV types were employed. When the data from these studies, which used different methodologies, were combined, HPV-1, -2, -3, -4 or -10 were found in 80/237 (34%) of transplant samples and in 6/16 (38%) of control samples [$p = 0.95$]. Mucosal HPV types 6/11 and 16/18 were found in 23/199 (11%) of transplant samples and in 0/16 (0%) of controls where probes detecting these HPV types were employed [$p = 0.32$]. HPV-5/8 was found in 22/314 (7%) of transplant samples and in 0/16 (0%) of controls [$p = 0.65$]. Similarly, one recent study found EV-related HPV types (not further characterized) in 14/50 (28%) of skin warts and common skin-associated HPV types in only 2/50 (4%) of skin warts [$p = 0.05$] (Shamanin et al., 1994a).

(ii) Verrucous keratoses (precancerous lesions)

Table 52 summarizes HPV DNA prevalence in case series (> 5 lesions) of verrucous keratoses. Only three case–control studies have been carried out and the numbers examined were small.

HPV DNA detection rates in transplant-associated verrucous keratoses in studies employing Southern blot or in-situ hybridization without amplification were 0–40%, with most studies detecting HPV DNA in approximately 20–30%. In studies employing PCR, detection rates were 0–73% but in three of these, in which multiple probes were employed, HPV DNA detection rates were between 24 and 73% (Shamanin et al., 1994a; Stark et al., 1994; Tieben et al., 1994).

Combining data from studies using probes designed to detect type-specific HPV, albeit using different methodologies showed that, overall, common skin-associated HPV types 1–4 and 10 were found in 27/219 (12%) of transplant samples compared to 4/23 (17%) of control samples [$p = 0.68$]. HPV types 5/8 were found in 16/292 (5.4%) of transplant samples and 2/36 (5.6%) of control [$p < 0.5$], and mucosal HPV types 6/11 and 16/18 were found in 23/231 (10%) of transplant samples and 0/36 (0%) of control samples [$p = 0.05$].

(iii) Squamous-cell carcinoma

Table 53 summarizes HPV DNA prevalence in case series of transplant-associated squamous-cell carcinoma. Only two case–control studies have been performed and the numbers examined are small.

HPV DNA detection rates for studies employing Southern blot and in-situ hybridization without amplification in transplant squamous-cell carcinomas ranged from 5–100%. Studies employing PCR identified HPV DNA in 0–81% of lesions. In one case–control study employing PCR and multiple probes, HPV DNA was found in 2/9 (22%) of control squamous-cell carcinomas compared with 10/30 (33%) of transplant-associated squamous-cell carcinomas (Stark et al., 1994).

Table 52. Prevalence of HPV DNA in verrucous keratoses of transplant recipients

Reference	Study area	Detection method (types included)	No. of cases	Overall HPV positivity (%)[a]	HPV-type specific positivity				Comments
					1–4/10	5/8	6/11 16/18	Others	
Rüdlinger et al. (1986)	United Kingdom	In-situ hybridization (1a, 2, 3, 4, 5/8, 6/11, 16)	11	1/11 (9)	1/11	0/11	0/11	–	Frozen tissue. No control samples examined
Barr et al. (1989)	United Kingdom	Dot blot (1, 2, 4, 5/8)	NA	NA	NA	7/44	NA	NA	–
Blessing et al. (1990)	United Kingdom	In-situ hybridization (4, 5/8)	19	5/19 (26)	2/19	3/19	–	–	Frozen tissue. No control samples examined
Euvrard et al. (1991)	France	In-situ hybridization (1, 2, 5, 16/18)	7	0/7 (0)	0/7	0/7	0/7	–	Frozen tissue
Viac et al. (1992)	France	In-situ hybridization (multiple probes)	11	4/11 (36)	2/11	0/11	0/11	Uncharacterized HPV types (2/11)	Frozen tissue
Euvrard et al. (1993)	France	In-situ hybridization (1, 2, 5, 16/18)	21	5/21 (24)	5/21	1/19	3/21	–	Multiple HPV types identified in single lesions. No control tissue examined
Soler et al. (1993)	France	Southern blot, in-situ hybridization and PCR (1, 2, 3, 4, 5/8, 6/11, 16/18)	18	11/18 (61)	4/18	1/18	15/18	–	Frozen tissue. Multiple HPV types found in single lesions
Trendfield et al. (1993)	Australia	Southern blot (1, 2, 3, 4, 5/8, 11, 16/18)	26	4/26 (15)	3/26	1/26	0/26	–	Frozen tissue
McGregor et al. (1994)	United Kingdom	PCR (5/8, 6/11, 16/18)	31 (transplant) 13 (non-transplant)	0/31 (0) 0/13 (0)	– –	0/31 0/13	0/31 0/13	–	Paraffin-embedded tissue
Pélisson et al. (1994)	France	In-situ hybridization (1, 2a, 3, 4, 5, 6a/11a, 16/18)	10 (transplant) 2 (non-transplant)	4/10 (40) 0/2 (0)	2/10 0/2	1/10 0/2	4/10 0/2	–	Frozen tissue. Multiple HPV types found in single lesions

Table 52 (contd)

Reference	Study area	Detection method (types included)	No. of cases	Overall HPV positivity (%)[a]	HPV type-specific detected				Comments
					1–4/10	5/8	6/11 16/18	Others	
Shamanin et al. (1994a)	United Kingdom	Southern blot and PCR (1–4, 10, 5/8, 6/11, 16/18 and others)	29	29/40 (73)	2/40	0/40	0/40	HPV-9, -15, -17, -20, -27, -29 and -49 found in 10/40 lesions. Uncharacterized HPV types found in 7/40 further lesions	Frozen tissue. No control samples studied
Stark et al. (1994)	United Kingdom	Southern blot and PCR (1, 2, 3, 4, 5/8, 6/11, 16/18)	46 (transplant) 21 (non-transplant)	11/46 (24) 4/21 (19)	5/46 3/21	2/46 2/21	1/46 0/21	Unknown HPV types (3/46)	Frozen tissue. No control samples examined
Tieben et al. (1994)	Netherlands	PCR and direct sequencing (multiple probes)	10	3/10 (30)	1/10	0/10	0/10	HPV type 36 (1/10). Uncharacterized HPV type (1/10)	Frozen tissue. No control samples

PCR, polymerase chain reaction; NA, not available
[a] Of those tested

Table 53. Prevalence of HPV DNA in squamous-cell carcinoma of transplant recipients

Reference	Study area	No. of cases	HPV detection method (types included)	Overall HPV positivity (%)ª	HPV type-specific positivity				Comments
					1–4/10	5/8	6/11 16/18	Other types	
Barr et al. (1989)	United Kingdom	25	Dot blot (1, 2, 4, 5/8)	16/25 (64)	1/25	15/25	–	–	Frozen tissue from five patients
Magee et al. (1989)	Texas, USA	8	In-situ hybridization (1–4, 16/18, 6/11)	8/8 (100)	0/8	–	8/8	–	–
Blessing et al. (1990)	United Kingdom	11	In-situ hybridization (4, 5/8)	2/11 (18)	2/11	0/11	–	–	Frozen tissue
Dyall-Smith et al. (1991)	United Kingdom	188	PCR amplification (1–4, 5, 7, 9, 11, 16/18, 19, 25)	0/188 (0)	0/188	0/188	0/188	–	Frozen tissue. No control SCC studied
Viac et al. (1992)	France	8	In-situ hybridization (multiple probes)	2/8 (25)	1/8	0/8	1/8	–	–
Euvrard et al. (1993)	France	46	In-situ hybridization (1, 2, 5, 16/18)	25/46 (54)	20/46	2/46	15/46	–	Frozen tissue. Multiple HPV types found in single lesions. No control samples studied
Purdie et al. (1993)	United Kingdom	10	Dot blot and Southern blot (1–4, 10, 5/8, 6/11, 16/18)	6/10 (60)	2/10	2/10	0/10	Unknown HPV types (4/10)	–
Smith et al. (1993)	Australia	20	PCR amplification (probes not specified)	0/20 (0)	–	–	–	–	–
Soler et al. (1993)	France	26	Southern blot, PCR and in-situ hybridization (1–4, 5/8, 6/11, 16/18)	21/26 (81)	0/26	6/26	20/26	–	Frozen tissue. Multiple HPV types found in single lesions
Trenfield et al. (1993)	Australia	40	Southern blot (multiple probes)	2/40 (5)	1/40	0/40	0/40	HPV-36 found in 1 SCC	Frozen tissue
Pélisson et al. (1994)	France	13	In-situ hybridization (1a, 2a, 5, 6a/11a, 16/18)	8/13 (62)	3/13	1/13	7/13	–	–
McGregor et al. (1994)	United Kingdom	14 transplant 22 non-transplant	PCR amplification (5/8, 6/11, 16/18)	0/14 (0) (transplant) 0/22 (0) (non-transplant)	– –	0/14 0/22	0/14 0/22	–	Frozen tissue. No control SCC studied Paraffin-embedded material

Table 53 (contd)

Reference	Study area	No. of cases	HPV detection method (types included)	Overall HPV positivity (%)[a]	HPV type-specific positivity			Other types	Comments
					1-4/10	5/8	6/11 16/18		
Shamanin et al. (1994a)	United Kingdom	23	Southern blot and PCR (1, 2, 3, 5, 7, 10, 37, 40)	17/23 (74)	0/23	0/23	0/23	HPV-27, -29 and -47 found in 5/23 SCC. Unknown types were found in a further 8/23 SCC.	Frozen tissue. No control samples examined
Stark et al. (1994)	United Kingdom	30 transplant patients 9 controls	Southern blot and PCR (1-4, 5/8, 6/11, 16/18)	10/30 (33) (transplant) 2/9 (22) (control)	3/30 1/9	0/30 1/9	2/30 0/9	Unknown HPV types identified in 6/30 SCC	Frozen samples
Tieben et al. (1994)	Netherlands	24	PCR and direct sequencing (multiple probes)	5/24 (21)	1/24	1/24	0/24	HPV-14 found in 2/24 SCC. Unknown types found in 2/24 SCC	Frozen tissue
Berkhout et al. (1995)	Netherlands	53	PCR (degenerate nested primer, direct sequencing)	43/53 (81)	0/53	0/53	0/53	HPV-24 (1) HPV-19 (1) HPV-20 (3) HPV-25 (2) HPV-15 (9) HPV-38 (1) HPV-23 (3) Undefined (15)	Multiple HPV types found in some lesions

PCR, polymerase chain reaction; SCC, squamous-cell carcinoma
[a] Of those types tested

Combining the data from these studies, as above, showed common skin-associated HPV types 1–4 and 10 were found in 34/452 (7%) of transplant and 1/9 (11%) of control samples. HPV-5/8 was found in 27/458 (6%) of transplant and 1/31 (3%) of non-transplant samples. Mucosal HPV types 6/11 and 16/18 were found in 53/430 (12%) of transplant and 0/31 (0%) of controls. In three studies in which multiple probes were employed, a number of other HPV types, including HPV-36, -27, -29, -47 and -14, were identified in some squamous-cell carcinomas (Shamanin et al., 1994a; Stark et al., 1994; Tieben et al., 1994). A study using nested primers specifically designed to detect EV HPV types found a broad spectrum of these types in 81% (43) of squamous-cell carcinomas, including HPV-15, -19, -20, -23, -24, -25 and -38. The significance of these findings and their role in transformation remains unclear (Berkhout et al., 1995).

(iv) Basal-cell carcinoma

Table 54 summarizes HPV DNA prevalence in a small number of case series and one case–control study of basal-cell carcinoma. Detection rates were between 0% and 100% but the numbers of tumours were very small. Combining the data from these studies, as above, showed common skin-associated HPV types 1–4 and 10 were found in 4/20 (20%) of transplant basal-cell carcinomas. HPV types 5/8 were not identified in any of 31 transplant basal-cell carcinomas or of 15 control basal-cell carcinomas. HPV types 16/18 were found in 3/31 (10%) of transplant basal-cell carcinomas in one study (Pélisson et al., 1994) and in none of 15 control basal-cell carcinomas in another study (McGregor et al., 1994).

(c) HPV infection and cancer at other sites

There are few reports of HPV infection in association with cancer at other sites in transplant recipients. Querci della Rovere et al. (1988) documented HPV-11 infection in a case of bladder cancer in a renal-transplant recipient. In two series of bladder cancer patients, HPV infection (HPV-16/18) was only found in one patient in each series (of 10 and 22 patients, respectively) who had received a renal transplant (Kitamura et al., 1988; Maloney et al., 1994).

HPV was identified in one malignant melanoma in an immunosuppressed patient but not in 35 other malignant melanoma specimens from immunocompetent patients (Scheurlen et al., 1986b). Other case reports documented HPV-16 in an oropharyngeal carcinoma following cardiac transplantation (Demetrick et al., 1990), HPV-16 in a carcinoma of the tongue (Lookingbill et al., 1987) and HPV-2 in a spinocerebellar tumour following renal transplantation (Sassolas et al., 1991). Koilocytosis and hyperkeratosis suggestive of HPV infection were reported in three cases of head and neck cancer following renal, cardiac and bone-marrow transplantation (Bradford et al., 1990).

2.5.3 Studies in HIV-infected persons

Infection with human immunodeficiency virus (HIV) leads to a profound alteration of the immune function that differs from that of most other immunosuppressive conditions in being increasingly severe over a period of a few to many years. There are several possible mechanisms by which HIV could affect the natural history of HPV and related neoplasia, see Figure 18. HIV-induced immunosuppression might reactivate latent HPV infection and lead to higher HPV

Table 54. Prevalence of HPV DNA in basal-cell carcinoma of transplant recipients

Reference	Study area	No. of cases	HPV detection method (including types)	Overall HPV positivity (%)[a]	HPV type-specific positivity 1–4/10	5/8	6/11, 16/18	Other types	Comments
Rüdlinger et al. (1986)	United Kingdom	1	Southern blot (1–4, 5/8, 6/11, 16)	0/1 (0)	0/1	0/1	0/1	–	–
Obalek et al. (1988)	–	2	Southern blot (1, 4, 5, 10, 11, 16/38)	2/2 (100)	2/2	0/2	0/2	–	–
Euvrard et al. (1993)	France	2	In-situ hybridization (mixed probe)	0/2 (0)	0/2	0/2	0/2	–	–
Trenfield et al. (1993)	Australia	11	Southern blot (1–4, 5/8, 11, 16/18)	1/11 (9)	1/11	0/11	0/11	–	–
McGregor et al. (1994)	United Kingdom	11 (transplant) 15 (non-transplant)	PCR amplification (5/8, 6/11, 16/18)	0/11 (0) (transplant) 0/15 (0) (non-transplant)	–	0/11 0/15	0/11 0/15	–	Paraffin embedded tissue
Pélisson et al. (1994)	France	4	In-situ hybridization (1, 2, 5, 6/11, 16/18)	3/4 (75)	1/4	0/4	3/4	–	Frozen tissue. No control BCC samples
Shamanin et al. (1994a)	United Kingdom	5	PCR and direct sequencing (degenerate primers designed to detect a range of cutaneous HPV types)	3/5 (60)	0/5	0/5	0/5	X	Frozen tissue
Tieben et al. (1994)	Netherlands	4	PCR (four consensus primers designed to detect cutaneous HPV types)	0/4 (0)	0/4	0/4	0/4	0/4	Frozen tissue

PCR, polymerase chain reaction; BCC, basal-cell carcinoma; X, uncharacterized HPV types
[a] Of those types tested

replication, and this would be important if a dose–response situation exists for the carcinogenic potential of HPV-infection. It is also possible that severe immunosuppression might influence directly the risk of progression from a premalignant to a malignant stage. Finally, it is theoretically possible that HIV could have a direct oncogenic potential but there is little evidence to support such a model of association.

Figure 18. Possible interactions between HIV-induced immunosuppresion and HPV infection in carcinogenesis

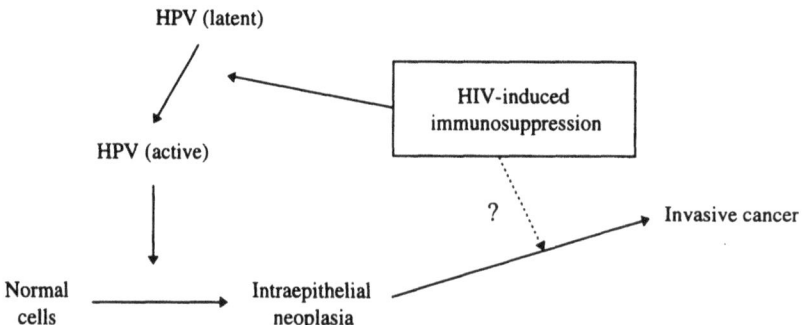

Research attempting to disentangle the potential relationship between HIV and HPV-associated malignancy has so far been primarily based on small cross-sectional and case–control studies of populations at particular risk of HIV-infection, with precancerous lesions rather than invasive neoplasm as the outcome of interest. The short existence of the HIV epidemic, the initial male predominance in many societies and the young populations at risk have, in particular, limited the possibilities for studying large numbers of HIV-infected women, especially those with cancer. The ability to control for confounding is particularly relevant while studying the influence of HIV on HPV-related malignancy. Not only are both HIV and most known high-risk types of HPV sexually transmitted, but HIV-infected persons have a lifestyle that for other reasons may increase their risk of certain cancers. The small sample size in many of the published studies among HIV-infected subjects limits their possibility to adequately control for behavioural covariates and risk factors associated with HIV infection.

(a) Studies of the uterine cervix

The influence of HIV on HPV expression and HPV-associated malignancy of the uterine cervix has been dealt with in a limited number of review papers (Palefsky, 1991; Rabkin & Blattner, 1991; Sillman & Sedlis, 1991; Northfelt & Palefsky, 1992; Braun, 1994; Stratton & Ciacco, 1994).

(i) Precancerous lesions

Table 55 summarizes the studies on precancerous lesions. In the late 1980s, the first case reports and case series were published suggesting an association between HIV-induced immuno-

Table 55. Prevalence of HPV in precancerous lesions of the uterine cervix in HIV-infected persons

Reference and study area	HIV positive, number and type	HIV negative, number and type	HPV prevalence %	Odds ratio (95% CI)	Cervical abnormality %	Odds ratio (95% CI)	HPV test (types)	Pathology reading	Comments
Byrne et al. (1989) United Kingdom	19 recruited from HIV+ STD-clinic attendees		95		3 CIN III 1 CIN II 1 atypia 1 SPI 1 HPV		Observed at colposcopy	Pap smear and biopsy	Prevalence of HPV in lower genital tract
Schrager et al. (1989) USA	35 IVDU and partners of IVDU	23 IVDU and partners of IVDU	HIV+, 26 HIV−, 4	7.6 (0.9–65)	Squamous atypia HIV+, 31 HIV−, 4	10 (1.2–85)	Cytological or histopathological findings	Pap smear	HIV-infected: fewer used barrier contraceptives, more had had STD.
Feingold et al. (1990) USA	35 IVDU and partners of IVDU	32 IVDU and partners of IVDU	HIV+, 49 HIV−, 25	2.8 (1.0–8.0)	SIL HIV+, 40 HIV−, 9	6.4 (1.6–25)	Southern blot (cervicovaginal lavage)	Pap smear	More non-whites among HIV-positive women
Schäfer et al. (1991) Germany	111 gynaecological in-patients or HIV infection	76 IVDU	HIV+, 48 HIV−, 20	[3.7 (1.9–7.3)]	Dysplasia or neoplasia HIV+, 41 HIV−, 9	[7.0 (2.9–17)]	Cytology	Pap smear	Crude odds-ratio
Vermund et al. (1991) USA	51	45	HIV+, 53 symptomatic, 70 asymptomatic, 22 HIV−, 22	[3.9 (1.6–9.6)]	SIL Symptomatic HIV+, 42 Asymptomatic HIV+, 17 HIV−, 13	[8.1 (2.9–22)] [1.0 (0.3–3.7)] 4.6 (0.8–28)	Southern blot (11, 16, 18) (lavage)	Pap smear	Extension of study by Feingold et al. (1990)
Kreiss et al. (1992) Nairobi, Kenya	147 prostitutes	51 prostitutes	HIV+, 37 HIV−, 24	1.7 (0.8–3.6)*	CIN Overall HIV+ HPV+, 26 HPV−, 24 HIV+ HPV+, 47 HPV−, 9 HIV− HPV+, 57 HPV−, 7	0.9 (0.2–3.5)* 9.4 (1.7–52) 17 (1.4–217)	Dot blot/Southern blot (6, 11, 16, 18, 31, 33, 35)	Cytology	*Adjusted for age and years of prostitution. Women with CIN and HPV: 6/11, 4 cases 16/18, 4 cases unknown, 5 cases

Table 55 (contd)

Reference and study area	HIV positive, number and type	HIV negative, number and type	HPV prevalence %	Odds ratio (95% CI)	Cervical abnormality %	Odds ratio (95% CI)	HPV test (types)	Pathology reading	Comments
Laga et al. (1992) Kinshasa, Zaire	47 prostitutes	48 prostitutes	HIV+, 38 HIV−, 8 HIV+/CIN+, 73 HIV+/CIN−, 30	6.8 (1.9–26.8) 6.2 [1.3–29]	CIN HIV+, 27 HIV−, 3	15 (1.8–95)	ViraType™ Southern blot (low stringency) (6,11,16,18,31,33, 35)	Cytology	13 Pap smears inadequate for interpretation
ter Meulen et al. (1992) Tanzania	46 gynaecological in-patients	313 gynaecological in-patients	Any type: HIV+, 78 HIV−, 56 Type 16/18 HIV+, 30 HIV−, 14	HPV (total)* 2.52 (p = 0.02) HPV 16/18 2.42 (p = 0.02)	HIV+, 2.4 HIV−, 2.8		PCR (consensus primer and type-specific, 16, 18)	Pap smear	*Adjusted for age
Conti et al. (1993) Italy	273 former IVDU	161 former IVDU			HIV+, 42 HIV−, 8	4.2 (2.1–8.4)* HPV−/HIV+ 1.2 [p > 0.05] HPV−/HIV− 11 (2.8–42) HPV+/HIV+ 64 (19–214)	Cytological diagnosis	Cytology confirmed by biopsy	Cross-sectional study, potential selection bias (inflated) *Adjusted for age and number of sexual partners CIN II–III/HIV+: CD4+ count< 500/mm³ versus CD4+ ≥ 500/mm³, 5.4 (2.6–11)
Maggwa et al. (1993) Nairobi, Kenya	205 attendees of family-planning clinic	3853 attendees of family-planning clinic			HIV+, 4.9 HIV−, 1.9	2.8 (1.3–5.9)		Cytology	Adjusted for age, sexual behaviour and demographic variables
Ho et al. (1994) New York, USA	97 IVDU, HIV-related diseases, or partners of IVDU	110 IVDU, HIV-related diseases, or partners of IVDU	All HPV types HIV−, 23 HIV+, 50 CD4+% > 20, 45 CD4+% ≤ 20, 61 Types 16,18,31,33, 35 HIV−, 6.4 HIV+, 14	3.3 (1.8–6.1) 2.8 (1.3–6.0) 5.3 (2.2–13) 3.5 (1.3–9.2)			Southern blot hybridization		Strong HPV signal HIV−, 1.0 HIV+ CD4+% > 20, 2.6 (0.62–11) CD4+% < 20, 5.9 (1.4–25) Includes some persons previously studied by Vermund et al. (1991).

Table 55 (contd)

Reference and study area	HIV positive, number and type	HIV negative, number and type	HPV prevalence %	Odds ratio (95% CI)	Cervical abnormality %	Odds ratio (95% CI)	HPV test (types)	Pathology reading	Comments
Klein et al. (1994) New York, USA	114 IVDU, or HIV-positive partners	139 IVDU, or HIV-positive partners			HIV−, 10 HIV+, 22 CD4% > 20, 17 CD4% ≤ 20, 35 *Multivariate analysis* HPV infection High-risk HPV Strong HPV signal Low CD4+	2.5 (1.2–5.1) 1.8 (0.7–4.6) 4.8 (2.0–12) 6.8 (2.9–15.7) 12 (4.1–34) 10.8 (3.5–33.7) 3.1 (1.0–9.5)	Southern blot hybridization	Cytology	No demographic or behavioural variables associated with SIL. Included persons studied by Vermund et al. (1990) and Ho et al. (1994)
Seck et al. (1994) Dakar, Senegal	HIV-1, 18 HIV-2, 17 from infectious disease clinic	58 women in infectious disease clinic	*HIV-1* STH, 19 PCR, 75 *HIV-2* STH, 47 PCR, 73 *HIV−* STH, 4 PCR, 2	6.4 (0.6–80) 11.5 (2.7–56) 24.1 (3.5–257) 10.5 (24–52)	*HIV-1 versus HIV* normal dysplasia *HIV-2 versus HIV* normal dysplasia	1 23.3 (2.9–205) 1 9.3 (1.1–79)	Southern transfer hybridization (6,11,16,18,31,33, 35) PCR (consensus primer)	Cytology	
Williams et al. (1994) San Francisco, USA	55 IVDU	59 IVDU	*Dot blot* HIV+, 19 HIV−, 5 *PCR* HIV+, 57 HIV−, 13	4.2 (1.0–25) 8.9 (3.2–27)	9/11 SIL in HIV+	6.1 (1.2–61)	ViraType™ and PCR	Cytology	Recruited from larger cohort (see also Table 56)
Wright et al. (1994a) New York, USA	398 attendees of AIDS clinics, STD-clinics, methadone clinics	357 same	HIV+, 61 HIV−, 36 $p < 0.01$		*CIN I* HIV−, 4 HIV+, 13 *CIN II–III* HIV−, 1 HIV+, 7	[4.3 (2.3–8.1)] [15 (3.6–64)]	PCR L1 consensus primers	Cytology + histology (biopsy)	Independent variables in multiple regression model for CIN risk: HPV-DNA, HIV-positivity, CD4+ < 200/mm³ and > 34 years of age

[ ] Calculated by the Working Group
CIN, cervical intraepithelial neoplasia; SIL, squamous intraepithelial lesion; IVDU, intravenous drug users; STH, Southern transfer hybridization; PCR, polymerase chain reaction; STD, sexually transmitted disease; SPI, subclinical papillomavirus infection; Pap, Papanicolaou; CD4+, CD4 cells

suppression and cervical intraepithelial neoplasia (Bradbeer, 1987). Henry et al. (1989) reported mild to moderate dysplasia with atypical condyloma in all of their first four consecutively identified HIV-positive women at a medical centre in Minnesota, USA.

Byrne et al. (1989) re-examined 19 of 36 women diagnosed with HIV-positivity after routine testing became available at St Mary's Hospital in London. Seven (37%) cervical smears were reported to be abnormal, out of which four (21%) were histologically verified as intraepithelial neoplasia (Table 55). Disease at more than one site was detected in half of the patients, and, overall, 18 (95%) showed evidence of clinical/subclinical HPV infection of the lower genital tract (including vagina, vulva, perineum). The disease would have remained undetected in more than half of the group had colposcopy not been undertaken. Nine of the women were intravenous drug abusers.

In an analysis of cervicovaginal smears with the cytopathologist blinded to the subject's viral status, a significantly higher percentage of cytological squamous atypia was documented in HIV-positive (11/35; 31%) compared to HIV-negative women (1/23; 4%) (Schrager et al., 1989). Furthermore, cytological or histopathological findings suggestive of HPV infection were observed in 26% of HIV-positive women compared to 4% of HIV-negative women. However, the controls in this study were not comparable to HIV-positive cases in terms of sexual behaviour, history of sexually transmitted diseases and frequency of use of barrier methods of contraception.

Vermund et al. (1991) extended a study by Feingold et al. (1990) on HPV-associated disease in intravenous-drug-using women or women with heterosexual contact with male drug users in the USA. In this study of 96 women, non-white subjects were disproportionately represented among HIV-infected women but other behavioural and sociodemographic characteristics were similar. Symptomatic HIV-positive women were more likely to be HPV positive by Southern blot hybridization (70%) than asymptomatic (22%) or HIV-seronegative women (22%). Among symptomatic HIV-positive women, a strong association between HPV and squamous intraepithelial lesions was documented [OR, 8.1 (95% CI, 2.9–22)] whereas the association was non-significant for the other two groups. These and other studies conducted in the late 1980s and early 1990s suggested that more severe HIV-induced immunosuppression might exacerbate HPV-mediated cervical cytological abnormalities (Maiman et al., 1991; Schäfer et al., 1991; Conti et al., 1993).

Kreiss et al. (1992) performed a nested case–control study of 147 HIV-positive and 51 HIV-negative women within a large cohort of prostitutes established in Nairobi but were unable to document significant differences with respect to the prevalence of HPV-DNA in the two groups (adjusted OR, 1.7 (95% CI, 0.8–3.6)). Papanicolaou smears were only available on the most recently enroled 63 women in the study. Based on cytological examination of this subset, CIN was unrelated to HIV seropositivity. Furthermore, among women with cervical HPV DNA, HIV infection was not associated with an increased prevalence of CIN (47% in HIV-positive versus 57% in HIV-negative women). [A strength of this study is that the populations studied were relatively homogeneous with respect to sexual behaviour and condom use.]

In contrast, in a somewhat smaller but otherwise similarly designed nested case–control study in Kinshasa, Zaire, Laga et al. (1992) found a significantly higher prevalence of HPV DNA in HIV-positive cases (18/47; 38%) compared to controls (4/48; 8%) (OR, 6.8 (95% CI,

1.9–26.8)). HPV was detected both by ViraType™ and Southern blotting. Pap smears were obtained on all women but 13 were inadequate for interpretation. Eleven (27%) HIV-positive women had CIN compared with one (13%) of the HIV-negative women (OR, 15 (95% CI, 1.8–95)). Eight (73%) of the 11 HIV-positive women who had CIN also had HPV DNA detected, compared to nine (30%) of 30 with no CIN ($p = 0.02$, Fisher's exact test). Cases and controls in this study did not differ on important demographic or sexual behavioural characteristics but clinical acquired immunodeficiency syndrome (AIDS) was observed more frequently (7% of HIV-positive cases) than in the study population reported by Kreiss et al. (1992) (0.7%).

In a cross-sectional study of 359 gynaecological in-patients without cancer from Tanzania (ter Meulen et al., 1992), 1/42 (2.4%) of HIV-positive women compared with 8/285 (2.8%) of HIV-negative women had an abnormal Pap-smear. None of the HIV-positive women were suspected of being severely immunosuppressed, owing to the lack of severe HIV-related symptoms. Nevertheless, HIV-positive women were 3.3 times more likely to be positive for HPV-16/18 (detected by PCR) than HIV-negative women (OR, 3.3; $p = 0.02$) after adjusting for differences in sexual behaviour and history of sexually transmitted diseases. [No analysis of the association between HPV and smear abnormality by HIV status was presented by the authors.]

In their large study of 4058 women attending two peri-urban family-planning clinics in Nairobi, Kenya, Maggwa et al. (1993) documented CIN on the Pap smears of 10 of 205 (4.9%) HIV-positive women, compared to 72 of 3853 (1.9%) HIV-seronegative women (OR, 2.7 (95% CI, 1.3–5.5)). This association remained after controlling for sexual behaviour and other risk factors. [HPV testing was not performed in this study.]

In a study of 673 Spanish prostitutes and 1182 non-prostitutes attending a family-planning clinic, the odds ratio for cervical intraepithelial neoplasia in HIV-positive prostitutes was 14.2 (95% CI, 4.8–42.4) compared to non-prostitute women [HIV status unknown] whereas there was no increased risk of CIN among HIV-negative prostitutes (OR, 1.2 (95% CI, 0.5–2.8)). Within the group of prostitutes, the odds ratio for CIN in HIV-positive compared to HIV-negative women was 12.7 (95% CI, 3.9–40.9) (de Sanjosé et al., 1993).

In a study of 93 women (58 HIV negative, 18 HIV-1 positive, 17 HIV-2 positive) from Senegal (Seck et al., 1994), detection of HPV-16, -18, -31, -33, -35 was significantly associated with HIV-1 and HIV-2 infection (HPV-16/18 versus HPV-negative: OR, 56 (95% CI, 26–121); HPV-31/33/35 versus HPV-negative: OR, 8.4 (95% CI, 2.2–32.4)). HIV infection (HIV-1 or HIV-2) was associated with evidence of dysplasia following adjustment for age and sexual behaviour variables (OR, 5.5 (95% CI, 1.0–30)). Among HIV-positive women with HPV DNA detected by PCR, dysplasia was demonstrated by cytological analyses in 2/6 (33%) with mild HIV-disease, and 7/10 (70%) with severe HIV-disease (OR, 4.7 (95% CI, 0.4–73)).

In a study of 33 HIV-1 infected women in the USA, Vernon et al. (1994) found frequent co-localization of HIV-1 and HPV in CIN lesions. HIV and HPV were each detected by PCR in 17 (52%) cervical biopsy samples. HIV and HPV were detected together in 10 (50%) of the 20 samples showing CIN, but in none of 13 samples showing normal histology or inflammatory atypia ($p = 0.002$, 1-tailed test).

Whereas most studies published so far have either used HIV-positivity per se or degree of severity of HIV-associated disease as a surrogate marker for level of immune status, more recent studies increasingly include an evaluation by level of $CD4^+$ cell count.

In a cross-sectional study of 434 female former intravenous drug abusers in Italy, Conti et al. (1993) found histological evidence of CIN in 115 of 273 (42%) HIV-positive women and in 13 of 161 (8%) HIV-negative women (OR, 4.2 (95% CI, 2.1–8.4), after adjustment for age and number of sexual partners). The prevalence of CIN increased with the stage of HIV infection with an OR of 5.4 (95% CI, 2.6–11) for women with a $CD4^+$ cell count < $500/mm^3$, compared with those with a count ≥ $500/mm^3$. There was an interaction between cytologically diagnosed HPV infection and HIV status with odds ratios for CIN of 1.2 (non-significant) in HPV-negative/HIV-positive women, 11 (95% CI, 2.8–42) in HPV-positive/HIV-negative women and 64 (95% CI, 19–214) in HPV-positive/HIV-positive women, when compared with HPV-negative/HIV-negative women. [The selection of study subjects may have inflated the prevalence of CIN.]

Ho et al. (1994) found in their analysis of 207 primarily intravenous drug using women that young age (OR, 2.5 (95% CI, 1.3–4.8)) and HIV-positivity (OR, 3.0 (95% CI, 1.5–5.7)) were the only independent demographic and behavioural factors to be associated with HPV DNA positivity as measured by Southern blot. The association with HIV was only changed marginally between the univariate and the multivariate analyses indicating limited confounding influence. Prevalence of HPV increased with decreasing $CD4^+$ cell level from 23% among immunocompetent HIV-negative subjects to 45% in mild-to-moderate immunosuppressive conditions (HIV-positivity and $CD4^+\% > 20$) and to 61% in severe immunosuppression ($CD4^+\% < 20$). HPV-16, -18, -31, -33 and -35 were not particularly strongly associated with HIV-positivity. A general increase in the number of detectable viral copies of HPV with increasing immunosuppression was indirectly supported by the finding of a significant association between strong Southern blot hybridization signal strength and increasing HIV-induced immunosuppression (see Table 55). Among 29 study subjects who did not have any sexual exposure in the previous year, 1/16 of HIV-seronegative women were HPV-positive (6.3%), compared with 8/13 of HIV-positive women (61.5%). This is in line with the hypothesis that HIV-induced immunosuppressed individuals may be prone to persistent HPV infection.

In a study in the USA of 253 women at risk of HIV infection because of intravenous drug abuse or through a partner who used intravenous drugs, Klein et al. (1994) identified SIL in 22% of HIV-positive women compared with 10% of HIV-negative women (OR, 2.5 (95% CI, 1.2–5.1)). In multivariate analyses, the presence of SIL was independently related to the presence of high-risk HPV types (12 (95% CI, 4.1–34)) and severe HIV-related immunosuppression (3.1 (95% CI, 1.0–9.5)).

Wright et al. (1994a) performed a cross-sectional study of 398 HIV-positive and 357 HIV-negative women recruited from HIV/AIDS clinics, STD clinics or methadone clinics in the USA. HIV-positive women were more likely to have a history of prostitution, intravenous drug usage, genital warts and genital herpes than HIV-negative women. Eighty (20%) of the HIV-positive women had CIN confirmed by biopsy (CIN I: 52 (13%), CIN II–III: 28 (7%) compared to 15 (4.2%) of HIV-negative women (CIN I: 13 (4%), CIN II–III: 2 (1%)). No invasive cancers were found. HPV DNA detected by PCR (*L1* consensus primer) was observed in 213 (61%) HIV-positive women compared to 114 (36%) HIV-negative women ($p < 0.01$). In multiple regression analysis, HPV DNA positivity, HIV positivity, $CD4^+$ cell count < $200/mm^3$, and age > 34 years were all found to be independently associated with CIN (all stages).

The influence of immunosuppression was further evaluated in a cross-sectional study by Williams et al. (1994) based on 114 intravenous drug users in San Francisco, USA. A close association between HIV, HPV and abnormal cervical cytology was observed, as shown in Table 56. In a multivariate model of risk factors for cervical epithelial abnormalities that excluded those showing only atypia with inflammation, both cervical HPV detected by dot blot (OR, 32 (95% CI, 2.9–354)) and positive HIV serostatus with $CD4^+$ cell count below $250/mm^3$ (OR, 127 (95% CI, 7.5–2133)) were independent predictors.

Table 56. Relation between human immunodeficiency virus serostatus, presence of cervical human papillomavirus, and cervical cytology

HPV/HIV	Cervical cytology		Odds ratio	95% CI	p
	Abnormal	Normal			
Dot blot					
HPV–/HIV–	0	47			
HPV–/HIV+	5	31	7.3	0.7–354	0.08
HPV+/HIV–	1	2	16	0.2–1254	0.2
HPV+/HIV+	4	4	38	2.7–1888	0.001
PCR					
HPV–/HIV–	0	41			
HPV–/HIV+	3	17	6.8	0.5–367	0.1
HPV+/HIV–	1	6	5.8	0.07–471	0.3
HPV+/HIV+	6	18	13	1.4–610	0.009

Adapted from Williams et al. (1994)

(ii) Progression of disease and treatment

Maiman et al. (1993) followed 44 HIV-positive and 125 HIV-negative women in New York for up to 43 months (mean 15 months). More HIV-positive women (39%) developed biopsy-proven recurrent CIN after treatment than HIV-negative women (9%; $p < 0.01$). CIN severity and lesion size were, however, similar in the two groups. Recurrent disease was associated with the degree of immunosuppression, occurring in 18% of women with a $CD4^+$ cell count $> 500/mm^3$ and in 45% of those with a $CD4^+$ cell count $< 500/mm^3$ ($p < 0.05$).

In Germany, Petry et al. (1994) carried out a prospective study of immunosuppressed women, who were either HIV-infected (n = 48) or transplant recipients (n = 52). The aim of the study was to evaluate progression from cervical HPV-positivity to CIN or from CIN I to CIN II–III. Women with cervical lesions were matched (1 : 2) with immunocompetent, HIV-negative controls and colposcopy, cytology and HPV DNA typing (ViraType™) performed at each visit. Progression was more common in the combined groups of immunosuppressed women (6/11, 55%) than in controls (2/21, 10%; $p = 0.01$, Wilcoxon test). All patients with a $CD4^+$ cell count of less than $400/mm^3$ or who had been immunosuppressed for more than three years suffered from progressive lesions. The cure rate among controls was 18/20 regardless of whether conization or laser-vaporization was used, but it was much lower (4/10) among immunocompromised patients. [Data for HIV-positive women and renal allograft recipients were not presented separately.]

It is possible, in theory, that CIN preceded HIV acquisition in these women, and that it may even have promoted HIV infection, as is the mechanism established for other sexually transmitted diseases with ulcerous lesions. Neither cross-sectional nor case–control studies will give us the necessary answer. However, the increased prevalence of CIN reported in late-stage HIV infection in other studies, together with the more frequent and more rapid recurrence of CIN lesions after treatment in HIV-positive individuals suggests that HIV infection precedes CIN rather than the reverse.

(iii) Invasive cervical cancer

Invasive cervical cancer (ICC) has, since January 1993, been included as an AIDS-defining illness in HIV-positive women (Centers for Disease Control, 1992), primarily because of the plausibility of an association. There are at present few data to substantiate an increased risk of ICC among HIV-infected women. Increased occurrence of ICC has not been observed in the USA among women at high risk for AIDS (Rabkin *et al.*, 1993; Wright *et al.*, 1994a). In a large linkage study between AIDS and cancer registries in seven health departments in the USA, which has been reported as an abstract, Coté *et al.* (1993) found ICC in AIDS patients to be only increased marginally over background levels. The lack of an increased risk of ICC may be explained partly by the late introduction of HIV in the female population. Possibly, HIV-infected women die before CIN progresses to ICC. Active-screening programmes among HIV-infected women may also reduce the likelihood of progression to ICC. HIV-infected women have a higher rate of sexually transmitted diseases than women in general, and are therefore more likely to be in close contact with the health-care system, both before and after their HIV infection.

Based on hospital records from Lusaka, Zambia, no evidence of an influence of the HIV-epidemic on ICC rates was documented (Rabkin & Blattner, 1991) despite nearly 10% of pregnant women and 18% of normal blood donors being HIV-infected by 1985 (Melbye *et al.*, 1986). [Life expectancy for an HIV-positive person in Africa is particularly low.]

(b) Studies of the anorectal region

General reviews covering aspects of anal cancer and HPV in HIV-infected individuals are sparse (Palefsky, 1991; Rabkin & Blattner, 1991). The most comprehensive and detailed review on the subject so far has been presented by Palefsky (1994).

The assessment of anorectal epithelial cytology poses special problems because of variability in the quality of the cellular presentation and faecal contamination. Furthermore, biopsy materials have, in the studies undertaken so far, only exceptionally been obtained to evaluate further the cytological results. A significant association between cytology and histopathology was observed in one study (Palefsky *et al.*, 1990), whereas Surawicz *et al.* (1993) reported that evaluation of 90 homosexual men referred for internal lesions from a cross-sectional community-based study by biopsy recorded a threefold higher prevalence of dysplasia than detected with cytology.

(i) Precancerous lesions

Table 57 summarizes the studies on precancerous lesions. In a prospective study of 61 homosexual men, cytological evidence of dysplasia with concomitant features of HPV infection was observed at least once in 24 men, and HPV without dysplasia on at least one occasion in a further 26 men (Frazer *et al.*, 1986). Twenty of the men were HIV positive and among these men a reduced $CD4^+/CD8^+$ ratio was associated with the presence of dysplasia.

HPV-6/11, -16/18 or -31, -33, -35 was found in anal swabs from 41 (39%) of 105 homosexual men from Washington DC and New York, USA (Caussy *et al.*, 1990a). This figure was 53% in HIV-infected subjects compared to 29% in HIV-negative subjects ($p = 0.01$). In HIV-infected subjects, a low $CD4^+$ cell count was independently associated with anal HPV detection whereas the number of partners and frequency of receptive anal intercourse was unimportant. Abnormal cytology was seen in 9/37 (24%) HIV-infected men compared to 4/55 (7%) HIV-negative men ($p = 0.03$) and was strongly associated with the detection of any HPV genotype by dot blot. None of 15 subjects with HPV detected only by PCR had anal epithelial abnormality.

Kiviat *et al.* (1990) reported 13/49 (27%) HIV-infected bisexual and homosexual men compared to 3/47 (6%) HIV-negative men to have detectable anal HPV by dot blot hybridization (OR, 10 (95% CI, 1.9–57)). [No data on anal cytology/histology were available.]

Anal HPV DNA was detected overall in 15% of 120 Danish homosexual men but in 61.1% of 33 men who were HIV-positive (Melbye *et al.*, 1990). As shown in Figure 19, HPV detection was closely associated with immunosuppression. Anal cytology was abnormal in 19.5% and correlated with HPV (OR, 6.1 (95% CI, 2.1–18)). Type-specific associations were found with HPV -31, -33 and -35 (OR, 8.5 (95% CI, 1.9–39)) and HPV-16/18 (OR, 3.1 (95% CI, 0.8–12)) but not HPV-6/11 (OR, 1.0 (0.11–9.7)). Overall, HPV was detected in 39% of subjects with abnormal cytology. HPV was found in all four subjects with an abnormal anal cytology and a $CD4^+/CD8^+$ ratio below 0.4, but in only three of 14 subjects (21.4%) with abnormal anal cytology and a ratio ≥ 1.3.

In their study of 97 HIV-positive homosexual men with CDC (Centers for Disease Control) group IV disease in San Francisco, USA, Palefsky *et al.* (1990) found HPV DNA (ViraPap™/Viratype™) in 54% while 39% had abnormal anal cytology (for details see Table 57). Anal intraepithelial neoplasia (AIN) was diagnosed in 15 specimens (15%). Abnormal cytology was significantly associated with anal HPV (OR, 4.6; $p = 0.003$) and, among those infected with two or more HPV types, 10/12 had abnormal anal cytology (OR, 39). $CD4^+$ cell counts obtained from medical records were inversely associated with cytological abnormality but did not contribute significantly to a multiple regression model that also included HPV.

Based on a sample of 112 Australian homosexual men presenting consecutively for routine screening for STDs and HIV, 19% showed evidence of mild to moderate dysplastic changes (AIN I or AIN II) (Law *et al.*, 1991). HPV DNA (6/11, 16/18) was detected by dot blot hybridization in 40% of anal smear samples (6/11 in 18%; 16/18 in 11%; both groups in 12%). There was a significant association between the detection of HPV-16/18 DNA and anal dysplasia but not between HPV infection or anal dysplasia and HIV-positivity, immune status, sexual practices or other STDs.

Table 57. Studies of precancerous lesions of the anorectal region in HIV-infected persons

Reference and study area	Number of HIV+ cases	Number of HIV− controls	HPV prevalence %	Odds ratio (95% CI)	Anorectal abnormality %	Odds ratio (95% CI)	HPV test (types)	Pathology reading	Comments
Frazer et al. (1986) Australia	20 homosexual men	41 homosexual men	HIV+, 80* HIV−, 53*	[3.5, 1.0–12]	HIV+, 45* HIV−, 15*	[4.8 (1.4–16)]	Cytological reading	Cytology	*Based on least abnormal smear obtained from each subject
Caussy et al. (1990a) USA	43 homosexual men	62 homosexual men	HIV+, 53 HIV−, 29	p = 0.01	HIV+, 24 HIV−, 7	p = 0.03	ViraType™ and PCR (6/11, 16, 18, 33)	Cytology (ASIL)	
Kiviat et al. (1990) USA	49 homo/-bisexual men	47 homo/-bisexual men	HIV+, 27 HIV−, 6	10 (1.9–57)			ViraPap™		
Melbye et al. (1990) Denmark	33 homosexual men	87 homosexual men	HIV+, 61.1 CD4 %; > 40, 10 40–31, 7.5 30–21, 13 20–11, 34 ≤ 10, 36		ASIL + HPV CD4+/CD8+ ratio ≥ 1.0, 5.9 [0.9–39] < 1.0, 30.0 (3.1–290)		ViraType™ (6/11, 16/18, 31,33,35)	Cytology (ASIL)	
Palefsky et al. (1990) San Francisco, USA	97 homosexual men with CDC group IV disease		All types, 54 HPV-6/11*, 23 HPV-16/-18*, 29 HPV-31, -33, -35*, 20		HIV+, 39 4 condylomas 19 atypias 11 AIN I 4 AIN II		ViraType™ (6/11, 16/18, 31, 33, 35)	Cytology and histology	*Alone or in combination with the other types
Law et al. (1991a) Australia	45 consecutive homosexual men for STD screening	67 consecutive homosexual men for STD screening	All men (HIV+, HIV−) HPV-6/11, 18 HPV-16/18, 11 Both, 12		All men (HIV+, HIV−) AIN I–II, 19 AIN I, 17 men AIN II, 4 men		Dot blot hybridization	Cytology	No correlation between HPV or dysplasia and HIV
Bernard et al. (1992) France	54 homosexual and IVDU men	54 male partners to women with cervical HPV or dysplasia	HIV+ All types, 67 HPV-6/11, 17 HPV-16/18, -31/33/35, 83 HIV− All types, 54 HPV-6/11, 62 HPV-16/18, -31/33/35, 38	All types [1.7 (0.8–3.8)]	HIV+ AIN (PIN) I, 9 AIN II–III, 24 HIV− AIN I, 20 AIN II–III, 6		In-situ hybridization		Link between CMV and high-risk HPV observed irrespective of HIV status

Table 57 (contd)

Reference and study area	Number of HIV+ cases	Number of HIV− controls	HPV prevalence %	Odds ratio (95% CI)	Anorectal abnormality %	Odds ratio (95% CI)	HPV test (types)	Pathology reading	Comments
Critchlow et al. (1992) USA	26 consecutive homosexual men for HIV testing	119 consecutive homosexual men for HIV testing	HIV+, 31 HIV−, 8	5.8 (1.1–30) adjusted for STD history, age, anorectal symptoms			Dot filter hybridization		HIV positivity did not influence type of HPV. HPV prevalence up with severity of HIV disease
Palefsky et al. (1992) San Francisco, USA	37 with stage IV HIV disease		Increased from 60 to 89		ASIL, 27–65 AIN, 8–32 AIN II–III, 0–16		ViraPap™/Type™	Cytology and anoscopy biopsy	Prospective study over an average of 17 months
Kiviat et al. (1993) USA	285 homosexual men seeking HIV testing	204 homosexual men seeking HIV testing	Southern blot HIV+, 55 HIV−, 23 PCR HIV+, 92 HIV−, 78	4.0 (2.7–6.2) 3.1 (1.6–5.8)	HIV+, 26 HIV−, 8 HIV+ only Atypia CD4+ < 200, 28 201–500, 25 501–800, 25 > 800, 30 ASIL CD4+ < 200, 36 201–500, 35 501–800, 25 > 800, 8	5.6 (3.0–10.5) HIV+ versus HIV− Atypia 4.2 (1.6–11) 3.3 (1.6–6.5) 2.7 (1.4–5.4) 2.6 (1.2–5.4 ASIL 9.9 (3.7–27) 8.7 (4.1–18) 5.1 (2.3–11) 1.3 (0.4–4.2)	Southern transfer hybridization and PCR (6/11, 16/18, 31/33/35)	Cytology Bethesda recommendation	OR for ASIL by level of HPV DNA: CD4+ count ≤ 500/mm³ versus > 500/mm³ STH+/PCR+ 2.6 (1.2–5.7) STH−/PCR+ 6.3 (0.8–72)
Brown et al. (1994) Indiana, USA	12 (10 men) from STD and gynaecology clinics	41 (27 men) from STD and gynaecology clinics	High risk HPVs: HIV+, 58 HIV−, 17	[6.8 (1.7–28)]			Hybrid Capture™		
Palefsky et al. (1994) San Francisco, USA	37 homosexual men from San Francisco General Hospital Cohort Study	28 homosexual men from San Francisco General Hospital Cohort Study	HIV+, 51 HIV−, 36	[4.6 (0.9–23)]	HIV+, 28 HIV−, 8		ViraPap™/Type™	Cytology	HPV and ASIL correlated with HIV+ and CD4+ count < 200/mm³ and current smoking

Table 57 (contd)

Reference and study area	Number of HIV+ cases	Number of HIV− controls	HPV prevalence %		Anorectal abnormality %	Odds ratio (95% CI)	HPV test (types)	Pathology reading	Comments
				Odds ratio (95% CI)					
Williams et al. (1994) San Francisco, USA	55 IVDU women	59 IVDU women	*Dot blot* HIV+, 32 HIV−, 14 *PCR* HIV+, 77 HIV−, 56		HIV+, 79	3.4 (0.9–16) *Dot blot* HPV−/HIV−, 1.0 HPV−/HIV+, 2.4 (0.4–16) HPV+/HIV−, 2.5 (0.04–38) HPV+/HIV+, 9.2 (1.6–64) (no association with PCR)	ViraPap™/Type™ and PCR	Cytology	Recruited from a larger cohort. No association between ASIL and CD4⁻ count

[ ] Calculated by the Working Group
PCR, polymerase chain reaction; CDC, Centers for Disease Control; STD, sexually transmitted diseases; IVDU, intravenous drug users; CMV, cytomegalovirus; ASIL, anal squamous intraepithelial lesions; DFH, dot-filter hybridization; AIN, anal intraepithelial neoplasia; PIN, penile intraepithelial neoplasia; STH, Southern transfer hybridization; CD4⁺, CD4⁻ cells; OR, odds ratio

Figure 19. Percentage of anal HPV DNA (ViraPap™/ViraType™) detected by level of CD4⁺/CD8⁺ markers in homosexual men

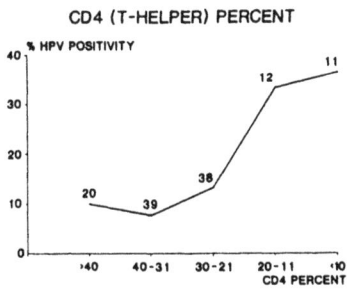

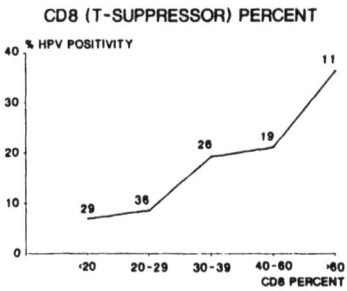

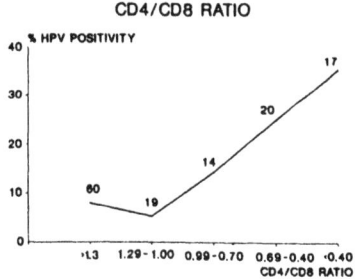

From Melbye et al. (1990)

Bernard et al. (1992) studied an equal number (54) of HIV-positive and HIV-negative men all presenting with anogenital lesions such as flat condyloma or condyloma acuminatum. Whereas most HIV-positive subjects were homosexual or intravenous drug users, the negative men were partners to women with genital HPV or dysplasia. High-risk HPV types (16/18, 31, 33, 35) were more common (83%) in HIV-positive persons. Low-risk types (6/11) were more common in HIV-negative subjects (62%). High-risk types of HPV were seen in 94% (15/16) of men with AIN(PIN) II–III compared to 6% for low-risk HPVs, whereas 50% and 37.5%, respectively, were reported in AIN(PIN) I. A significant association between high-risk HPVs and the detection of cytomegalovirus in the same lesion was observed irrespective of HIV status.

Critchlow et al. (1992) reported a significant association between HIV-infection and anal HPV DNA as measured by dot filter hybridization after adjustment for STD history, age and current anorectal disease (OR, 5.8 (95% CI, 1.1–30)). HIV-infection did not influence type of HPV detected but severity of HIV-related disease was positively related to HPV prevalence.

In a larger and more-recent study by the same group (Kiviat et al., 1993), a random sample of 285 HIV-positive and 204 HIV-negative homosexual men seeking HIV testing in Seattle, USA, was surveyed. HPV DNA was detected by Southern blot hybridization in 55% and 23% of HIV-positive and HIV-negative men, respectively (OR, 4.0 (95% CI, 2.7–6.2)) and by PCR in 92% and 78%, respectively (OR, 3.1 (95% CI, 1.6–5.8)). Each specific group of HPV DNA types surveyed was more common in HIV-infected men (Table 58). Detection of HPV by both Southern blot hybridization and PCR (assumed to indicate a high level of HPV) was significantly associated with anal intraepithelial lesions. However, after adjustment for level of detectable HPV DNA, severely immunosuppressed HIV-positive men (CD4$^+$ cell count < 500/mm^3) were at higher risk of anal intraepithelial lesions than men with a CD4$^+$ cell count of more than 500/mm^3 (OR, 2.9 (95% CI, 1.4–6.2)). [This finding indicates a possible independent role of immunosuppression in addition to HPV.]

Sixty-six of 299 (22%) HIV-positive and 24 of 213 (11%) HIV-negative men from the above-mentioned study were referred for biopsies of internal anorectal lesions (Surawicz et al., 1993). Of 78 men with HPV-associated internal lesions, only 36% had dysplasia diagnosed by cytology, while 92% had dysplasia evaluated by histology (27% high grade). Their findings of correlation of anal abnormalities with histological diagnosis are presented in Table 59. HIV-status did not influence the prevalence of high-grade lesions (27% and 25% in HIV-positive and HIV-negative men, respectively). Both high-risk and low-risk HPV types were common in many of the biopsy specimens but high-risk types 16/18/45 were more common among HIV-positive men (48%) than HIV-negative men (21%; $p = 0.08$).

In a study of 62 subjects with condylomata acuminata in the USA (Brown et al., 1994), seven of 12 (58%) HIV-positive subjects (10 men) were positive for high-risk HPVs (HPV-16, -18, -31, -33, 35, -45, -51, -52 and -56) by Hybrid Capture^{TM} compared with seven of 41 (17%) immunocompetent subjects [crude OR, 6.8 (95% CI, 1.7–28)]. All subjects were positive for low-risk HPV types (6, 11, 42–44), except one of the HIV-positive patients who was only positive for high-risk HPVs.

In a study of 37 HIV-positive and 28 HIV-negative homosexual men, Palefsky et al. (1994) found both anal intraepithelial lesions and the presence of HPV to be closely associated with HIV positivity in men with CD4$^+$ cell count below 200/mm^3. Furthermore, a multivariate analysis indicated a possible influence of current smoking.

Breese et al. (1995) conducted a cross-sectional and follow-up study of 93 HIV-positive and 116 HIV-negative homosexual/bisexual men in the USA. Subjects were tested for anogenital HPV types 6/11, 16/18 and 31/33/35 (ViraPap^{TM}/ViraType^{TM}) at baseline and, for a subset

Table 58. Prevalence of anal HPV DNA in HIV-positive and HIV-negative homosexual men as detected by dot-filter hybridization, low- and high-stringency Southern transfer hybridization, and PCR

	HIV+ (%)	HIV− (%)	Odds ratio	95% CI
Dot blot	(n = 304)	(n = 211)		
Any HPV	52	18	5.1	3.3–7.9
Southern	(n = 285)	(n = 204)		
Any HPV	55	23	4.0	2.7–6.2
HPV-16, -18	21	7	5.0	2.6–9.6
HPV-31, -33, -35	15	3	8.7	3.5–26
HPV-6, -11	21	7	5.0	2.6–9.6
Unclassified HPV	16	8	3.7	1.7–6.3
Multiple HPV	15	3	8.5	3.4–25.2
PCR	(n = 241)	(n = 152)		
Any HPV	92	78	3.1	1.6–5.8
HPV-16, -18	53	38	3.6	1.8–7.2
HPV-31, -33, -35	43	15	7.4	3.4–16
HPV-6, -11	47	39	3.1	1.6–6.2
Unclassified HPV	19	22	2.2	1.0–4.9
Multiple HPV	44	23	4.9	2.4–10

From Kiviat *et al.* (1993)
PCR, polymerase chain reaction

Table 59. Correlation of anal abnormalities with histological diagnosis

Anoscopic abnormalities	Negative	Low-grade (AIN I)	High-grade (AIN II–III)	Total
Discrete warts	3	26	8	37[a]
Circumferential ring of warts	2	14	7	23
Flat white epithelium	1	11	6	18
Normal or non-HPV-associated findings	7	0	1	8[a]
Total	13	51	22	86[a]

From Surawicz *et al.* (1993); AIN, anal intraepithelial neoplasia
[a] Biopsies from 2 HIV-seronegative men in each of these categories were unsatisfactory

of men, six months later. Overall 20 (17%) HIV-negative and 57 (61%) HIV-positive men were positive for HPV ($p < 0.001$). HPV-16/18 DNA was detected most frequently, accounting for 51% and 65% of infections in HIV negative and HIV positive men, respectively. HPV was more common in men with AIDS related complex (ARC)/AIDS (74%) than in asymptomatic HIV-positive men (53%, $p = 0.08$); the prevalence of infection increased significantly with declining

CD4⁺ cell count ($p < 0.05$). Persistent HPV infection after an initial positive test was also more common in men with ARC/AIDS (95%) than asymptomatic HIV-positive men (62%) or HIV-negative men (61%).

Several studies among women are under way, but so far the only one published in this area is by Williams *et al.* (1994). In their study of 114 intravenous drug users, these investigators found anal HPV to be twice as common as cervical HPV and associated with HIV-positivity by both dot blot (OR, 2.5 (95% CI, 0.9–7)) and PCR (OR, 2.6 (95% CI, 1.0–6.8)). Overall, anal intraepithelial lesions were seen in 14% (15/109) of the women of which 11 were HIV-infected (OR, 3.4 (95% CI, 0.9–16)). ASIL was closely associated with simultaneous high-level (dot blot-positive) HPV DNA and HIV positivity (OR, 9.2 (95% CI, 1.6–64)), but no association was found with level of CD4⁺ cell count.

(ii) Progression of disease

In San Francisco, USA, Palefsky *et al.* (1992) followed 37 homosexual men with stage IV HIV-disease prospectively for an average of 17 months and found the prevalence of anal epithelial abnormalities to increase from 27% to 65% over this period. The percentage of men with AIN increased from 8 to 32% and high grade AIN from 0 to 16%. HPV DNA as detected by ViraPap™/ViraType™ technique increased from 60 to 89%. Among subjects who had no cytological abnormality at the start of the study, 11 of 12 (92%) who were HPV-positive and 5 of 13 (38%) who were HPV-negative developed anal disease during follow-up ($p = 0.02$).

(iii) Invasive anal cancer

Reports from Denmark, Sweden and the USA have shown significant increases in the incidence of epidermoid anal cancer, not only during the AIDS era, but over the last 30 years (Goldman *et al.*, 1989; Frisch *et al.*, 1993; Melbye *et al.*, 1994a). The increase has been more pronounced in women than in men and in urban areas than in rural areas. Furthermore, black people are at higher risk than whites and never-married men at higher risk than ever-married men. Interestingly, the increased risk of anal cancer in never-married men has been documented as far back as the 1940s and 1950s (Frisch *et al.*, 1993). These trends show that important behavioural and environmental changes were taking place before the beginning of the AIDS epidemic. However, data from the Surveillance, Epidemiology and End Results Programme (SEER) in the USA have shown a remarkable increase in incidence among men in the San Francisco Bay area in the last decade (1973–75: 0.5 per 10^5; 1988–89: 1.2 per 10^6; $p < 0.001$). Furthermore, the relative risk of anal cancer among never-married men compared to ever married men increased from 6.7 (95% CI, 4.7–9.5) in 1979–84 to 10 (95% CI, 7.5–14) in 1985–89 (Melbye *et al.*, 1994a).

Melbye *et al.* (1994b) used a linkage between AIDS (50 050 reports) and cancer (859 398 reports) registries in seven health departments in the USA to investigate the association between HIV infection and epidermoid anal cancer. Compared to general population rates, the relative risk of anal cancer at and after AIDS diagnosis (11 cases) was 84 (95% CI, 46–152) among homosexual men and 38 (95% CI, 9.4–151) among non-homosexual men (two cases). The relative risk of anal cancer was 14 (95% CI, 6.6–29) in the period two to five years before AIDS and 27 (95% CI, 16–47) during the two years before AIDS diagnosis (p for trend = 0.004) (Table 60).

Table 60. Relative risk (observed/expected ratio) of epidermoid anal and anorectal cancer among AIDS patients compared with population controls matched for age, sex, and race

Time from AIDS diagnosis	No. of cases		Relative risk (95% CI)
	Observed	Expected	
2–5 years before	7	0.502	14 (6.6–29)
0.25–2 years before	13	0.475	27 (16–47)
0.25 years before or after	9	0.113	80 (41.4–153)
0.25–0.75 years after	3	0.072	42 (13.4–129)
> 0.75–2.25 years after	4	0.082	49 (18.3–130)

From Melbye et al. (1994b)

3. Molecular Mechanisms of Carcinogenesis

3.1 Experimental data supporting the carcinogenicity of specific HPV genotypes and analysing the mechanism of HPV-linked carcinogenesis

3.1.1 Low-risk and high-risk HPV infections

Shortly after the isolation and characterization of the most prevalent HPV types found in genital warts (HPV-6 and -11) (Gissmann & zur Hausen, 1980; Gissmann *et al.*, 1982) and cervical cancer (HPV-16 and -18) (Dürst *et al.*, 1983; Boshart *et al.*, 1984), the concept of low-risk and high-risk HPV infections for malignant conversion was introduced (zur Hausen, 1985). Initially it was based exclusively on the high prevalence of type 16/18 viruses in malignant tumours and the rarity of cancer biopsies containing HPV-6 or -11.

During subsequent years, functional differences between both subgroups of papillomaviruses became apparent, which will be described below. Increased chromosomal abnormalities and concomitant aneuploidy were observed in high-risk HPVs selectively (Fu *et al.*, 1988; Claas *et al.*, 1992). In analogy to several other DNA tumour virus systems, oncoproteins of high-risk HPVs showed specific interactions with cellular proteins engaged in the regulation of proliferation.

The terminology of high-risk HPV types in this section is restricted to those genital virus types that perturb normal growth and genomic stability of primary human cells *in vitro*. It is likely, however, that a number of other types, found less frequently in anogenital cancers, also share these properties, although they have not yet been analysed experimentally to the same extent.

3.1.2 Chromosomal instability of high-risk HPV-infected cells

The induction of chromosomal instability had been observed initially in cells infected with SV40, polyomavirus or oncogenic adenoviruses and could be attributed to functions of the T antigen or the adenovirus E1A oncoprotein (Caparossi & Bacchetti, 1990; Drews *et al.*, 1992; Woods *et al.*, 1994; Laurent *et al.*, 1995). Based on in-vitro data demonstrating the induction of chromosomal instability by the overexpression of high-risk HPV genes and in other oncogenic DNA virus systems, it was proposed that high-risk HPVs could act as solitary carcinogens (zur Hausen, 1991). The gradual accumulation of mutations within latently infected host cells and of chromosomal abnormalities resulting from the function of viral oncoproteins would lead to a selection of clones with specific cellular DNA modifications. In a detailed study, White *et al.* (1994) reported that the expression in human cells of HPV-16 *E6*, and, to a lesser extent and through a different mechanism, HPV-16 *E7*, results in an accumulation of genetic alterations within those cells carrying the respective gene (Hashida & Yasumoto, 1991). The expression of HPV-6 *E6* or *E7* genes did not lead to detectable modifications of host cell DNA.

These data may point to a critical mechanistic difference between low- and high-risk HPV infections. In high-risk infections, time may be a sufficient factor to permit the accumulation of mutational changes due to the function of viral oncoproteins, and may suffice for the gradual progression towards malignant conversion in the absence of other cofactors (zur Hausen, 1991). However, additional genotoxic cofactors may accelerate this process. Infections with low-risk viruses, in contrast, would lead to cancer only in exceptional circumstances where other factors contribute mechanistically to modifications of the host-cell genome. Interestingly, cancers containing high-risk HPVs are aneuploid and regularly progress to metastatic growth, whereas those containing low-risk HPV genotypes frequently reveal polyploidy, grow invasively and metastasize rarely (reviewed in zur Hausen, 1991).

3.1.3 Immortalization and transformation of cells by HPVs

Immortalization of cells is defined as continuous in-vitro growth of primary cells, whereas transformation is defined as the ability to induce tumours in immunocompromised hosts.

Organotypic cultures initiated from immortalized cells reveal a histological pattern virtually indistinguishable from intraepithelial neoplastic lesions (reviewed in McDougall, 1994), indicating that HPV-immortalized keratinocytes are a useful model for the analysis of the role of HPVs in cervical neoplasia. Furthermore, immortalized cell lines containing high-risk HPVs have been established from genital intraepithelial neoplasms (Schneider-Maunoury et al., 1987; Stanley et al., 1989; Bedell et al., 1991). Based on these studies, it has been suggested that HPV-immortalized cells correspond to the clinical pattern of intraepithelial neoplasia (zur Hausen & de Villiers, 1995).

(a) Contribution of viral and cellular genes

HPVs can induce immortalization in primary cultures of human and rodent cells. There is a good correlation between the clinical classification of high risk and low risk of a given HPV type and its immortalization potential *in vitro*. In human cells, immortalization is restricted to high-risk viruses, whereas in rodent cells, low-risk HPV types also possess weak immortalizing potential.

In the first published transformation assay for a high-risk HPV, NIH 3T3 cells were transfected with recombinant full length HPV-16 DNA and a selectable marker, and transformed foci were obtained after drug selection (Yasumoto et al., 1986). Similar assays were subsequently developed with several other rodent cell lines including Rat-3Y1 and Rat-1 cells (Bedell et al., 1987; Watanabe & Yoshiike, 1988). Mutational analyses revealed that the HPV *E7* gene codes for the major transforming function with *E6* contributing to the formation of soft agar clones (Phelps et al., 1988; Vousden et al., 1988; Sedman et al., 1991).

Subsequently it was discovered that the HPV *E7* gene can cooperate with the *ras* oncogene to transform primary baby rat kidney cells (Matlashewski et al., 1987; Phelps et al., 1988; Storey et al., 1988). The *E6* gene can cooperate with *ras* and immortalize baby mouse kidney cells (Storey & Banks, 1993).

Potentially more relevant to the biology of the human papillomaviruses was the finding that high-risk HPVs could induce immortalization of primary human cells, including primary human genital keratinocytes (Dürst et al., 1987a; Pirisi et al., 1987; Pirisi et al., 1988; Kaur &

McDougall, 1988; Pirisi *et al.*, 1988; Schlegel *et al.*, 1988; Woodworth *et al.*, 1988). The immortalized cell lines developed a fully transformed phenotype only after prolonged passage in tissue culture (Hurlin *et al.*, 1991; Pecoraro *et al.*, 1991; Pei *et al.*, 1993) or transfection with an activated viral Ha-*ras* gene (DiPaolo *et al.*, 1989; Dürst *et al.*, 1989). Co-transfection of primary human foreskin keratinocytes with HPV-18 and v-*fos* gave rise to cell lines producing non-invasive tumours in immunocompromised mice (Pei *et al.*, 1993). In one study, HPV-immortalized human keratinocytes were induced to tumorigenic progression by treatment with *N*-methyl-*N*-nitrosourea (see IARC, 1987a) (Klingelhutz *et al.*, 1993). These cells showed chromosome 18q deletions involving the tumour suppressor gene *DCC*. The cells also showed aberrations of chromosome 5q, also detected in primary cervical cancers, but this was not associated with detectable alterations in the expression of the *APC* gene associated with the development of adenopolyposis coli. These results support the hypothesis that additional cellular mutations may be required for malignant progression (zur Hausen, 1986, 1994).

Mutational analyses showed that both *E6* and *E7* were required for efficient immortalization of primary human genital tract keratinocytes (Hawley-Nelson *et al.*, 1989; Münger *et al.*, 1989a; Hudson *et al.*, 1990). In organotypic cultures of keratinocytes, *E6/E7* expression caused alterations in terminal differentiation resulting in histopathological abnormalities that are similar to those seen in preneoplastic lesions *in vivo* (McCance *et al.*, 1988; Hudson *et al.*, 1990; reviewed by McDougall, 1994).

Epithelial cells derived from different anatomical regions were immortalized by HPVs and in most cases *E6* and *E7* together were required for efficient immortalization although, under certain conditions, the HPV *E6* or *E7* genes alone were found to have a low immortalization potential (Halbert *et al.*, 1991). One exception is mammary epithelial cells, in which early passage cells could be immortalized by the *E7* gene alone (Wazer *et al.*, 1995) and relatively late passage cultures were immortalized by the HPV *E6* gene alone (Band *et al.*, 1990, 1991).

The requirement for viral oncoprotein expression to maintain the immortalized state was initially demonstrated in tissue culture cells immortalized by temperature-sensitive mutants of SV40 and polyomaviruses (Brugge & Butel, 1975; Martin & Chou, 1975; Randa *et al.*, 1989; Strauss *et al.*, 1990). The additional involvement of cellular genes was suggested by the low efficiency of immortalization induced by these viruses and the fact that the majority of infected cells, although expressing viral oncoproteins, continued to have a finite lifespan (Whitaker *et al.*, 1992). In addition, senescing somatic cell hybrids continued to transcribe HPV-18 *E6/E7* RNAs (Chen *et al.*, 1993b). The existence of at least four complementation groups for senescence in cells immortalized either by SV40 or high-risk HPV genes, respectively (Pereira-Smith & Smith, 1981; Whitaker *et al.*, 1992; Chen *et al.*, 1993b; Duncan *et al.*, 1993), underlines the importance of loss of specific cellular gene functions in the process of immortalization (for review, see zur Hausen & de Villiers, 1995). The specific host cell genes involved in this process have not yet been identified.

(b) Chromosomal abnormalities in HPV-immortalized cells

Chromosomal abnormalities and alterations in ploidy are regularly detected in HPV-immortalized cell lines, with some evidence for additional specific changes during oncogenic progression. Cells immortalized following the introduction of HPV sequences frequently show alterations involving chromosome 1 (Smith *et al.*, 1989), which may contribute to the escape from normal differentiation pathways and the acquisition of a growth advantage. HPV-immortalized cells also frequently show abnormalities of chromosome 3 (Smith *et al.*, 1989), non-random loss of chromosomes 11, 19 (Popescu & DiPaolo, 1990), 5, 7, 8, 12, 16 and 22 (Smith *et al.*, 1989) and abnormalities in chromosome 10 (Crook *et al.*, 1990; Pei *et al.*, 1991). Cytogenetic analysis of HPV-18-immortalized foreskin keratinocytes showed that loss of chromosomes 21 and Y and alterations in chromosome 5q correlated with the spontaneous progression to tumorigenicity following continuous propagation in culture (Hurlin *et al.*, 1991). Treatment of the same cell line with *N*-methyl-*N*-nitrosourea also induced tumorigenic progression, which was associated with 5q+, 18q– and loss of Y (Klingelhutz *et al.*, 1993).

Chromosomal alterations occurring in tumours are described later.

(c) Transcriptional modulation by HPV oncoproteins

Neither HPV E6 nor E7 are DNA-binding proteins, yet they both can influence transcription from certain promoters. The HPV-16 E7 protein was first shown to be able to activate transcriptionally the adenovirus *E2* promoter (Phelps *et al.*, 1988). In the murine fibroblast cell line NIH 3T3, the E6 protein can also activate this promoter efficiently (Sedman *et al.*, 1991). Promoter mapping studies showed that binding sites for the E2F transcription factors were required for the E7-mediated transcriptional activation of the adenovirus *E2* promoter, thereby establishing a functional similarity between E7 and the 12S mRNA-encoded adenovirus E1A protein (Phelps *et al.*, 1991). These studies provided the first evidence that E7 can interfere with the regulation of viral and cellular genes mediated by members of the E2F family of transcription factors.

Conversely, the E6 protein was found to be able to modulate the expression of several basic promoters that contain a TATA box only (Lamberti *et al.*, 1990; Desaintes *et al.*, 1992). In addition, the HPV E6 protein can also interfere with the transcriptional activation and repression functions of the p53 tumour suppressor protein/transcription factor (Lechner *et al.*, 1992; Mietz *et al.*, 1992). p53-independent transcriptional repression by HPV-16 E6 also has been reported (Etscheid *et al.*, 1994). The modulation of cyclin A expression by viral oncoproteins has been reported recently (Oshima *et al.*, 1993; Spitkowsky *et al.*, 1994).

(d) Positive and negative transforming functions of HPV

The *E2*, *E5*, *E6* and *E7* open-reading frames of several HPV genotypes contribute to the immortalization/transformation function of the viruses. The expression of *E6* and *E7*, but not *E2* or *E5*, is regularly maintained after integration of the viral genome during carcinogenic progression (Schwartz *et al.*, 1985). Expression of *E6* and *E7* appears to be necessary for the induction as well as the maintenance of the transformed state (von Knebel-Doeberitz *et al.*, 1988; Crook *et al.*, 1989; von Knebel-Doeberitz *et al.*, 1992, 1994).

(i) HPV E5

The *E5* genes from both low-risk and high-risk HPVs encode short hydrophobic peptides (Bubb *et al.*, 1988; Halbert & Galloway, 1988) that have mitogenic activity in a number of cell types including primary human foreskin keratinocytes and synergize with the epidermal growth factor (EGF) (Leechanachai *et al.*, 1992; Pim *et al.*, 1992; Straight *et al.*, 1993; Bouvard *et al.*,

1994). The number of EGF receptors was found to be increased two- to five-fold and enhanced receptor recycling was also detected in HPV *E5*-expressing human keratinocytes. Similarly, EGF-induced receptor phosphorylation was significantly increased in *E5*-expressing cells (Straight *et al.*, 1993). Like BPV-1 E5 proteins (Burkhardt *et al.*, 1989; Goldstein & Schlegel, 1990; Goldstein *et al.*, 1991), HPV E5 proteins were detected in the Golgi apparatus, the endoplasmatic reticulum, as well as in nuclear membranes, and they are able to form complexes with the 16 kDa subunit of a vacuolar ATPase (Conrad *et al.*, 1993). The E5 oncoprotein of HPV-16 inhibited the acidification of endosomes in human keratinocytes (Straight et al., 1995). Therefore, the HPV E5 proteins, like the BPV-1 E5 (Martin *et al.*, 1989; Petti *et al.*, 1991), appear to interfere with growth-factor-mediated signal transduction. According to this model, the E5 protein may endow HPV-infected cells with an initial growth advantage by interfering with the integration of positive and negative extracellular growth signals. This might lead to an enhanced responsiveness to positive extracellular signals of HPV-infected cells.

(ii) HPV E6

The HPV *E6* open-reading frames encode zinc-binding nuclear proteins of approximately 150 amino acids in length with a rather basic isoelectric point. They contain two pairs of Cys–X–X–Cys-sequence motives with a characteristic spacing of 29 amino acids (Cole & Danos, 1987). These cysteine-rich sequences have been implicated in zinc binding (Barbosa *et al.*, 1989). One biochemical function for the E6 proteins was provided by the discovery that, like the SV40 T antigen and the Ad5 E1B 55 kDa protein (Lane & Crawford, 1979; Linzer & Levine, 1979), high-risk HPV E6 proteins can interact specifically with the p53 tumour suppressor protein (Werness *et al.*, 1990; Crook *et al.*, 1991b).

It was observed that the levels of p53 in HPV-positive cells were very low (Matlashewski *et al.*, 1986b). This led to the suggestion that, unlike SV40 T antigen and the E1B 55 kDa protein, which inactivate p53 by sequestering it in stable complexes, the E6 proteins may inactivate p53 through degradation (Werness *et al.*, 1990). This hypothesis was supported by invitro studies that showed that the interaction between p53 and a high-risk HPV E6 protein resulted in the rapid degradation of p53 through the ubiquitin-mediated proteolysis pathway (Scheffner *et al.*, 1990; Crook *et al.*, 1991b). Biochemical studies showed that a 100 kDa host cellular protein designated E6-AP mediates the interaction between E6 and p53 (Huibregtse *et al.*, 1991, 1993). The E6/E6-AP complex acts as a ubiquitin ligase and therefore plays a direct enzymatic role in the ubiquitination reaction of p53 (Scheffner *et al.*, 1993). The E6/E6-AP functional inactivation of p53 is therefore mediated by a ubiquitin cascade with the E6/E6-AP complex directly conjugating ubiquitin to p53 (Scheffner *et al.*, 1995). As a consequence, the protein levels and the metabolic half-life of p53 in high-risk HPV E6-expressing cells are decreased (Hubbert *et al.*, 1992; Lechner *et al.*, 1992; Band *et al.*, 1993).

The interaction between the HPV E6 protein and p53 causes the functional inactivation of p53. The p53 tumour-suppressor protein has the properties of a sequence specific transcriptional activator (Kern *et al.*, 1991; El-Deiry *et al.*, 1992; Funk *et al.*, 1992; Pietenpol *et al.*, 1994) and this activity plays a pivotal role in p53-mediated tumour suppression. It has been shown that the high-risk HPV E6 proteins, like SV40 T antigen, are able to abrogate the transcriptional activation and repression potential of p53 (Lechner *et al.*, 1992; Mietz *et al.*, 1992; Hoppe-Seyler & Butz, 1993), which supports the notion that the regulatory function of p53 is disrupted in high-risk HPV-infected cells. The functional importance of the interaction between high-risk HPV E6 and p53 was further corroborated by studies that analysed a p53-controlled G1/S cell cycle checkpoint. The intracellular p53 levels rapidly increase in response to DNA damage, resulting either in cell-cycle arrest or apoptosis (reviewed by Lane, 1992). The augmented levels of p53 induce the expression of negative growth regulators including the cyclin-dependent kinase inhibitor $p21^{cip1}$ leading to a growth arrest at the G1/S boundary (El-Deiry et al., 1993; Harper et al., 1993; Xiong et al., 1993). The integrity of this checkpoint appears to contribute critically to the ability of a normal cell either to repair the damaged DNA prior to initiation of DNA replication or undergo apoptosis. This checkpoint is not functional in cells transfected transiently with high-risk HPV E6 (Kessis et al., 1993a; Foster et al., 1994; Gu et al., 1994; Canman et al., 1995), which is manifested by genomic instability (Livingstone et al., 1992). However, in HPV-positive cervical carcinoma cell lines, functional p53 protein has been detected (Butz et al., 1995).

Since the ability of HPV E6 to bind and/or degrade p53 does not seem to account completely for the biological activities of E6 (Sedmann et al., 1992; Ishiwatari et al., 1994), several laboratories are in the process of defining additional cellular targets of the HPV E6 protein using various biochemical and genetic screening methods. These studies have been hampered somewhat by the absence of definitive structure–function studies. Cellular proteins associated with E6 have been identified, but with the exception of the E6-AP protein (Huibregtse et al., 1993), their identity and biological importance are unknown (Keen et al., 1994).

(iii) HPV E7

HPV *E7* genes encode zinc-binding nuclear phosphoproteins, of approximately 100 amino acids in size, that have an acidic isoelectric point. The amino terminal domain of the HPV E7 protein is strikingly similar to regions of the Ad E1A proteins and the SV40 T antigen (Figge et al., 1988; Phelps et al., 1988). The conserved regions of the three DNA tumour virus oncoproteins participate in the binding of the pocket proteins, a family of structurally related cellular proteins that includes the retinoblastoma tumour-suppressor protein (pRB), p107 and p130 (DeCaprio et al., 1988; Whyte et al., 1988; Dyson et al., 1989). The pocket protein binding site was mapped to a short peptide sequence located in the amino terminal domain of E7 (Münger et al., 1989b; Barbosa et al., 1990; Jones et al., 1990b). Co-precipitation experiments showed that HPV-16 E7, like SV40 T antigen, binds preferentially to the hypophosphorylated form of pRB *in vivo* (Imai et al., 1991; Dyson et al., 1992). Cell cycle analyses have revealed that the state of phosphorylation of pRB is regulated in a cell-cycle-dependent manner. In the G0 and G1 phases of the cell cycle, when pRB is active as a growth suppressor, it is in a hypophosphorylated form. Upon cell cycle progression, pRB becomes phosphorylated at multiple serine residues by one or more cyclin-dependent kinases at the G1/S boundary. Consequently, pRB is present in a hyperphosphorylated form during S, G2 and early M phases, and is dephosphorylated in late M phase (reviewed by Weinberg, 1995). Complex formation between E7 and the pocket proteins results in their functional inactivation thereby dysregulating progression of the cell cycle into S phase. The ability to form complexes with the pocket proteins may therefore contribute to the ability of the HPV E7 protein to induce DNA synthesis (Sato et al., 1989b; Banks et al., 1990).

Members of the E2F family of transcription factors are regarded as modulators of pocket protein function (reviewed by Nevins, 1992). When bound to the G0/G1 specific hypophosphorylated form of pRB, E2F acts as a transcriptional repressor. Upon G1/S-specific phosphorylation of pRB, the E2F/pRB complex is disrupted and E2F has transcriptional activation function (Weintraub et al., 1992). E2F/pocket protein complexes are detected by electrophoretic mobility shift assays using nuclear protein extracts and an E2F binding site oligonucleotide as a probe. In high-risk HPV E7-expressing cell lines, the E2F/pocket protein complexes are functionally compromised (Chellappan et al., 1992; Pagano et al., 1992) — the HPV E7 protein can disrupt pRB/E2F complex and interact with the cyclin A/E2F complex without efficiently disrupting it (Arroyo et al., 1993). The interaction of E7 with the cyclin A/E2F complex leads to its functional inactivation resulting in the transcriptional activation of responsive promoters (Lam et al., 1994).

The regulation of the transcriptional activity of E2F by the pocket proteins may be an important step for ordered G1/S transition and the disruption of this regulatory circuit by the E7 protein in HPV-infected cells is thought to contribute critically to carcinogenic progression. In agreement with this model, it has been shown that overexpression of E2F leads to cell cycle progression and morphological changes characteristic of cellular transformation (Johnson et al., 1994; Singh et al., 1994). E7 expression can abrogate at least some of the growth-suppression functions of p53 (reviewed in Farthing & Vousden, 1994), although wild-type p53 expression can inhibit transformation by E7 (Crook et al., 1991c, 1994). In cells with an intact p53 pathway, overexpression of E2F induces apoptosis (Qin et al., 1994; Wu & Levine, 1994) and it seems likely that E6 expression is important in the abrogation of this function.

Like Ad E1A, HPV-16 E7 is able to bind cyclin A as well as a histone H1 kinase (Dyson et al., 1992; Davies et al., 1993; Tommasino et al., 1993). Interestingly, the pocket protein p107 can serve as a substrate for this protein kinase activity (Davies et al., 1993). Whether this is a direct interaction or is mediated by an adaptor protein is unclear at present.

Several mutagenic analyses of E7 have helped define the molecular determinants for the multiple biological and biochemical properties of E7. The ability of E7 to interact efficiently with the pocket proteins was found to be critical for many of the biological and biochemical properties of E7 (Edmonds & Vousden, 1989; Storey et al., 1990; Watanabe et al., 1990; Phelps et al., 1992). This was illustrated clearly by studies of chimeric high-risk/low-risk HPV E7 proteins, which showed that the differences in transformation efficiencies in rodent cells correlated directly with the relative binding efficiency to retinoblastoma protein. Sequence comparisons revealed a single consistent amino acid sequence difference in the pRB binding sites between the high-risk and the low-risk E7 proteins (Asp 21 in HPV-16 E7 corresponding to Gly 22 in HPV-6 E7). Mutation of the corresponding residues in E7 showed that this difference is largely responsible for the differential transforming capacity of the low-risk and the high-risk E7 proteins (Heck et al., 1992; Sang & Barbosa, 1992a). The relevance of these findings, however, may be limited to E7 proteins encoded by HPVs that are associated with anogenital tract lesions since the E7 protein encoded by HPV-1, an HPV type associated with benign plantar warts, also efficiently interacts with pRB (Ciccolini et al., 1994; Schmitt et al., 1994).

Several studies have provided evidence for the presence of additional regions that, independent of or in addition to pRB binding, are important for E7 function in cellular immortalization and transformation. Mutations in the amino terminal CR1 homology domain of E7 interfere with its transformation potential independent of pRB binding (Edmonds & Vousden, 1989; Phelps *et al.*, 1992; Brokaw *et al.*, 1994) and pRB-binding-deficient E7 mutants, in the context of the whole genome, are able to induce cellular immortalization of primary human genital epithelial cells (Jewers *et al.*, 1992). It has also been shown in the CRPV system that CRPV mutations in the pRB binding site did not result in the prevention of papillomas (Defeo-Jones *et al.*, 1993). The pRB binding function of E7 is necessary for the immortalization of human cells, when only E6 and E7 proteins are expressed (Melillo *et al.*, 1994).

The specific contributions of the cysteine-rich carboxyl-terminus of E7 are poorly understood. Mutations in the carboxyl-terminal half of E7 that interfere with any of the functions of E7 generally also affect the intracellular stability of the protein, suggesting that the integrity of the carboxyl-terminus is important for its intracellular stability (Phelps *et al.*, 1992; McIntyre *et al.*, 1993). There are several studies that suggest specific contributions of the carboxyl-terminus to E7 functions. Binding of E7 to pRB abrogates the nonspecific DNA-binding properties of pRB and studies with truncated E7 polypeptides suggest that, in addition to the pRB binding site, carboxyl-terminal sequences are also necessary for this activity (Stirdivant *et al.*, 1992). Similarly, the ability of E7 to disrupt the complex between the cellular transcription factor E2F and pRB requires additional sequences in the carboxyl-terminus of E7 (Hwang *et al.*, 1993; Wu *et al.*, 1993). It has been suggested that this region of E7 constitutes an independent low-affinity binding site for pRB (Patrick *et al.*, 1994). The only mutation that rendered E7 incompetent for immortalization was located in the carboxyl-terminus (Jewers *et al.*, 1992). The HPV E7 protein can form dimeric or multimeric complexes through carboxyl-terminal sequences. The biological implications of this property of E7 are not clear (Roth *et al.*, 1992; McIntyre *et al.*, 1993).

(iv) HPV E2

Expression of the HPV *E2* gene is frequently disrupted as a result of the integration of the viral genome during carcinogenic progression. HPV *E2* gene encodes DNA-binding proteins that can repress transcription from the HPV promoter(s) that govern expression of the *E6* and *E7* oncogenes (Thierry & Yaniv, 1987; Romanczuk *et al.*, 1991; Thierry & Howley, 1991). HPV genomes in which *E2* expression is disrupted have higher levels of *E6/E7* expression (Sang & Barbosa, 1992b) and an enhanced immortalization activity as compared to a wild type genome (Romanczuk & Howley, 1992). In accord with these results, the re-establishment of *E2* expression in cervical carcinoma cell lines results in growth suppression, which is at least in part mediated via the repression of the HPV *E6/E7* promoter (Thierry & Yaniv, 1987; Hwang *et al.*, 1993).

(e) HPV-targeted cellular proteins in cervical carcinogenesis

(i) p53

The most intensively studied genetic alterations in cervical cancers are those affecting the tumour suppressor gene *p53*. Alteration in *p53* is a common event in the development of most major carcinomas, suggesting that loss of normal p53 function is an important step during carcinogenesis (Hollstein *et al.*, 1991). The observation that one of the HPV-encoded oncoproteins, E6, can interact with, and functionally inactivate, the p53 protein (see above) suggested that somatic alteration within the *p53* gene may not be a necessary step during the development of HPV-associated cancers. A large number of studies have attempted to address this question by analysing the status of the *p53* gene in HPV-positive and HPV-negative cancers and cancer cell lines. Results from the cancer cell lines were very striking and reproducible between different groups. No *p53* mutations were detected in a total of 11 independently derived HPV-positive cell lines, whilst three separate HPV-negative cervical carcinoma cell lines showed evidence of point mutation at a hot spot region within the *p53* gene, two at codon 273 and one at codon 245 (Crook *et al.*, 1991d; Scheffner *et al.*, 1991; Iwasaka *et al.*, 1993). This inverse relationship between *p53* mutation and HPV infection was interpreted as evidence supporting the importance of loss of p53 function in the development of these tumours and the functional significance of the E6/p53 interaction. Subsequent studies in primary cancer biopsies have been less clear. In 16 independent analyses of HPV-associated genital cancers, eight tumours with evidence of *p53* mutation were detected in a total of 375 cancers (2%) (Crook *et al.*, 1991d, 1992; Fujita *et al.*, 1992; Lo *et al.*, 1992; Tsuda & Hirohashi, 1992; Chen *et al.*, 1993c; Choo & Chong, 1993; Helland *et al.*, 1993; Paquette *et al.*, 1993; Busby-Earle *et al.*, 1994; Chen *et al.*, 1994a; Jiko *et al.*, 1994; Kurvinen *et al.*, 1994; Lee *et al.*, 1994; Pao *et al.*, 1994b; Park *et al.*, 1994). The observation that *p53* mutations are extremely rare in HPV-positive cancers is not in dispute. The detection of *p53* point mutations in apparently HPV-negative cancers has been less consistent. Some studies reported a relatively high incidence of *p53* mutations in these tumors, although most found a low incidence of mutation, regardless of the HPV type. Overall, 146 HPV-negative tumours were analysed and *p53* mutations identified in 24 (16%). Four studies investigating head and neck tumours identified a total of six *p53* mutations in 27 HPV-positive cancers (22%) and 32 *p53* point mutations in 81 HPV-negative cancers (40%) (Brachman *et al.*, 1992; Lee *et al.*, 1993; Chang *et al.*, 1994; Snijders *et al.*, 1994b).

Analysis of p53 protein levels, as an indication of *p53* abnormalities, also fails to provide a good consensus; some studies showed a correlation between absence of HPV sequences and p53 protein detection (Tervahauta *et al.*, 1993), which is not detected by others (Cooper *et al.*, 1993). These studies are more difficult to interpret than those describing direct sequencing of the *p53* gene within the tumour cells, since the correlation between p53 levels and abnormalities within the protein is not perfect. One study in which both protein levels and *p53* sequence was determined revealed a point mutation in only one of eight cervical cancers with immunohistochemical p53 staining (Busby-Earle *et al.*, 1994). Loss of heterozygosity on chromosome 17p is associated with HPV-negative cancers (Kaelbling *et al.*, 1992), although the importance of this may be related to the loss of another gene in this region of chromosome 17, rather than *p53* itself.

The identification of tumours apparently lacking both HPV and *p53* mutations suggests that other pathways or different genetic lesions are involved in the development of these cancers (Park *et al.*, 1994). Studies of p53 function have shown that the activity of the p53 protein can be regulated by interaction with cell proteins. One of these, termed MDM2, is transcriptionally activated by p53 itself and binds to p53 within the activation domain, inhibiting p53 activity and providing a feedback mechanism for the modulation of p53 function. Some tumours that do not show frequent evidence of somatic mutation within the p53 protein itself have been shown to carry amplifications of the *MDM2* gene, although one study of HPV-negative cervical cancers failed to detect these amplifications (Kessis *et al.*, 1993b).

Several tumours have also been identified that are positive for both *p53* mutations and HPV. Some studies show an association of *p53* mutations with more aggressive cervical cancers, although this is not always seen (Chen *et al.*, 1994a; Jiko *et al.*, 1994). A small study of metastases from HPV-positive primary cancers suggested the possibility that the acquisition of *p53* mutations may contribute to the further progression of an HPV-associated primary cancer. *p53* Mutations have been identified as a late-stage event in other tumour types and under experimental conditions certain forms of mutant *p53* display transforming activities that are independent of the loss of wild-type growth suppressor function. It is therefore postulated that the interaction of E6 with the wild-type p53 protein in HPV-infected cervical cells results in the loss of protein function, whereas expression of a mutant p53 protein might provide an additional oncogenic signal at later stages of progression (Crook & Vousden, 1992). Some other studies have failed to detect *p53* mutations in HPV-positive metastases (Stanley & Sarkar, 1994) and not enough tumours have been examined to determine whether this genetic event contributes significantly to metastatic progression in these cancers. Transfection of HPV-16-immortalized and HPV-18-immortalized human cervical cell lines with a dominantly transforming mouse mutant p53 resulted in enhanced growth rates of the human cell lines and an increase in the efficiency of anchorage and independent colony formation; however, cells expressing the mutant p53 protein did not become tumorigenic (Chen *et al.*, 1993c).

(ii) pRB

Like p53, pRB is a tumour suppressor whose function is frequently lost during the development of several types of human cancer (Weinberg, 1995). The HPV-encoded oncoprotein E7 has been shown to interact with, and inactivate the function of pRB (see section above). Analysis of cervical carcinoma cells lines for alterations in the *pRB* gene revealed mutations only in the two HPV-negative lines studied, with wild-type present in the six HPV-positive lines (Scheffner *et al.*, 1991). This suggests an inverse correlation between HPV positivity and *pRB* mutation, similar to that postulated for HPV and *p53*. Further analyses of primary tumour material have been hampered because of the large size of the *pRB* gene, but one study of 12 HPV-negative small-cell cervical cancers failed to find any evidence of *pRB* mutation (Pao *et al.*, 1994b). Alterations of the cyclin dependent kinase inhibitor p16, which are frequently seen in other pRB-positive cell lines, are not detected in the HPV-positive cervical carcinoma lines, again supporting a functional significance of the E7/pRB interaction in these cells. Deletions of chromosome 9p21, containing the p16 locus, are also rarely seen in cervical cancer (reviewed in Stanley & Sarkar, 1994).

3.1.4 Experimental evidence for a role of high-risk HPVs in malignant conversion and in human cervical cancers

(a) Requirement for HPV gene expression for invasive growth and the malignant phenotype

A low level of HPV *E6/E7* expression was noted in the proliferative layer of low-grade CIN in comparison with more advanced lesions (Dürst *et al.*, 1991; Iftner *et al.*, 1992; Stoler *et al.*, 1992).

Two sets of experimental data reveal the requirement of HPV *E6/E7* gene expression for the invasive phenotype of human cells after heterografting these cells into immunocompromised mice. Cells immortalized by HPV-16 reduce E6/E7 transcription substantially upon heterografting (Dürst et al., 1991). Similarly, non-malignant hybrid cells produced by cell fusion of HPV-18-containing HeLa cells and human fibroblasts or human keratinocytes, which expressed significant levels of viral oncoproteins when kept in tissue culture, revealed a substantial transcriptional repression of these genes within three days of transplantation into the nude mouse system (Bartsch et al., 1992). Malignant revertants obtained from these lines or the parental HeLa cells fail to reveal this transcriptional down-regulation.

The requirement for high expression levels of viral oncoproteins for the malignant phenotype is further underlined by experiments using inducible *E6/E7* antisense constructs, in the human cervical carcinoma cell line C4-1 (von Knebel-Doeberitz et al., 1988, 1992). By inducing the antisense transcription, cell growth was impaired and carcinogenicity abolished. In a specific cervical cancer cell line, SW 752, HPV-18 *E6/E7* transcription could be switched off by the addition of dexamethasone. These cells ceased to grow in culture and were no longer carcinogenic in nude mice receiving dexamethasone. Reconstitution of either *E6* or *E7* expression by an hormone-inducible promoter restored the carcinogenicity (von Knebel-Doeberitz et al., 1994).

The selective down-regulation of HPV transcription in immortalized cells and not in malignant cells can be reproduced under tissue culture conditions by 5-azacytidine treatment or by the addition of human or murine macrophages (Rösl et al., 1988, 1994; Kleine et al., 1995). In the latter two studies it was demonstrated that the production of TNFα by macrophages was induced by a cytokine (MCP-1) selectively produced by non-malignant cells; TNFα mediates the down-regulation of HPV-16 and -18 transcription in these cells. This suggests that the transition from immortalization to malignant conversion involved the modification of genes engaged in the control of HPV transcription and which are activated by a paracrine regulatory pathway.

(b) Integration of HPV sequences

During the normal HPV life cycle, viral DNA is maintained episomally in the nucleus of the infected cell. The detection of integrated viral DNA sequences in cervical neoplasia (Schwartz et al., 1985) is frequently associated with malignant progression, integration being more common in carcinomas than in cervical intraepithelial neoplasia (Cullen et al., 1991), with some studies reporting integration in high-grade dysplasia (Lehn et al., 1988; Fukushima et al., 1990). The persistence of both episomal and integrated copies of the HPV genome in some cervical cancers has been reported (Kristiansen et al., 1994b) and most studies identify at least some carcinomas with only episomal viral DNA (Das et al., 1992b). Similar integration of HPV sequences is reported in HPV-associated vulval carcinomas (Venuti & Marcante, 1989). The consequences of integration and potential contribution to tumour progression may reflect perturbations in viral and host gene expression.

(i) Effects of integration on viral gene expression

Many studies agree that integration of viral sequences can result in partial loss of the viral genome and loss of expression of several viral open-reading frames (Wilczynski et al., 1988b). The *E6* and *E7* genes, however, are almost always found to be expressed in HPV-associated cancers (van den Brule et al., 1991b). Integration is postulated to deregulate *E6* and *E7* expression through loss of viral transcriptional regulators such as E2 and/or escape from intracellular control through transcriptional initiation of these viral regions from flanking cellular promoters (Rösl et al., 1991). However, a significant proportion of cervical tumours arise without evidence for integration of HPV sequences, and recent studies suggest that loss of the E2 regulatory region is not the only mechanism to perturb E6/E7 expression. A specific binding site for the transcription factor YY1 in the HPV-18 promoter was shown to be involved in the regulation of E6/E7 gene transcription (Bauknecht et al., 1992). Analysis of the viral promoters in malignant tumours harbouring episomal HPV-16 sequences only, showed that three of six cases carried a mutation in the YY1 binding site and that this resulted in enhanced activity of the E6/E7 promoter (Dong et al., 1994). Several papers examining individual tumours report evidence of modifications within the locus control region of both HPV-16-associated (Tidy et al., 1989) and HPV-6-associated tumours (reviewed in Kitasato et al., 1994) containing episomal viral DNA. Integration may also result in increased stability of the E6/E7 in mRNA (Jeon & Lambert, 1995), giving cells with integrated viral sequences a selective growth advantage (Jeon et al., 1995).

(ii) Effects of integration on cell gene expression

Another potential oncogenic consequence of HPV integration is the transcriptional activation of cellular proto-oncogenes by viral promoters. Although several reports show integration of the HPV sequences close to proto-oncogenes such as *myc* at chromosome 8q24 (Dürst et al., 1987b; Couturier et al., 1991), there is no firm evidence for consistency in the integration site with respect to any one specific chromosomal location (Mincheva et al., 1987). However, several studies have suggested that the integration may occur preferentially at fragile sites, frequently within the location of a proto-oncogene (Dürst et al., 1987b; Popescu et al., 1989).

Integration *per se* is not sufficient for malignant conversion. Somatic cell hybridizations have produced a non-malignant phenotype of hybrid cells in spite of the persistence of integrated viral DNA and the continued expression of viral oncoproteins (Saxon et al., 1986; Koi et al., 1989).

(c) Chromosomal abnormalities in HPV-associated cancers

(i) Primary tumours

Cytogenetic analyses of cervical carcinomas have demonstrated non-random alterations of several chromosomes. Chromosome 1 is commonly involved in structural or numerical alterations in cervical cancers (Atkin, 1986), with frequent loss of heterozygosity in the short arm of chromosome 1 at 1p36 (Wong et al., 1993). These changes were found in both HPV-positive and HPV-negative cancers and were not related to the stage of the tumour, which suggests that they did not contribute to the progression of the established tumour. This is supported by the detection of chromosome 1 aberrations in early premalignant cervical lesions (Atkin et al., 1983). Another common region of loss of heterozygosity is on the short arm of chromosome 3, identified as 3p14 and 3p25 (Chung et al., 1992), 3p21-22 (Karlsen et al., 1994) or 3p14-21 and 3p22-24.1 (Yokota et al., 1989). As with the alterations on chromosome 1, loss of genetic material at these loci was seen in both HPV-positive and HPV-negative women and, although HPV integration has been reported occasionally in these regions (Mincheva et al., 1987), there was no correlation between HPV infection and chromosome 3p deletion. Loss of heterozygosity on chromosome 3 was found in both invasive cancers and cervical premalignancies, suggesting that like chromosome 1, these alterations play a role in tumour development. The detection of numerical and structural changes in chromosome 1 may provide a method to study premalignant stages in cervical smears (Segers et al., 1994). A recent study has also described loss of heterozygosity for one or more markers on chromosome 11 in 14/32 patients, with evidence for the existence of a cervical cancer-related tumour suppressor gene at 11q22-11q24 (Hampton et al., 1994). This correlates with the earlier observation that the tumorigenicity of the HPV-18-expressing cervical carcinoma cell line HeLa and of the HPV-16-expressing cell line SiHa can be suppressed by the addition of a normal human chromosome 11 in somatic cell hybrids (Saxon et al., 1986; Koi et al., 1989). A potential candidate for a tumour suppressor gene in this region has been reported (Lichy et al., 1992). Interestingly, only human embryonic fibroblasts with a deletion on chromosome 11 were susceptible to HPV-16-mediated transformation. The region deleted in these cells was between 11p11.11-11p15.1, which may indicate the possible location of another tumour suppressor gene active in controlling malignant development of HPV-infected cells on this chromosome (Smits et al., 1988). Cells with this chromosomal deletion reveal an upregulation of the regulatory subunit of the protein phosphatase 2A, which in turn leads to an upregulation of transfected E6/E7 transcription (Smits et al., 1992b). Other regions sustaining loss of heterozygosity in cervical cancer include 9q, 10q and 17p (Jones et al., 1994), 4q, 5p, 5q, 11p and 18p (Mitra et al., 1994) and 1p, 1q, 2q, 3q, 5q, 6p, 6q, 9q, 10q, 11p, 11q, 17p and 17q (Sreekantaiah et al., 1991).

(d) Alterations of specific proto-oncogenes

(i) ras

Analysis of cervical tumours for mutational activation of the Ha- or Ki-*ras* genes generally revealed no evidence that *ras* point mutation is an important step in the development of these cancers (Willis et al., 1993), although one study reported mutations in Ha-*ras* in 7/29 advanced-stage tumours (Riou et al., 1988). Anal cancers, which show an HPV association very similar to that seen with cervical cancers, and vulvar cancers also failed to display evidence of frequent *ras* mutation (Hiorns et al., 1990; Tate et al., 1994). Cancers at other sites which are less strongly linked to HPV infection, such as head and neck tumours or prostate cancers, show a significantly higher incidence of *ras* mutations, with some evidence of association with late-stage disease (Anwar et al., 1992a, 1993).

(ii) myc

Reports of c-*myc* amplification or overexpression in cervical cancers are not consistent. Several studies report alterations in c-*myc* in a significant proportion of cervical cancers, some up to 90% (Riou et al., 1984; Ocadiz et al., 1987). However, other studies fail to find amplification of c-*myc* sequences in any of the tumours examined (Yokota et al., 1989). The latter study examined only stage I and II tumours and this discrepancy may be related to the stage of the tumours under investigation. Overexpression of c-*myc* RNA has also been associated with aggressive disease, with c-*myc*-positive tumours showing a higher incidence of metastasis and recurrence (Riou et al., 1992). c-*myc* Protein was detected in invasive carcinomas but not lower-grade cervical lesions in some studies (Devictor et al., 1993), while other studies failed to find evidence for myc expressed-protein in cervical neoplasia (Hughes et al., 1989).

Introduction of v-*myc* into HPV-immortalized human cervical epithelial cells did not result in the generation of tumorigenic lines (DiPaolo *et al.*, 1989). Elevated levels of c-*myc* expression have been detected in HPV-positive cervical carcinoma cell lines (Dürst *et al.*, 1987b) and amplification and overexpression of c-*myc* sequences in an HPV-16-containing cervical cell line was associated with an increased growth rate and resistance to differentiation, although in this case the potential acquisition of a tumorigenic phenotype was not examined (Crook *et al.*, 1990).

(iii) Other alterations

HPV-immortalized human keratinocytes, induced to tumorigenic progression following treatment with *N*-methyl-*N*-nitrosourea, showed chromosome 18q deletions and were subsequently shown to have undergone a deletion of the tumour-suppressor gene *DCC* (Klingelhutz *et al.*, 1993).

The role of other oncogenes in cervical cancers has been less extensively studied. Analysis of the c-*erb*B-2 gene provided some evidence that amplification and overexpression of this gene may be associated with advanced tumours with a poor prognosis (Kihana *et al.*, 1994). *LA-1* oncogene amplification may also play a role in cervical cancer development (Sharma *et al.*, 1994).

Analysis of the loss of heterozygosity frequently observed on chromosome 3p has implicated a role for the loss of the *raf-1* gene and the retinoic acid receptor, as in the development of cervical cancers (Yokota *et al.*, 1989; Chung *et al.*, 1992), although the significance of this to the biology of these tumours is not known.

A study of DNA hypomethylation in biopsy specimens from 41 patients with varying degrees of cervical abnormalities showed a progressive increase during progression through premalignant to malignant lesions (Kim *et al.*, 1994). The HPV status of the lesions examined in this study was not determined, so further studies of the relationship, if any, between HPV infection and DNA hypomethylation are warranted. At least one cervical cell line (CaSki) exists in which even HPV genomes are hypermethylated rather than hypomethylated (Rösl *et al.*, 1993).

3.1.5 Interactions between HPV and environmental agents

Although there is compelling epidemiological and molecular evidence to link papillomaviruses to the etiology of squamous-cell carcinomas, additional factors contribute to this multistage process.

(a) Interaction with other viruses

Early suspicions of a role of herpes simplex virus (HSV) infections in cancer of the cervix were based on seroepidemiological studies (Rawls *et al.*, 1968; Nahmias *et al.*, 1970). Subsequently, in-vitro transformation studies of hamster cells by HSV-1 and HSV-2 have been reported (Duff & Rapp, 1971). In subsequent years, the value of these studies has been questioned (reviewed in zur Hausen, 1975, 1983), particularly after a large prospective study failed to provide support for the early suspicion (Vonka *et al.*, 1984).

The concept that HSV and HPV may act as syncarcinogens (zur Hausen, 1982) has not been supported by a case–control study conducted by Muñoz *et al.* (1995) in Spain and Colombia, yet finds some support from in-vitro transformation studies. HPV-16-immortalized human foreskin keratinocytes transfected with a recombinant plasmid bearing the HSV-2 fragment Bg/II N yielded tumorigenic clones, whereas the parental HPV-immortalized cell lines were incapable of inducing tumours. Southern blot analysis of the viral sequences present in the transformed cell lines indicated that while HPV-16 genomes were maintained in an unchanged integrated state, a complete loss of HSV-2 sequences was observed in the tumour-derived cell lines (DiPaolo et al., 1990). HSV-2 morphological transformation region III has been reported to induce rearrangements of HPV-18 DNA sequences in immortalized human keratinocytes and chromosomal changes in HPV-16-immortalized human cell lines (Dhanwada et al., 1993). A previous report showed stimulation of HPV-18 transcription by HSV-1 DNA fragments (Gius & Laimins, 1989).

Significantly, herpes-group viruses, as well as vaccinia virus and adenoviruses, can induce amplification of papovavirus DNA contained in various cell lines, a process also observed in some of these lines after treatment with chemical or physical inhibitors (Lavi, 1982; Schlehofer et al., 1983a; Matz et al., 1985). HSV-1 infection of a BPV-1 transformed mouse cell line caused amplification of the BPV-1 DNA sequences (Schmitt et al., 1989).

Papillomavirus expression *in vitro* can also be influenced by other viruses including human immunodeficiency virus (HIV) (see section 2.5.3) and human herpesvirus 6 (HHV-6). HHV-6, a T-lymphotropic virus, widely distributed in the general population, can transactivate the long terminal repeat (LTR) of HIV. Recently, human exocervical cells immortalized with HPV-16 and HPV-positive cervical carcinoma cell lines were successfully infected with HHV-6, as demonstrated by expression of the early–late antigens of HHV-6 and maintenance of the viral genome (Chen et al., 1994b). HHV-6-infected cervical carcinoma cell lines were more tumorigenic in nude mice when compared to the parental counterparts; however, HPV-16-immortalized cells bearing HHV-6 episomes did not induce tumours in mice. The level of HPV *E6* and *E7* mRNAs was increased by HHV-6 in the infected carcinoma cell lines, possibly through the same mechanism by which HHV-6 transactivates the HIV-1 LTR. HHV-6 DNA was detected in six out of 72 cases of squamous-cell carcinoma and CIN in China, but it was absent from normal cervical tissues. HPV-16 was also found in four of the HHV-6-positive samples (two carcinomas, two CIN III) (Chen et al., 1994b). The relevance of these interactions *in vivo* awaits further investigation.

Herpes-dependent and herpes-independent parvoviruses have been shown to interfere negatively with oncogenes (Toolan & Ledinko, 1968). In this context, the observed inhibition of DNA amplification by adeno-associated viruses (AAV) seems to be of relevance (Schlehofer et al., 1983b). Recently, AAV-2 has been shown to inhibit HPV-16-induced oncogenic transformation '*in vitro*'. This inhibition is mediated by the AAV *Rep78* gene, possibly at the level of transcription of the viral oncogenes (Hermonat, 1994). This could explain the tumour suppressor properties of AAV and corroborate the seroepidemiological findings of higher titres of anti-adeno-associated virus antibodies in the normal population compared to cancer patients (Sprecher-Goldberger et al., 1971; Mayor et al., 1976; Georg-Fries et al., 1984).

(b) Hormones and antioestrogens

Several studies show that hormones interact at the molecular level with papillomavirus genomes and modify their expression. The upstream regulatory region of papillomaviruses contained glucocorticoid responsive elements, as shown by the enhancement of HPV-16 transcription upon dexamethasone treatment of cells in culture (Chan *et al.*, 1988). This was also shown in transgenic mice containing the HPV-18 long terminal repeat linked to the *Escherichia coli* β-galactosidase gene (Cid *et al.*, 1993). Transformation of mouse primary cells by HPV-16 in combination with an activated oncogene has been shown to be dependent on glucocorticoids: cells became transformed and tumorigenic in the presence of dexamethasone (Crook *et al.*, 1988; Pater *et al.*, 1988). Furthermore, these experiments could be reproduced in the presence of progesterone and progestins; the latter are pharmacologically active components in oral contraceptives (Pater *et al.*, 1990). This effect could be inhibited by RU486, a synthetic antagonist of these hormones (Pater & Pater, 1991).

Dexamethasone has been shown to interfere differentially with the transcription of HPV *E6* and *E7* genes in HPV-18-positive cervical carcinoma cell lines as follows: enhanced gene transcription, associated with growth stimulation, was observed in the two cell lines C4-1 and C4-2; no effect was seen in HeLa cells, whereas a marked reduction in transcription, accompanied by growth retardation, was observed with SW 756 (von Knebel-Doeberitz *et al.*, 1991). These results may be explained by *cis* effects exerted by flanking host cell DNA sequences differing among the individual cell lines tested. Recently, the levels of the HPV-18-E7 protein in HeLa and C4-1 cell lines have been shown to be increased by hydrocortisone, while progesterone, oestrogen or testosterone had no effect (Selvey *et al.*, 1994). No progesterone or oestrogen receptors were detected in these carcinoma cell lines, but HPV-16 expression was markedly increased in human ectocervical cells exposed to glucocorticoid or progesterone (Mittal *et al.*, 1993a). This effect was inhibited by the anti-progestin RU486 and was shown to be dependent upon three hormone-responsive elements present in the viral regulatory region (Mittal *et al.*, 1993b).

Oestrogen and progesterone receptors were measured in normal cervical tissues and HPV-affected tissues from the cervix, vulva and penis (Monsonego *et al.*, 1991). While penile samples did not contain hormone receptors, cervical lesions had high levels, with high-grade lesions exhibiting the highest values, whereas low levels were detected in the vulvar tumours. Among the cervical tissues, squamous carcinomas had low levels of progesterone and an absence of oestrogen receptors. No association was found between levels of receptors and oral contraceptive use. Elevated progesterone receptor levels were more significantly correlated with HPV-16, -18-positive cervical lesions than to HPV-negative samples. Immunocytochemical localization of the receptors showed that they were evenly distributed in the connective tissue, but never detected in the epithelial cells. This is in contrast to what has been observed in cell culture and suggests an indirect effect of hormones on the HPV-infected cells. Additional studies are required to establish the relevance of the association between hormones and HPV during malignant transformation *in vivo*.

Oestrogen metabolism was measured in laryngeal papillomas, benign tumours that are known to be linked to HPV-6 and -11 infection, and in which oestrogen binding is known to be increased (Newfield *et al.*, 1993). Increased tumour risk is associated with increased 16-α-hydroxylation, while reduced risk is related to 2-hydroxylation. Explant cultures of laryngeal papillomas were shown to have an increased 16-α-hydroxylation of oestradiol-17β (see IARC, 1987b) when compared to normal laryngeal cells. Oestradiol-17β and 16-α-hydroxyoestrone increased the proliferation of laryngeal papilloma cells; on the other hand, the alternative metabolite 2-hydroxyoestrone had an anti-proliferative effect on these cells. Since indole-3-carbinol is a potent inducer of 2-hydroxylation of oestradiol-17β, this compound was added to laryngeal cell cultures and shown to inhibit oestradiol-17β-induced cell proliferation, similar to the effect observed with 2-hydroxyoestrone. Further experiments have shown that dietary indole-3-carbinol reduced the development of tumours in infected laryngeal tissue xenografts in nude mice.

The chemotherapeutic agent tamoxifen has been shown to stimulate the proliferation of an HPV-16-positive cervical carcinoma cell line (Hwang et al., 1992). At low concentrations, this drug was shown to increase both the HPV-16 mRNA and E7 levels, which may account for the higher proliferation rates observed. On the other hand, the growth of this HPV-16-positive cell line was inhibited by higher concentrations of tamoxifen, as seen in a wide variety of tissues and cell lines.

(c) Chemicals

The pioneering studies of Rous and his associates demonstrated that the tarring of skin or treatment of skin with other chemical carcinogens accelerates greatly the emergence of CRPV-induced papillomas and their malignant conversion (Rous & Kidd, 1938). Studies conducted by M.S. Campo and W.F. Jarrett and their colleagues revealed the interaction of BPV infection and exposure to bracken fern (see IARC, 1987c) in the induction of malignant tumours in bovines (see section 4). The contribution of bracken fern is due to both its carcinogenic and immuno-suppressive properties (see section 4).

Mutagens and immunosuppressants, such as those present in bracken fern or derived from the constituents of tobacco smoke (see IARC, 1986), may co-operate with the papillomavirus in the induction of malignancies in different ways (Jackson et al., 1993). Several reports describe the interaction between BPV and chemical cofactors in the induction of malignant tumours (see section 4). A recent observation of extensive papillomatosis of the hairy skin spreading from oral mucosa in an iatrogenically immunosuppressed dog provides further support for reactivation of latent papillomavirus infections (in this case, canine oral papillomavirus (COPV)) and expansion in the tissue tropism of the virus (Sundberg et al., 1994).

Treatment of a mouse BPV-1-transformed cell line with N-methyl-N'-nitro-N-nitroso-guanidine (MNNG) (see IARC, 1987d) led to the amplification of both episomal and integrated sequences of BPV-1 DNA (Schmitt et al., 1989). 12-O-Tetradecanoylphorbol 13-acetate (TPA), on the other hand, was ineffective, either alone or in combination with MNNG. Amplification of BPV DNA by initiating agents may be an important event in the co-operative effects between viral genomes and other carcinogens.

Constituents of tobacco smoke and its derived nitroso compounds have been shown to be potent carcinogens in different experimental systems (see IARC, 1986). Higher levels of these compounds were detected in cervical secretions of smokers compared with nonsmokers (Sasson et al., 1985; Schiffman et al., 1987). Mutagenic activity in cervical cells was demonstrated to be similar to that observed in human lung tissue (Phillips & Nishe, 1993), which points to a possible role of these compounds in cervical carcinogenesis. When exposed to either benzo[a]-pyrene or ethyl methanesulfonate, HPV-16-immortalized human oral keratocytes were able to proliferate in higher calcium concentration, whereas normal and non-carcinogen exposed cells differentiated terminally under these conditions (Li et al., 1992). Moreover, they acquired the ability to induce squamous-cell carcinomas in 20–50% of the injected animals. These carcinomas eventually regressed and it was noted that they had a wild-type c-Ha-ras and p53. When compared to their normal counterparts, these cells expressed higher levels of E6/E7 mRNAs and transforming growth factor (TGF)-α, which may have accounted for their enhanced growth capacity both in vitro and in vivo. Further experiments have shown that exposure to N-nitrosamines and MNNG leads to very similar results, with higher transcription of c-myc and EGF receptor genes (Kim et al., 1993a).

Normal and HPV-18-immortalized human foreskin keratinocytes were treated with N-methyl-N-nitrosourea either alone, or followed by 12-O-tetradecanoylphorbol 13-acetate, and injected into nude mice (Garrett et al., 1993). Even after prolonged incubation in the animals, tumours were never generated by the chemically treated normal cells or the HPV-18-immortalized cells treated only with N-methyl-N-nitrosourea. On the other hand, poorly differentiated squamous-cell carcinomas were observed when the HPV-18 immortalized cells were exposed to both chemicals. Cell lines derived from the tumours exhibited the same copy numbers of HPV-18 DNA as found in the parental lines before chemical exposure, and no indication of alteration in the ras gene was detected. However, karyotypic analysis revealed several chromosomal alterations, including a deletion in 18q affecting the DCC (deleted in colon cancer) tumour suppressor gene locus, frequently deleted in colon carcinomas (see section 3.1.3). Low amounts of DCC mRNA were also found in HPV-immortalized and chemically transformed human oral keratinocytes (Kim et al., 1993b).

(d) Radiation

Ultraviolet (UV) radiation (see IARC, 1992) and X-radiation are known to induce mutations in cellular DNA, and exposure to UV radiation can alter immune function (Kripke & Morison, 1985). Mutations could also increase the expression of viral oncoproteins, through direct interference with viral or cellular factors that down-regulate viral transcription or replication. In general, non-melanoma skin cancers arise in body areas exposed to sunlight. This accounts for skin cancers in immunocompetent as well as immunosuppressed patients and epidermodysplasia, a very rare hereditary condition predisposing to HPV infection, and to the subsequent development of cancers within the papillomas. Since these skin cancers, particularly in immunosuppressed patients, have recently been shown to contain in part novel HPV types (Shamanin et al., 1994a; Berkhout et al., 1995), the localization of these cancers could suggest an interaction between sunlight and papillomavirus infections.

Experiments performed in the hairless mouse *Mus musculus* HRA/Skh suggest the participation of UV radiation in the induction of papillomas and carcinomas in association with a papillomavirus closely related to *Mastomys natalensis* papillomavirus (MnPV) (Tilbrook et al., 1989).

A 16-fold increase in the risk of malignant transformation has been reported after X-ray irradiation therapy for multiple laryngeal papillomas, with a latency period of 5–40 years (summarized in Lindeberg & Elbrond, 1991). Verrucous carcinomas of the larynx present as exophytic warty tumours, some of which have been shown to contain not only HPV-16 DNA, but also low-risk HPV DNAs that are found more frequently in laryngeal papillomatosis (Byrne et al., 1987; Kashima et al., 1988; Brandsma & Abrahamson, 1989). A recent report shows relatively high frequencies of anaplastic transformation after irradiation of primary laryngeal carcinomas, and recommends a surgical approach to the treatment of these tumours (Hagen et al., 1993).

The effect of radiation of HPV-containing human epithelial cells provides a useful model to study genetic alterations contributing to transformation. The exposure of HPV-16-immortalized human foreskin cells to X-irradiation resulted in malignant conversion after approximately 100 additional tissue culture passages (Dürst et al., 1995). Human bronchial epithelial cells, immortalized with HPV-18, were exposed to ionizing radiation. The derived cell lines showed several chromosomal alterations, but they were not tumorigenic in nude mice, despite their ability to grow in soft agar (Willey et al., 1993). The effect of different doses of radon-simulated α-particles was tested on HPV-18-immortalized bronchial cells (Hei et al., 1994). Cells were irradiated with a single radiation dose and maintained in culture for a period of up to three months, after which they became tumorigenic. No mutation in the K-, H- or N-*ras* genes was found in four of these tumours. Since HPV DNA is occasionally found in bronchogenic carcinomas (Stremlau et al., 1985), it may be important to assess the risk of environmental or occupational radon exposure on the progression of HPV lesions of the respiratory epithelium.

3.1.6 HPV in mice

(a) HPV recombinant retrovirus

Sasagawa et al. (1992b) infected the mouse vagina with a retrovirus carrying the *E6* and *E7* oncogenes of HPV-16. Infection resulted in the onset of both low- and high-grade dysplasia: 11/39 mice developed low-grade dysplasia and 22/39 developed high-grade dysplasia. Eight of 30 mice infected with the carrier retrovirus alone developed only low-grade dysplasia. Progression to cancer occurred in 6/15 mice treated with the carcinogen MNNG and in 2/13 mice treated with TPA. Therefore, HPV-16, like animal papilloma viruses (see section 4.2.5) (Gaukroger et al., 1993), can synergize with both a carcinogen and a tumour promoter.

(b) HPV transgenic mice

Studies in transgenic mice can be loosely divided into three groups: (i) those in which the HPV genome, subgenomic regions of the HPVs or other genes are expressed from the homologous HPV promoter elements; (ii) those in which the HPV genome or subgenomic regions are expressed from promoters to target expression toward organs other than the skin or to achieve diffuse expression in the transgene; (iii) those in which expression of the HPV genome or subgenomic regions is targeted toward the skin.

(i) Transgenic animals with the HPV control region

Choo *et al.* (1992) generated transgenic animals with the SV40 T antigen fused to the HPV-18 long control region. Low-level expression of T antigen was detected in several tissues, including the stomach and large intestine but not in the skin or in the anogenital area. In a more recent study, Comerford *et al.* (1995) expressed the *E6* and *E7* genes from the homologous HPV-18 control region and found that these transgenic mice developed genital tract disease after a prolonged latency period: 41% of the female transgenic mice developed mesenchymal cervical lesions and tumours. The transgenic males exhibited enlarged seminal vesicles and preputial glands at an age of 10 weeks. This study, in contrast to Choo *et al.* (1992), therefore suggests that the HPV-18 long control region does indeed contain elements that target the expression of a transgene to the urogenital tract. The two studies were performed in a slightly different genetic background which might, at least in part, account for the different findings.

(ii) Transgenic animals with non-skin-specific expression of the HPV oncogenes

Kondoh *et al.* (1991) produced transgenic mice with the HPV-16 *E6* and *E7* oncogenes under the control of the mouse mammary tumour virus (MMTV) long terminal repeat. At eight to 10 months after birth, the male mice developed testicular germ-cell tumours of the seminoma type.

Arbeit *et al.* (1993) used the HPV-16 *E6* and *E7* genes expressed from a human β-actin promoter to generate transgenic mice. A large number of mice developed neuroepithelial tumours starting at 10 weeks after birth. Expression of the HPV oncoprotein E7 was detected in the tumours but not in normal tissues of the mice. The tumour suppressor genes *pRB* and *p53*, were expressed in the tumours in their wild-type forms.

Particularly perspicacious with respect to the delineation of HPV oncogene function *in vivo* have been studies in which the expression of the HPV oncogenes was targeted to the mouse ocular lens by using the murine crystallin promoter. HPV *E6* and *E7* induced hyperproliferation and inhibition of differentiation, and adult mice displayed microphthalmia and cataracts with a very high penetrance. One particular mouse line, with a very-high level of transgene expression, developed lenticular eye tumours (Griep *et al.*, 1993). Additional studies with mice transgenic for *E6* or *E7* alone showed that both oncogenes had a distinct phenotype: *E7* transgenic mice developed cataracts and microphthalmia, and the retinoblastoma protein binding site on E7 was found to be important for this phenotype. The HPV *E6* transgenic mice had cataracts only. The normal apoptosis and denucleation programme in differentiating lens fibre cells was disrupted in *E6* transgenic animals but lens tumours developed exclusively in *E6/E7* double transgenic mice. These studies clearly demonstrated that the *E6* and *E7* genes play important roles in cellular transformation *in vivo* (Pan & Griep, 1994). Similar results in mice transgenic for *E7* expression in a *p53* nullizygous background underline the relevance of the *E6–p53* interaction in cancer development (Howes *et al.*, 1994).

One of the *E6/E7* transgenic mice lines (Griep *et al.*, 1993) also developed epidermal cancers at a very-high incidence. Development of these lesions correlated with the expression of *E6* and *E7* and often occurred at sites of wounding (Lambert *et al.*, 1993).

(iii) Transgenic animals with skin-specific expression of the HPV oncogenes

Skin targeted expression of the HPV oncogenes is achieved by using keratin promoters.

E6 and *E7* expressed from the human keratin K1 promoter leads to the formation of wart-like lesions in older mice. Specific mutational activation of the *ras* oncogene was observed in the papillomas, illustrating that additional cellular events may have to occur in addition to an HPV infection for an overt lesion to occur (Greenhalgh *et al.*, 1994).

The human keratin 14 promoter was used to target HPV oncogene expression to the basal layer of the skin. Progressive epithelial neoplasia was observed in the transgenic animals and lesions appeared at multiple sites, including pinnal and truncal skin, face, snout and eyelids and anus. The phenotype progressed through discernible stages: mild hyperplasia was followed by hyperplasia and progressed to dysplasia and papillomatosis. The step-wise development of disease implicated additional cellular events to be necessary for carcinogenic progression (Arbeit *et al.*, 1994).

Expression of the early region genes of HPV-16 from the bovine keratin K10 promoter resulted in generalized epidermal hyperplasia with a marked increase of proliferating cells in the basal and superbasal layers of the skin. Expression of c-*myc* and TGF α was also enhanced, and negative growth regulatory functions of TGF β were at least in part abrogated in the skin of transgenic mice (Auewarakul *et al.*, 1994).

Transgenic mice with the HPV-16 early region expressed from the bovine keratin K6 promoter developed stomach cancer consisting of multiple malignant carcinoids originating from the neuroendocrine enterochromaffin-like cells at the squamocolumnar epithelial junction. These tumours again developed after prolonged asymptomatic expression of the HPV genome indicating the necessity for additional mutations to occur (Searle *et al.*, 1994).

3.2 Immune mechanisms and HPV-associated neoplasia

HPVs are exclusively intraepithelial pathogens with a replication cycle that is time dependent and differentiation dependent. Productive infections are chronic and the lesions may persist for many months. The viruses are not cytolytic and no inflammation accompanies infection and replication, a phenomenon that may retard the initiation of or even prevent an effective immune response. This said, the central questions are therefore whether natural infection with HPV induces an immune response to any viral protein and if so what is the nature of this response, when and how does it occur and how does it influence HPV-associated oncogenesis. The serological data are given in section 1.2.

3.2.1 Immunosuppression

Evidence from immunosuppressed individuals suggests strongly that the immune system is important in the pathogenesis of HPV-induced disease and malignant progression (Lutzner, 1985). Generalized warts have been reported in individuals with inherited immune deficiencies, specifically those in whom the T-cell arm of the response is in deficit (Lawlor *et al.*, 1974). Cutaneous and genital warts are one of the most frequent viral complications in patients immunosuppressed as a consequence of renal transplantation and these lesions are refractory to most therapeutic strategies (Benton *et al.*, 1992). Renal allograft recipients are at significantly increased risk for the development of cutaneous neoplasms but there are conflicting reports of the role of HPV in this (see section 2.5.2).

Individuals immunosuppressed as a consequence of HIV infection show similar trends with respect to anogenital neoplasia (Braun, 1994). The role of HIV infection in the pathogenesis of HPV-associated cervical neoplasia is not clear despite extensive investigation (see section 2.5.3). Unfortunately, the data from many studies are incomplete because either the HPV status of the HIV-infected individuals was not ascertained, the sample size was too small, the relevant control groups were not included, the evaluation of immune function was not attempted or clinical disease grading was not reported.

Overall, however, the evidence from transplant recipients, inherited immunodeficiencies and HIV-infected individuals suggests that it is the absolute deficit in $CD4^+$ cells that is important in HPV infection and associated neoplastic progression. This implies a central role for $CD4^+$ cell-mediated mechanisms in the control of HPV infection. The role of the humoral response in HPV infection remains open to debate. Disorders of humoral immunity do not result in an increased susceptibility to HPV-induced lesions (Lutzner, 1985), which suggests that antibody has little to do with the maintenance of HPV infections. There is persuasive evidence from animal studies in rabbits and cattle that antibodies directed against the major capsid protein L1 are protective (Campo, 1994).

3.2.2 Histological studies

The involution and regression of benign cutaneous and genital warts is accompanied by a noticeable histological reaction characteristic of a delayed type hypersensitivity response with a pronounced influx of mononuclear cells dominated by $CD4^+$ cells and macrophages (Stanley *et al.*, 1994). Immunohistological studies have shown that non-regressing anogenital warts are characterized by a relative lack of immune activity: mononuclear cells are present predominantly in the stroma and the few intraepithelial lymphocytes are mainly $CD8^+$ cells. Spontaneously regressing lesions are characterized by a mononuclear cell infiltrate dominated by $CD4^+$, $CD45RO^+$ T cells and macrophages (Stanley *et al.*, 1995). The wart keratinocytes express HLA-DR and ICAM-1 and endothelial cells in the stromal capillaries immediately underneath the infected epithelium express the adhesion molecules E selectin and VCAM and the cytokine RANTES. Interestingly, no statistical difference in the numbers of Langerhans' cells in either active warts or regressing warts was observed in this study (Stanley *et al.*, 1995), although the morphology of Langerhans' cells in active warts was characterized by a loss of dendritic arborizations, a phenomenon reported also in HPV-associated cervical lesions (Barton *et al.*, 1988; Hughes *et al.*, 1988; Morelli *et al.*, 1994). A similar immune infiltrate and expression of MHC class II antigen in keratinoytes were also observed in regressing CRPV warts (Okabayashi *et al.*, 1991).

The situation in cervical lesions differs from that of genital warts and is related to the grade of disease and neoplastic status. Low-grade cervical lesions (CIN I) are to a large extent immunologically quiescent. There is general agreement that there is a reduction in the number of Langerhans' cells (Morris *et al.*, 1983; Tay *et al.*, 1987a; Hawthorn *et al.*, 1988) and changes in Langerhans' cell morphology (Hughes *et al.*, 1988) have been described. High-grade intraepithelial cervical lesions are also characterized by a reduction in Langerhans' cells (Tay *et al.*, 1987a; Hawthorn *et al.*, 1988; Viac *et al.*, 1990). Several groups have investigated T-cell numbers in lesions with varying results. Tay *et al.* (1987b) described a significant reduction in intraepithelial T-cell numbers in all grades of CIN with a preferential decline in the CD4$^+$ subset. Morris et al. (1983) showed a reduction in intraepithelial T cells in low-grade lesions but an increase in the CD8$^+$ subset in CIN III. Similarly, Viac et al. (1990) reported increased numbers of both stromal and epithelial lymphocytes in CIN II–III with a dominance of CD8$^+$ cells in the epithelium but equivalent numbers of CD4$^+$ and CD8$^+$ cells in the stroma.

Surveillance and defence against viral infection and tumours are mediated via both MHC-restricted and non-restricted effector mechanisms. Nearly all of the latter are mediated via large granular lymphocytes and include natural killer cells. Large granular lymphocytes with the national killer (NK) phenotype CD56$^+$,CD16$^+$,CD3$^-$,CD2^{variable},CD57^{variable} are rarely found within the normal cervical squamous epithelium or CIN (Syrjanen et al., 1986; Viac et al., 1990; McKenzie et al., 1991) although they are present in the stroma and the endocervix. A separate and small subset of large granular lymphocytes, CD56$^+$,CD3$^+$,CD2$^+$,CD16$^-$, is found within the ectocervical epithelium, and this subset dominates the intraepithelial population in high-grade CIN (McKenzie et al., 1991).

Increased numbers of T cells are seen locally in squamous-cell carcinoma of the cervix (Ferguson et al., 1985; Hilders et al., 1993; Ghosh et al., 1994) with a dominance of the CD8$^+$ subset. These CD8$^+$ tumour-infiltrating cells can cause effective and specific in-vitro killing of autologous tumour targets (Okada et al., 1989). However, bulk cultures of tumour-infiltrating cells generated from cervical squamous-cell carcinomas showed non-MHC-restricted cytotoxicity in the majority of cases (Ghosh et al., 1994). T-cell clones isolated from two cases had the phenotype CD3$^+$,CD4$^+$,CD56$^+$/CD56$^-$ and showed low cytotoxicity to autologous tumour cells (Ghosh & Moore, 1992).

3.2.3 Cell-mediated immunity

(a) Helper T-cell responses

Although the histological evidence indicates that HPV-associated lesions elicit an immune response, the target antigens in this response are unknown. However, there is evidence from both experimental animal models and humans that viral proteins can be immune targets. Murine keratinocytes expressing HPV-16 *E6* or *E7* can be grafted onto the flanks of syngeneic immunocompetent mice to reform a differentiated epithelium. Subsequent challenge of the recipients by intradermal inoculation in the ear with a recombinant vaccinia virus expressing HPV-16 *E6* or *E7* results in a delayed-type hypersensitivity response (McLean et al., 1993; Chambers et al., 1994a). This response is CD4$^+$ cell-dependent (McLean et al., 1993). Intradermal challenge with HPV-16 E7 protein also elicits a delayed-type hypersensitivity response provided that a nonspecific inflammatory stimulus, such as the phorbol ester TPA, is applied to the ear in concert with the protein challenge (Chambers et al., 1994b), which illustrates the crucial role of inflammation, at least in this model system. The ability to prime the immune system and elicit a delayed-type hypersensitivity response is critical and is dependent upon antigen dose in this model. Thus, there is a threshold graft inoculum of HPV-16 expressing keratinocytes, below which, although an epithelium reforms, a delayed-type hypersensitivity response cannot be elicited despite repeated antigen challenge (Chambers et al., 1994b). A delayed-type hypersensitivity response has also been detected in regressor rabbits against the structural proteins of

CRPV (Hopfl et al., 1993) and in CIN patients against the L1 protein of HPV-16 (Hopfl et al., 1991).

Using synthetic peptides and fusion proteins in lymphoproliferation assays, murine helper T-cell epitopes in HPV-16 E7 have been determined in several studies (Davies et al., 1990; Comerford et al., 1991; Tindle et al., 1991; Shepherd et al., 1992). A public T_h epitope (DRAHYNI) which provides cognate help for B cells in all strains tested has been located at aminoacids 48–54 in HPV-16 E7 (Tindle et al., 1991). However, it does not appear to hold this property in humans (Tindle & Frazer, 1994). As this latter observation shows, peptides recognized by the murine T-cell response repertoire may not have the same identity for humans.

The analysis of T-cell responses for HPV proteins has been hampered by the heterogeneity of the circulating T-cell population. In one of the first studies to be reported, Strang et al. (1990) showed proliferative responses to peptides from the E6 and L1 proteins of HPV-16 when peripheral blood mononuclear cells from healthy donors were tested. Peptide-specific clones and T-cell lines were then used to define the HLA restriction of these responses. Using a similar approach, three T_h epitopes in HPV-16 E7 were identified that were recognized in association with at least two different HLA haplotypes (Altmann et al., 1992). In a study using overlapping peptides spanning the entire HPV-16 E7 protein, lymphoproliferative responses to a carboxyl-terminal peptide 72–97 were significantly related to ongoing infection with HPV-16 and related types (Kadish et al., 1994). Specific T-cell responses to HPV-16 L1 have been detected in patients with cervical dysplasias (Shepherd et al., 1994). In this context, it is of interest that T-cell responses to structural proteins of CRPV have been shown to increase in the papilloma–carcinoma conversion with a dramatic increase in the response to L2 (Selvakumar et al., 1994).

(b) Cytotoxic T-cell responses

Cell-mediated cytotoxicity is a phenomenon mediated via a range of cells which include $CD4^+$ and $CD8^+$ cells, LAK cells and NK cells. Classically, cytotoxic T cells are class I restricted $CD8^+$ cells and the role of these cells in HPV infection is under intense investigation. Since transformed cells from HPV-associated cancers consistently express the E6 and E7 viral proteins, these would represent targets for cytotoxic T cells *a priori*. Various investigators have attempted to determine the immunogenicity of these proteins in rodents in experiments in which cells transfected with HPV genes are used as tumour challenge. Using this approach it has been shown that HPV-16 E6 and E7 can act as tumour rejection antigens (Chen et al., 1991; Meneguzzi et al., 1991; Chen et al., 1992a). In an extension of these studies, it was shown that HPV-16 E7-transfected melanoma cells grew progressively in the immunocompetent host, but that transfection of these cells with B7 (the counter receptor for CD28) induced rejection of both the B7 transfectant and the parental E7 expressing line (Chen et al., 1992b); $CD8^+$ antitumour cytotoxic T cells could be isolated from protected mice (Chen et al., 1992b). Evidence for the induction of HPV-16 E7-specific cytotoxic T cells has come from the studies of Feltkamp et al. (1993), in which vaccination with a synthetic peptide of the HPV-16 E7 sequence, amino acids 49–57, protected against challenge with HPV-16-transformed tumour cells and induced cytotoxic T cells which lysed tumour cells *in vitro*.

However, in other studies the E6 and E7 proteins have been weakly immunogenic (Gao et al., 1994; Sadovnikova et al., 1994). Thus, mice immunized with HPV-16 E6- or E7-

transfected cells did not generate detectable cytotoxic T-cell responses, which were only seen in mice immunized with E6 or E7 recombinant vaccinia virus. These studies also illustrate the limitations of predictive peptide motifs. Thus, a motif-positive peptide of HPV-16 E6 that showed strong MHC class I binding in the RMA-S assay was not recognized by anti-E6 cytotoxic T cells generated by an E6 recombinant vaccinia virus. Instead, these T cells recognized a motif-negative peptide that showed weak class I binding (Gao et al., 1994). Similar observations were made for HPV-16 E7 (Sadovnikova et al., 1994).

Nevertheless, motif predictions have been useful in humans. Tarpey et al. (1994) used the HLA A2.1 motif to locate putative cytotoxic T-cell epitopes in HPV-11 E7. Of the three nonapeptides tested, one primed cytotoxic T cells to recognize and lyse cells infected by HPV-11 E7 recombinant vaccinia virus. Potential HLA-A T-cell epitopes in HPV-16 E6 and E7 have been identified for five HLA-A alleles using a set of overlapping nonapeptides and T2 binding assays (Kast et al., 1994). However, the authenticity of these peptides as cytotoxic T-cell targets remains to be proven.

An alternative strategy for defining cytotoxic T-cell targets in humans is to use mice transgenic for a human HLA allele, immunized with recombinant HPV proteins to generate cytotoxic T-cell precursors *in vivo*. This approach has been taken by Beverley et al. (1994) using HLA-A2 transgenics and HPV-16 E6. Their preliminary data suggest that an E6 epitope can be presented by HLA-A2. However, as these workers point out, there is a paradox between the murine and human systems. The murine experiments show that E6 and E7 contain cytotoxic T-cell epitopes and conventional immunization procedures generate T cells against them, but, to date, there are no reports of human cytotoxic T cells that recognize HPV antigens in association with HLA-A2 or any other HLA allele. It is worth re-emphasizing that HPV is an exclusively intraepithelial pathogen; viral gene expression is confined to keratinocytes, which are incapable of delivering accessory signals to T cells — a situation that could induce tolerance rather than prime an active immune response (Bal et al., 1990; Chambers et al., 1994b).

3.2.4 Major histocompatibility complex (MHC) expression

(a) MHC class I

Loss or downregulation of class I MHC expression is a well recognized mechanism whereby viruses escape immune detection, and the expression of MHC molecules in relation to HPV-associated neoplasms has been closely investigated (Stern & Duggan Keen, 1994). Immunohistological studies on cryostat sections using the monoclonal antibody W6/32 provided little evidence for class I modulation in benign HPV lesions or CIN (Viac et al., 1990; Glew et al., 1993a). Similar results were obtained by Torres et al. (1993) using the monoclonal antibody HC10 in the analysis of paraffin sections from a large series of premalignant cervical lesions. However, in an extensive study analysing HLA expression in paraffin-embedded material using a polyclonal antibody RaHC and the monoclonal antibody HC10, disturbed HLA class I heavy chain expression was found in all grades of CIN and cancer of the cervix (Cromme et al., 1993a). The monoclonal antibody W6/32 recognizes monomorphic determinants of the heterodimeric HLA class I molecule; the monoclonal antibody HC10 recognizes HLA, B and C locus products preferentially; RaHC is specific for HLA A, B and C heavy chains. The differences in staining patterns observed in these studies could reflect allele-specific downregulation, which would be detectable by loss of staining with HC10 and RaHC, or alternatively the presence of incomplete or modified heavy chains, which would stain positively with W6/32 but not with HC10/RaHC. They may also reflect the inadequacies of assessing HLA expression by immunohistochemistry on small biopsies where fixation and processing artifacts could distort the analysis.

There is no dispute that class I expression is downregulated in cervical squamous-cell carcinoma (Connor & Stern, 1990; Cromme *et al.*, 1993a; Glew *et al.*, 1993a; Torres *et al.*, 1993; Hilders *et al.*, 1994). These changes occur in both HPV-positive and HPV-negative lesions and have been shown, in a proportion of tumours, to be controlled post-transcriptionally (Cromme *et al.*, 1993b). In HPV-16/18-positive tumours, this post-transcriptional loss of HLA class I expression is related to the loss of peptide transport due to downregulation of expression of TAP-1 protein (Cromme *et al.*, 1994). This is an important observation, but it is unlikely that all class I downregulation in cervical cancer is due to this single mechanism. Connor & Stern (1990) observed that loss of $\beta2$ microglobulin was often accompanied by the absence of HLA heavy chains and this suggests that the regulation of several MHC-associated gene products may be altered in invasive cancers. Whatever the mechanism of downregulation, these changes may be of central importance functionally, since the absence of class I or allele-specific downregulation would be expected to interfere with T-cell recognition of target antigens (whether of host or viral origin) and disable cytotoxic T-cell effector mechanisms. In support of this, there is evidence from preliminary studies that patients with early cervical cancers with downregulated class I have a poorer clinical outcome (Connor *et al.*, 1993).

(b) MHC class II

Normal ectocervical epithelium does not express class II antigens, although HLA-DR expression has been reported in the transformation zone (Roncalli *et al.*, 1988). The expression of class II by HPV-infected keratinocytes in low-grade cervical lesions is variable with some studies finding no expression (Hughes *et al.*, 1988; Warhol & Gee, 1989) and other patchy focal expression (Fais *et al.*, 1991; Coleman & Stanley, 1994). Class II expression is seen in high-grade CIN, although the extent of expression varies from patchy HLA-DR positivity (Ferguson *et al.*, 1985) to diffuse extensive staining (Glew *et al.*, 1992; Cromme *et al.*, 1993a; Coleman & Stanley, 1994). Expression of class II molecules occurs in at least 80% of cervical cancers (Glew *et al.*, 1992; Cromme *et al.*, 1993a; Glew *et al.*, 1993a). Glew *et al.* (1992) postulated that such expression in high-grade CIN and cervical cancer is a reflection of the transformation of squamous metaplastic cells, which they have shown to be class II-positive. An alternative explanation is that this expression is in part induced rather than constitutive. This explanation is supported by the observation of increased numbers of T cells in the subepithelial stroma of HLA-DR-positive as compared to HLA-DR-negative CIN (Coleman & Stanley, 1994) and an increase in tumour-infiltrating cells in DR-positive regions of cervical squamous-cell carcinomas (Hilders *et al.*, 1994). In addition, no constitutive expression of HLA-DR could be shown on fully transformed HPV-16-expressing keratinocytes *in vitro*, although it could be induced by γ-interferon (Coleman & Stanley, 1994). A large proportion of high-grade CIN express ICAM-1, as well as HLA-DR, although co-expression of these molecules is not inevitable and an ICAM-1 positive lesion can be HLA-DR negative (Stanley *et al.*, 1994b). Evidence from in-vitro studies with HPV-16-expressing keratinocyte cell lines indicates that this expression in high-grade lesions is constitutive rather than induced (Coleman *et al.*, 1993b), suggesting that ICAM-1 expression *in vivo* in CIN III is unlikely to be a virally induced phenomenon but rather a consequence of neoplastic transformation *per se*.

3.2.5 HLA polymorphisms: association with cervical cancer risk

The recognition of foreign as opposed to self antigen depends upon the recognition by the T-cell receptor of subtle changes in the MHC/peptide complex as presented on the cell surface. Fundamentally many immune responses are controlled by genes of the MHC complex and, crucially, there is evidence that host resistance or susceptibility to pathogens is dependent in part on the dynamic interaction between the host MHC and permissivity for the presentation of pathogen peptides (Parham, 1994). For any one protein, different alleles of the MHC will present different peptides to the immune system. Thus, the loss or upregulation of different alleles could influence the natural history of HPV infection and the risk of neoplastic progression. If this were the case, then it could be reflected in different HLA frequencies in patients with cervical carcinoma when compared to the appropriate normal population.

Associations between HLA haplotype and cervical carcinoma have been reported in recent studies. Using serological typing, Wank and Thomssen (1991) showed association with HLA-DQw3 and increased risk for cervical cancer but decreased risk in association with DR6 in a German patient group. A similar association but with a smaller relative risk was found in a Norwegian study (Helland *et al.*, 1992). Serological typing does not discriminate alleles as precisely as molecular typing, and typing by PCR and single-strand oligonucleotide probes in the German group revealed that DQB1*0301 and *0303 were the risk alleles for cervical cancer (Wank *et al.*, 1993). However, in a study in the United Kingdom of 57 patients with cervical squamous-cell carcinoma and 857 controls using molecular and serological typing, no such association was found (Glew *et al.*, 1993b).

Gregoire *et al.* (1994) showed an association between DQB1*0303 and cervical cancer risk in African American women but could not show an association between HPV type in the tumour and HLA. This is in contrast to the recent studies of Odunsi *et al.* (1995) who found a strong association between HLA DQB1*0301 and CIN and HPV. Apple *et al.* (1994) investigated the role of the HLA class II loci and HPV type in cervical cancer. This case–control study included biopsies from 98 Hispanic patients with cervical cancer, and cervical scrapes from 220 Hispanic control women with normal Pap smears. All patients were from the same geographic area in the South West of the USA. In this group, certain HLA class II haplotypes, including DB1*150 – DQB1*0602, were significantly associated with HPV-16-containing cancer, whereas DR13 haplotypes were negatively associated. If the type specificity of these associations are confirmed, this may be of fundamental importance since it implies that specific HLA class II haplotypes influence the response to HPV-encoded epitopes and the risk of neoplastic progression. It is of interest that class II haplotypes have been implicated when MHC class I is downregulated in the majority of cervical squamous-cell carcinomas. The high frequency of HLA-B locus downregulation seen in both premalignant and malignant lesions (Cromme *et al.*, 1993a) raises the suspicion that these locus products may be important for the presentation of target host or HPV peptides. Evidence in support of this has recently been presented (Ellis *et al.*, 1995). In this study, potential cytotoxic T-cell epitopes in HPV-16 E6 for HLA-B7 were identified by T2 binding assays. Sequence analysis of the E6 region from HPV-16 isolates derived from HLA-B7 cervical cancer patients identified a consistent mutation in the N-terminal corresponding to two of the B7 binding epitopes. The mutation, a single base change from guanosine to adenosine results in a change in the amino acid sequence from arginine to glycine in the binding peptide at position 3. This amino acid substitution does not affect binding, but does alter the residues exposed to the T-cell receptor and would be likely to alter the affinity of the TCR/MHC peptide binding. It seems likely that the mutant is a true HPV-16 viral variant with a wide geographical distribution, implying that the HLA-B7 allele is important in the immunological control of HPV-16 infection in a manner analogous to other HLA alleles involved in antiviral surveillance (Gavioli *et al.*, 1993). A role for HLA haplotype and susceptibility to HPV-associated cancer is strongly supported by data from the rabbit, with the observation that regression or progression of papillomas induced by CRPV is linked respectively to the MHC DR and DQ phenotypes of the animals (Han *et al.*, 1992).

4. Studies of Cancer in Animals

Due to the species specificity of papillomaviruses, infection of experimental animals with HPVs is not possible. However, understanding the natural history and carcinogenic potential of HPVs is assisted by the study of several animal papillomaviruses.

In the analysis of the association of animal papillomavirus with naturally occurring or experimentally induced neoplasia in various species, benign tumours (warts) rather than cancer are often taken as the end-point, often on the grounds that: (i) the incidence of warts is higher than that of cancer and it is therefore easier to monitor; (ii) it is difficult to follow the course of disease in wild animals; (iii) domestic animals, such as cattle, are usually killed before the onset of malignancy; and (iv) papillomavirus-associated cancer may ultimately derive from warts exposed to the action of cofactors, and thus the presence of warts can be considered as an indication of possible incipient neoplastic progression. All of the reported genomic sequences of animal papillomaviruses are available in the EMBL and GeneBank data.

For each of the animal papillomaviruses included in this section, naturally occurring warts and their progression to cancer are described first, followed by experimental production of tumours in natural and in heterologous hosts.

4.1 Non-human primate papillomaviruses

Two different types of papillomavirus were isolated from papillomas of the colobus monkey (*Colobus guereza*): CgPV-1 from a penile papilloma and CgPV-2 from a cutaneous papilloma (O'Banion *et al.*, 1987; Kloster *et al.*, 1988). A different papillomavirus was isolated from 5/8 cases of focal epithelial hyperplasia in the pygmy chimpanzee (*Pan paniscus*) and called PCPV (Van Ranst *et al.*, 1991). This virus is related to HPV-13 which induces focal epithelial hyperplasia in humans.

Rhesus monkey genital papillomavirus

Kloster *et al.* (1988) isolated and cloned an integrated papillomavirus genome from a lymph node metastasis of a penile squamous-cell carcinoma in a rhesus monkey (*Maccaca mulatta*). The viral DNA was designated RhPV-1 and used as a probe in a retrospective study of a rhesus colony (Ostrow *et al.*, 1990). The authors analysed individuals that had either mated directly with the 'index male' or with intermediate sexual partners. They analysed by PCR biopsies or scrapes from 30 females, one male and the index male, all belonging to the same group, from four mature females from a different group and from seven virgin females. The direct (6/12) and indirect (15/18) mates of the index male were found to be positive for viral DNA, clinical lesions or histopathology (Figure 20). One intermediate male analysed by PCR was positive for RhPV-1 DNA and four intermediate males were all clinically positive (Figure 20). The lesions displayed various degrees of atypia, ranging from koilocytosis, CIN I, koilocytosis plus CIN I, to invasive squamous-cell carcinomas of the penis and the cervix. The virgin females and those from the outside group showed no RhPV-1 infection. These results strongly linked, in a causal way, infection by RhPV-1 with genital neoplasia.

Figure 20. RhPV-1 transmission and mating relationships in rhesus monkeys

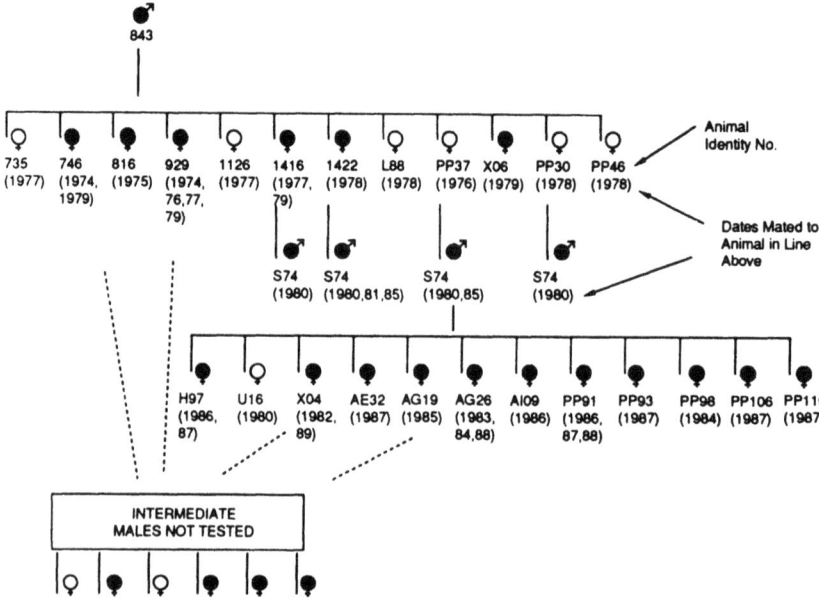

The most direct sexual relationships are shown with the dates of interactions. Filled symbols represent animals for which at least one clinical, histopathological or molecular result indicate papillomavirus infection. Open symbols represent negative individuals. Virgin females and females mated outside the group are not shown. Reproduced from Ostrow et al. (1990) with the permission of the authors.

In a recent study, Ostrow et al. (1995) analysed a number of fresh or archival genital tissues of rhesus monkeys from three geographically distinct regions for evidence of papillomavirus infection. By PCR, sequences related to RhPV-1 DNA were found in 12/59 (20%) animals from the three areas. The serological status of the animals was also investigated and 34/59 (57.6%) animals were positive for at least one RhPV-1 antigen. Most of the RhPV-1 DNA-positive animals were also serologically positive (8/10 tested cases), whereas most serologically positive animals were RhPV-1 DNA negative (23/31 tested cases). Histopathological analysis showed that the vast majority of cervical smears and biopsies were clinically normal, with the occasional presence of mild-to-moderate chronic inflammation and focal squamous metaplasia. Four cases showed features of papillomavirus infection; of these one was classified as CIN I, and another was the only case concordant with seropositivity; all cases were RhPV-1 DNA negative. The situation parallels HPV infection in humans, where the detection of seropositivity is higher than the detection of viral DNA.

4.2 Bovine papillomavirus

4.2.1 Heterogeneity of bovine papillomavirus

Bovine papillomaviruses (BPVs) make up a heterogeneous group of viruses with worldwide distribution. They induce papillomatosis of the skin, the genital and paragenital area, the eye, the alimentary canal and the bladder. Six types (BPV-1 to -6) have been described in detail (Jarrett *et al.*, 1984a), but many more remain to be identified and isolated. The six well-characterized BPVs fall into two subgroups, A and B, depending on the size of the viral genome and the degree of their molecular and immunological relationship. The molecular and immunological differences between the members of the two subgroups underlie biological differences. Thus, subgroup A members (BPV-1, BPV-2 and BPV-5) induce fibropapillomas, warts with fibroblastic and epithelial components, whereas subgroup B members (BPV-4 and BPV-6) induce purely epithelial papillomas (Campo *et al.*, 1980; Jarrett *et al.*, 1984a); BPV-3 has been found in epithelial papillomas (Pfister *et al.*, 1979a) (Table 61).

Table 61. Bovine papillomaviruses and their tumours

Subgroup	Virus type	Associated tumours
A	BPV-1	Fibropapillomas of the paragenital areas
	BPV-2	Fibropapillomas of the skin
		Fibropapillomas of the alimentary canal[a]
	BPV-5	Fibropapillomas of teats and udders
B	BPV-3	Papillomas of skin
	BPV-4	Papillomas of the alimentary canal
	BPV-6	Papillomas of teats and udders

[a]Alimentary canal fibropapillomas do not produce virus
From Pfister *et al.* (1979a), Campo *et al.* (1980, 1981) and Jarrett *et al.* (1984a)

4.2.2 BPV-1

BPV-1 induces primarily fibropapilloma of the penis of bulls and of the teats and udders of cows and can also infect adjacent skin and the muzzle, leading to the same histological lesions (Campo *et al.*, 1981). BPV-1 has been used extensively in transmission experiments, where the 'take' in cattle can be up to 100% (Jarrett, 1985). Olson *et al.* (1969) were the first to perform transmission experiments with BPV and, although at that time the multiplicity of BPV was not known, it is reasonable to assume that the virus was either BPV-1 or BPV-2, as it was extracted from fibropapillomas of the skin. In addition to transmitting BPV to skin, Gordon and Olson (1968) induced meningiomas in 17/19 calves (89.5%) by injection of the virus into the brain. The latency period was nine months and the take in the brain was the same as that in the skin.

A review of early transmission experiments both in homologous and heterologous hosts is given in Olson (1987).

(a) BPV-1 in hamsters

Inoculation of BPV-1 into Syrian hamsters (*Mesocricetus auratus*) induced subcutaneous fibromas and fibrosarcomas, chondromas of the ear and meningiomas of the brain, depending on the site of injection; metastases to internal organs were relatively frequent particularly in the lungs (10% of the animals) (Olson et al., 1969). In a typical experiment, Pfister et al. (1981b) extracted BPV-1 from an udder fibropapilloma of a cow and inoculated approximately 10^9 viral particles/ml subcutaneously in the back of six two-month-old hamsters. Two of the animals developed fibrosarcomas at the site of injection, with a latency period of about 14 months. Both fibrosarcomas contained viral DNA, which was present in multiple episomal copies, but not structural viral antigens or virus particles. Both tumours were transplantable to other hamsters.

(b) BPV-1 in transgenic mice

BPV-1 transgenic mice have been generated by Lacey et al. (1986). A partial tandem duplication of the BPV-1 genome was used, containing two copies of the early transforming region and one of the late structural genes. Two transgenic mice were obtained, one of which died soon after birth. The other mouse had approximately five copies of integrated viral DNA in head-to-tail tandem structures. The heterozygous progeny of this mouse were used to generate homozygous animals. The homozygotes were normal during development and early adulthood. However, when about eight months old, all animals developed skin tumours, initially benign fibromas, in multiple body locations. Fibromas also developed on the tails of heterozygotes where they had been clipped for DNA analysis. The fibromas became malignant and invasive with age. No virion or viral structural antigen was detected in the fibromas or fibrosarcomas. Whereas in young normal mice and in normal skin the viral DNA was integrated into the cellular DNA, in the tumours the viral DNA was episomal and amplified. Viral transcription activity increased during tumour progression from fibroma to fibrosarcoma (Bossy-Wetzel et al., 1992; Christofori & Hanahan, 1994).

4.2.3 BPV-2

BPV-2 induces typical skin warts of the neck and shoulder in cattle (Campo et al., 1981). The histology of these skin warts is similar to that of BPV-1 warts (Jarrett, 1985). BPV-2 is also found in fibropapillomas of the oesophagus and rumen (Jarrett et al., 1984b), but these tumours, contrary to the fibropapillomas of the skin, do not produce virus and appear to be the result of abortive infection. Transmission experiments of BPV-2 to the skin have a take of 100% (Jarrett, 1985).

(a) BPV-2 in bladder cancers

In a study in Scotland, 30% of the cattle with squamous-cell carcinoma (80 animals) of the upper alimentary tract had concurrent bladder tumours. Animals can have more than one type of bladder tumour. Haemangioendotheliomas were found in 23%, transitional-cell carcinomas in 8%, fibromas in 4% and adenocarcinomas in 1% (Jarrett et al., 1978a). The same histological types of bladder tumours, in addition to papillomas and squamous-cell carcinomas, have been found in other parts of the world in association with a diet of bracken fern (Pamukcu, 1963; Rosenberger, 1971). Bracken fern contains mutagenic (Evans *et al.*, 1982a) and immunosuppressive compounds (Evans *et al.*, 1982b).

Injection of a 10% suspension of bovine wart tissue in the urinary bladder of two- to three-month-old calves induced fibromas and polyps in 13/15 animals (Olson *et al.*, 1959). The calves were killed from 40 to 80 days after inoculation and no malignant progression was observed. In another experiment (Olson *et al.*, 1965), suspensions of six naturally occurring bladder tumours (2 haemangiomas, 1 haemangioma plus papilloma, 2 papillomas, 1 papilloma plus adenocarcinoma plus squamous carcinoma — this latter case was accompanied by metastasis to the iliac node) were inoculated in the skin, the vagina and the urinary bladder of young calves. Of 17 innoculated calves, 10 developed skin fibropapillomas, seven developed fibropapillomas of the vagina and five developed polyps and fibromas of the urinary bladder. These experiments demonstrated both the presence of BPV in tumours of the urinary bladder and the ability of the virus to induce bladder tumours. At the time, the heterogeneity of BPV was not known and the identity of the virus used in the above experiments is uncertain.

Campo *et al.* (1992) reported that the virus involved in bladder cancer in cattle was BPV-2. Multiple copies of episomal BPV-2 DNA were found in 7/15 biopsies (46%) of naturally occurring bladder tumours from animals from bracken fern-infested areas. Eight of 10 normal bladder biopsies were negative and, of the remaining two biopsies, one was positive for BPV-2 DNA and the other for an unidentified papillomavirus. In an experiment designed to reproduce the papilloma–carcinoma syndrome of the upper alimentary canal (see below), further evidence was obtained of the involvement of BPV-2 and of its synergism with bracken fern in the induction of urinary bladder malignancies. Calves approximately three to five months old were immunosuppressed either by treatment with azathioprine (see IARC, 1987e) (10 animals) or by a diet of bracken fern (12 animals) (Table 62). Some of the animals were infected with BPV-4 (see below), but not with BPV-2. All the immunosuppressed calves developed urinary bladder tumours starting approximately two years after the beginning of the experiment. However, in the animals immunosuppressed with azathioprine, the tumours were benign haemangiomas, whereas in the animals fed with bracken fern, the tumours were malignant and representative of the whole range of naturally occurring bladder cancers. Bladder biopsies were analysed for the presence of BPV DNA in three animals from the azathioprine group and in 10 animals from the bracken fern group. BPV-2 DNA was found in tumour biopsies of 9/13 animals, including the haemangiomas of the azathioprine-treated animals (Table 62). The negative biopsies were from four animals of the bracken fern group. In the cases with multiple tumour types, the tumours were either all positive or all negative. As in the natural bladder cancers, no virus or structural viral antigens was detected in the experimental tumours. It was concluded that immunosuppression favoured the establishment of premalignant viral lesions, but mutagens present in the fern promoted their malignant progression.

(b) BPV-2 latency

The above experiment also suggested the presence of latent BPV-2, which could be reactivated by immunosuppressive treatment, as in the bladder and/or by skin damage (Campo *et al.*,

Table 62. Bladder cancers, alimentary canal tumours and viral latency in experimental calves

Group	Animal	Treatment	Bladder cancer	Alimentary papilloma	Alimentary cancer	Site of skin warts
1	1	BPV-4		Yes		
	2			Yes		
	3			Yes		
	4			Yes		
	5			Yes		
	6			Yes		Bleeding site (BPV-1)
2	7	BPV-4 +	Yes (BPV-2)	Yes (++)		Scarification site (BPV-1)
	8	azathioprine	Yes (BPV-2)	Yes (++)		Scarification site (BPV-1)
	9	(2 mg/kg	Yes (ND)	Yes (++)		
	10	bw/day)	Yes (ND)	Yes (++)		
	11		Yes (ND)	Yes (++)		
	12		Yes (BPV-2)	Yes (++)		
3	13	Azathioprine	Yes (ND)			Scratch on neck (BPV-2)
	14	(2 mg/kg	Yes (ND)			
	15	bw/day)	Yes (ND)			
	16		Yes (ND)			Lips (BPV-2)
4	17	None				
	18					
	19					
	20					
5	21	Bracken fern	Yes (BPV-2)			
	22		Yes (BPV-2)			
	23		Yes (no BPV)			
	24		Yes (ND)			
	25		Yes (BPV-2)			Scratch on neck (BPV-2)
	26		Yes (no BPV)			
6	27	BPV-4 +	Yes (BPV-2)	Yes (+)		
	28	bracken fern	Yes (BPV-2)	Yes (+)		
	29		Yes (ND)	Yes (+)		
	30		Yes (no BPV)	Yes (+)	Yes (no BPV)	
	31		Yes (no BPV)	Yes (+)	Yes (no BPV)	
	32		Yes (BPV-2)	Yes (+)		
7	33	Quercetin	No			Scarification site (BPV-1)
	34		No			Scarification site (BPV-1)
8	35	BPV-4 +	No	Yes		Scarification site (BPV-1)
	36	quercetin	No	Yes		Scarification site (BPV-1)

From Campo *et al.* (1992, 1994a,b)
Degree of alimentary papillomatosis is indicated by +
ND, not determined

1994a). Four of 10 of the azathioprine-treated animals developed skin warts; two of the warts contained BPV-1 and two BPV-2. One of the 12 bracken fern-fed animals developed a BPV-2 wart. All the warts developed at sites of damaged skin (Table 62). All of four animals that had been administered the flavonoid quercetin (see IARC, 1987f) but were fully immunocompetent developed BPV-1 warts at the site of damaged skin (Table 62), indicating that wounding, with the attendant cell proliferation, is sufficient for reactivation of latent virus.

(c) BPV-2 in hamsters

A 10% suspension of a BPV-2 fibropapilloma taken from the neck of a cow was injected into the back of one hamster. After two years, a fibropapilloma developed at the injection site, which contained multiple episomal copies of BPV-2 DNA but no virus or structural viral antigens (Moar *et al.*, 1981).

4.2.4 BPV-3

BPV-3 was isolated from an epithelial skin papilloma of a calf in Australia (Pfister *et al.*, 1979b). Nothing is known about its natural history and no transmission experiment has been performed.

4.2.5 BPV-4

BPV-4 is the causative agent of alimentary tract papillomas (Campo *et al.*, 1980). In a survey of 7746 cattle from local abattoirs, Jarrett *et al.* (1978b) found alimentary canal tumours in 19% of the animals. Of these, 78% had epithelial squamous papillomas and 22% had fibropapillomas; 79% of the affected animals had papillomas at one site and the remaining 21% at more than one site. The epithelial papillomas were productive for and induced by BPV-4 (Campo *et al.*, 1980), whereas BPV-2 DNA, but not the virus, was present in the fibropapillomas (Jarrett *et al.*, 1984b).

(a) BPV-4 and alimentary tract cancer

In the above abattoir survey, 80 cases of squamous-cell carcinomas of the upper alimentary canal (7% tongue, 4% palate, 8% pharynx, 41% oesophagus and groove, 30% (sic) rumen) were observed in animals from the so-called cancer farms, the grazing ground of which was infested with bracken fern: 96% of the animals with cancers had papillomas and 13% of the animals with papillomas had squamous-cell carcinomas; all the histological stages from papillomas to squamous carcinomas were observed (Jarrett, 1978): 36% of the animals with upper alimentary cancers had metastases (liver and/or spleen), 56% had large intestine tumours (polyps, adenomas and adenocarcinomas) and 30% had urinary bladder cancers. In a survey of 366 cattle from the cancer farms, 39% had squamous oral papillomas; of these, 24% had papillomas at one site and 65% had widespread papillomas at multiple sites (Jarrett, 1978; Jarrett *et al.*, 1978a,b).

The papilloma–carcinoma syndrome was reproduced experimentally by Campo *et al.* (1994b) in an experiment that lasted 13 years. Of 32 calves three to five months old, six were infected in the palate with BPV-4, six were infected with BPV-4 and immunosuppressed with azathioprine, four were immunosuppressed with azathioprine, six were kept on a diet of bracken fern, six were infected with BPV-4 and fed bracken fern and four were kept as controls

(Table 62). All calves infected with BPV-4 developed squamous papillomas at the sites of intramucosal injection into the palate. However, the animals immunosuppressed either by azathioprine or by bracken-fern developed florid and persistent papillomatosis with papillomas that spread from the inoculation site, particularly in the azathioprine-treated animals. The last surviving animal from the BPV-4-and-bracken-fern group still had papillomas 13 years after infection and these had spread from the mouth to the lower oesophagus and the rumen. The virus-infected azathioprine-treated animals had to be killed on humanitarian grounds and no progression from papilloma to carcinoma was observed. Two of six animals from the virus-and-bracken-fern group developed cancers of the upper alimentary canal and the lower intestine, six and 10 years, respectively, after the start of the experiment. The two animals had typical papillomas, foci of carcinoma in the oesophagus infiltrating the subjacent tissue and polyps, adenomas and adenocarcinomas of the duodenum, jejunum and colon. No malignancy of the alimentary tract was detected in animals of the other groups. As already observed for the naturally occurring alimentary canal cancers (Campo et al., 1985), no BPV-4 DNA could be detected in the experimental cancers. It was concluded from this experiment that immunosuppression prevented rejection of papillomas and allowed their expansion, while other compounds present in the bracken fern promoted their neoplastic progression.

(b) BPV-4 in mouse xenografts

The tumorigenic potential of BPV-4 has been studied in nude mice xenografts. Chips of bovine fetal palate tissue infected with BPV-4 were implanted in nude mice either under the kidney capsule or subcutaneously and induced virus-producing papillomas in 19/21 mice within 22 weeks. One of the xenograft papillomas underwent spontaneous transformation to a squamous-cell carcinoma which infiltrated the kidney with metastasis to the spleen (Gaukroger et al., 1989, 1991). The malignant cells were confirmed to be of bovine origin by MHC typing and by the nucleotide sequence of the bovine *ras* gene. No BPV-4 DNA was detected either in the primary or in the metastatic cancer. Spontaneous conversion of papillomas in the xenograft system is a very rare event as it was observed only once out of approximately 100 papilloma-bearing mice generated in different experiments. In a further experiment, neoplastic progression was greatly accelerated by the implantation in the recipient mice of slow releasing pellets of either 7,12-dimethylbenz[*a*]anthracene (DMBA) or 12-*O*-tetradecanoylphorbol 13-acetate (TPA). When the mice were exposed to DMBA, the progression of BPV-4 papillomas to carcinomas was observed in 13/20 (65%) implants and when mice were exposed to TPA, in 4/33 (12%) implants. No tumours (papillomas or carcinomas) were found in mice receiving implants of the chemicals alone (DMBA, 0/10; TPA, 0/25). It was concluded that BPV-4 could synergize with both a classical tumour initiator and a classical tumour promoter (Gaukroger et al., 1993).

(c) BPV-4 in hamsters

Six young hamsters were injected with a 10% suspension of a BPV-4 papilloma in the right buccal pouch and intradermally on the skin of the back. One hamster developed a liposarcoma at the site of injection on the back 20 months later. The tumour showed no evidence of fibrocytic transformation, which was in agreement with the inability of the virus to transform fibroblasts *in vivo*; it was positive for viral DNA, which was present in multiple episomal copies, but not for virions or structural antigens (Moar et al., 1986).

4.2.6 BPV-5 and BPV-6

BPV-5 induces 'rice grain' fibropapillomas on the teats and udders of cattle, so called because of their appearance (Campo *et al*, 1981). BPV-6 also induces epithelial papillomas (Jarrett *et al.*, 1984a). These two viruses have not been found in any other body location so far and the tumours produced have not been reported to undergo malignant conversion, although the BPV-6 papillomas are very persistent and natural regression has not been observed (Jarrett, 1985).

In a survey of 1657 cattle from local abattoirs (Lindholm *et al.*, 1984), 37.3% of the animals were found to have at least one teat or udder papilloma. Of the affected animals, 28.4% had BPV-1 warts, 88.5% had BPV-5 warts and 92.3% had BPV-6 warts; 58.6% had double infections with BPV-5 and BPV-6 and 22.9% had triple infections with BPV-1, BPV-5 and BPV-6; 13.9% were infected by only one virus — most often BPV-6 (8.7%) followed by BPV-5 (4.4%) and then by BPV-1 (0.8%). BPV-6 is the most frequent infection of the udder and teats of cattle (Table 63).

Table 63. Incidence (%) of BPV types in teat and udder papillomas

Multiplicity of papillomas	BPV-1	BPV-5	BPV-6
Single	0.8	4.4	8.7
Double — BPV-1 with...	–	2.6	2.1
Double — BPV-5 with...	2.6	–	58.6
Triple	22.9	22.9	22.9
Overall	28.4	88.5	92.3

From Lindholm et al. (1984)

4.2.7 Bovine ocular squamous-cell carcinoma (OSCC)

In Australia, some herds of cattle are commonly affected by OSCC (Spradbrow & Hoffman, 1980). The carcinomas derive from papillomas, and malignant transformation of papillomas is particularly noticeable in lightly pigmented animals, implicating ultraviolet light as a co-carcinogen. Viral particles, strongly resembling papillomavirus, were detected in 8/25 early lesions, including one conjunctival plaque, five conjunctival papillomas, one eyelid papilloma and one eyelid keratinized horn (Ford *et al.*, 1982). The viral DNA has not been cloned, so it is not known which BPV type is responsible for the precursor lesions of OSCC.

4.2.8 Bovine skin carcinoma

Australian herds are commonly affected also by skin cancer (Spradbrow *et al.*, 1987). As in the case of OSCC, the cancers derive from precursor lesions. Thirteen cattle, four to 15 years old, were studied. All animals had lesions of different degrees of severity, from early lesions, such as cutaneous horns with acanthosis and hyperkeratosis, to advanced lesions, such as squamous-cell carcinomas and basal-cell carcinomas. Four animals were observed for three years and in two of these progression of early lesions to squamous-cell cancer was observed. Viral DNA, hybridizing to BPV-1 in low stringency conditions, was found in 10/11 keratotic lesions and in 5/8 neoplasias, two of which were squamous cancers and three basal-cell carcinomas. The viral DNA has not been cloned, so the virus type cannot be defined; the virus has not been isolated and no transmission experiments have been done. However, as for OSCC, progression of early lesions to carcinomas has been observed and it was concluded that a type of papillomavirus, in conjunction with ultraviolet light, was responsible for the skin cancers.

4.2.9 BPV in equine sarcoids

Sarcoids are commonly found in horses (*Equus equus*) and donkeys (*Equus asinus*). Equine sarcoids are locally invasive non-metastatic fibropapillomas that are rarely rejected by the host. The histological similarity between equine sarcoids and bovine fibromas suggested a link between BPV and the equine disease. Infection of horses with bovine papilloma material induced sarcoids similar to those occurring naturally (Olson & Cook, 1951) but the experimental sarcoids regressed contrary to the natural ones.

Lancaster *et al.* (1977) were the first to detect BPV DNA in natural equine sarcoids. Neither the natural nor the experimental sarcoids contained virus or structural viral antigens. More recent analyses of these equine neoplasms confirmed those original findings (Table 64).

Table 64. DNA positivity for BPV types in equine sarcoids

Reference	BPV-1 (%)	BPV-2 (%)	Overall (%)
Angelos *et al.* (1991)	66.7	21.2	87.9
Otten *et al.* (1993)[a]	92.7	7.3	100
Bloch *et al.* (1994)	60.4	13.3	73.7
Reid *et al.* (1994)[b]	83.3	16.7	100

[a] Survey includes 32 horses and two donkeys.
[b] Survey includes 18 donkeys.

Angelos *et al.* (1991) found BPV DNA in 12/13 sarcoids from horses from New York State and in 17/20 sarcoids from horses from Switzerland. The viral DNA was BPV-1-like in 22 biopsies and BPV-2-like in seven biopsies. BPV DNA was also found in one biopsy each of fibrosarcoma, fibropapilloma and pyogranulomatous dermatitis. No biopsy showed a restriction enzyme pattern of viral DNA identical to reference BPV-1 or BPV-2 DNA, indicating the presence of BPV subtypes or variants.

Bloch *et al.* (1994) conducted a retrospective analysis of equine sarcoids by polymerase chain reaction (PCR) on DNA from formalin-fixed paraffin embedded sections of archival samples. They detected BPV DNA in 56/76 (74%) samples; of these 82% were BPV-1-like and 18% were BPV-2-like.

Reid and Smith (1992) and Reid et al. (1994) analysed 24 sarcoid samples from six horses and 18 donkeys by PCR. These authors found that all the biopsies contained BPV DNA and that again BPV-1-like sequences were more prevalent than BPV-2-like sequences. There was no correlation between viral type, clinical type and anatomic location of the lesions or sex of the animals.

The virtual absence in these surveys of BPV-1 or BPV-2 DNA sequences with restriction patterns identical to those of the reference genomes might suggest that particular variants or subtypes of BPV infect horses specifically. However this was not confirmed in another study. Otten et al. (1993) analysed by PCR 58 sarcoids from 32 horses and two donkeys. They found BPV-1 DNA in 55 biopsies and BPV-2 DNA in three biopsies. One horse had two sarcoids, one with BPV-1 DNA and the other with BPV-2 DNA. The BPV sequences in the sarcoids had the same restriction enzyme patterns found in BPV-1 and BPV-2 isolates from cutaneous bovine papillomas in cattle from the same geographical area, and the relative incidence of BPV-1 and BPV-2 infection was the same in cattle and horses, suggesting that the BPV variants found in equine sarcoids are not specific for horses. The involvement of BPV in equine sarcoids is the only known instance of naturally occurring infection in which papillomaviruses cross species barriers.

4.3 Equine papillomavirus (EqPV)

In addition to sarcoids, horses can develop cutaneous, genital, oral and ocular papillomas (Olson, 1987). Paraffin sections from 135 equine neoplasms were analysed for the presence of viral structural antigen (Junge et al., 1984). The tumours were 45 papillomas from penis, vulva, skin, eye and oral cavity and 90 carcinomas from eyelid, cornea, genital area, oral cavity, maxillary sinus and skin. Antigen was detected in seven cutaneous and five genital papillomas but not in the carcinomas.

A papillomavirus, EqPV, has been isolated from cases of cutaneous papillomas of one poney and one horse (O'Banion et al., 1986). The same viral type was found in papillomas of the muzzle and the leg but not in penile papillomas from four different horses; the authors concluded that the latter were possibly caused by a different equine papillomavirus.

4.4 Papillomaviruses in cervidae

Papillomavirus was isolated from fibropapillomas of European elk (*Alces a. alces*) (EEPV or EPV; Moreno-Lopez et al., 1981), reindeer (*Rangifer tarandus*) (RPV; Moreno-Lopez et al., 1987), red deer (*Cervus elaphus*) (RDPV; Moar & Jarrett, 1985), mule deer (*Odocoileus hemionus*) and white-tailed deer (*Odocoileus virginianus*) (deer fibromavirus subtypes a and b respectively; Groff et al., 1983). EEPV and RPV induced fibrosarcomas after experimental infection of young Syrian hamsters by subcutaneous injection (Stenlund et al., 1983; Moreno-Lopez et al., 1987). The cervidae papillomaviruses have recently been shown to contain a novel open-reading frame encoding transforming activity (Eriksson et al., 1994).

4.5 Ovine papillomatosis

Norval et al. (1985) found that 25/200 sheep from local Scottish abattoirs had rumenal fibropapillomas. One animal had a squamous-cell carcinoma. Six of 10 biopsies of the rumenal tumours had few cells (1–3) positive for common antigen (Table 65).

Table 65. Papillomavirus in tumours of sheep

Reference	Lesion	Viral DNA[a]	Viral antigen[a,b]	Virus[a]
Norval et al. (1985)	Rumenal fibropapilloma	0/30[c]	6/10	0/20
Vanselow et al. (1982)	Cutaneous papillomas	ND	ND	2/3
Vanselow & Spradbrow (1983)	Hyperkeratotic scales	ND	ND	0/1
Trenfield et al. (1990)	Cutaneous and vulvar lesions[d]	11/83	ND	ND
Tilbrook et al. (1992)	Perineal squamous-cell carcinomas and papillomas	20/26	0/17	ND
Hayward et al. (1993)	Cutaneous filiform papillomas	1/1	9/9	Yes (NR)

[a]Positive lesions/analysed lesions
[b]Common structural antigen
[c]Only tested with HPV-1 DNA
[d]Keratinized horns, papillomas and fibropapillomas
ND, not determined; NR, not reported

Other surveys of sheep were performed in Australia (Table 65). Vanselow et al. (1982) reported the isolation of a papillomavirus from the cutaneous papillomas of two Merino sheep. Two more sheep with papillomas were followed for several months and during the observation period the papillomas progressed to squamous-cell carcinomas. The same authors (Vanselow & Spradbrow, 1983) reported on another Merino sheep with squamous-cell carcinomas on a lower eyelid and on the vulva. Hyperkeratotic lesions in which virions were detected were present near both cancers but virus was not isolated.

In a later survey, Trenfield et al. (1990) analysed 67 ear lesions (cutaneous horns, papillomas, fibropapillomas) from 51 sheep and 16 lesions from other skin sites from 15 sheep. Ten ear lesions and one vulvar lesion were analysed for viral DNA using BPV-1 DNA as a probe. The vulvar lesion and 8/10 of the ear lesions were positive. The viral DNA gave a BPV-2 restriction pattern with eight enzymes and a BPV-1 restriction pattern with two enzymes, reminiscent of the situation found in horses (see section 4.2.9).

A similar survey was performed by Tilbrook et al. (1992). Five of 10 premalignant biopsies and 15/16 squamous-cell carcinomas, all from the perineal region of sheep, were found to contain papillomavirus-like DNA, by using both BPV probes and HPV probes.

The occurrence of filiform squamous papillomas on sheep was reported by Hayward et al. (1993), also in Australia. These papillomas were not of the fibropapilloma type but histologically resembled verruca vulgaris; they were present in less than 1% ($N = 2660$) of young sheep, always on the lower fore legs. Papillomavirus was visualized by electron microscopy and viral DNA was detected by hybridization with an HPV-16 DNA probe. All papillomas analysed were positive for the common viral antigen.

4.6 Cottontail rabbit papillomavirus (CRPV)

CRPV was the first papillomavirus to be identified and isolated, and the CRPV system was the first in which progression from benign papillomas to malignant carcinomas was observed and the synergism between virus and cofactors was documented (Rous & Beard, 1934; Rous & Kidd, 1938; Rous & Friedwald, 1944). In nature, CRPV infects primarily cottontail rabbits (*Sylvilagus floridanus*) and occasionally jackrabbits (*Lepus californicus*). The first phase of infection lasts from one to six weeks, during which papillomas (cutaneous horns) grow. Ninety-five to 100% of the infected animals develop papillomas. In 71% of the animals, the papillomas are permanently benign, in 6% of the animals the papillomas regress and in 23% of the animals the papillomas progress to squamous cancer within 12–18 months. Experimental infection of the domestic rabbit (*Oryctalagus cunniculus*) follows a different course. After one to six weeks of growth, 95–100% of rabbits have papillomas. Papilloma regression takes place in 10–40% of the rabbits after one to three months; in 20–30% of the rabbits, the papillomas remain permanently benign, but in 40–60% of the animals they progress to squamous-cell carcinomas in six to 12 months (Kreider, 1980; Wettstein, 1987). In domestic rabbits, therefore, more papillomas progress more rapidly to cancer than in cottontail rabbits, implicating the genetic background of the host in malignant conversion. Infectious virus is found in cottontail rabbit papillomas but not generally in domestic rabbit papillomas or in cancers in either species; however, viral DNA is present in the nonproductive lesions.

4.6.1 CRPV and co-carcinogens

The progression rate of papillomas induced by CRPV is influenced by other carcinogens (Rous & Kidd, 1938; Rous & Friedwald, 1944). When tar was applied to the skin of the ears of rabbits, hyperplastic skin and papillomas developed. The skin reverted to normal and the papillomas regressed or remained indolent when tar treatment was suspended. Only 1/90 tar-treated rabbits developed a carcinoma after two years of treatment. On the contrary, infection with CRPV of tar-treated rabbits either by scarification of hyperplastic skin or tar papillomas or by intravenous inoculation of virus resulted in the rapid appearance of highly malignant cancers in more than half of 70 rabbits (Rous & Kidd, 1938). In an experiment typical of a large series, eight rabbits had tar applied to the ears for 89 days, were infected with CRPV by intravenous injection and by scarification and then tarred again twice weekly for 25 days. Large numbers of papillomas developed rapidly on tarred skin in all rabbits; the papillomas continued growing even when tar treatment was discontinued. In 2/5 rabbits, the papillomas progressed to squamous and anaplastic carcinomas; in one rabbit, there was metastasis to local lymph nodes. None of five control rabbits that had been tarred but not infected with CRPV developed malignancies, although they did develop tar papillomas (Rous & Kidd, 1938).

Rapid malignant progression was observed also when CRPV papillomas were treated with carcinogens. Eight rabbits were infected with CRPV by scarification on six patches of skin, three patches on either side of each animal. Seven days later, healing was complete and each animal was swabbed on one of the three patches on one side with methylcholanthrene, tar plus methylcholanthrene or tar alone; the patches on the other side were swabbed with solvents only or left untreated; areas of skin not infected with CRPV were swabbed with carcinogens. All sites inoculated with the virus developed papillomas after 14 days, but the papillomas were larger and faster growing in the carcinogen-treated areas. Cancer started to appear as early as 63 days in two animals on sites treated with methylcholanthrene and with tar plus methylcholanthrene in one of the animals. After 85 days, all eight rabbits had developed cancers in the carcinogen-treated areas; these ranged from malignant papillomas to squamous-cell carcinomas, cystic squamous carcinomas and highly anaplastic carcinomas. Two rabbits had metastases to lymph nodes. There were more cancers in areas treated with methylcholanthrene and tar plus methylcholanthrene than in areas treated with tar. During the observation period, no cancer developed from untreated papillomas or from noninfected skin treated with carcinogens. From their extensive series of experiments, the authors concluded that CRPV and carcinogens synergize powerfully in inducing malignant conversion of papillomas (Rous & Friedwald, 1944).

4.6.2 CRPV latency

In an experiment designed to study latency and reactivation of CRPV, Amella et al. (1994) infected rabbits with serial dilutions of CRPV. With undiluted virus, 6/7 injection sites in seven rabbits developed papillomas. With virus diluted from 1:2 to 1:8, 8/8 sites in eight animals developed papillomas. With virus diluted from 1:10 to 1:100, 9/34 sites in 18 animals developed papillomas, while with virus diluted from 1:1000 to 1:100 000, none of 14 sites in 14 animals developed papillomas. However, 6/6 biopsies of the negative sites contained viral DNA detected by PCR. Virus was used at a dilution of 1:20 in order to generate papillomas only in a subset of sites. After virus injection, 24/43 sites (55.8%) were mildly irritated by subtherapeutic photodynamic therapy; 2/19 of the nonirritated sites (10.5%) developed papillomas, which contrasts with 11/24 of the irritated sites (45.8%) which did. PCR of injection sites that did not develop papillomas showed the presence of viral DNA. It was concluded that infection with low doses of virus results in the establishment of viral latency, and that virus can be reactivated by skin injury (see also section 4.2.8).

4.6.3 CRPV in transgenic rabbits

CRPV in conjunction with activated *ras* has been used to generate transgenic rabbits (Peng et al., 1993). Three transgenic rabbits were obtained. Two rabbits had only CRPV DNA and one had both CRPV DNA and activated *ras*. The two CRPV transgenic rabbits were phenotypically normal up to two weeks after birth; then they started developing epidermal hyperkeratosis. Small papillomas appeared when the animals were 20–30 days old that developed and spread all over the body. The rabbits died of pneumonia and septicaemia at 40 and 75 days, respectively. No malignant changes were detected in the papillomas. The third rabbit, transgenic for both CRPV DNA and *ras*, had thickened skin at birth and died at day 3. It was covered by epidermal papillomas that had already undergone highly malignant progression. The entire skin was described by the authors as 'an extended squamous carcinoma'. No neoplasia was detected in other organs. Integrated CRPV DNA was detected in all tissues but it was episomal and greatly amplified in tumours in all three rabbits. In contrast, there was no difference in *ras* transgene copy number between normal and tumour tissues. CRPV DNA was transcribed in papillomas and carcinomas but not in normal tissue, while *ras* was transcribed only in the cancers. It was concluded by the authors that CRPV-induced papillomas and that the rapid progression of papillomas to carcinomas was due to synergism between CRPV oncogenes and activated *ras*.

4.7 Domestic rabbit oral papillomavirus

Oral papillomas were found in 31% of 51 New Zealand white rabbits from two commercial sources. The virus was isolated and inoculated into the tongue and vulva of three noninfected rabbits. All rabbits developed papillomas of the tongue but not of the vulva, demonstrating site specificity. No cross-immunity was observed between skin (CRPV) and oral virus and it was concluded that the viruses have separate identities. When the oral papillomavirus was inoculated into baby hamsters, 9/10 hamsters developed fibromas (Sunberg *et al.*, 1985).

4.8 *Mastomys natalensis* papillomavirus (MnPV)

Mastomys natalensis is a common rodent in southern Africa. Colonies have been established in several laboratories. The animals of the Giessen colony and the Heidelberg colony harbour a latent papillomavirus, MnPV (Amtmann *et al.*, 1984; Amtmann & Wayss, 1987; Tan *et al.*, 1994b). Certain strains of the animals develop keratoacanthomas and papillomas of the skin, in an age-dependent manner. The tumours never appear in animals younger than 50 weeks old, but by 16 months of age 80% of the animals have tumours. Occasionally, the benign lesions progress to malignant cancers in older animals. The rate of malignant progression depends on the genetic susceptibility of the host — in the Heidelberg colony progression is only sporadic, while in the Giessen colony 11% of the animals undergo progression. The viral genome increases dramatically in copy number during tumour formation, from approximately 0.1 copy per cell in 16-week-old animals to more than 3000 copies per cell in 80-week-old animals. Amtmann *et al.* (1984) showed that treatment of the skin with TPA increased DNA copy number and lowered the age at tumour appearance to as early as 14 weeks. The same result was obtained when the skin was irritated with sandpaper (Siegsmund *et al.*, 1991).

4.9 Mouse papillomavirus (MmPV)

The only known mouse papillomavirus was isolated from a zoo colony of European harvest mice (*Micromys minutus*) (Sundberg *et al.*, 1988). Adult mice of each sex developed acanthomas, papillomas, inverted papillomas, sebaceous carcinomas and pulmonary keratinaceous cysts. The virus (MmPV) was detected in two papillomas, viral DNA in 28/28 biopsies, both benign and malignant, and structural antigen in 20/31 biopsies. The MmPV could be transmitted to one of two harvest mice but not to laboratory mice (CAF or C3H strains) or to wild deer mice (*Peromyscus maniculatus gambeli*).

4.10 Canine oral papillomavirus (COPV)

Dogs can be affected by oral papillomatosis, particularly if kept in kennels in large numbers. The incubation period of the oral papillomas varies from four to 10 weeks and regression usually follows in three to 14 weeks (Olson, 1987). Progression to squamous cancer is rare (Watrach *et al.*, 1970). Recently, three identical isolates of a papillomavirus, COPV, were isolated from oral papillomas from three dogs (*Canis familiaris*) and one coyote (*Canis latrans*). The COPV isolated from the coyote was transmitted to 2/3 dogs. One of the dog isolates was transmitted to 2/3 dogs and a second dog isolate to 1/3 dogs. The third dog isolate was not tested (Sundberg *et al.*, 1991).

Several thousands of kennel beagles were prophylactically vaccinated with a suspension of live COPV at 10–14 weeks of age. The vaccine was injected into the gluteal muscles. The great majority of dogs were protected from natural infection, but 5/500 dogs kept in the authors' laboratory and 7/4000 dogs kept in the breeder's kennels developed cancers at the site of vaccine inoculation. The cancers comprised 10 highly invasive squamous-cell carcinomas, one basal-cell epithelioma and one epidermal pseudocarcinomatous hyperplasia. Five of 12 cancers were positive for COPV structural antigen, but all were negative for virus. The biopsies were not analysed for viral DNA. As COPV does not naturally infect the skin, it was concluded that the cancers had been induced by the live virus in the vaccine (Bregman *et al.*, 1987).

4.11 Feline papillomas

Two Persian cats, 10 and 13 years old, respectively, both under steroid immunosuppressive therapy, developed sessile hyperkeratotic skin lesions, that were positive for papillomavirus, common viral structural antigen and viral DNA (Carney *et al.*, 1990). Both cats were negative for feline leukaemia virus (FeLV) and feline immunodeficiency virus (FIV). Transmission of the papillomavirus was attempted but was unsuccessful. The viral DNA was not cloned. In another study, one six-year-old cat positive for FIV developed wart-like lesions on the skin. The lesions were positive for papillomavirus and for viral structural antigen (Egberink *et al.*, 1992). It was concluded that cats display clinical papillomavirus lesions when immunosuppressed either by FIV infection or by therapy.

4.12 Avian papillomavirus

A papillomavirus (FPV) was isolated from a leg papilloma of a chaffinch (*Fringilla coelebs*) (Osterhaus *et al.*, 1977) but could not be transmitted to other finches or hamsters (Moreno-Lopez *et al.*, 1984).

5. Summary of Data Reported and Evaluation

5.1 HPV infection

Papillomaviruses are small, non-enveloped, viruses that contain a double-stranded, circular 8 kb DNA genome. They are highly host-specific, cannot be propagated in tissue culture and, with the exception of some ungulate papillomaviruses, infect only epithelial cells. Of the types described, more than 70 are human papillomaviruses (HPV) and approximately 20 are animal papillomaviruses. The types are classified according to their nucleotide sequences and form five taxonomic groups. These groups are not phenotypically homogeneous. Two of these groups contain most of the HPVs.

The papillomavirus genome can be divided into three regions. The long control region contains *cis*-responsive elements, which are required for the regulation of gene expression and DNA replication. The early region codes for proteins involved in the regulation of viral transcription (E2), viral DNA replication (E1 and E2), cell proliferation (E5, E6 and E7) and, possibly, some late steps in the viral life cycle (E4). The late region contains two genes, which code for the capsid proteins L1 and L2.

Several advances have recently been made in understanding the immune response to HPVs. Seroreactive and T-cell epitopes of HPV proteins have been identified using a variety of techniques. In most instances, it is unclear if these epitopes are recognized in the course of natural infection. Using ELISA (enzyme-linked immunosorbent assay), based upon HPV virus-like particles synthesized by the expression of HPV late genes in recombinant vectors, antibodies reactive to the virus capsid have been found in a proportion of patients with HPV infections and HPV-related diseases. Antibodies to early HPV proteins have also been detected in patients with HPV-associated diseases as well as in healthy individuals. It remains to be seen whether accurate and reliable immunological assays that measure exposure to HPVs can be developed.

Over the last five years, there has been substantial improvement in the methods used to detect HPV DNA. Different assays are now available that can detect small amounts of HPV DNA, quantify the amount of viral DNA in clinical specimens, identify a broad spectrum of genital and cutaneous HPV types, test for selected HPV types and localize the viral genome and viral transcripts to individual cells.

Polymerase chain reaction (PCR) amplification has provided sensitive and specific assays for a broad spectrum of HPV DNAs. Using consensus or general primers, a large number of HPV DNAs can be amplified in a single reaction. Detection systems using oligonucleotide probes permit identification of individual HPV types in a fashion suitable for large-scale studies. Nucleotide sequences of PCR products can also be compared with databases of HPV genomic sequences for unequivocal identification of HPV types. Some commercially available non-PCR-based assays provide standardized reagents, test separately for high-risk and low-risk HPV types, and quantify HPV DNA levels in clinical specimens. Future investigations will determine whether HPV DNA assays are valuable in screening for cervical cancer and its precursors and in the management of women with cervical cytological abnormalities.

Genital HPVs are transmitted primarily through sexual contact with infected cervical, vaginal, vulvar, penile or anal epithelium. Perinatal transmission, digital and oral transfer, and auto-inoculation of genital HPV types have also been documented. Transmission of all HPV types is probably more efficient in the presence of an abraded epithelial surface.

The prevalence of genital HPV infection is highest among sexually active young adults and is similar for men and women. Shortly after sexual debut, risk of infection with each new sexual contact is high. HPV infections are common throughout the world. Recent data suggest that there may be geographic differences in the prevalence of specific HPV types and variants.

Prevalent HPV infections have been studied extensively but little is known about the incidence and natural history of primary infections. Findings from a variety of studies suggest that after infection, most individuals do not develop clinical signs or symptoms. The natural history of specific viral types may be different. Only a small percentage of infected individuals will develop HPV-associated cancer.

Morphological changes occur in the epithelium of the lower genital tract and anus in response to infection with HPV. The cytological and histological alterations that occur as a result of a productive infection reflect the cytopathic effects of the virus on epithelial cells and include nuclear atypia, an increased mitotic rate and koilocytosis. The productive phase of HPV infection is generally pronounced in what is referred to as low-grade cervical intraepithelial neoplasia (CIN). Following HPV infection, a cancer precursor state may develop. This is accompanied by an increase in nuclear atypia and mitotic rate, as well as architectural disorganization. Such lesions are generally aneuploid and frequently contain abnormal mitotic figures. These precursor lesions are referred to as high-grade CIN.

The presence of CIN adjacent to areas of invasive cancer, the cytological and histological similarities between CIN and invasive cancer, and the observation of tongues of early invasion arising directly from CIN are compelling pathological evidence that CIN is a precursor to invasive cancer.

Genital HPVs are the etiological agents for condylomata, recurrent respiratory papillomas and some papillomas at other mucosal surfaces. Cutaneous HPVs cause skin warts. Benign HPV disease is treated by chemical and physical agents or by surgical removal. Excisional therapy is preferred for treatment of HPV-associated intraepithelial neoplasia, especially for treatment of high-grade lesions. Non-invasive treatment strategies of proven efficacy are not available for these lesions. However, immunization strategies are being devised and in the future these may help prevent or control HPV-associated diseases.

5.2 Studies of cancer in humans

There is compelling epidemiological evidence that some HPV types are human carcinogens. In methodologically sound studies, HPVs are found in over 90% of all invasive cervical cancers and in a high proportion of certain other anogenital cancers. Carcinogenicity in humans has been most firmly established for HPV-16, but strong evidence of carcinogenicity also exists for certain other HPV types.

Case series from many areas of the world have established that a high proportion (~50%) of cervical cancers and high-grade CIN lesions contain HPV-16 DNA. Almost 100 case–control studies have been reported that examine the relationship between HPV and cervical neoplasia. Almost all have found positive associations. Among the most informative studies, strong associations (prevalence odds ratios > 20) with HPV-16 DNA have been observed with remarkable consistency for invasive cancer and high-grade CIN, ruling out the possibility that this association can be explained by chance, bias or confounding.

Currently available prospective data indicate that HPV-16 infection precedes high-grade CIN and predicts an elevated risk of developing it, although the relative risks observed are lower than the prevalence odds ratios generated by case–control studies. The epidemiological data regarding HPV-16 and cervical neoplasia are consistent with the established epidemiological risk factors (e.g. sexual behaviour) and with the biological data cited below.

On the basis of strong and consistent case–control study results, a causal role for HPV-16 in anal cancer is highly likely. The lack of prospective data is partially mitigated by similarities between cervical and anal anatomy, pathology, and risk factors.

Based on more-limited case series and case–control data, HPV-16 infection is likely to have a causal role in the etiology of poorly keratinized squamous-cell cancers of the vulva associated with adjacent vulvar intraepithelial neoplasia (VIN), and in carcinoma of the penis. The epidemiological data linking HPV-16 to the risk of other cancers are currently inadequate.

After HPV-16, HPV-18 is the type most clearly shown by epidemiological data to be a human carcinogen. The evidence is limited to the cervix, in which HPV-18 appears to be strongly linked to a substantial minority of squamous cancers and approximately half of the adenocarcinomas.

Additional anogenital HPV types are implicated as human carcinogens of the cervix (including, at least, HPV types 31, 33, 35, 39, 45, 51, 52, 56 and 58). Among these types, the epidemiological evidence is strongest for HPV-31 and -33. However, full evaluation is hampered by the low prevalence of individual types.

Although there are rare case reports of tumours containing HPV-6 or -11 DNA, the epidemiological data suggest that HPV-6 and -11 are not human carcinogens for the cervix. The epidemiological evidence for carcinogenicity of HPV-6 and -11 at non-cervical sites is judged to be inadequate. There are no adequate epidemiological studies of other anogenital HPV types.

In addition to the epidemiological studies conducted in the general population, some studies of HPV and cancer have been conducted in special populations. An increasing number of studies have shown women immunosuppressed by human immunodeficiency virus (HIV) infection to be at higher risk of HPV-associated cervical intraepithelial neoplasia, but, so far, an increased risk of invasive cervical cancer has not been established. Many studies have shown a high prevalence and viral load of anal HPV in immunosuppressed HIV-infected individuals. There is increasing evidence for a direct effect of immunosuppression on the development of HPV-associated AIN (anal intraepithelial neoplasia) and anal cancer.

To date, case series have not shown a high prevalence of HPV infection in skin cancer patients in the general population, with the exception of two rare types of skin neoplasms (periungual squamous-cell carcinoma and periungual and palmoplantar Bowen's disease) in which HPV-16 and/or -18 have been consistently found. In contrast, HPVs are recovered frequently from skin cancers in immunocompromised individuals. In a total of nine studies, HPV DNA was found in a high proportion (~60%) of squamous-cell carcinomas of the skin in epidermodysplasia verruciformis (EV) patients; HPV-5 was the predominant type. The prevalence of HPV infection varies widely in case series of skin cancer among transplant patients. A broad range of HPV types has been found, with no particular HPV type predominating.

5.3 Molecular mechanisms of carcinogenesis

Molecular studies have identified mechanisms utilized by high-risk HPV types that contribute to carcinogenesis. DNA and transcripts of specific HPV types are regularly detected in biopsies from cervical cancer and in its precursor lesions. Specific viral oncogenes have been identified that differ functionally between cancer-linked HPVs and those preferentially found in genital warts, leading to their classification as high-risk and low-risk HPVs, respectively. Besides growth promotion, high-risk HPVs induce chromosomal instability and could therefore act as solitary carcinogens. High-risk HPVs immortalize human and rodent cells *in vitro*, which can subsequently convert to malignant growth either spontaneously or after exposure to other carcinogens. In several HPV-positive cervical carcinoma cell lines of human origin, the malignant phenotype has been shown to depend on the activity of viral oncogenes. The E6 and E7 oncoproteins of the high-risk HPVs interfere with the functions of negative cellular regulators, including the tumour-suppressor proteins p53 and pRB, respectively. The activity of these viral oncogenes in transgenic animals supports the importance of the viral–host protein interactions in tumorigenesis.

The importance of deregulation of HPV oncogene expression to the malignant progression of HPV-infected cells is well supported. This commonly occurs following integration of the viral genome, but other mechanisms, such as alterations within the host cell genome and in the viral promoter, have been identified. Chromosomal abnormalities occur during tumour progression, indicating that alterations in cellular genes contribute to this process. The cellular genes that are affected by these chromosomal abnormalities have not been identified. The status of the *p53* tumour suppressor gene has been most extensively studied; somatic mutations within this gene occur only very rarely in HPV-positive cancers. The incidence of *p53* mutations in apparently HPV-negative cancers appears to be somewhat higher, although many studies fail to find such alterations in either HPV-positive or -negative cancers.

Cofactors may play a role in HPV-linked carcinogenesis. Herpes-group viruses were initially implicated. There exist no convincing epidemiological data in support of this hypothesis, although some experimental findings show that HPV-immortalized cell lines can be transformed by segments of the herpes simplex virus (HSV) type 2 or the human herpesvirus type 6 genome. HSV infections lead to efficient amplification of latent papovavirus genomes. Glucocorticoid hormones and progesterone may co-operate with HPV infections by activating early gene transcription. The effects of chemical or physical carcinogens on progression of papillomavirus-induced lesions have been documented in a number of studies.

Regression of HPV-induced warts is accompanied histologically by a response characteristic of a $CD4^+$-cell-dependent delayed-type hypersensitivity reaction; animal models support this observation. The increased prevalence of HPV infections in immunosuppressed individuals (such as those undergoing organ transplantation, those with HIV infection or those with inherited T-cell immunodeficiencies) further supports a role for $CD4^+$ cells in the control of HPV infection. The association between the duration and degree of immunosuppression and the increased risk for HPV-associated neoplasia supports the notion that viral DNA persistence is important for neoplastic transformation and progression. Preliminary evidence suggests that some HPV-infected individuals make a serum-neutralizing antibody in response to viral proteins.

The oncoproteins of HPV-16 can act as tumour rejection antigens in animal models and induce HPV-16 specific cytotoxic T cells. Conventional immunization strategies can induce such cytotoxic T cells. Although there is no evidence for HPV-16-specific cytotoxic T cells in humans with HPV-associated disease, the animal models suggest that effective presentation of HPV oncoproteins to the immune system is potentially immunotherapeutic. However, in HPV-associated cervical neoplasia, there is an overall downregulation of HLA class I molecules, raising doubts about the potential effectiveness of such therapies. The presentation by HLA-B7 of an HPV-16 E6 variant peptide may be a biological mechanism for immune escape by the virus. A role for major histocompatibility complex (MHC) haplotypes in susceptibility to, or protection from papillomavirus-associated neoplasia is supported by data from rabbits and from humans.

5.4 Studies of cancer in animals

Although there is no established animal model for any of the HPVs, several of the animal papillomaviruses are associated with the development of malignant lesions both in the natural and heterologous hosts. Experimental studies of cottontail rabbit papillomavirus (CRPV) in domestic rabbits clearly demonstrate a direct causal relationship between infection by this virus and development of cancer. There is also strong evidence supporting a causal role for bovine papillomavirus (BPV)-2 in the development of bladder cancer and BPV-4 in alimentary tract cancer in cattle, although malignant progression has not been documented in the absence of additional carcinogens. Synergy in carcinogenesis between papillomaviruses and other factors is evident in the rabbit (experimentally applied chemical carcinogens) and cattle models (naturally occurring immunosuppressants and mutagens). Carcinogenic activity of other animal papillomaviruses has not been established, although malignant progression of virus-associated lesions has been reported in several cases.

The rhesus monkey model provides evidence for the sexual transmission of RhPV. The rabbit and the cattle systems are of value in the study of viral latency.

5.5 Evaluation

There is *sufficient evidence* in humans for the carcinogenicity of human papillomavirus (HPV) types 16 and 18.

There is *evidence suggesting lack of carcinogenicity* to the cervix in humans of HPV types 6 and 11.

There is *limited evidence* in humans for the carcinogenicity of some other HPV types.

HPVs cannot infect animals. Some animal papillomaviruses cause cancer in their natural hosts.

Overall evaluation

HPV types 16 and 18 are *carcinogenic to humans (Group 1)*.

HPV types 31 and 33 are *probably carcinogenic to humans (Group 2A)*.

Some HPV types other than 16, 18, 31 and 33 are *possibly carcinogenic to humans (Group 2B)*.

The carcinogenicity of HPV types 16 and 18 is supported by experimental evidence that proteins of these viruses interfere with the functions of cellular regulatory pathways.

6. References

Aareleid, T., Pukkala, E., Thomson, H. & Hakama, M. (1993) Cervical cancer incidence and mortality trends in Finland and Estonia: a screened vs. an unscreened population. *Eur. J. Cancer,* **29A**, 745–749

Abdelsayed, R.A. (1991) Study of human papillomavirus in oral epithelial dysplasia and epidermoid carcinoma in the absence of tobacco and alcohol use. *Oral Surg. oral Med. oral Pathol.,* **71**, 730–732

Abramson, A.L., Brandsma, J., Steinberg, B. & Winkler, B. (1985) Verrucous carcinoma of the larynx: possible human papillomavirus etiology. *Arch. Otolaryngol. Head Neck Surg.,* **111**, 709–715

Abramson, A.L., Steinberg, B.M. & Winkler, B. (1987) Laryngeal papillomatosis: clinical, histopathologic and molecular studies. *Laryngoscope,* **97**, 678–685

Abramson, A.L., Shikowitz, M.J., Mullooly, V.M., Steinberg, B.M., Amella, C.A. & Rothstein, H.R. (1992) Clinical effects of photodynamic therapy on recurrent laryngeal papillomas. *Arch. Otolaryngol. Head Neck Surg.,* **118**, 25–29

Acs, J., Hildesheim, A., Reeves, W.C., Brenes, M., Brinton, L., Lavery, C., de la Guardia, M.E., Godoy, J. & Rawls, W.E. (1989) Regional distribution of human papillomavirus DNA and other risk factors for invasive cervical cancer in Panama. *Cancer Res.,* **49**, 5725–5729

Adam, E., Kaufman, R.H., Adler-Storthz, K., Melnick, J.L. & Dreesman, G.R. (1985) A prospective study of association of herpes simplex virus and human papillomavirus infection with cervical neoplasia in women exposed to diethylstilbestrol *in utero. Int. J. Cancer,* **35**, 19–26

Alberico, S., Facca, M.C., Di Bonito, L., Millo, R., Casaccia, R. & Mandruzzato, G.P. (1988) Frequency of cervico-vaginal infections (*Trichomonas vaginalis*; *Chlamydia trachomatis* -CHL-; herpes simplex virus -HSV-; human papilloma virus -HPV-) in cervical intraepithelial neoplasia. *Eur. J. gynaecol. Oncol.,* **9**, 252–257

Alloub, M.I., Barr, B.B.B., McLaren, K.M., Smith, I.W., Bunney, M.H. & Smart, G.E. (1989) Human papillomavirus infection and cervical intraepithelial neoplasia in women with renal allografts. *Br. med. J.,* **298**, 153–156

Almeida, J.D., Oriel, J.D. & Stannard, L.M. (1969) Characterization of the virus found in human genital warts. *Microbios,* **3**, 225–232

Altmann, A., Jochmus-Kudielka, I., Frank, R., Gausepohl, H., Moebius, U., Gissmann, L. & Meuer, S.C. (1992) Definition of immunogenic determinants of the human papillomavirus type 16 nucleoprotein E7. *Eur. J. Cancer,* **28**, 326–333

Amburgey, C.F., VanEenwyk, J., Davis, F.G., Bowen, P.E., Persky, V. & Goldberg, J. (1993) Undernutrition as a risk factor for cervical intraepithelial neoplasia: a case–control analysis. *Nutr. Cancer,* **20**, 51–60

Amella, C.A., Lofgren, L.A., Ronn, A.M., Nouri, M., Shikowitz, M.J. & Steinberg, B.M. (1994) Latent infection induced with cottontail rabbit papillomavirus: a model for human papillomavirus latency. *Am. J. Pathol.,* **144**, 1167–1171

Amortegui, A.J., Meyer, M.P., McIntyre-Seltman, K. & Locker, J. (1990) Detection of human papillomavirus DNA in cervical lesions by in situ hybridization using biotinylated DNA probes. *Int. J. gynecol. Pathol.*, **9**, 306–315

Amtmann, E. & Wayss, K. (1987) The *Mastomys natalensis* papillomavirus. In: Selzman, N.P. & Howley, P.M., eds, *The Papillomaviruses*, New York, Plenum Press, pp. 187–198

Amtmann, E., Volm, M. & Wayss, K. (1984) Tumour induction in the rodent *Mastomys natalensis* by activation of endogenous papilloma virus genomes. *Nature*, **308**, 291–292

Andersen, E.S. & Husth, M. (1992) Cryosurgery for cervical intraepithelial neoplasia. *Gynecol. Oncol.*, **45**, 240–242

Andersen, W.A., Franquemont, D.W., Williams, J., Taylor, P.T. & Crum, C.P. (1991) Vulvar squamous cell carcinoma and papillomaviruses: two separate entities? *Am. J. Obstet. Gynecol.*, **165**, 329–335

Anderson, S.M., Brooke, P.K., Van Eyck, S.L., Noell, H. & Frable, W.J. (1993) Distribution of human papillomavirus types in genital lesions from two temporally distinct populations determined by in situ hybridization. *Hum. Pathol.*, **24**, 547–553

Andersson-Ellström, A., Dillner, J., Hagmar, B., Schiller, J. & Forssman, L. (1994) No serological evidence for non-sexual spread of HPV16 (Letter to the Editor). *Lancet*, **344**, 1435

Androphy, E.J., Dvoretsky, I. & Lowy, D.R. (1985) X-linked inheritance of epidermodysplasia verruciformis: genetic and virologic studies of a kindred. *Arch. Dermatol.*, **121**, 864–868

Angelos, J.A., Marti, E., Lazary, S. & Carmichael, L.E. (1991) Characterization of BPV-like DNA in equine sarcoids. *Arch. Virol.*, **119**, 95–109

Anisimová, E., Barták, P., Vlcek, D., Hirsch, I., Bricháček, B. & Vonka, V. (1990) Presence and type specificity of papillomavirus antibodies demonstrable by immunoelectron microscopy tests in samples from patients with warts. *J. gen. Virol.*, **71**, 419–422

Anwar, K., Nakakuki, K., Shiraishi, T., Naiki, H., Yatani, R. & Inuzuka, M. (1992a) Presence of *ras* oncogene mutations and human papillomavirus DNA in human prostate carcinomas. *Cancer Res.*, **52**, 5991–5996

Anwar, K., Naiki, H., Nakakuki, K. & Inuzuka, M. (1992b) High frequency of human papillomavirus infection in carcinoma of the urinary bladder. *Cancer*, **70**, 1967–1973

Anwar, K., Nakakuki, K., Naiki, H. & Inuzuka, M. (1993) *ras* Gene mutations and HPV infection are common in human laryngeal carcinoma. *Int. J. Cancer*, **53**, 22–28

Aparicio-Duque, R., Mittal, K.R., Chan, W. & Schinella, R. (1991) Cloacogenic carcinoma of the anal canal and associated viral lesions: an in situ hybridization study for human papilloma virus. *Cancer*, **68**, 2422–2425

Apple, R.J., Erlich, H.A., Klitz, W., Manos, M.M., Becker, T.M. & Wheeler, C.M. (1994) HLA DR-DQ associations with cervical carcinoma show papillomavirus-type specificity. *Nat. Genet.*, **6**, 157–162

Apt, D., Chong, T., Liu, Y. & Bernard, H.-U. (1993) Nuclear factor I and epithelial cell-specific transcription of human papillomavirus type 16. *J. Virol.*, **67**, 4455–4463

Apt, D., Liu, Y. & Bernard, H.-U. (1994) Cloning and functional analysis of spliced isoforms of human nuclear factor I-X: interference with transcriptional activation by NFI/CTF in a cell-type specific manner. *Nucleic Acids Res.*, **22**, 3825–3833

Aral, S.O. & Holmes, K.K. (1995) Epidemiology of sexual behavior and sexually transmitted diseases. In: Holmes, K.K., Mardh, P.-A., Sparling, P.F., Wiesner, P.J., Cates, W., Lemon, S.M. & Stamm, W.E., eds, *Sexually Transmitted Diseases*, 2nd ed., New York, McGraw-Hill, pp. 19–36

REFERENCES

Arbeit, J.M., Münger, K., Howley, P.M. & Hanahan, D. (1993) Neuroepithelial carcinomas in mice transgenic with human papillomavirus type 16 E6/E7 ORFs. *Am. J. Pathol.*, **142**, 1187–1197

Arbeit, J.M., Münger, K., Howley, P.M. & Hanahan, D. (1994) Progressive squamous epithelial neoplasia in K14-human papillomavirus type 16 transgenic mice. *J. Virol.*, **68**, 4358–4368

Arends, M.J., Donaldson, Y.K., Duval, E., Wyllie, A.H. & Bird, C.C. (1993) Human papillomavirus type 18 associates with more advanced cervical neoplasia than human papillomavirus type 16. *Hum. Pathol.*, **24**, 432–437

Armbruster-Moraes, E., Ioshimoto, L.M., Leao, E. & Zugaib, M. (1993) Detection of human papillomavirus deoxyribonucleic acid sequences in amniotic fluid during different periods of pregnancy (Letter to the Editor). *Am. J. Obstet. Gynecol.*, **169**, 1074–1075

Arndt, O., Zeise, K., Bauer, I. & Brock, J. (1992) Type 6/11 and 16/18 squamous epithelial cancers of the upper respiratory tract and digestive system: an in situ hybridization study. *Laryngo-Rhino-Otologie*, **71**, 500–504 (in German)

Arndt, O., Zeise, K., Bauer, I. & Brock, J. (1993) Correlation between chronic hyperplastic laryngitis and infection with human papillomaviruses. *HNO*, **41**, 123–127 (in German)

Arroyo, M., Bagchi, S. & Raychaudhuri, P. (1993) Association of the human papillomavirus type 16 E7 protein with the S-phase-specific E2F-cyclin A complex. *Mol. cell. Biol.*, **13**, 6537–6546

Asato, T., Nakajima, Y., Nagamine, M., Nakashima, Y., Takei, H., Maehama, T., Yamashiro, T., Higashi, M., Nakayama, M. & Kanazawa, K. (1994) Correlation between the progression of cervical dysplasia and the prevalence of human papillomavirus. *J. infect. Dis.*, **169**, 940–941

Ashinoff, R., Li, J.J., Jacobson, M., Friedman-Kien, A.E. & Geronemus, R.G. (1991) Detection of human papillomavirus DNA in squamous cell carcinoma of the nail bed and finger determined by polymerase chain reaction. *Arch. Dermatol.*, **127**, 1813–1818

Atkin, N.B. (1986) Chromosome 1 aberrations in cancer. *Cancer Genet. Cytogenet.*, **21**, 279–285

Atkin, N.B., Baker, M.C. & Ferti Passantonopoulou, A. (1983) Chromosome changes in early gynecologic malignancies. *Acta cytol.*, **27**, 450–453

Auborn, K.J. & Steinberg, B.M. (1991) A key DNA-protein interaction determines the function of the 5′URR enhancer in human papillomavirus type 11. *Virology*, **181**, 132–138

Auewarakul, P., Gissmann, L. & Cid-Arregui, A. (1994) Targeted expression of the E6 and E7 oncogenes of human papillomavirus type 16 in the epidermis of transgenic mice elicits generalized epidermal hyperplasia involving autocrine factors. *Mol. cell. Biol.*, **14**, 8250–8258

Azocar, J., Abad, S.M.J., Acosta, H., Hernandez, R., Gallegos, M., Pifano, E., Blanch, R. & Kramar, A. (1990) Prevalence of cervical dysplasia and HPV infection according to sexual behavior. *Int. J. Cancer*, **45**, 622–625

Badaracco, G., Giovinazzi, R., Sedati, A., Venuti, A. & Marcante, M.L. (1992) A follow-up study on human papillomavirus types 16 and 18 infections and cervical neoplasia. *J. exp. clin. Cancer Res.*, **11**, 259–262

Baggish, M.S. (1982) Management of cervical intraepithelial neoplasia by carbon dioxide laser. *Obstet. Gynecol.*, **60**, 378–384

Baird, P.J. (1983) Serological evidence for the association of papillomavirus and cervical neoplasia. *Lancet*, **ii**, 17–18

Baken, L.A., Koutsky, L.A., Kuypers, J., Kosorok, M.R., Lee, S.-K., Kiviat, N.B. & Holmes, K.K. (1995) Genital human papillomavirus infection among male and female sex partners: prevalence and type-specific concordance. *J. infect. Dis.*, **171**, 429–432

Baker, C.C. & Howley, P.M. (1987) Differential promoter utilization by the bovine papillomavirus in transformed cells and productively infected wart tissues. *EMBO J.*, **6**, 1027–1035

Baker, D.A., Douglas, J.M., Jr, Buntin, D.M., Micha, J.P., Beutner, K.R. & Patsner, B. (1990) Topical podofilox for the treatment of condylomata acuminata in women. *Obstet. Gynecol.*, **76**, 656–659

Baker, T.S., Newcomb, W.W., Olson, N.H., Cowsert, L.M., Olson, C. & Brown, J.C. (1991) Structures of bovine and human papillomaviruses: analysis by cryoelectron microscopy and three-dimensional image reconstruction. *Biophys. J.*, **60**, 1445–1456

Bal, V., McIndoe, A., Denton, G., Hudson, D., Lombardi, G., Lamb, J. & Lechler, R. (1990) Antigen presentation by keratinocytes induces tolerance in human T cells. *Eur. J. Immunol.*, **20**, 1893–1897

Band, V., Zajchowski, D., Kulesa, V. & Sager, R. (1990) Human papilloma virus DNAs immortalize normal human mammary epithelial cells and reduce their growth factor requirements. *Proc. natl Acad. Sci. USA*, **87**, 463–467

Band, V., De Caprio, J.A., Delmolino, L., Kulesa, V. & Sager, R. (1991) Loss of p53 protein in human papillomavirus type 16 E6-immortalized human mammary epithelial cells. *J. Virol.*, **65**, 6671–6676

Band, V., Dalal, S., Delmolino, L. & Androphy, E.J. (1993) Enhanced degradation of p53 protein in HPV-6 and BPV-1 E6-immortalized human mammary epithelial cells. *EMBO J.*, **12**, 1847–1852

Banks, L., Matlashewski, G., Pim, D., Churcher, M., Roberts, C. & Crawford, L. (1987) Expression of human papillomavirus type 6 and type 16 capsid proteins in bacteria and their antigenic characterization. *J. gen. Virol.*, **68**, 3081–3089

Banks, L., Edmonds, C. & Vousden, K.H. (1990) Ability of the HPV16 E7 protein to bind RB and induce DNA synthesis is not sufficient for efficient transforming activity in NIH3T3 cells. *Oncogene*, **5**, 1383–1389

Barbosa, M.S., Lowy, D.R. & Schiller, J.T. (1989) Papillomavirus polypeptides E6 and E7 are zinc-binding proteins. *J. Virol.*, **63**, 1404–1407

Barbosa, M.S., Edmonds, C., Fisher, C., Schiller, J.T., Lowy, D.R. & Vousden, K.H. (1990) The region of the HPV E7 oncoprotein homologous to adenovirus E1a and SV40 large T antigen contains separate domains for Rb binding and casein kinase II phosphorylation. *EMBO J.*, **9**, 153–160

Barnes, W., Delgado, G., Kurman, R.J., Petrilli, E.S., Smith, D.M., Ahmed, S., Lorincz, A.T., Temple, G.F., Jenson, A.B. & Lancaster, W.D. (1988) Possible prognostic significance of human papillomavirus type in cervical cancer. *Gynecol. Oncol.*, **29**, 267–273

Barr, B.B., Benton, E.C., McLaren, K., Bunney, M.H., Smith, I.W., Blessing, K. & Hunter, J.A.A. (1989) Human papilloma virus infection and skin cancer in renal allograft recipients. *Lancet.*, **i**, 124–129

Barrasso, R. (1992) HPV-related genital lesions in men. In: Muñoz, N., Bosch, F.X., Shah, K.V. & Meheus, A., eds, *The Epidemiology of Cervical Cancer and Human Papillomavirus* (IARC Scientific Publications No. 119), Lyon, IARC, pp. 85–92

Barrasso, R., de Brux, J., Croissant, O. & Orth, G. (1987a) High prevalence of papillomavirus-associated penile intraepithelial neoplasia in sexual partners of women with cervical intraepithelial neoplasia. *N. Engl. J. Med.*, **317**, 916–923

Barrasso, R., Coupez, F., Ionesco, M. & de Brux, J. (1987b) Human papilloma viruses and cervical intraepithelial neoplasia: the role of colposcopy. *Gynecol. Oncol.*, **27**, 197–207

Barrett, T.J., Silbar, J.D. & McGinley, J.P. (1954) Genital warts — a venereal disease. *J. Am. med. Assoc.*, **154**, 333–334

Barton, S.E., Maddox, P.H., Jenkins, D., Edwards, R., Cuzick, J. & Singer, A. (1988) Effect of cigarette smoking on cervical epithelial immunity: a mechanism for neoplastic change? *Lancet*, **ii**, 652–654

Bartsch, D., Boye, B., Baust, C., zur Hausen, H. & Schwarz, E. (1992) Retinoic acid-mediated repression of human papillomavirus 18 transcription and different ligand regulation of the retinoic acid receptor β gene in nontumorigenic and tumorigenic HeLa hybrid cells. *EMBO J.*, **11**, 2283–2291

Bauer, H.M., Ting, Y., Greer, C.E., Chambers, J.C., Tashiro, C.J., Chimera, J., Reingold, A. & Manos, M.M. (1991) Genital human papillomavirus infection in female university students as determined by a PCR-based method. *J. Am. med. Assoc.*, **265**, 472–477

Bauer, H.M., Hildesheim, A., Schiffman, M.H., Glass, A.G., Rush, B.B., Scott, D.R., Cadell, D.M., Kurman, R.J. & Manos, M.M. (1993) Determinants of genital human papillomavirus infection in low-risk women in Portland, Oregon. *Sex. transm. Dis.*, **20**, 274–278

Bauknecht, T., Angel, P., Royer, H.-D. & zur Hausen, H. (1992) Identification of a negative regulatory domain in the human papillomavirus type 18 promoter: interaction with the transcription repressor YY1. *EMBO J.*, **11**, 4607–4617

Bauknecht, T., Jundt, F., Herr, I., Oehler, T., Delius, H., Shi, Y., Angel, P. & zur Hausen, H. (1995) A switch region determines the cell type-positive or negative action of YY1 on the activity of the human papillomavirus type 18 promoter. *J. Virol.*, **69**, 1–12

Bavin, P.J., Giles, J.A., Deery, A., Crow, J., Griffiths, P.D., Emery, V.C. & Walker, P.G. (1993) Use of semi-quantitative PCR for human papillomavirus DNA type 16 to identify women with high grade cervical disease in a population presenting with a mildly dyskaryotic smear report. *Br. J. Cancer*, **67**, 602–605

Beaudenon, S., Praetorius, F., Kremsdorf, D., Lutzner, M., Worsaae, N., Pehau-Arnaudet, G. & Orth, G. (1987) A new type of human papillomavirus associated with oral focal epithelial hyperplasia. *J. invest. Dermatol.*, **88**, 130–135

Becker, T.M., Stone, K.M. & Alexander, E.R. (1987) Genital human papillomavirus infection: a growing concern. *Obstet. gynecol. Clin. North Am.*, **14**, 389–396

Becker, T.M., Wheeler, C.M., McGough, N.S., Jordan, S.W., Dorin, M. & Miller, J. (1991) Cervical papillomavirus infection and cervical dysplasia in Hispanic, native American, and non-Hispanic white women in New Mexico. *Am. J. public Health*, **81**, 582–586

Becker, T.M., Wheeler, C.M., McGough, N.S., Parmenter, C.A., Jordan, S.W., Stidley, C.A., McPherson, R.S. & Dorin, M.H. (1994) Sexually transmitted diseases and other risk factors for cervical dysplasia among southwestern Hispanic and non-Hispanic white women. *J. Am. med. Assoc.*, **271**, 1181–1188

Beckmann, A.M., Daling, J.R., Sherman, K.J., Maden, C., Miller, B.A., Coates, R.J., Kiviat, N.B., Myerson, D., Weiss, N.S., Hislop, T.G., Beagrie, M. & McDougall, J.K (1989) Human papillomavirus infection and anal cancer. *Int. J. Cancer*, **43**, 1042–1049

Beckmann, A.M., Acker, R., Christiansen, A.E. & Sherman, K.J. (1991a) Human papillomavirus infection in women with multicentric squamous cell neoplasia. *Am. J. Obstet. Gynecol.*, **165**, 1431–1437

Beckmann, A.M., Sherman, K.J., Saran, L. & Weiss, N.S. (1991b) Genital-type human papillomavirus infection is not associated with surface epithelial ovarian carcinoma. *Gynecol. Oncol.*, **43**, 247–251

Bedell, M.A., Jones, K.H. & Laimins, L.A. (1987) The E6-E7 region of human papillomavirus type 18 is sufficient for transformation of NIH 3T3 and rat-1 cells. *J. Virol.*, **61**, 3635–3640

Bedell, M.A., Hudson, J.B., Golub, T.R., Turyk, M.E., Hosken, M., Wilbanks, G.D. & Laimins, L.A. (1991) Amplification of human papillomavirus genomes *in vitro* is dependent on epithelial differentiation. *J. Virol.*, **65**, 2254–2260

Bejui-Thivolet, F., Chardonnet, Y. & Patricot, L.M. (1990a) Human papillomavirus type 11 DNA in papillary squamous cell lung carcinoma. *Virchows Arch. A*, **417**, 457–461

Bejui-Thivolet, F., Liagre, N., Chignol, M.C., Chardonnet, Y. & Patricot, L.M. (1990b) Detection of human papillomavirus DNA in squamous bronchial metaplasia and squamous cell carcinomas of the lung by in situ hybridization using biotinylated probes in paraffin-embedded specimens. *Hum. Pathol.*, **21**, 111–116

Benamouzig, R., Pigot, F., Quiroga, G., Validire, P., Chaussade, S., Catalan, F. & Couturier, D. (1992) Human papillomavirus infection in esophageal squamous-cell carcinoma in western countries. *Int. J. Cancer*, **50**, 549–552

Bender, H.G., Degen, K.W. & Beck, L. (1988) Human papilloma virus findings in the perimeter of vulvo-vaginal malignancies. *Eur. J. gynaecol. Oncol.*, **9**, 287–290

Benton, C., Shahidulhah, H. & Hunter, J.A.A. (1992) Human papillomaviruses in the immunosuppressed. *Papillomavirus Rep.*, **3**, 23–26

Beral, V., Hermon, C., Muñoz, N. & Devesa, S.S. (1994) Cervical cancer. *Cancer Surv.*, **19/20**, 265–285

Bergeron, C., Naghashfar, Z., Canaan, C., Shah, K.V., Fu, Y. & Ferenczy, A. (1987a) Human papillomavirus type 16 in intraepithelial neoplasia (Bowenoid papulosis) and coexistent invasive carcinoma of the vulva. *Int. J. Gynecol. Pathol.*, **6**, 1–11

Bergeron, C., Ferenczy, A., Shah, K.V. & Naghashfar, Z. (1987b) Multicentric human papillomavirus infections of the female genital tract: correlation of viral types with abnormal mitotic figures, colposcopic presentation, and location. *Obstet. Gynecol.*, **69**, 736–742

Bergeron, C., Barrasso, R., Beaudenon, S., Flamant, P., Croissant, O. & Orth, G. (1992) Human papillomaviruses associated with cervical intraepithelial neoplasia: great diversity and distinct distribution in low- and high-grade lesions. *Am. J. surg. Pathol.*, **16**, 641–649

Bergman, A., Bhatia, N.N. & Broen, E.M. (1984) Cryotherapy for treatment of genital condylomata during pregnancy. *J. reprod. Med.*, **29**, 432–435

Berkhout, R.J.M., Tieben, L.M., Smits, H.L., Bouwes Bavinck, J.N., Vermeer, B.J. & ter Schegget, J. (1995) Nested PCR approach for detection and typing of epidermodysplasia verruciformis-associated human papillomavirus types in cutaneous cancers from renal transplant recipients. *J. clin. Microbiol.*, **33**, 690–695

Bernard, H.-U., Oltersdorf, T. & Seedorf, K. (1987) Expression of the human papillomavirus type 18 E7 gene by a cassette-vector system for the transcription and translation of open reading frames in eukaryotic cells. *EMBO J.*, **6**, 133–138

Bernard, C., Mougin, C., Madoz, L., Drobacheff, C., Van Landuyt, H., Laurent, R. & Lab, M. (1992) Viral co-infections in human papillomavirus-associated anogenital lesions according to the serostatus for the human immunodeficiency virus. *Int. J. Cancer*, **52**, 731–737

Bernard, H.-U., Chan, S.-Y., Manos, M.M., Ong, C.-K., Villa, L.L., Delius, H., Peyton, C.L., Bauer, H.M. & Wheeler, C.M. (1994a) Identification and assessment of known and novel human papillomaviruses by polymerase chain reaction amplification, restriction fragment length polymorphisms, nucleotide sequence, and phylogenetic algorithms. *J. infect. Dis.*, **170**, 1077–1085

Bernard, H.-U., Chan, S.-Y. & Delius, H. (1994b) Evolution of papillomaviruses. *Curr. Top. Microbiol. Immunol.*, **186**, 33–54

Bernard, C., Mougin, C., Bettinger, D., Didier, J.M. & Lab, M. (1994c) Detection of human papillomavirus by in-situ polymerase chain-reaction in paraffin-embedded cervical biopsies. *Mol. cell. Probes*, **8**, 337–343

Beutner, K.R., Becker, T.M. & Stone, K.M. (1991) Epidemiology of human papillomavirus infections. *Dermatol. Clin.*, **9**, 211–218

Beverley, P.C.L., Sadovnikova, E., Zhu, X., Hickling, J., Gao, L., Chain, B., Collins, L., Crawford, L., Vousden, K. & Strauss, H.J. (1994) Strategies for studying mouse and human immune responses to human papillomavirus type 16. In: *Vaccines Against Virally Induced Cancers (Ciba Foundation Symposium 187)*, Chichester, John Wiley & Sons, pp. 78–96

Bigrigg, M.A., Codling, B.W., Pearson, P., Read, M.D. & Swingler, G.A. (1990) Colposcopic diagnosis and treatment of cervical dysplasia at a single clinic visit. Experience of low-voltage diathermy loop in 1000 patients. *Lancet*, **336**, 229–231

Billaudel, S., Aillet, G., Tardivel, P., Besse, B., Sagot, P., Le Guyader, F., Mensier, A. & Lopes, P. (1991) Typing of papillomaviruses in cervical dysplasias: its value in treatment. *J. Gynecol. Obstet. Biol. Reprod. (Paris)*, **20**, 941–945 (in French)

Birkeland, S.A., Storm, H.H., Lamm, L.U., Barlow, L., Blohmé, I., Forsberg, B., Eklund, B., Fjeldborg, O., Friedberg, M., Frödin, L., Glattre, E., Halvorsen, S., Holm, N.V., Jakobsen, A., Jørgensen, H.E., Ladefoged, J., Lindholm, T., Lundgren, G. & Pukkala, E (1995) Cancer risk after renal transplantation in the Nordic countries, 1964–1986. *Int. J. Cancer*, **60**, 183–189

Bjersing, L., Rogo, K., Evander, M., Gerdes, U., Stendahl, U. & Wadell, G. (1991) HPV 18 and cervical adenocarcinomas. *Anticancer Res.*, **11**, 123–127

Blauvelt, A., Duarte, A.M., Pruksachatkunakorn, C., Leonardi, C.L. & Schachner, L.A. (1992) Human papillomavirus type 6 infection involving cutaneous nongenital sites. *J. Am. Acad. Dermatol.*, **27**, 876–879

Blessing, K., McLaren, K.M., Benton, E.C., Bar, B.B., Bunney, M.H., Smith, I.W. & Beveridge, G.W. (1989) Histopathology of skin lesions in renal allograft recipients — an assessment of viral features and dysplasia. *Histopathology*, **14**, 129–139

Blessing, K., McLaren, K.M., Morris, R., Barr, B.B., Benton, E.C., Alloub, M., Bunney, M.H., Smith, I.W., Smart, G.E. & Bird, C.C. (1990) Detection of human papillomavirus in skin and genital lesions of renal allograft recipients by in situ hybridization. *Histopathology*, **16**, 181–185

Bleul, C., Müller, M., Frank, R., Gausepohl, H., Koldovsky, U., Mgaya, H.N., Luande, J., Pawlita, M., ter Meulen, J., Viscidi, R. & Gissmann, L. (1991) Human papillomavirus type 18 E6 and E7 antibodies in human sera: increased anti-E7 prevalence in cervical cancer patients. *J. clin. Microbiol.*, **29**, 1579–1588

Blitz, I.L. & Laimins, L.A. (1991) The 68-kilodalton E1 protein of bovine papillomavirus is a DNA binding phosphoprotein which associates with the E2 transcriptional activator *in vitro*. *J. Virol.*, **65**, 649–656

Bloch, N., Breen, M. & Spradbrow, P.B. (1994) Genomic sequences of bovine papillomaviruses in formalin-fixed sarcoids from Australian horses revealed by polymerase chain reaction. *Vet. Microbiol.*, **41**, 163–172

Blomfield, P.L., Buxton, J., Dunn, J. & Luesley, D.M. (1993) Pregnancy outcome after large loop excision of the cervical transformation zone. *Am. J. Obstet. Gynecol.*, **169**, 620–625

Bloss, J.D., Liao, S.-Y., Wilczynski, S.P., Macri, C., Walker, J., Peake, M. & Berman, M.L. (1991) Clinical and histologic features of vulvar carcinomas analyzed for human papillomavirus status: evidence that squamous-cell carcinoma of the vulva has more than one etiology. *Hum. Pathol.*, **22**, 711–718

Bonnez, W., Da Rin, C., Rose, R.C. & Reichman, R.C. (1991) Use of human papillomavirus type 11 virions in an ELISA to detect specific antibodies in humans with condylomata acuminata. *J. gen. Virol.*, **72**, 1343–1347

Bonnez, W., Kashima, H.K., Leventhal, B., Mounts, P., Rose, R.C., Reichman, R.C. & Shah, K.V. (1992) Antibody response to human papillomavirus (HPV) type 11 in children with juvenile-onset recurrent respiratory papillomatosis (RRP). *Virology*, **188**, 384–387

Bonnez, W., Da Rin, C., Rose, R.C., Tyring, S.K. & Reichman, R.C. (1993) Evolution of the antibody response to human papillomavirus type 11 (HPV-11) in patients with condyloma acuminatum according to treatment response. *J. med. Virol.*, **39**, 340–344

Bonnez, W., Rose, R.C., Borkhuis, C., Da Rin, C. & Reichman, R.C. (1994a) Evaluation of temperature sensitivity of human papillomavirus type 11 by using the human xenograft severe combined immunodeficiency mouse model. *J. clin. Microbiol.*, **32**, 1575–1577

Bonnez, W., Elswick, R.K., Jr, Bailey-Farchione, A., Hallahan, D., Bell, R., Isenberg, R., Stoler, M.H. & Reichman, R.C. (1994b) Efficacy and safety of 0.5% podofilox solution in the treatment and suppression of anogenital warts. *Am. J. Med.*, **96**, 420–425

Borg, A.J., Medley, G. & Garland, S.M. (1993) Prevalence of HPV in a Melbourne female STD population: comparison of RNA and DNA probes in detecting HPV by dot blot hybridization. *Int. J. sex transm. Dis. AIDS*, **4**, 159–164

Bornstein, J., Kaufman, R.H., Adam, E. & Adler-Storthz, K. (1988) Multicentric intraepithelial neoplasia involving the vulva: clinical features and association with human papillomavirus and herpes simplex virus. *Cancer*, **62**, 1601–1604

Bosch, F.X. & Cardis, E. (1990) Cancer incidence correlations: genital, urinary and some tobacco-related cancers. *Int. J. Cancer*, **46**, 178–184

Bosch, F.X. & Muñoz, N. (1989) Human papillomavirus and cervical neoplasia: a critical review of the epidemiological evidence. In: Muñoz, N., Bosch, P.X. & Jensen, O.M., eds, *Human Papillomavirus and Cervical Cancer* (IARC Scientific Publications No. 94), Lyon, IARC, pp. 135–151

Bosch, F.X., Muñoz, N., de Sanjosé, S., Izarzugaza, I., Gili, M., Viladiu, P., Tormo, M.J., Moreo, P., Ascunce, N., Gonzalez, L.C., Tafur, L., Kaldor, J.M., Guerrero, E., Aristizabal, N., Santamaria, M., Alonso de Ruiz, P. & Shah, K.V. (1992) Risk factors for cervical cancer in Colombia and Spain. *Int. J. Cancer*, **52**, 750–758

Bosch, F.X., Muñoz, N., de Sanjosé, S., Navarro, C., Moreo, P., Ascunce, N., Gonzalez, L.C., Tafur, L., Gili, M., Larrañaga, I., Viladiu, P., Daniel, R.W., de Ruiz, P.A., Aristizabal, N., Santamaria, M., Guerrero, E. & Shah, K.V. (1993) Human papillomavirus and cervical intraepithelial neoplasia grade III/carcinoma *in situ*: a case–control study in Spain and Colombia. *Cancer Epidemiol. Biomarkers Prev.*, **2**, 415–422

Bosch, F.X., Muñoz, N., de Sanjosé, S., Guerrero, E., Gaffari, A.M., Kaldor, J., Castellsagué, X. & Shah, K.V. (1994a) Importance of human papillomavirus endemicity in the incidence of cervical cancer: an extention of the hypothesis on sexual behavior. *Cancer Epidemiol. Biomarkers Prev.*, **3**, 375–379

Bosch, F.X., de Sanjosé, S. & Muñoz, N. (1994b) Correspondence re: M. Schiffman and A. Schatzkin, test reliability is critically important to molecular epidemiology: an example from studies of human papillomavirus infection and cervical neoplasia. Cancer Res. (suppl.), 54: 1944s–1947s, 1994 (Letter to the Editor). *Cancer Res.*, **54**, 6288–6289

Bosch, F.X., Manos, M.M., Muñoz, N., Sherman, M., Jansen, A.M., Peto, J., Schiffman, M.H., Moreno, V., Kurman, R., Shah, K.V. & International Biological Study on Cervical Cancer (IBSCC) Study Group (1995) Prevalence of human papillomavirus in cervical cancer: a worldwide perspective. *J. natl Cancer Inst.*, **87**, 796–802

Boshart, M., Gissmann, L., Ikenberg, H., Kleinheinz, A., Scheurlen, W. & zur Hausen, H. (1984) A new type of papillomavirus DNA and its prevalence in genital cancer biopsies and in cell lines derived from cervical cancer. *EMBO J.*, **3**, 1151–1157

Bossy-Wetzel, E., Bravo, R. & Hanahan, D. (1992) Transcription factors *junB* and *c-jun* are selectively up-regulated and functionally implicated in fibrosarcoma development. *Genes Dev.*, **6**, 2340–2351

Bouvard, V., Matlashewski, G., Gu, Z.-M., Storey, A. & Banks, L. (1994) The human papillomavirus type 16 E5 gene cooperates with the E7 gene to stimulate proliferation of primary cells and increases viral gene expression. *Virology*, **203**, 73–80

Boyle, C.A., Lowell, D.M., Kelsey, J.L., LiVolsi, V.A. & Boyle, K.E. (1989) Cervical intraepithelial neoplasia among women with papillomavirus infection compared to women with *Trichomonas* infection. *Cancer*, **64**, 168–172

Brachman, D.G., Graves, D., Vokes, E., Beckett, M., Haraf, D., Montag, A., Dunphy, E., Mick, R., Yandell, D. & Weichselbaum, R.R. (1992) Occurrence of *p53* gene deletions and human papillomavirus infection in human head and neck cancer. *Cancer Res.*, **52**, 4832–4836

Bradford, C.R., Hoffman, H.T., Wolf, G.T., Carey, T.E., Baker, S.R. & McClatchey, K.D. (1990) Squamous carcinoma of the head and neck in organ transplant recipients: possible role of oncogenic virus. *Laryngoscope*, **100**, 190–194

Bradbeer, C. (1987) Is infection with HIV a risk factor for cervical intraepithelial neoplasia? (Letter to the Editor). *Lancet*, **ii**, 1277–1278

Brandenberger, A.W., Rüdlinger, R., Hänggi, W., Bersinger, N.A. & Dreher, E. (1992) Detection of human papillomavirus in vulvar carcinoma: a study by in situ hybridisation. *Arch. Gynecol. Obstet.*, **252**, 31–35

Brandsma, J.L. & Abramson, A.L. (1989) Association of papillomavirus with cancers of the head and neck. *Arch. Otolaryngol. Head Neck Surg.*, **115**, 621–625

Brandsma, J.L., Steinberg, B.M., Abramson, A.L. & Winkler, B. (1986) Presence of human papillomavirus type 16 related sequences in verrucous carcinoma of the larynx. *Cancer Res.*, **46**, 2185–2188

Brandsma, J.L., Burk, R.D., Lancaster, W.D., Pfister, H. & Schiffman, M.H. (1989) Inter-laboratory variation as an explanation for varying prevalence estimates of human papillomavirus infection. *Int. J. Cancer*, **43**, 260–262

Brandwein, M.S., Nuovo, G.J. & Biller, H. (1993) Analysis of prevalence of human papillomavirus in laryngeal carcinomas: study of 40 cases using polymerase chain reaction and consensus primers. *Ann. Otol. Rhinol. Laryngol.*, **102**, 309–313

Braun, L. (1994) Role of human immunodeficiency virus infection in the pathogenesis of human papillomavirus-associated cervical neoplasia. *Am. J. Pathol.*, **144**, 209–214

Braun, L., Farmer, E.R. & Shah, K.V. (1983) Immunoperoxidase localization of papillomavirus antigen in cutaneous warts and bowenoid papulosis. *J. med. Virol.*, **12**, 187–193

Bream, G.L., Ohmstede, C.-A. & Phelps, W.C. (1993) Characterization of human papillomavirus type 11 E1 and E2 proteins expressed in insect cells. *J. Virol.*, **67**, 2655–2663

Breese, P.L., Judson, F.N., Penley, K.A. & Douglas, J.M., Jr (1995) Anal human papillomavirus infection among homosexual and bisexual men: prevalence of type-specific infection and association with human immunodeficiency virus. *Sex. transm. Dis.*, **22**, 7–14

Bregman, C.L., Hirth, R.S., Sundberg, J.P. & Christensen, E.F. (1987) Cutaneous neoplasms in dogs associated with canine oral papillomavirus vaccine. *Vet. Pathol.*, **24**, 477–487

Brenes, M.M., De Lao, S.L., Gómez, B. & Reeves, W.C. (1987) Controlled study of cases of uterine cervix cancer and infection with human papillomavirus in Latin America. *Rev. med. Panama*, **12**, 173–181 (in Spanish)

Brinton, L.A., Nasca, P.C., Mallin, K., Baptiste, M.S., Wilbanks, G.D. & Richart, R.M. (1990) Case–control study of cancer of the vulva. *Obstet. Gynecol.*, **75**, 859–866

Brinton, L.A., Li, J.-Y., Rong, S.-D., Huang, S., Xiao, B.S., Shi, B.-G., Zhu, Z.-J., Schiffman, M.H. & Dawsey, S. (1991) Risk factors for penile cancer: results from a case–control study in China. *Int. J. Cancer*, **47**, 504–509

Brisson, J., Morin, C., Fortier, M., Roy, M., Bouchard, C., Leclerc, J., Christen, A., Guimont, C., Penault, F. & Meisels, A. (1994) Risk factors for cervical intraepithelial neoplasia: differences between low- and high-grade lesions. *Am. J. Epidemiol.*, **140**, 700–710

Broders, A.C. (1932) Carcinoma *in situ* contrasted with benign penetrating epithelium. *J. Am. med. Assoc.*, **99**, 1670–1674

Brokaw, J.L., Yee, C.L. & Münger, K. (1994) A mutational analysis of the amino terminal domain of the human papillomavirus type 16 E7 oncoprotein. *Virology*, **205**, 603–607

Brown, D.R., Bryan, J.J., Cramer, H., Katz, B.P., Handy, V. & Fife, K.H. (1994) Detection of multiple human papillomavirus types in condylomata acuminata from immunosuppressed patients. *J. infect. Dis.*, **170**, 759–765

Browne, H.M., Churcher, M.J., Stanley, M.A., Smith, G.L. & Minson, A.C. (1988) Analysis of the L1 gene product of human papillomavirus type 16 by expression in a vaccinia virus recombinant. *J. gen. Virol.*, **69**, 1263–1273

Brugge, J.S. & Butel, J.S. (1975) Role of simian virus 40 gene A function in maintenance of transformation. *J. Virol.*, **15**, 619–635

van den Brule, A.J.C., Meijer, C.J.L.M., Bakels, V., Kenemans, P. & Walboomers, J.M.M. (1990) Rapid detection of human papillomavirus in cervical scrapes by combined general primer-mediated and type-specific polymerase chain reaction. *J. clin. Microbiol.*, **28**, 2739–2743

van den Brule, A.J.C., Walboomers, J.M.M., Du Maine, M., Kenemans, P. & Meijer, C.J.L.M. (1991a) Difference in prevalence of human papillomavirus genotypes in cytomorphologically normal cervical smears is associated with a history of cervical intraepithelial neoplasia. *Int. J. Cancer*, **48**, 404–408

van den Brule, A.J.C., Cromme, F.V., Snijders, P.J.F., Smit, L., Oudejans, C.B.M., Baak, J.P.A., Meijer, C.J.L.M. & Walboomers, J.M.M. (1991b) Nonradioactive RNA in situ hybridization detection of human papillomavirus 16-E7 transcripts in squamous-cell carcinomas of the uterine cervix using confocal laser scan microscopy. *Am. J. Pathol.*, **139**, 1037–1045 van den Brule, A.J.C., Snijders, P.F.J., Meijer, C.J.L.M. & Walboomers, J.M.M. (1993) PCR-based detection of genital HPV genotypes: an update and future perspectives. *Papillomavirus Rep.*, **4**, 95–99

Brunham, R.C. & Plummer, F.A. (1990) A general model of sexually transmitted disease epidemiology and its implications for control. *Med. Clin. North Am.*, **74**, 1339–1352

Bryan, R.L., Bevan, I.S., Crocker, J. & Young, L.S. (1990) Detection of HPV 6 and 11 in tumours of the upper respiratory tract using the polymerase chain reaction. *Clin. Otolaryngol.*, **15**, 177–180

Bryant, P., Davies, P. & Wilson, D. (1991) Detection of human papillomavirus DNA in cancer of the urinary bladder by in situ hybridisation. *Br. J. Urol.*, **68**, 49–52

Bubb, V., McCance, D.J. & Schlegel, R. (1988) DNA sequence of the HPV-16 E5 ORF and the structural conservation of its encoded protein. *Virology*, **163**, 243–246

Burger, M.P.M., Hollema, H., Pieters, W.J.L.M. & Quint, W.G.V. (1995) Predictive value of human papillomavirus type for histological diagnosis of women with cervical abnormalities. *Br. med. J.*, **310**, 94–95

Burkhardt, A., Willingham, M., Gay, C., Jeang, K.-T. & Schlegel, R. (1989) The E5 oncoprotein of bovine papillomavirus is oriented asymmetrically in Golgi and plasma membranes. *Virology*, **170**, 334–339

Busby-Earle, R.M.C., Steel, C.M., Williams, A.R.W., Cohen, B. & Bird, C.C. (1994) p53 Mutations in cervical carcinogenesis — low frequency and lack of correlation with human papillomavirus status. *Br. J. Cancer*, **69**, 732–737

Buscema, J., Naghashfar, Z., Sawada, E., Daniel, R., Woodruff, J.D. & Shah, K.V. (1988) The predominance of human papillomavirus type 16 in vulvar neoplasia. *Obstet. Gynecol.*, **71**, 601–606

Butterworth, C.E., Jr, Hatch, K.D., Macaluso, M., Cole, P., Sauberlich, H.E., Soong, S.J., Borst, M. & Baker, V.V. (1992) Folate deficiency and cervical dysplasia. *J. Am. med. Assoc.*, **267**, 528–533

Butz, K., Shahabeddin, L., Geisen, C., Spitkovsky, D., Ullmann, A. & Hoppe-Seyler, F. (1995) Functional p53 protein in human papillomavirus-positive cancer cells. *Oncogens*, **10**, 927–936

Byrne, J.C., Tsao, M.-S., Fraser, R.S. & Howley, P.M. (1987) Human papillomavirus-11 DNA in a patient with chronic laryngotracheobronchial papillomatosis and metastatic squamous-cell carcinoma of the lung. *New Engl. J. Med.*, **317**, 873–878

Byrne, M.A., Taylor-Robinson, D., Munday, P.E. & Harris, J.R.W. (1989) The common occurrence of human papillomavirus infection and intraepithelial neoplasia in women infected by HIV. *AIDS*, **3**, 379–382

Byrne, M.A., Parry, G.C.N., Morse, A., Taylor-Robinson, D., Malcolm, A.D.B. & Coleman, D.V. (1990) A prospective study of human papillomavirus infection of the cervix. *Cytopathology*, **1**, 329–337

Campion, M.J., McCance, D.J., Cuzick, J. & Singer, A. (1986) Progressive potential of mild cervical atypia: prospective cytological, colposcopic, and virological study. *Lancet*, **ii**, 237–240

Campo, M.S. (1991) Vaccination against papillomavirus. *Cancer Cells*, **3**, 421–426

Campo, M.S. (1994) Towards vaccines for papillomavirus. In: Stern, P.L. & Stanley, M.A., eds, *Human Papillomaviruses and Cervical Cancer*, Oxford, Oxford University Press, pp. 177–191

Campo, M.S., Moar, M.H., Jarrett, W.F.H. & Laird, H.M. (1980) A new papillomavirus associated with alimentary cancer in cattle. *Nature*, **286**, 180–182

Campo, M.S., Moar, M.H., Laird, H.M. & Jarrett, W.F.H. (1981) Molecular heterogeneity and lesion site specificity of cutaneous bovine papillomaviruses. *Virology*, **113**, 323–335

Campo, M.S., Moar, M.H., Sartirana, M.L., Kennedy, I.M. & Jarrett, W.F.H. (1985) The presence of bovine papillomavirus type 4 DNA is not required for the progression to, or the maintenance of, the malignant state in cancers of the alimentary canal in cattle. *EMBO J.*, **4**, 1819–1825

Campo, M.S., Jarrett, W.F.H., Barron, R.J., O'Neil, B.W. & Smith, K.T. (1992) Association of bovine papillomavirus type 2 and bracken fern with bladder cancer in cattle. *Cancer Res.*, **52**, 6898–6904

Campo, M.S., Grindlay, G.J., O'Neil, B.W., Chandrachud, L.M., McGarvie, G.M. & Jarrett, W.F.H. (1993) Prophylactic and therapeutic vaccination against a mucosal papillomavirus. *J. gen. Virol.*, **74**, 945–953

Campo, M.S., Jarrett, W.F.H., O'Neil, W. & Barron, R.J. (1994a) Latent papillomavirus infection in cattle. *Res. vet. Sci.*, **56**, 151–157

Campo, M.S., O'Neil, B.W., Barron, R.J. & Jarrett, W.F.H. (1994b) Experimental reproduction of the papilloma-carcinoma complex of the alimentary canal in cattle. *Carcinogenesis*, **15**, 1597–1601

Canman, C.E., Gilmer, T.M., Coutts, S.B. & Kastan, M.B. (1995) Growth factor modulation of p53-mediated growth arrest versus apoptosis. *Genes Dev.*, **9**, 600–611

Caparossi, D. & Bacchetti, S. (1990) Definition of adenovirus type 5 functions involved in the induction of chromosomal aberrations in human cells. *J. gen. Virol.*, **71**, 801–808

Carey, F.A., Salter, D.M., Kerr, K.M. & Lamb, D. (1990) An investigation into the role of human papillomavirus in endobronchial papillary squamous tumours. *Respir. Med.*, **84**, 445–447

Carney, H.C., England, J.J., Hodgin, E.C., Whiteley, H.E., Adkison, D.L. & Sundberg, J.P. (1990) Papillomavirus infection of aged Persian cats. *J. Vet. diagn. Invest.*, **2**, 294–299

Carson, L.F., Twiggs, L.B., Okagaki, T., Clark, B.A., Ostrow, R.S. & Faras, A.J. (1988) Human papillomavirus DNA in adenosquamous carcinoma and squamous cell carcinoma of the vulva. *Obstet. Gynecol.*, **72**, 63–67

Carter, J.J., Yaegashi, N., Jenison, S.A. & Galloway, D.A. (1991) Expression of human papillomavirus proteins in yeast *Saccharomyces cerevisiae*. *Virology*, **182**, 513–521

Carter, J.J., Hagensee, M.B., Lee, S.K., McKnight, B., Koutsky, L.A. & Galloway, D.A. (1994) Use of HPV-1 capsids produced by recombinant vaccinia viruses in an ELISA to detect serum antibodies in people with foot warts. *Virology*, **199**, 284–291

Carter, J.J., Wipf, G.C., Hagensee, M.E., McKnight, B., Habel, L.A., Lee, S.-K., Kuypers, J., Kiviat, N., Daling, J.R., Koutsky, L.A., Watts, H., Holmes, K.K. & Galloway, D.A. (1995) Use of human papillomavirus type 6 capsids to detect antibodies in people with genital warts. *J. infect. Dis.* (in press)

Cason, J., Kambo, P.K., Best, J.M. & McCance, D.J. (1992) Detection of antibodies to a linear epitope on the major coat protein (L1) of human papillomavirus type-16 (HPV-16) in sera from patients with cervical intraepithelial neoplasia and children. *Int. J. Cancer*, **50**, 349–355

Caussy, D., Goedert, J.J., Palefsky, J., Gonzales, J., Rabkin, C.S., DiGioia, R.A., Sanchez, W.C., Grossman, R.J., Colclough, G., Wiktor, S.Z., Krämer, A., Biggar, R.J. & Blattner, W.A. (1990a) Interaction of human immunodeficiency and papilloma viruses: association with anal epithelial abnormality in homosexual men. *Int. J. Cancer*, **46**, 214–219

Caussy, D., Marrett, L.D., Worth, A.J., McBride, M. & Rawls, W.E. (1990b) Human papillomavirus and cervical intraepithelial neoplasia in women who subsequently had invasive cancer. *Can. med. Assoc. J.*, **142**, 311–317

Centers for Disease Control (1992) 1993 revised classification system for HIV infection and expanded surveillance case definition for AIDS among adolescents and adults. *MMWR*, **41/RR-17**, 1–19

Chambers, M.A., Stacey, S.N., Arrand, J.R. & Stanley, M.A. (1994a) Delayed-type hypersensitivity response to human papillomavirus type 16 E6 protein in a mouse model. *J. gen. Virol.*, **75**, 165–169

Chambers, M.A., Wei, Z., Coleman, N., Nash, A.A. & Stanley, M.A. (1994b) 'Natural' presentation of human papillomavirus type-16 E7 protein to immunocompetent mice results in antigen-specific sensitization or sustained unresponsiveness. *Eur. J. Immunol.*, **24**, 738–745

Chan, W.-K., Gloss, B. & Bernard, H.-U. (1988) Human papillomavirus-16 and genital cancer: are tests for the viral gene expression in vitro indicators for risk factors *in vivo*? *Ann. Acad. Med. Singapore*, **17**, 232–237

Chan, W.-K., Klock, G. & Bernard, H.-U. (1989) Progesterone and glucocorticoid response elements occur in the long control regions of several human papillomaviruses involved in anogenital neoplasia. *J. Virol.*, **63**, 3261–3269

Chan, W.-K., Chong, T., Bernard, H.-U. & Klock, G. (1990) Transcription of the transforming genes of the oncogenic human papillomavirus-16 is stimulated by tumor promotors through AP1 binding sites. *Nucleic Acids Res.*, **18**, 763–769

Chan, S.-Y., Bernard, H.-U., Ong, C.-K., Chan, S.-P., Hofmann, B. & Delius, H. (1992a) Phylogenetic analysis of 48 papillomavirus types and 28 subtypes and variants: a showcase for the molecular evolution of DNA viruses. *J. Virol.*, **66**, 5714–5725

Chan, S.-Y., Ho, L., Ong, C.-K., Chow, V., Drescher, B., Dürst, M., ter Meulen, J., Villa, L., Luande, J., Mgaya, H.N. & Bernard, H.-U. (1992b) Molecular variants of human papillomavirus type 16 from four continents suggest ancient pandemic spread of the virus and its coevolution with humankind. *J. Virol.*, **66**, 2057–2066

Chan, S.-Y., Tan, C.-H., Delius, H. & Bernard, H.-U. (1994a) Human papillomavirus type 2c is identical to human papillomavirus type 27. *Virology*, **201**, 397–398

Chan, K.W., Lam, K.Y., Chan, A.C.L., Lau, P. & Srivastava, G. (1994b) Prevalence of human papillomavirus types 16 and 18 in penile carcinoma: a study of 41 cases using PCR. *J. clin. Pathol.*, **47**, 823–826

Chan, S.-Y., Delius, H., Halpern, A.L. & Bernard, H.-U. (1995) Analysis of genomic sequences of 95 papilloma virus types: uniting typing, phylogeny and taxonomy. *J. Virol.*, **69**, 3074–3083

Chandrachud, L.M., Grindlay, G.J., McGarvie, G.M., O'Neil, B.W., Wagner, E.R., Jarrett, W.F.H. & Campo, M.S. (1995) Vaccination of cattle with the N-terminus of L2 is necessary and sufficient for preventing infection by BPV-4. *Virology* (in press)

Chang, K.-W., Chang, C.-S., Lai, K.-S., Chou, M.-J. & Choo, K.-B. (1989) High prevalence of human papillomavirus infection and possible association with betel quid chewing and smoking in oral epidermoid carcinomas in Taiwan. *J. med. Virol.*, **28**, 57–61

Chang, F., Syrjänen, S., Nuutinen, J., Kärjä, J. & Syrjänen, K. (1990a) Detection of human papillomavirus (HPV) DNA in oral squamous cell carcinomas by in situ hybridization and polymerase chain reaction. *Arch. dermatol. Res.*, **282**, 493–497

Chang, F., Syrjänen, S., Shen, Q., Ji, H.X. & Syrjänen, K. (1990b) Human papillomavirus (HPV) DNA in esophageal precancer lesions and squamous cell carcinomas from China. *Int. J. Cancer*, **45**, 21–25

Chang, F., Syrjänen, S., Shen, Q., Ji, H. & Syrjänen, K. (1990c) Detection of human papillomavirus (HPV) in genital warts and carcinomas by DNA in situ hybridization in Chinese patients. *Cytopathology*, **1**, 97–103

Chang, F., Syrjänen, S., Shen, Q., Wang, L., Wang, D. & Syrjänen, K. (1992) Human papillomavirus involvement in esophageal precancerous lesions and squamous cell carcinomas as evidenced by microscopy and different DNA techniques. *Scand. J. Gastroenterol.*, **27**, 553–563

Chang, F., Syrjänen, S., Shen, Q., Wang, L. & Syrjänen, K. (1993) Screening for human papillomavirus infections in esophageal squamous cell carcinomas by in situ hybridization. *Cancer*, **72**, 2525–2530

Chang, F., Syrjänen, S., Tervahauta, A., Kurvinen, K., Wang, L. & Syrjänen, K. (1994) Frequent mutaions of p53 gene in oesophageal squamous cell carcinomas with and without human papillomavirus (HPV) involvement suggests the dominant role of environmental carcinogens in oesophageal carcinogenesis. *Br. J. Cancer*, **70**, 346–351

Chellappan, S., Kraus, V.B., Kroger, B., Münger, K., Howley, P.M., Phelps, W.C. & Nevins, J.R. (1992) Adenovirus E1A, simian virus 40 tumor antigen, and human papillomavirus E7 protein share the capacity to disrupt the interaction between transcription factor E2F and the retinoblastoma gene product. *Proc. natl Acad. Sci. USA*, **89**, 4549–4553

Chen, L.P., Thomas, E.K., Hu, S.-L., Hellström, I. & Hellström, K.E. (1991) Human papillomavirus type 16 nucleoprotein E7 is a tumor rejection antigen. *Proc. natl Acad. Sci. USA*, **88**, 110–114

Chen, L.P., Mizuno, M.T., Singhal, M.C., Hu, S.-L., Galloway, D.A., Hellström, I. & Hellström, K.E. (1992a) Induction of cytotoxic T lymphocytes specific for a syngeneic tumor expressing the E6 oncoprotein of human papillomavirus type 16. *J. Immunol.*, **148**, 2617–2621

Chen, L., Ashe, S., Brady, W.A., Hellström, I., Hellström, K.E., Ledbetter, J.A., McGowan, P. & Linsley, P.S. (1992b) Costimulation of antitumor immunity by the B7 counterreceptor for the T lymphocyte molecules CD28 and CTLA-4. *Cell*, **71**, 1093–1102

Chen, S.-L., Han, C.P., Tsao, Y.P., Lee, J.W. & Yin, C.S. (1993a) Identification and typing of human papillomavirus in cervical cancers in Taiwan. *Cancer*, **72**, 1939–1945

Chen, L., Ashe, S., Singhal, M.C., Galloway, D.A., Hellström, I. & Hellström, K.E. (1993b) Metastatic conversion of cells by expression of human papillomavirus type 16 *E6* and *E7* genes. *Proc. natl Acad. Sci. USA*, **90**, 6523–6527

Chen, T.-M., Chen, C.-A., Hsieh, C.-Y., Chang, D.-Y., Chen, Y.-H. & Defendi, V. (1993c) The state of p53 in primary human cervical carcinomas and its effects in human papillomavirus-immortalized human cervical cells. *Oncogene*, **8**, 1511–1518

Chen, T.-M., Pecoraro, G. & Defendi, V. (1993d) Genetic analysis of in vitro progression of human papillomavirus-transfected human cervical cells. *Cancer Res.*, **53**, 1167–1171

Chen, C.-A., Chen, T.-M., Wu, C.-C., Chang, C.-F. & Hsieh, C.-Y. (1994a) Human papillomavirus DNA and p53 status in stage IB bulky cervical cancer. *J. Cancer Res. clin. Oncol.*, **120**, 678–682

Chen, M., Popescu, N., Woodworth, C., Berneman, Z., Corbellino, M., Lusso, P., Ablashi, D.V. & DiPaolo, J.A. (1994b) Human herpesvirus 6 infects cervical epithelial cells and transactivates human papillomavirus gene expression. *J. Virol.*, **68**, 1173–1178

Chetsanga, C., Malmstrom, P.U., Gyllensten, U., Moreno-Lopez, J., Dinter, Z. & Pettersson, U. (1992) Low incidence of human papillomavirus type 16 DNA in bladder tumor detected by the polymerase chain reaction. *Cancer*, **69**, 1208–1211

Chin, M.T., Broker, T.R. & Chow, L.T. (1989) Identification of a novel constitutive enhancer element and an associated binding protein: implications for human papillomavirus type 11 enhancer regulation. *J. Virol.*, **63**, 2967–2976

Chong, T., Chan, W.-K. & Bernard, H.-U. (1990) Transcriptional activation of human papillomavirus 16 by nuclear factor I, AP1, steroid receptors and a possibly novel transcription factor, PVF: a model for the composition of genital papillomavirus enhancers. *Nucleic Acids Res.*, **18**, 465–470

Chong, T., Apt, D., Gloss, B., Isa, M. & Bernard, H.-U. (1991) The enhancer of human papillomavirus type 16: binding sites for the ubiquitous transcription factors oct-1, NFA, TEF-2, NFl, and AP-1 participate in epithelial cell-specific transcription. *J. Virol.*, **65**, 5933–5943

Choo, K.-B. & Chong, K.Y. (1993) Absence of mutation in the p53 and retinoblastoma susceptibility genes in primary cervical carcinomas. *Virology*, **193**, 1042–1046

Choo, Y.C., Seto, W.H., Hsu, C., Merigan, T.C., Tan, Y.H., Ma, H.K. & Ng, N.H. (1986) Cervical intraepithelial neoplasia treated by perilesional injection of interferon. *Br. J. Obstet. Gynaecol.*, **93**, 372–379

Choo, K.-B., Shen, H.-D., Leung, W.-Y. & Lee, Y.-N. (1988) A distinct difference in the prevalence of papillomavirus infection in cytologically normal and neoplastic cells of the uterine cervix. *Chin. med. J. (Taipei)*, **42**, 1–6

Choo, K.-B., Chong, K.Y., Liew, L.-N., Hsu, H.-C. & Cheng, W.T. (1992) Unregulated and basal transcriptional activities of the regulatory sequence of the type 18 human papillomavirus genome in transgenic mice. *J. Virol.*, **188**, 378–383

Chow, L.T., Nasseri, M., Wolinsky, S.M. & Broker, T.R. (1987a) Human papillomavirus types 6 and 11 mRNAs from genital condylomata acuminata. *J. Virol.*, **61**, 2581–2588

Chow, L.T., Reilly, S.S., Broker, T.S. & Taichman, L.B. (1987b) Identification and mapping of human papillomavirus type 1 RNA transcripts recovered from plantar warts and infected epithelial cell cultures. *J. Virol.*, **61**, 1913–1918

Christensen, N.D. & Kreider, J.W. (1990) Antibody-mediated neutralization *in vivo* of infectious papillomaviruses. *J. Virol.*, **64**, 3151–3156

Christensen, N.D. & Kreider, J.W. (1991) Neutralization of CRPV infectivity by monoclonal antibodies that identify conformational epitopes on intact virions. *Virus Res.*, **21**, 169–179

Christensen, N.D. & Kreider, J.W. (1993) Monoclonal antibody neutralization of BPV-1. *Virus Res.*, **28**, 195–202

Christensen, P.-H., Jørgensen, K. & Grøntved, A. (1984) Juvenile papillomatosis of the larynx. A 45 years' follow up from the county of Funen, Denmark. *Acta otolaryngol. (Stockh.)*, **Suppl. 412**, 37–39

Christensen, N.D., Kreider, J.W., Cladel, N.M., Patrick, S.D. & Welsh, P.A. (1990) Monoclonal antibody-mediated neutralization of infectious human papillomavirus type 11. *J. Virol.*, **64**, 5678–5681

Christensen, N.D., Kreider, J.W., Kan, N.C. & DiAngelo, S.L. (1991) The open reading frame L2 of cottontail rabbit papillomavirus contains antibody-inducing neutralizing epitopes. *Virology*, **181**, 572–579

Christensen, N.D., Kreider, J.W., Shah, K.V. & Rando, R.F. (1992) Detection of human serum antibodies that neutralize infectious human papillomavirus type 11 virions. *J. gen. Virol.*, **73**, 1261–1267

Christensen, N.D., Höpfl, R., DiAngelo, S.L., Cladel, N.M., Patrick, S.D., Welsh, P.A., Budgeon, L.R., Reed, C.A. & Kreider, J.W. (1994a) Assembled baculovirus-expressed human papillomavirus type 11 L1 capsid protein virus-like particles are recognized by neutralizing monoclonal antibodies and induce high titres of neutralizing antibodies. *J. gen. Virol.*, **75**, 2271–2276

Christensen, N.D., Kirnbauer, R., Schiller, J.T., Ghim, S.-J., Schlegel, R., Jenson, A.B. & Kreider, J.W. (1994b) Human papillomavirus types 6 and 11 have antigenically distinct strongly immunogenic conformationally dependent neutralizing epitopes. *Virology*, **205**, 329–335

Christofori, G. & Hanaham, D. (1994) Molecular dissection of multi-stage tumorigenesis in transgenic mice. *Semin. Cancer Biol.*, **5**, 3–12

Chuang, T.-Y., Perry, H.O., Kurland, L.T. & Ilstrup, D.M. (1984) Condyloma acuminatum in Rochester, Minn, 1950–1978. I. Epidemiology and clinical features. *Arch. Dermatol.*, **120**, 469–475

Chung, G.T., Huang, D.P., Lo, K.W., Chan, M.K. & Wong, F.W. (1992) Genetic lesion in the carcinogenesis of cervical cancer. *Anticancer Res.*, **12**, 1485–1490

Ciccolini, F., Di Pasquale, G., Carlotti, F., Crawford, L. & Tommasino, M. (1994) Functional studies of E7 proteins from different HPV types. *Oncogene*, **9**, 2633–2638

Cid, A., Auewarakul, P., Garcia-Carranca, A., Ovseiovich, R., Gaissert, H. & Gissmann, L. (1993) Cell-type-specific activity of the human papillomavirus type 18 upstream regulatory region in transgenic mice and its modulation by tetradecanoyl phorbol acetate and glucocorticoids. *J. Virol.*, **67**, 6742–6752

Claas, E.C.J., Quint, W.G.V., Pieters, W.J.L.M., Burger, M.P.M., Oosterhuis, W.J. & Lindeman, J. (1992) Human papillomavirus and the three group metaphase figure as markers of an increased risk for the development of cervical carcinoma. *Am. J. Pathol.*, **140**, 497–502

Clertant, P. & Seif, I. (1984) A common function for polyoma virus large-T and papillomavirus E1 proteins? *Nature*, **311**, 276–279

Coker, A.L., Jenkins, G.R., Busnardo, M.S., Chambers, J.C., Levine, L.Z. & Pirisi, L. (1993) Human papillomaviruses and cervical neoplasia in South Carolina. *Cancer Epidemiol. Biomarkers Prev.*, **2**, 207–212

Cole, S.T. & Danos, O. (1987) Nucleotide sequence and comparative analysis of the human papillomavirus type 18 genome: phylogeny of papillomaviruses and repeated structure of the E6 and E7 gene products. *J. mol. Biol.*, **193**, 599–608

Coleman, N. & Stanley, M.A. (1994) Analysis of HLA-DR expression on keratinocytes in cervical neoplasia. *Int. J. Cancer*, **56**, 314–319

Coleman, M., Estève, J., Damiecki, P., Arslan, A. & Renard, H. (1993a) *Time Trends in Cancer Incidence and Mortality* (IARC Scientific Publications No.121), Lyon, IARC

Coleman, N., Greenfield, I.M., Hare, J., Kruger-Gray, H., Chain, B.M. & Stanley, M.A. (1993b) Characterization and functional analysis of the expression of intercellular adhesion molecule-1 in human papillomavirus-related disease of cervical keratinocytes. *Am. J. Pathol.*, **143**, 355–367

Colgan, T.J., Percy, M.E., Suri, M., Shier, R.M., Andrews, D.F. & Lickrish, G.M. (1989) Human papillomavirus infection of morphologically normal cervical epithelium adjacent to squamous dysplasia and invasive carcinoma. *Hum. Pathol.*, **20**, 316–319

Collins, J.E., Jenkins, D. & McCance, D.J. (1988) Detection of human papillomavirus DNA sequences by in situ DNA-DNA hybridisation in cervical intraepithelial neoplasia and invasive carcinoma: a retrospective study. *J. clin. Pathol.*, **41**, 289–295

Comerford, S.A., McCance, D.J., Dougan, G. & Tite, J.P. (1991) Identification of T- and B-cell epitopes of the E7 protein of human papillomavirus type 16. *J. Virol.*, **65**, 4681–4690

Comerford, S.A., Maika, S.D., Laimins, L.A., Messing, A., Elsässer, H.-P. & Hammer, R.E. (1995) E6 and E7 expression from the HPV 18 LCR: development of genital hyperplasia and neoplasia in transgenic mice. *Oncogene*, **10**, 587–597

Condylomata International Collaborative Study Group (1993a) Recurrent condylomata acuminata treated with recombinant interferon alpha-2a: a multicenter double-blind placebo-controlled clinical trial. *Acta derm. venereol. (Stockh.)*, **73**, 223–226

Condylomata International Collaborative Study Group (1993b) Randomized placebo-controlled double-blind combined therapy with laser surgery and systemic interferon-α2a in the treatment of anogenital condylomata acuminata. *J. infect. Dis.*, **167**, 824–829

Connor, M.E. & Stern, P.L. (1990) Loss of MHC class-I expression in cervical carcinomas. *Int. J. Cancer.*, **46**, 1029–1034

Connor, M.E., Davidson, S.E., Stern, P.L., Arrand, J.R. & West, C.M.L. (1993) Evaluation of multiple biological parameters in cervical carcinoma: high macrophage infiltration in HPV-associated tumors. *Int. J. Gynecol. Cancer*, **32**, 103–109

Conrad, M., Bubb, V.J. & Schlegel, R. (1993) The human papillomavirus type 6 and 16 E5 proteins are membrane-associated proteins which associate with the 16-kilodalton pore-forming protein. *J. Virol.*, **67**, 6170–6178

Conti, M., Agarossi, A., Parazzini, F., Muggiasca, M.L., Boschini, A., Negri, E. & Casolati, E. (1993) HPV, HIV infection, and risk of cervical intraepithelial neoplasia in former intravenous drug abusers. *Gynecol. Oncol.*, **49**, 344–348

Cook, L.S., Koutsky, L.A. & Holmes, K.K. (1993) Clinical presentation of genital warts among circumcised and uncircumcised heterosexual men attending an urban STD clinic. *Genitourin. Med.*, **69**, 262–264

Cooper, K., Herrington, C.S., Graham, A.K., Evans, M.F. & McGee, J.O'D. (1991a) In situ human papillomavirus (HPV) genotyping of cervical intraepithelial neoplasia in South African and British patients: evidence for putative HPV integration *in vivo*. *J. clin. Pathol.*, **44**, 400–405

Cooper, K., Herrington, C.S., Graham, A.K., Evans, M.F. & McGee, J. O'D. (1991b) In situ evidence for HPV 16, 18, 33 integration in cervical squamous cell cancer in Britain and South Africa. *J. clin. Pathol.*, **44**, 406–409

Cooper, K., Herrington, C.S., Lo, E.S.-F., Evans, M.F. & McGee, J.O'D. (1992) Integration of human papillomavirus types 16 and 18 in cervical adenocarcinoma. *J. clin. Pathol.*, **45**, 382–384

Cooper, K., Herrington, C.S., Evans, M.F., Gatter, K.C. & McGee, J.O'D. (1993) p53 antigen in cervical condylomata, intraepithelial neoplasia, and carcinoma: relationship to HPV infection and integration. *J. Pathol.*, **171**, 27–34

Coppleson, M. (1991) Colposcopic features of papillomaviral infection and premalignancy in the female lower genital tract. *Dermatol. Clin.*, **9**, 251–266

Corbitt, G., Zarod, A.P., Arrand, J.R., Longson, M. & Farrington, W.T. (1988) Human papillomavirus (HPV) genotypes associated with laryngeal papilloma. *J. clin Pathol.*, **41**, 284–288

Cordiner, J.W., Sharp, F. & Briggs, J.D. (1980) Cervical intraepithelial neoplasia in immunosuppressed women after renal transplantation. *Scott. med. J.*, **25**, 275–277

Cornelissen, M.T.E., Bots, T., Briët, M.A., Jebbink, M.F., Struyk, A.P.H.B., van den Tweel, J.G., Greer, C.E., Smits, H.L. & ter Schegget, J. (1992) Detection of human papillomavirus types by the polymerase chain reaction and the differentiation between high-risk and low-risk cervical lesions. *Virchows Arch. B.*, **62**, 167–171

Coté, T., Schiffman, M., Biggar, R., Goedert, J., Blattner, W. and the NACMR Study Group (1993) Invasive cervical cancer among women with AIDS: results of registry linkage (Meeting Abstract). *Proc. Ann. Meet. Am. Assoc. Cancer Res.*, **34**, A1546

Couturier, J., Sastre-Garau, X., Schneider-Maunoury, S., Labib, A. & Orth, G. (1991) Integration of papillomavirus DNA near *myc* genes in genital carcinomas and its consequences for proto-oncogene expression. *J. Virol.*, **65**, 4534–4538

Cox, J.T., Lörincz, A.T., Schiffman, M.H., Sherman, M.E., Cullen, A. & Kurman, R.J. (1995) Human papillomavirus testing by hybrid capture appears to be useful in triaging women with a cytologic diagnosis of atypical squamous cells of undetermined significance. *Am. J. Obstet. Gynecol.*, **172**, 946–954

Crawford, L.V. & Crawford, E.M. (1963) A comparative study of polyoma and papillomaviruses. *Virology*, **21**, 258–263

Cripe, T.P., Haugen, T.H., Turk, J.P., Tabatabai, F., Schmid, P.G., Dürst, M., Gissmann, L., Roman, A. & Turek, L.P. (1987) Transcriptional regulation of the human papillomavirus-16 E6-E7 promoter by a keratinocyte-dependent enhancer, and by viral E2 *trans*-activator and repressor gene products: implications for cervical carcinogenesis. *EMBO J.*, **6**, 3745–3753

Critchlow, C.W. & Koutsky, L.A. (1995) Epidemiology of human papillomavirus infection. In: Mindel, A., ed., *Genital Warts. Human Papillomavirus Infection*, London, Edward Arnold, pp. 53–81

Critchlow, C.W., Holmes, K.K., Wood, R., Krueger, L., Dunphy, C., Vernon, D.A., Daling, J.R. & Kiviat, N.B. (1992) Association of human immunodeficiency virus and anal human papillomavirus infection among homosexual men. *Arch. intern. Med.*, **152**, 1673–1676

Croissant, O., Breitburd, F. & Orth, G. (1985) Specificity of cytopathic effect of cutaneous human papillomaviruses. *Clin. Dermatol.*, **3**, 43–55

Cromme, F.V., Meijer, C.J., Snijders, P.J.F., Uyterlinde, A., Kenemans, P., Helmerhorst, T., Stern, P.L., van den Brule, A.J.F. & Walboomers, J.M.M. (1993a) Analysis of MHC class I and II expression in relation to presence of HPV genotypes in premalignant and malignant cervical lesions. *Br. J. Cancer*, **67**, 1372–1380

Cromme, F.V., Snijders, P.J., van den Brule, A.J.C., Kenemans, P., Meijer, C.J.L.M. & Walboomers, J.M.M. (1993b) MHC class I expression in HPV 16 positive cervical carcinomas is post-transcriptionally controlled and independent from c-*myc* overexpression. *Oncogene*, **8**, 2969–2975

Cromme, F.V., Airey, J., Heemels, M.-T., Ploegh, H.L., Keating, P.J., Stern, P.L., Meijer, C.J.L.M. & Walboomers, J.M.M. (1994) Loss of transporter protein, encoded by the TAP-1 gene, is highly correlated with loss of HLA expression in cervical carcinomas. *J. exp. Med.*, **179**, 335–340

Crook, T. & Vousden, K.H. (1992) Properties of p53 mutations detected in primary and secondary cervical cancers suggest mechanisms of metastasis and involvement of environmental carcinogens. *EMBO J.*, **11**, 3935–3940

Crook, T., Storey, A., Almond, N., Osborn, K. & Crawford, L. (1988) Human papillomavirus type 16 cooperates with activated *ras* and *fos* oncogenes in the hormone-dependent transformation of primary mouse cells. *Proc. natl Acad. Sci. USA*, **85**, 8820–8824

Crook, T., Morgenstern, J.P., Crawford, L. & Banks, L. (1989) Continued expression of HPV-16 E7 protein is required for maintenance of the transformed phenotype of cells co-transformed by HPV-16 plus EJ-*ras*. *EMBO J.*, **8**, 513–519

Crook, T., Greenfield, I., Howard, J. & Stanley, M. (1990) Alterations in growth properties of human papilloma virus type 16 immortalised human cervical keratinocyte cell line correlate with amplification and overexpression of c-*myc* oncogene. *Oncogene*, **5**, 619–622

Crook, T., Wrede, D., Tidy, J., Scholefield, J., Crawford, L. & Vousden, K.H. (1991a) Status of c-*myc*, *p53* and retinoblastoma genes in human papillomavirus positive and negative squamous cell carcinomas of the anus. *Oncogene*, **6**, 1251–1257

Crook, T., Tidy, J.A. & Vousden, K.H. (1991b) Degradation of p53 can be targeted by HPV E6 sequences distinct from those required for p53 binding and trans-activation. *Cell,* **67**, 547–556

Crook, T., Fisher, C. & Vousden, K.H. (1991c) Modulation of immortalizing properties of human papillomavirus type 16 E7 by p53 expression. *J. Virol.,* **65**, 505–510

Crook, T., Wrede, D. & Vousden, K.H. (1991d) p53 Point mutation in HPV negative human cervical carcinoma cell lines. *Oncogene,* **6**, 873–875

Crook, T., Wrede, D., Tidy, J.A., Mason, W.P., Evans, D.J. & Vousden, K.H. (1992) Clonal p53 mutation in primary cervical cancer: association with human-papillomavirus-negative tumours. *Lancet,* **339**, 1070–1073

Crook, T., Marston, N.J., Sara, E.A. & Vousden, K.H. (1994) Transcriptional activation by p53 correlates with suppression of growth but not transformation. *Cell,* **79**, 817–827

Cruickshank, M.E., Flannelly, G., Campbell, D.M. & Kitchener, H.C. (1995) Fertility and pregnancy outcome following large loop excision of the cervical transformation zone. *Br. J. Obstet. Gynaecol.,* **102**, 467–470

Crum, C.P. & Levine, R.U. (1984) Human papillomavirus infection and cervical neoplasia: new perspectives. *Int. J. gynecol. Pathol.,* **3**, 376–388

Crum, C.P., Barber, S. & Roche, J.K. (1991) Pathobiology of papillomavirus-related cervical diseases: prospects for immunodiagnosis. *Clin. Microbiol. Rev.,* **4**, 270–285

Cubie, H.A., Norval, M., Crawford, L., Banks, L. & Crook, T. (1989) Lymphoproliferative response to fusion proteins of human papillomaviruses in patients with cervical intraepithelial neoplasia. *Epidemiol. Infect.,* **103**, 625–632

Cullen, A.P., Reid, R., Campion, M. & Lörincz, A.T. (1991) Analysis of the physical state of different human papillomavirus DNAs in intraepithelial and invasive cervical neoplasm. *J. Virol.,* **65**, 606–612

Cullen, T.S. (1900) *Cancer of the Uterus*, New York, Appleton & Co.

Cuthill, S., Sibbet, G.J. & Campo, M.S. (1993) Characterization of a nuclear factor, papilloma enhancer binding factor-1, that binds the long control region of human papillomavirus type 16 and contributes to enhancer activity. *Mol. Carcinog.,* **8**, 96–104

Cuzick, J. (1995) Human papillomavirus infection of the prostate. *Cancer Surv.,* **23**, 91–95

Cuzick, J. & Boyle, P. (1988) Trends in cervix cancer mortality. *Cancer Surv.,* **7**, 417–439

Cuzick, J., Singer, A., De Stavola, B.L. & Chomet, J. (1990) Case–control study of risk factors for cervical intraepithelial neoplasia in young women. *Eur. J. Cancer,* **26**, 684–690

Cuzick, J., Terry, G., Ho, L., Hollingworth, T. & Anderson, M. (1994) Type-specific human papillomavirus DNA in abnormal smears as a predictor of high-grade cervical intraepithelial neoplasia. *Br. J. Cancer,* **69**, 167–171

Cuzick, J., Szarewski, A., Terry, G., Ho, L., Hanby, A., Maddox, P., Anderson, M., Kocjan, G., Steele, S.J. & Guillebaud, J. (1995) HPV testing in primary cervical screening. *Lancet* (in press)

Czeglédy, J., Gergely, L., Hernádi, Z. & Póka, R. (1989) Detection of human papillomavirus deoxyribonucleic acid in the female genital tract. *Med. Microbiol. Immunol. (Berl.),* **178**, 309–314

Czeglédy, J., Rogo, K.O., Evander, M. & Wadell, G. (1992a) High-risk human papillomavirus types in cytologically normal cervical scrapes from Kenya. *Med. Microbiol. Immunol. (Berl.),* **180**, 321–326

Czeglédy, J., Póka, R., Veress, G. & Gergely, L. (1992b) Amplification of human papillomavirus type 16 transforming genes from cervical cancer biopsies and lymph nodes of Hungarian patients. *J. clin. Microbiol.,* **30**, 233–236

Czerwenka, K.F. & Schön, H.J. (1989) The importance of papillomavirus infections in cervical cancer and their preneoplastic stage including different associated genital lesions. *Gynäkol. Rundsch.*, **29** (Suppl. 3), 44–53 (in German)

Daling, J.R. & Sherman, K.J. (1992) Relationship between human papillomavirus infection and tumours of anogenital sites other than the cervix. In: Muñoz, N., Bosch, F.X., Shah, K.V. & Meheus, A., eds, *The Epidemiology of Cervical Cancer and Human Papillomavirus* (IARC Scientific Publications No. 119), Lyon, IARC, pp. 223–241

Daling, J.R., Weiss, N.S., Hislop, T.G., Maden, C., Coates, R.J., Sherman, K.J., Ashley, R.L., Beagrie, M., Ryan, J.A. & Corey, L. (1987) Sexual practices, sexually transmitted diseases, and the incidence of anal cancer. *N. Engl. J. Med.*, **317**, 973–977

Das, B.C., Sharma, J.K., Gopalkrishna, V., Das, D.K., Singh, V., Gissmann, L., zur Hausen, H. & Luthra, U.K. (1992a) A high frequency of human papillomavirus DNA sequences in cervical carcinomas of Indian women as revealed by Southern blot hybridization and polymerase chain reaction. *J. med. Virol.*, **36**, 239–245

Das, B.C., Sharma, J.K., Gopalakrishna, V. & Luthra, U.K. (1992b) Analysis by polymerase chain reaction of the physical state of human papillomavirus type 16 DNA in cervical preneoplastic and neoplastic lesions. *J. gen. Virol.*, **73**, 2327–2336

David, M., Sohl, S., Krause, H., Farkic, M. & Neuhaus, R. (1993) Changes in cervix cytology in women with liver transplants treated with immunosuppressive therapy. *Zentralbl. Gynakol.*, **115**, 362–365 (in German)

Davidson, M., Schnitzer, P.G., Bulkow, L.R., Parkinson, A.J., Schloss, M.L., Fitzgerald, M.A., Knight, J.A., Murphy, C.M., Kiviat, N.B., Toomey, K.E., Reeves, W.C., Schmid, D.S. & Stamm, W.E. (1994) The prevalence of cervical infection with human papillomaviruses and cervical dysplasia in Alaska native women. *J. infect. Dis.*, **169**, 792–800

Davies, D.H., Hill, C.M., Rothbard, J.B. & Chain, B.M. (1990) Definition of murine T helper cell determinants in the major capsid protein of human papillomavirus type 16. *J. gen. Virol.*, **71**, 2691–2698

Davies, R., Hicks, R., Crook, T., Morris, J. & Vousden, K. (1993) Human papillomavirus type 16 E7 associates with a histone H1 kinase and with p107 through sequences necessary for transformation. *J. Virol.*, **67**, 2521–2528

Deau, M.-C., Favre, M. & Orth, G. (1991) Genetic heterogeneity among human papillomaviruses (HPV) associated with epidermodysplasia verruciformis: evidence for multiple allelic forms of HPV 5 and HPV 8 E6 genes. *Virology*, **184**, 492–503

Deau, M.-C., Favre, M., Jablonska, S., Rueda, L.-A. & Orth, G. (1993) Genetic heterogeneity of oncogenic human papillomavirus type 5 (HPV 5) and phylogeny of HPV 5 variants associated with epidermodysplasia verruciformis. *J. clin. Microbiol.*, **31**, 2918–2926

DeCaprio, J.A., Ludlow, J.W., Figge, J., Shew, J.-Y., Huang, C.-M., Lee, W.-H., Marsilio, E., Paucha, E. & Livingston, D.M. (1988) SV40 large tumor antigen forms a specific complex with the product of the retinoblastoma susceptibility gene. *Cell*, **54**, 275–283

Defeo-Jones, D., Vuocolo, G.A., Haskell, K.M., Hanobik, M.G., Kiefer, D.M., McAvoy, E.M., Ivey-Hoyle, M., Brandsma, J.L., Oliff, A. & Jones, R.E. (1993) Papillomavirus E7 protein binding to the retinoblastoma protein is not required for viral induction of warts. *J. Virol.*, **67**, 716–725

Delius, H. & Hofmann, B. (1994) Primer-directed sequencing of human papillomavirus types. *Curr. Top. Microbiol. Immunol.*, **186**, 13–31

Della Torre, G., Pilotti, S., de Palo, G. & Rilke, F. (1978) Viral particles in cervical condylomatous lesions. *Tumori*, **64**, 549–553

Del Mistro, A., Braunstein, J.D., Halwer, M. & Koss, L.G. (1987) Identification of human papillomavirus types in male urethral condylomata acuminata by in situ hybridization. *Hum. Pathol.*, **18**, 936–940

Delvenne, P., Fontaine, M.-A., Delvenne, C., Nikkels, A. & Boniver, J. (1994) Detection of human papillomaviruses in paraffin-embedded biopsies of cervical intraepithelial lesions: analysis by immunohistochemistry, in situ hybridization, and the polymerase chain reaction. *Mod. Pathol.*, **7**, 113–119

Demeter, T., Kulski, J.K., Sterrett, G.F. & Pixley, E.C. (1987) Detection of DNA of human papillomavirus types 6/11 and 16/18 in cell scrapings of the uterine cervix by filter in situ hybridisation: correlation with cytology, colposcopy and histology. *Eur. J. Epidemiol.*, **3**, 404–413

Demeter, L.M., Stoler, M.H., Bonnez, W., Corey, L., Pappas, P., Strussenberg, J. & Reichman, R.C. (1993) Penile intraepithelial neoplasia: clinical presentation and an analysis of the physical state of human papillomavirus DNA. *J. infect. Dis.*, **168**, 38–46

Demetrick, D.J., Inoue, M., Lester, W.M., Kingma, I., Duggan, M.A. & Paul, L.C. (1990) Human papillomavirus type 16 associated with oral squamous carcinoma in a cardiac transplant recipient. *Cancer*, **66**, 1726–1731

Desaintes, C., Hallez, S., Van Alphen, P. & Burny, A. (1992) Transcriptional activation of several heterologous promoters by the E6 protein of human papillomavirus type 16. *J. Virol.*, **66**, 325–333

Devictor, B., Bonnier, P., Piana, L., Andrac, L., Lavaut, M.-N., Allasia, C. & Charpin, C. (1993) c-*myc* Protein and Ki-67 antigen immunodetection in patients with uterine cervix neoplasia: correlation of microcytophotometric analysis and histological data. *Gynecol. Oncol.*, **49**, 284–290

Dhanwada, K.R., Garrett, L.R., Smith, P., Thompson, K.D., Doster, A. & Jones, C. (1993) Characterization of human keratinocytes transformed by high risk human papillomavirus types 16 or 18 and herpes simplex virus type. *J. gen. Virol.*, **74**, 955–963

Dickens, P., Srivastava, G. & Liu, Y.T. (1992) Human papillomavirus 16/18 and nasopharyngeal carcinoma. *J. clin. Pathol.*, **45**, 81–82

Dillner, J. (1990) Mapping of linear epitopes of human papillomavirus type 16: the E1, E2, E4, E5, E6 and E7 open reading frames. *Int. J. Cancer*, **46**, 703–711

Dillner, J. (1994) Antibody responses to defined HPV epitopes in cervical neoplasia. *Papillomavirus Rep.*, **5**, 35–41

Dillner, J., Dillner, L., Robb, J., Willems, J., Jones, I., Lancaster, W., Smith, R. & Lerner, R. (1989a) A synthetic peptide defines a serologic IgA response to a human papillomavirus-encoded nuclear antigen expressed in virus-carrying cervical neoplasia. *Proc. natl Acad. Sci. USA*, **86**, 3838–3841

Dillner, L., Bekassy, Z., Jonsson, N., Moreno-Lopez, J. & Blomberg, J. (1989b) Detection of IgA antibodies against human papillomavirus in cervical secretions from patients with cervical intraepithelial neoplasia. *Int. J. Cancer*, **43**, 36–40

Dillner, J., Dillner, L., Utter, G., Eklund, C., Rotola, A., Costa, S. & DiLuca, D. (1990a) Mapping of linear epitopes of human papillomavirus type 16: the L1 and L2 open reading frames. *Int. J. Cancer*, **45**, 529–535

Dillner, L., Moreno-Lopez, J. & Dillner, J. (1990b) Serological responses to papillomavirus group-specific antigens in women with neoplasia of the cervix uteri. *J. clin. Microbiol.*, **28**, 624–627

Dillner, L., Heino, P., Moreno-Lopez, J. & Dillner, J. (1991) Antigenic and immunogenic epitopes shared by human papillomavirus type 16 and bovine, canine, and avian papillomaviruses. *J. Virol.*, **65**, 6862–6871

Dillner, L., Fredriksson, A., Persson, E., Forslund, O., Hansson, B.-G. & Dillner, J. (1993) Antibodies against papillomavirus antigens in cervical secretions from condyloma patients. *J. clin. Microbiol.*, **31**, 192–197

Dillner, J., Lenner, P., Lehtinen, M., Eklund, C., Heino, P., Wiklund, F., Hallmans, G. & Stendahl, U. (1994) A population-based seroepidemiological study of cervical cancer. *Cancer Res.*, **54**, 134–141

Dillner, J., Wiklund, F., Lenner, P., Eklund, C., Frederiksson Shanazarian, V., Schiller, J.T., Hibma, M., Hallmans, G. & Stendahl, U. (1995) Antibodies against linear and conformational epitopes of human papillomavirus type 16 that independently associate with incident cervical cancer. *Int. J. Cancer*, **60**, 377–382

Di Lonardo, A., Venuti, A. & Marcante, M.L. (1992) Human papillomavirus in breast cancer. *Breast Cancer Res. Treat.*, **21**, 95–100

DiLorenzo, T.P., Tamsen, A., Abramson, A.L. & Steinberg, B.M. (1992) Human papillomavirus type 6a DNA in the lung carcinoma of a patient with recurrent laryngeal papillomatosis is characterized by a partial duplication. *J. gen. Virol.*, **73**, 423–428

Di Luca, D., Pilotti, S., Stefanon, B., Rotola, A., Monini, P., Tognon, M., De Palo, G., Rilke, F. & Cassai, E. (1986) Human papillomavirus type 16 DNA in genital tumours: a pathological and molecular analysis. *J. gen. Virol.*, **67**, 583–589

DiPaolo, J.A., Woodworth, C.D., Popescu, N.C., Notario, V. & Doniger, J. (1989) Induction of human cervical squamous cell carcinoma by sequential transfection with human papillomavirus 16 DNA and viral Harvey *ras*. *Oncogene*, **4**, 395–399

DiPaolo, J.A., Woodworth, C.D., Popescu, N.C., Koval, D.L., Lopez, J.V. & Doniger, J. (1990) HSV-2-induced tumorigenicity in HPV16-immortalized human genital keratinocytes. *Virology*, **177**, 777–779

Dong, X.-P., Stubenrauch, F., Beyer-Finkler, E. & Pfister, H. (1994) Prevalence of deletions of YY1-binding sites in episomal HPV 16 DNA from cervical cancers. *Int. J. Cancer*, **58**, 803–808

Donnan, S.P.B., Wong, F.W.S., Ho, S.C., Lau, E.M., Takashi, K. & Estève, J. (1989) Reproductive and sexual risk factors and human papilloma virus infection in cervical cancer among Hong Kong Chinese. *Int. J. Epidemiol.*, **18**, 32–36

Doorbar, J. (1991) An emerging function for E4. *Papillomavirus Rep.*, **2**, 145–147

Doorbar, J. & Gallimore, P.H. (1987) Identification of proteins encoded by the L1 and L2 open reading frames of human papillomavirus 1a. *J. Virol.*, **61**, 2793–2799

Doorbar, J., Ely, S., Sterling, J., McLean, C. & Crawford, L. (1991) Specific interaction between HPV-16 E1-E4 and cytokeratins results in collapse of the epithelial cell intermediate filament network. *Nature*, **352**, 824–827

van Doornum, G.J., Hooykaas, C., Juffermans, L.H.J., van der Lans, S.M.G.A., van der Linden, M.M.D., Coutinho, R.A. & Quint, W.G. (1992) Prevalence of human papillomavirus infections among heterosexual men and women with multiple sexual partners. *J. med. Virol.*, **37**, 13–21

Dorsey, J.H. & Diggs, E.S. (1979) Microsurgical conization of the cervix by carbon dioxide laser. *Obstet. Gynecol.*, **54**, 565–570

Dostatni, N., Lambert, P.F., Sousa, R., Ham, J., Howley, P.M. & Yaniv, M. (1991) The functional BPV-1 E2 *trans*-activating protein can act as a repressor by preventing formation of the initiation complex. *Genes Dev.*, **5**, 1657–1671

Downey, G.P., Bavin, P.J., Deery, A.R.S., Crow, J., Griffiths, P.D., Emery, V.C. & Walker, P.G. (1994) Relation between human papillomavirus type 16 and potential for progression of minor-grade cervical disease. *Lancet*, **344**, 432–435

Doyle, D.J., Henderson, L.A., LeJeune, F.E., Jr & Miller, R.H. (1994) Changes in human papillomavirus typing of recurrent respiratory papillomatosis progressing to malignant neoplasm. *Arch. Otolaryngol. Head Neck Surg.*, **120**, 1273–1276

Drews, R.E., Chan, V.T.-W. & Schnipper, L.E. (1992) Oncogenes result in genomic alterations that activate a transcriptionally silent dominantly selectable reporter gene (neo). *Mol. cell. Biol.*, **12**, 198–206

Duff, R. & Rapp, F. (1971) Oncogenic transformation of hamster cells after exposure to herpes simplex virus type 2. *Nature New Biol.*, **233**, 48–50

Duggan, M.A., Inoue, M., McGregor, S.E., Gabos, S., Nation, J.G., Robertson, D.I. & Stuart, G.C.E. (1990) Nonisotopic human papillomavirus DNA typing of cervical smears obtained at the initial colposcopic examination. *Cancer*, **66**, 745–751

Duggan, M.A., Boras, V.F., Inoue, M. & McGregor, S.E. (1991) Human papillomavirus DNA in anal carcinomas. Comparison of in situ and dot blot hybridization. *Am. J. clin. Pathol.*, **96**, 318–325

Duggan, M.A., Benoit, J.L., McGregor, S.E., Nation, J.G., Inoue, M. & Stuart, G.C.E. (1993) The human papillomavirus status of 114 endocervical adenocarcinoma cases by dot blot hybridization. *Hum. Pathol.*, **24**, 121–125

Duncan, E.L., Whitaker, N.J., Moy, E.L. & Reddel, R.R. (1993) Assignment of SV40-immortalized cells to more than one complementation group for immortalization. *Exp. Cell Res.*, **205**, 337–344

Dürst, M., Gissmann, L., Ikenberg, H. & zur Hausen, H. (1983) A papillomavirus DNA from a cervical carcinoma and its prevalence in cancer biopsy samples from different geographic regions. *Proc. natl Acad. Sci. USA*, **80**, 3812–3815

Dürst, M., Dzarlieva-Petrusevska, R.T., Boukamp, P., Fusenig, N.E. & Gissmann, L. (1987a) Molecular and cytogenetic analysis of immortalized human primary keratinocytes obtained after transfection with human papillomavirus type 16 DNA. *Oncogene*, **1**, 251–256

Dürst, M., Croce, C.M., Gissmann, L., Schwarz, E. & Huebner, K. (1987b) Papillomavirus sequences integrate near cellular oncogenes in some cervical carcinomas. *Proc. natl Acad. Sci. USA*, **84**, 1070–1074

Dürst, M., Gallahan, D., Jay, G. & Rhim, J.S. (1989) Glucorticoid-enhanced neoplastic transformation of human keratinocytes by human papillomavirus type 16 and an activated *ras* oncogene. *Virology*, **173**, 767–771

Dürst, M., Bosch, F.X., Glitz, D., Schneider, A. & zur Hausen, H. (1991) Inverse relationship between human papillomvirus (HPV) type 16 early gene expression and cell differentiation in nude mouse epithelial cysts and tumors induced by HPV-positive human cell lines. *J. Virol.*, **65**, 796–804

Dürst, M., Glitz, D., Schneider, A. & zur Hausen, H. (1992) Human papillomavirus 16 (HPV 16) gene expression and DNA replication in cervical neoplasia: analysis by in situ hybridization. *Virology*, **189**, 132–140

Dürst, M., Winkenbach, S., Wanschura, S., zur Hausen, H. & Bullerdiek, J. (1995) Malignant progression of an HPV 16-immortalized human keratinocyte cell line (HPK IA) *in vitro*. *Cancer Genet. Cytogenet.* (in press)

Dyall-Smith, D., Trowell, H., Mark, A. & Dyall-Smith, M. (1991) Cutaneous squamous cell carcinomas and papillomaviruses in renal transplant recipients: a clinical and molecular biological study. *J. dermatol. Sci.*, **2**, 139–146

Dyson, N., Howley, P.M., Münger, K. & Harlow, E. (1989) The human papilloma virus-16 E7 oncoprotein is able to bind to the retinoblastoma gene product. *Science*, **243**, 934–937

Dyson, N., Guida, P., Münger, K. & Harlow, E. (1992) Homologous sequences in adenovirus E1A and human papillomavirus E7 proteins mediate interaction with the same set of cellular proteins. *J. Virol.*, **66**, 6893–6902

Edmonds, C. & Vousden, K.H. (1989) A point mutational analysis of human papillomavirus type 16 E7 protein. *J. Virol.*, **63**, 2650–2656

Effert, P.J., Frye, R.A., Neubauer, A., Liu, E.T. & Walther, P.J. (1992) Human papillomavirus types 16 and 18 are not involved in human prostate carcinogenesis: analysis of archival human prostate cancer specimens by differential polymerase chain reaction. *J. Urol.*, **147**, 192–196

Egawa, K., Inaba, Y., Yoshimura, K. & Ono, T. (1993a) Varied clinical morphology of HPV-1-induced warts, depending on anatomical factors. *Br. J. Dermatol.*, **128**, 271–276

Egawa, K., Shibasaki, Y. & de Villiers, E.-M. (1993b) Double infection with human papillomavirus 1 and human papillomavirus 63 in single cells of a lesion displaying only an human papillomavirus 63-induced cytopathogenic effect. *Lab. Invest.*, **69**, 583–588

Egawa, K., Honda, Y., Inaba, Y., Kojo, Y., Ono, T. & de Villiers, E.-M. (1994) Multiple plantar epidermoid cysts harboring carcinoembryonic antigen and human papillomavirus DNA sequences. *J. Am. Acad. Dermatol.*, **30**, 494–496

Egberink, H.F., Berrocal, A., Bax, H.A.D., van den Ingh, T.S.G.A.M., Walter, J.H. & Horzinek, M.C. (1992) Papillomavirus associated skin lesions in a cat seropositive for feline immunodeficiency virus. *Vet. Microbiol.*, **31**, 117–125

El-Deiry, W.S., Kern, S.E., Pietenpol, J.A., Kinzler, K.W. & Vogelstein, B. (1992) Definition of a consensus binding site for p53. *Nat. Genet.*, **1**, 45–49

El-Deiry, W.S., Tokino, T., Velculescu, V.E., Levy, D.B., Parsons, R., Trent, J.M., Lin, D., Mercer, W.E., Kinzler, K.W. & Vogelstein, B. (1993) WAF1, a potential mediator of p53 tumor suppression. *Cell*, **75**, 817–825

Eliezri, Y.D., Silverstein, S.J. & Nuovo, G.J. (1990) Occurrence of human papillomavirus type 16 DNA in cutaneous squamous and basal cell neoplasms. *J. Am. Acad. Dermatol.*, **23**, 836–842

Ellis, J.R.M., Keating, P.J., Baird, J., Hounsell, E.F., Renouf, D.V., Rowe, M., Hopkins, D., Duggan-Keen, M.F., Bartholomew, J.S., Young, L.S. & Stern, P.L. (1995) The association of an HPV 16 oncogene variant with HLA-B7 has implications for vaccine design in cervical cancer. *Nat. Med.*, **1**, 464–470

Eluf-Neto, J., Booth, M., Muñoz, N., Bosch, F.X., Meijer, C.J.L.M. & Walboomers, J.M.M. (1994) Human papillomavirus and invasive cervical cancer in Brazil. *Br. J. Cancer*, **69**, 114–119

Engels, H., Nyongo, A., Temmerman, M., Quint, W.G.V., Van Marck, E. & Eylenbosch, W.J. (1992) Cervical cancer screening and detection of genital HPV-infection and chlamydial infection by PCR in different groups of Kenyan women. *Ann. Soc. belg. Méd. trop.*, **72**, 53–62

Eriksson, A., Stewart, A.C., Moreno-Lopez, J. & Pettersson, U. (1994) The genomes of the animal papillomaviruses European elk papillomavirus, deer papillomavirus, and reindeer papillomavirus contain a novel transforming gene (E9) near the early polyadenylation site. *J. Virol.*, **68**, 8365–8373

Eron, L.J., Judson, F., Tucker, S., Prawer, S., Mills, J., Murphy, K., Hickey, M., Rogers, M., Flannigan, S., Hien, N., Katz, H.I., Goldman, S., Gottlieb, A., Adams, K., Burton, P., Tanner, D., Taylor, E. & Peets, E. (1986) Interferon therapy for condylomata acuminata. *N. Engl. J. Med.*, **315**, 1059–1064

Eron, L.J., Alder, M.B., O'Rourke, J.M., Rittweger, K., DePamphilis, J. & Pizzuti, D.J. (1993) Recurrence of condylomata acuminata following cryotherapy is not prevented by systemically administered interferon. *Genitourin. Med.*, **69**, 91–93

Eschle, D., Dürst, M., ter Meulen, J., Luande, J., Eberhardt, H.C., Pawlita, M. & Gissmann, L. (1992) Geographical dependence of sequence variation in the E7 gene of human papillomavirus type 16. *J. gen. Virol.*, **73**, 1829–1832

Etscheid, B.G., Foster, S.A. & Galloway, D.A. (1994) The E6 protein of human papillomavirus type 16 functions as a transcriptional repressor in a mechanism independent of the tumor suppressor protein, p53. *Virology*, **205**, 583–585

Euvrard, S., Chardonnet, Y., Dureau, G., Hermier, C. & Thivolet, J. (1991) Human papillomavirus type 1-associated squamous cell carcinoma in a heart transplant recipient. *Arch. Dermatol.*, **127**, 559–564

Euvrard, S., Chardonnet, Y., Pouteil-Noble, C., Kanitakis, J., Chignol, M.C., Thivolet, J. & Touraine, J.L. (1993) Association of skin malignancies with various and multiple carcinogenic and noncarcinogenic human papillomaviruses in renal transplant recipients. *Cancer*, **72**, 2198–2206

Evander, M., Edlund, K., Gustafsson, Å., Jonsson, M., Karlsson, X., Rylander, E. & Wadell, G. (1995) Human papillomavirus infection is transient in young women: a population-based cohort study. *J. infect. Dis.*, **171**, 1026–1030

Evans, A.S. & Monaghan, J.M. (1985) Spontaneous resolution of cervical warty atypia: the relevance of clinical and nuclear DNA features: a prospective study. *Br. J. Obstet. Gynaecol.*, **92**, 165–169

Evans, I.A., Prorok, J.H., Cole, R.C., Al-Salmani, M.H., Al-Samarrai, A.M.H., Patel, M.C. & Smith, R.M.M. (1982a) The carcinogenic, mutagenic and teratogenic toxicity of bracken. *Proc. R. Soc. Edinburgh*, **81B**, 65–77

Evans, W.C., Patel, M.C. & Koohy, Y. (1982b) Acute bracken poisoning in homogastric and ruminant animals. *Proc. R. Soc. Edinburgh*, **81B**, 29–64

Evans, B.A., Bond, R.A. & MacRae, K.D. (1992) A colposcopic case–control study of cervical squamous intraepithelial lesions in women with anogenital warts. *Genitourin. Med.*, **68**, 300–304

Eversole, L.R., Laipis, P.J. & Green, T.L. (1987a) Human papillomavirus type 2 DNA in oral and labial verruca vulgaris. *J. cutan. Pathol.*, **14**, 319–325

Eversole, L.R., Laipis, P.J., Merrell, P. & Choi, E. (1987b) Demonstration of human papillomavirus DNA in oral condyloma acuminatum. *J. oral Pathol.*, **16**, 266–272

Fairley, C.K., Chen, S., Tabrizi, S.N., Leeton, K., Quinn, M.A. & Garland, S.M. (1992) The absence of genital human papillomavirus DNA in virginal women. *Int. J. STD AIDS*, **3**, 414–417

Fairley, C.K., Chen, S., Tabrizi, S.N., McNeil, J., Becker, G., Walker, R., Atkins, R.C., Thomson, N., Allan, P., Woodburn, C. & Garland, S.M. (1994a) Prevalence of HPV DNA in cervical specimens in women with renal transplants: a comparison with dialysis-dependent patients and patients with renal impairment. *Nephrol. Dial. Transplant.*, **9**, 416–420

Fairley, C.K., Sheil, A.G.R., McNeil, J.-J., Ugoni, A.M., Disney, A.P.S., Giles, G.G. & Amiss, N. (1994b) The risk of ano-genital malignancies in dialysis and transplant patients. *Clin. Nephrol.*, **41**, 101–105

Fais, S., Delle Fratte, F., Mancini, F., Cioni, V., Guadagno, M., Vetrano, G. & Pallone, F. (1991) Human cervical epithelial cells that express HLA-DR associated with viral infection and activated mononuclear cell infiltrate. *J. clin. Pathol.*, **44**, 290–292

Falcinelli, C., Luzi, P., Alberti, P., Cosmi, E.V. & Anceschi, M.M. (1993) Human papilloma virus infection and Ki-*ras* oncogene in paraffin-embedded squamous carcinomas of the cervix. *Gynecol. obstet. Invest.*, **36**, 185–188

Fanjul, A., Dawson, M.I., Hobbs, P.D., Jong, L., Cameron, J.F., Harlev, E., Graupner, G., Lu, X.-P. & Pfahl, M. (1994) A new class of retinoids with selective inhibition of AP-1 inhibits proliferation. *Nature*, **372**, 107–111

Farnsworth, A., Laverty, C. & Stoler, M.H. (1989) Human papillomavirus messenger RNA expression in adenocarcinoma *in situ* of the uterine cervix. *Int. J. gynecol. Pathol.*, **8**, 321–330

Farthing, A.J. & Vousden, K.H. (1994) Functions of human papillomavirus E6 and E7 oncoproteins. *Trends Microbiol.*, **2**, 170–174

Favre, M., Breitburd, F., Croissant, O. & Orth, G. (1975) Structural polypeptides of rabbit, bovine, and human papillomaviruses. *J. Virol.*, **15**, 1239–1247

Favre, M., Obalek, S., Jablonska, S. & Orth, G. (1989) Human papillomavirus type 49, a type isolated from flat warts of renal transplant patients. *J. Virol.*, **63**, 4909

Feingold, A.R., Vermund, S.H., Burk, R.D., Kelley, K.F., Schrager, L.K., Schreiber, K., Munk, G., Friedland, G.H. & Klein, R.S. (1990) Cervical cytologic abnormalities and papillomavirus in women infected with human immunodeficiency virus. *J. acquir. Immune Defic. Syndr.*, **3**, 896–903

Felix, J.C., Cote, R.J., Kramer, E.E.W., Saigo, P. & Goldman, G.H. (1993) Carcinomas of Bartholin's gland: histogenesis and the etiological role of human papillomavirus. *Am. J. Pathol.*, **142**, 925–933

Feltkamp, M.C., Smits, H.L., Vierboom, M.P.M., Minnaar, R.P., de Jongh, B.M., Drijfhout, J.W., ter Schegget, J., Melief, C.J.M. & Kast, W.M. (1993) Vaccination with cytotoxic T lymphocyte epitope-containing peptide protects against a tumor induced by human papillomavirus type 16-transformed cells. *Eur. J. Immunol.*, **23**, 2242–2249

Ferenczy, A., Bergeron, C. & Richart, R.M. (1990) Carbon dioxide laser energy disperses human papillomavirus deoxyribonucleic acid onto treatment fields. *Am. J. Obstet. Gynecol.*, **163**, 1271–1274

Ferenczy, A., Choukroun, D., Falcone, T. & Franco, E. (1995) The effect of cervical loop electrosurgical excision on subsequent pregnancy outcome: north american experience. *Am. J. Obstet. Gynecol.*, **172**, 1246–1250

Ferguson, A., Moore, M. & Fox, H. (1985) Expression of MHC products and leucocyte differentiation antigens in gynaecological neoplasms: an immunohistological analysis of the tumour cells and infiltrating leucocytes. *Br. J. Cancer*, **52**, 551–563

Figge, J., Webster, T., Smith, T.F. & Paucha, E. (1988) Prediction of similar transforming regions in simian virus 40 large T, adenovirus E1A, and *myc* oncoproteins. *J. Virol.*, **62**, 1814–1818

Finch, J.T. & Klug, A. (1965) The structure of viruses of the papilloma-polyoma type. III. Structure of rabbit papilloma virus, with an appendix on the topography of contrast in negative-staining for electron-microscopy. *J. mol. Biol.*, **13**, 1–12

Fletcher, A., Metaxas, N., Grubb, C. & Chamberlain, J. (1990) Four and a half year follow up of women with dyskaryotic cervical smears. *Br. med. J.*, **301**, 641–644

Ford, J.N., Jennings, P.A., Spradbrow, P.B. & Francis, J. (1982) Evidence for papillomaviruses in ocular lesions in cattle. *Res. vet. Sci.*, **32**, 257–259

Foster, S.A., Demers, G.W., Etscheid, B.G. & Galloway, D.A. (1994) The ability of human papillomavirus E6 proteins to target p53 for degradation *in vivo* correlates with their ability to abrogate actinomycin D-induced growth arrest. *J. Virol.*, **68**, 5698–5705

Franceschi, S., Doll, R., Gallwey, J., La Vecchia, C., Peto, R. & Spriggs, A.I. (1983) Genital warts and cervical neoplasia: an epidemiological study. *Br. J. Cancer*, **48**, 621–628

Franco, E.L. (1992) Measurement errors in epidemiological studies of human papillomavirus and cervical cancer. In: Muñoz, N., Bosch, F.X., Shah, K.V. & Meheus, A., eds, *The Epidemiology of Cervical Cancer and Human Papillomavirus* (IARC Scientific Publications No. 119), Lyon, IARC, pp. 181–197

Franco, E.L., Campos Filho, N., Villa, L.L. & Torloni, H. (1988) Correlation patterns of cancer relative frequencies with some socioeconomic and demographic indicators in Brazil: an ecologic study. *Int. J. Cancer*, **41**, 24–29

Frazer, I.H., Medley, G., Crapper, R.M., Brown, T.C. & Mackay, I.R. (1986) Association between anorectal dysplasia, human papillomavirus, and human immunodeficiency virus infection in homosexual men. *Lancet*, **ii**, 657–660

Fredericks, B.D., Balkin, A., Daniel, H.W., Schonrock, J., Ward, B. & Frazer, I.H. (1993) Transmission of human papillomaviruses from mother to child. *Aust. N. Z. J. Obstet. Gynaecol.*, **33**, 30–32

Friedman-Kien, A.E., Eron, L.J., Conant, M., Growdon, W., Badiak, H., Bradstreet, P.W., Fedorczyk, D., Trout, J.R. & Plasse, T.F. (1988) Natural interferon alfa for treatment of condylomata acuminata. *J. Am. med. Assoc.*, **259**, 533–538

Frisch, M., Melbye, M. & Møller, H. (1993) Trends in incidence of anal cancer in Denmark. *Br. med. J.*, **306**, 419–422

Frisch, M., Friis, S., Jørgensen, B.B., Krüger Kjaer, S. & Melbye, M. (1995) Decline in the incidence of penis cancer in an uncircumcised population (Denmark 1943–90). *Br. med. J.* (in press)

Fu, Y.S. & Reagan, J.W., eds (1989) *Pathology of the Uterine Cervix, Vagina, and Vulva*, Philadelphia, W.B. Saunders

Fu, Y.S., Reagan, J. & Richart, R.M. (1981) Definition of precursors. *Gynecol. Oncol.*, **12** (Suppl.), S220–S231

Fu, Y.S., Braun, L., Shah, K.V., Lawrence, W.D. & Robboy, S.J. (1983) Histologic, nuclear DNA, and human papillomavirus studies of cervical condylomata. *Cancer*, **52**, 1705–1711

Fu, Y.S., Huang, I., Beaudenon, S., Ionesco, M., Barrasso, R., de Brux, J. & Orth, G. (1988) Correlative study of human papillomavirus, DNA, histopathology, and morphometry in cervical condyloma and intraepithelial neoplasia. *Int. J. gynecol. Pathol.*, **7**, 297–307

Fuchs, P.G., Girardi, F. & Pfister, H. (1988) Human papillomavirus DNA in normal, metaplastic, preneoplastic and neoplastic epithelia of the cervix uteri. *Int. J. Cancer*, **41**, 41–45

Fuchs, P.G., Girardi, F. & Pfister, H. (1989) Human papillomavirus 16 DNA in cervical cancers and in lymph nodes of cervical cancer patients: a diagnostic marker for early metastases? *Int. J. Cancer*, **43**, 41–44

Fujii, T., Crum, C.P., Winkler, B., Fu, Y.S. & Richart, R.M. (1984) Human papillomavirus infection and cervical intraepithelial neoplasia: histopathology and DNA content. *Obstet. Gynecol.*, **63**, 99–104

Fujita, M., Inoue, M., Tanizawa, O., Iwamoto, S. & Enomoto, T. (1992) Alterations of the *p53* gene in human primary cervical carcinoma with and without human papillomavirus infection. *Cancer Res.*, **52**, 5323–5328

Fukushima, M., Yamakawa, Y., Shimano, S., Hashimoto, M., Sawada, Y. & Fujinaga, K. (1990) The physical state of human papillomavirus 16 DNA in cervical carcinoma and cervical intraepithelial neoplasia. *Cancer*, **66**, 2155–2161

Fulcheri, E., Baracchini, P., Gerbaldo, D. & Lapertosa, G. (1993) Human papillomavirus in cervical adenocarcinoma: an in situ hybridization study. *Pathologica*, **85**, 37–45

Funk, W.D., Pak, D.T., Karas, R.H., Wright, W.E. & Shay, J.W. (1992) A transcriptionally active DNA-binding site for human p53 protein complexes. *Mol. cell. Biol.*, **12**, 2866–2871

Furihata, M., Ohtsuki, Y., Ogoshi, S., Takahashi, A., Tamiya, T. & Ogata, T. (1993a) Prognostic significance of human papillomavirus genomes (type-16, -18) and aberrant expression of p53 protein in human esophageal cancer. *Int. J. Cancer*, **54**, 226–230

Furihata, M., Inoue, K., Ohtsuki, Y., Hashimoto, H., Terao, N. & Fujita, Y. (1993b) High-risk human papillomavirus infections and overexpression of p53 protein as prognostic indicators in transitional cell carcinoma of the urinary bladder. *Cancer Res.*, **53**, 4823–4827

Furth, P.A. & Baker, C.C. (1991) An element in the bovine papillomavirus late 3′ untranslated region reduces polyadenylated cytoplasmic RNA levels. *J. Virol.*, **65**, 5806–5812

Furuta, Y., Shinohara, T., Sano, K., Nagashima, K., Inoue, K., Tanaka, K. & Inuyama, Y. (1991) Molecular pathologic study of human papillomavirus infection in inverted papilloma and squamous cell carcinoma of the nasal cavities and paranasal sinuses. *Laryngoscope*, **101**, 79–85

Furuta, Y., Takasu, T., Asai, T., Shinohara, T., Sawa, H., Nagashima, K. & Inuyama, Y. (1992) Detection of human papillomavirus DNA in carcinomas of the nasal cavities and paranasal sinuses by polymerase chain reaction. *Cancer*, **69**, 353–357

Gaarenstroom, K.N., Melkert, P., Walboomers, J.M.M., van den Brule, A.J.C., Van Bommel, P.F.J. & Meyer, C.J.L.M. (1994) Human papillomavirus DNA and genotypes: prognostic factors for progression of cervical intraepithelial neoplasia. *Int. J. Gynecol. Cancer*, **4**, 73–78

Galloway, D.A. (1992) Serological assays for the detection of HPV antibodies. In: Muñoz, N., Bosch, F.X., Shah, K.V. & Meheus, A., eds, *The Epidemiology of Cervical Cancer and Human Papillomavirus* (IARC Scientific Publications No. 119), Lyon, IARC, pp. 147–161

Galloway, D.A. & McDougall, J.K. (1989) Human papillomaviruses and carcinomas. *Adv. Virus Res.*, **37**, 125–171

Gao, L., Chain, B., Sinclair, C., Crawford, L., Zhou, J., Morris, J., Zhu, X. & Stauss, H. (1994) Immune response to human papillomavirus type 16 E6 gene in a live vaccinia vector. *J. gen. Virol.*, **75**, 157–164

Garcia-Carranca, A., Thierry, F. & Yaniv, M. (1988) Interplay of viral and cellular proteins along the long control region of human papillomavirus type 18. *J. Virol.*, **62**, 4321–4330

Garden, J.M., O'Banion, M.K., Shelnitz, L.S., Pinski, K.S., Bakus, A.D., Reichmann, M.E. & Sundberg, J.P. (1988) Papillomavirus in the vapor of carbon dioxide laser-treated verrucae. *J. Am. med. Assoc.*, **259**, 1199–1202

Garrett, L.R., Perez-Reyes, N., Smith, P.P. & McDougall, J.K. (1993) Interaction of HPV-18 and nitrosomethylurea in the induction of squamous cell carcinoma. *Carcinogenesis*, **14**, 329–332

Garuti, G., Boselli, F., Genazzani, G. & Genazzani, A.R. (1991) Prevalence of different types of human papillomavirus in cervical infection of north Italian women. *Eur. J. Obstet. Gynecol. reprod. Biol.*, **39**, 227–233

Garven, T.C., Thelmo, W.L., Victor, J. & Pertschuk, L. (1991) Verrucous carcinoma of the leg positive for HPV DNA 11 and 18: a case report. *Hum. Pathol.*, **22**, 1170–1173

Gassenmaier, A. & Hornstein, O.P. (1988) Presence of human papillomavirus DNA in benign and precancerous oral leukoplakias and squamous cell carcinomas. *Dermatologica*, **176**, 224–233

Gassenmaier, A., Fuchs, P., Schell, H. & Pfister, H. (1986) Papillomavirus DNA in warts of immunosuppressed renal allograft recipients. *Arch. dermatol. Res.*, **278**, 219–223

Gaukroger, J.M., Bradley, A., O'Neil, B.W., Smith, K.T., Campo, M.S. & Jarrett, W.F.H. (1989) Induction of virus-producing tumours in athymic nude mice by bovine papillomavirus type 4. *Vet. Rec.*, **125**, 391–392

Gaukroger, J.M., Chandrachud, L., Jarrett, W.F.H., McGarvie, G.E., Yeudall, W.A., McCaffery, R.E., Smith, K.T. & Campo, M.S. (1991) Malignant transformation of a papilloma induced by bovine papillomavirus type 4 in the nude mouse renal capsule. *J. gen. Virol.*, **72**, 1165–1168

Gaukroger, J.M., Bradley, A., Chandrachud, L., Jarrett, W.F.H. & Campo, M.S. (1993) Interaction between bovine papillomavirus type 4 and cocarcinogens in the production of malignant tumours. *J. gen. Virol.*, **74**, 2275–2280

Gauthier, J.-M., Dillner, J. & Yaniv, M. (1991) Structural analysis of the human papillomavirus type 16-E2 transactivator with antipeptide antibodies reveals a high mobility region linking the transactivation and the DNA-binding domains. *Nucleic Acids Res.*, **19**, 7073–7079

Gavioli, R., Kurilla, M.G., de Campos Lima, P.O., Wallace, L.E., Dolcetti, R., Murray, R.J., Rickinson, A.B. & Masucci, M.G. (1993) Multiple HLA A11-restricted cytotoxic T-lymphocyte epitopes of different immunogenicities in the Epstein-Barr virus-encoded nuclear antigen 4. *J. Virol.*, **67**, 1572–1578

Gentile, G., Formelli, G., Orsoni, G., Rinaldi, A.M. & Busacchi, P. (1991) Immunosuppression and human genital papillomavirus infection. *Eur. J. gynaecol. Oncol.*, **12**, 79–81

Georg-Fries, B., Biederlack, S., Wolf, J. & zur Hausen, H. (1984) Analysis of proteins, helper dependence and seroepidemiology of a human parvovirus. *Virology*, **134**, 64–71

Ghim, S., Christensen, N.D., Kreider, J.W. & Jenson, A.B. (1991) Comparison of neutralization of BPV-1 infection of C127 cells and bovine fetal skin xenografts. *Int. J. Cancer*, **49**, 285–289

Ghim, S.-J., Jenson, A.B. & Schlegel, R. (1992) HPV-1 L1 protein expressed in cos cells displays conformational epitopes found on intact virions. *Virology*, **190**, 548–552

Ghim, S.-J., Newsome, J., Jenson, A.B. & Schlegel, R. (1995) Formalin-inactivated oral papilloma extracts and recombinant L1 vaccines protect completely against mucosal papillomavirus infection: a canine model. *Vaccine* (in press)

Ghosh, A.K. & Moore, M. (1992) Tumour-infiltrating lymphocytes in cervical carcinoma. *Eur. J. Cancer*, **28A**, 1910–1916

Ghosh, A.K., Smith, N.K., Stacey, S.N., Glew, S.S., Connor, M.E., Arrand, J.R. & Stern, P.L. (1993) Serological response to HPV 16 in cervical dysplasia and neoplasia: correlation of antibodies to E6 with cervical cancer. *Int. J. Cancer*, **53**, 591–596

Ghosh, A.K., Glenville, S., Bartholomew, J. & Stern, P.L. (1994) Analysis of tumour-infiltrating lymphocytes in cervical carcinoma. In: Stanley, M.A., ed., *Immunology of Human Papillomaviruses*, New York, Plenum, pp. 249–253

Girardi, F., Heydarfadai, M., Koroschetz, F., Pickel, H. & Winter, R. (1994) Cold-knife conization versus loop excision: histopathologic and clinical results of a randomized trial. *Gynecol. Oncol.*, **55**, 368–370

Giri, I. & Yaniv, M. (1988) Structural and mutational analysis of E2 *trans*-activating proteins of papillomaviruses reveals three distinct functional domains. *EMBO J.*, **7**, 2823–2829

Gissmann, L. & Müller, M. (1994) The current role of HPV-serology. In: Stanley, M. & Stern, P., eds, *Human Papillomaviruses and Cervical Cancer*, Oxford, Oxford University Press, pp. 132–145

Gissmann, L. & zur Hausen, H. (1980) Partial characterization of viral DNA from human genital warts (condylomata acuminata). *Int. J. Cancer*, **25**, 605–609

Gissmann, L., de Villiers, E.-M. & zur Hausen, H. (1982) Analysis of human genital warts (condylomata acuminata) and other genital tumors for human papillomavirus type 6 DNA. *Int. J. Cancer*, **29**, 143–146

Gissmann, L., Wolnik, L., Ikenberg, H., Koldovsky, U., Schnürch, H.G. & zur Hausen, H. (1983) Human papillomavirus types 6 and 11 DNA sequences in genital and laryngeal papillomas and in some cervical cancers. *Proc. natl Acad. Sci. USA*, **80**, 560–563

Gitsch, G., Kainz, C., Pohanka, E., Reinthaller, A., Kovarik, J., Tatra, G. & Breitenecker, G. (1992) Human papillomavirus infection of the uterine cervix in immune suppressed women after kidney transplantation. *Geburtsh. Frauenheilk.*, **52**, 764–766 (in German)

Gius, D. & Laimins, L.A. (1989) Activation of human papillomavirus type 18 gene expression by herpes simplex virus type 1 viral transactivators and a phorbol ester. *J. Virol.*, **63**, 555–563

Glew, S.S., Duggan-Keen, M., Cabrera, T. & Stern, P.L. (1992) HLA class II antigen expression in human papillomavirus-associated cervical cancer. *Cancer Res.*, **52**, 4009–4016

Glew, S.S., Connor, M.E., Snijders, P.J., Stanbridge, C.M., Buckley, C.H., Walboomers, J.M.M., Meijer, C.J.L.M. & Stern, P.L. (1993a) HLA expression in pre-invasive cervical neoplasia in relation to human papilloma virus infection. *Eur. J. Cancer*, **29A**, 1963–1970

Glew, S.S., Duggan-Keen, M., Ghosh, A.K., Ivinson, A., Sinnott, P., Davidson, J., Dyer, P.A. & Stern, P.L. (1993b) Lack of association of HLA polymorphisms with human papillomavirus-related cervical cancer. *Hum. Immunol.*, **37**, 157–164

Gloss, B., Bernard, H.-U., Seedorf, K. & Klock, G. (1987) The upstream regulatory region of the human papillomavirus-16 contains an E2 protein-independent enhancer which is specific for cervical carcinoma cells and regulated by glucocorticoid hormones. *EMBO J.*, **6**, 3735–3743

Gloss, B., Chong, T. & Bernard, H.-U. (1989) Numerous nuclear proteins bind the long control region of human papillomavirus type 16: a subset of 6 of 23 DNase I-protected segments coincides with the location of the cell-type-specific enhancer. *J. Virol.*, **63**, 1142–1152

Goff, B.A., Muntz, H.G., Bell, D.A., Wertheim, I. & Rice, L.W. (1993) Human papillomavirus typing in patients with Papanicolaou smears showing squamous atypia. *Gynecol. Oncol.*, **48**, 384–388

Goldman, S., Glimelius, B., Nilsson, B. & Påhlman, L. (1989) Incidence of anal epidermoid carcinoma in Sweden 1970–1984. *Acta chir. scand.*, **155**, 191–197

Goldstein, D.J. & Schlegel, R. (1990) The E5 oncoprotein of bovine papillomavirus binds to a 16 kDa cellular protein. *EMBO J.*, **9**, 137–145

Goldstein, D.J., Finbow, M.E., Andresson, T., McLean, P., Smith, K., Bubb, V. & Schlegel, R. (1991) Bovine papillomavirus E5 oncoprotein binds to the 16K component of vacuolar H^+-ATPases. *Nature*, **352**, 347–349

González-Garay, M.L., Barrera-Saldaña, H.A., Avilés, L.B., Alvarez-Salas, L.M. & Gariglio, P. (1992) Prevalence in two mexican cities of human papillomavirus DNA sequences in cervical cancer. *Rev. invest. Clín.*, **44**, 491–499

Gordon, D.E. & Olson, C. (1968) Meningiomas and fibroblastic neoplasia in calves induced with the bovine papilloma virus. *Cancer Res.*, **28**, 2423–2431

Gordon, M. & Palusci, V.J. (1989) HPV type 16 periungual carcinoma (Letter to the Editor). *J. Am. med. Assoc.*, **262**, 3407–3408

Gram, I.T., Macaluso, M., Churchill, J. & Stalsberg, H. (1992) *Trichomonas vaginalis* (TV) and human papillomavirus (HPV) infection and the incidence of cervical intraepithelial neoplasia (CIN) grade III. *Cancer Causes Control*, **3**, 231–236

Gravitt, P.E. & Manos, M.M. (1992) Polymerase chain reaction-based methods for the detection of human papillomavirus DNA. In: Muñoz, N., Bosch, F.X., Shah, K.V. & Meheus, A., eds, *The Epidemiology of Cervical Cancer and Human Papillomavirus* (IARC Scientific Publications No. 119), Lyon, IARC, pp. 121–133

Gravitt, P., Hakenewerth, A. & Stoerker, J. (1991) A direct comparison of methods proposed for use in widespread screening of human papillomavirus infections. *Mol. cell. Probes*, **5**, 65–72

Greenhalgh, D.A., Wang, X.-J., Rothnagel, J.A., Eckhardt, J.N., Quintanilla, M.I., Barber, J.L., Bundman, D.S., Longley, M.A., Schlegel, R. & Roop, D.R. (1994) Transgenic mice expressing targeted HPV-18 E6 and E7 oncogenes in the epidermis develop verrucous lesions and spontaneous, *ras*Ha-activated papillomas. *Cell Growth Differ.*, **5**, 667–675

Greer, R.O., Jr, Eversole, L.R. & Crosby, L.K. (1990) Detection of human papillomavirus-genomic DNA in oral epithelial dysplasias, oral smokeless tobacco-associated leukoplakias, and epithelial malignancies. *J. oral maxillofac. Surg.*, **48**, 1201–1205

Gregoire, L., Lawrence, W.D., Kukuruga, D., Eisenbrey, A.B. & Lancaster, W.D. (1994) Association between HLA-DQB1 alleles and risk for cervical cancer in African-American women. *Int. J. Cancer*, **57**, 504–507

Griep, A.E., Herber, R., Jeon, S., Lohse, J.K., Dubielzig, R.R. & Lambert, P.F. (1993) Tumorigenicity by human papillomavirus type 16 E6 and E7 in transgenic mice correlates with alterations in epithelial cell growth and differentiation. *J. Virol.*, **67**, 1373–1384

Griffin, N.R., Bevan, I.S., Lewis, F.A., Wells, M. & Young, L.S. (1990) Demonstration of multiple HPV types in normal cervix and in cervical squamous cell carcinoma using the polymerase chain reaction on paraffin wax embedded material. *J. clin. Pathol.*, **43**, 52–56

Griffin, N.R., Dockey, D., Lewis, F.A. & Wells, M. (1991) Demonstration of low frequency of human papillomavirus DNA in cervical adenocarcinoma and adenocarcinoma *in situ* by the polymerase chain reaction and in situ hybridization. *Int. J. gynecol. Pathol.*, **10**, 36–43

Grimmel, M., de Villiers, E.M., Neumann, C., Pawlita, M. & zur Hausen, H. (1988) Characterization of a new human papillomavirus (HPV 41) from disseminated warts and detection of its DNA in some skin carcinomas. *Int. J. Cancer*, **41**, 5–9

Groff, D.E., Sundberg, J.P. & Lancaster, W.D. (1983) Extrachromosomal deer fibromavirus DNA in deer fibromas and virus-transformed mouse cells. *Virology*, **131**, 546–550

Gross, G., Pfister, H., Hagedorn, M. & Gissmann, L. (1982) Correlation between human papillomavirus (HPV) type and histology of warts. *J. invest. Dermatol.*, **78**, 160–164

Grunebaum, A.N., Sedlis, A., Sillman, F., Fruchter, R., Stanek, A. & Boyce, J. (1983) Association of human papillomavirus infection with cervical intraepithelial neoplasia. *Obstet. Gynecol.*, **62**, 448–455

Grussendorf-Conen, E.I., Deutz, F.J. & de Villiers, E.-M. (1987) Detection of human papillomavirus-6 in primary carcinoma of the urethra in men. *Cancer*, **60**, 1832–1835

Gu, Z., Pim, D., Labrecque, S., Banks, L. & Matlashewski, G. (1994) DNA damage induced p53 mediated transcription is inhibited by human papillomavirus type 18 E6. *Oncogene*, **9**, 629–633

Guerin-Reverchon, I., Chardonnet, Y., Viac, J., Chouvet, B., Chignol, M.C. & Thivolet, J. (1990) Human papillomavirus infection and filaggrin expression in paraffin-embedded bipsy specimens of extragenital Bowen's disease and genital bowenoid papulosis. *J. Cancer Res. clin. Oncol.*, **116**, 295–300

Guerrero, E., Daniel, R.W., Bosch, F.X., Castellsagué, X., Muñoz, N., Gili, M., Viladiu, P., Navarro, C., Zubiri, M.L., Ascunce, N., Gonzalez, L.C., Tafur, L., Izarzugaza, I. & Shah, K.V. (1992) Comparison of ViraPap, Southern hybridization, and polymerase chain reaction methods for human papillomavirus indentification in an epidemiological investigation of cervical cancer. *J. clin. Microbiol.*, **30**, 2951–2959

Guijon, F.B., Paraskevas, M. & Brunham, R. (1985) The association of sexually transmitted diseases with cervical intraepithelial neoplasia: a case–control study. *Am. J. Obstet. Gynecol.*, **151**, 185–190

Guillou, L., Sahli, R., Chaubert, P., Monnier, P., Cuttat, J.-F. & Costa, J. (1991) Squamous cell carcinoma of the lung in a nonsmoking, nonirradiated patient with juvenile laryngotracheal papillomatosis. Evidence of human papillomavirus-11 DNA in both carcinoma and papillomas. *Am. J. surg. Pathol.*, **15**, 891–898

Guitart, J., Bergfeld, W.F., Tuthill, R.J., Tubbs, R.R., Zienowicz, R. & Fleegler, E.J. (1990) Squamous cell carcinoma of the nail bed: a clinicopathological study of 12 cases. *Br. J. Dermatol.*, **123**, 215–222

Gupta, J., Pilotti, S., Shah, K.V., De Palo, G. & Rilke, F. (1987) Human papillomavirus-associated early vulvar neoplasia investigated by in situ hybridization. *Am. J. surg. Pathol.*, **11**, 430–434

Gutman, L.T., St Claire, K.K., Everett, V.D., Ingram, D.L., Soper, J., Johnston, W.W., Mulvaney, G.G. & Phelps, W.C. (1994) Cervical-vaginal and intraanal human papillomavirus infection of young girls with external genital warts. *J. infect. Dis.*, **170**, 339–344

Hagen, B. & Skjeldestad, F.E. (1993) The outcome of pregnancy after CO_2 laser conisation of the cervix. *Br. J. Obstet. Gynaecol.*, **100**, 717–720

Hagen, P., Lyons, G.D. & Haindel, C. (1993) Verrucous carcinoma of the larynx: role of human papillomavirus, radiation, and surgery. *Laryngoscope*, **103**, 253–257

Hagensee, M.E., Yaegashi, N. & Galloway, D.A. (1993) Self-assembly of human papillomavirus type 1 capsids by expression of the L1 protein alone or by coexpression of the L1 and L2 capsid proteins. *J. Virol.*, **67**, 315–322

Hakama, M., Magnus, K. & Pettersson, F. (1991) Effect of organized screening on the risk of cervical cancer in the Nordic countries. In: Miller, A.B., Chamberlain, J., Day, N.E., Hakama, M. & Prorok, P.C., eds, *Cancer Screening*, Cambridge, Cambridge University Press, pp. 152–162

Halbert, C.L. & Galloway, D.A. (1988) Identification of the E5 open reading frame of human papillomavirus type 16. *J. Virol.*, **62**, 1071–1075

Halbert, C.L., Demers, G.W. & Galloway, D.A. (1991) The E7 gene of human papillomavirus type 16 is sufficient for immortalization of human epithelial cells. *J. Virol.*, **65**, 473–478

Halpert, R., Fruchter, R.G., Sedlis, A., Butt, K., Boyce, J.G. & Sillman, F.H. (1986) Human papillomavirus and lower genital neoplasia in renal transplant patients. *Obstet. Gynecol.*, **68**, 251–258

Ham, J., Dostatni, N., Gauthier, J.-M. & Yaniv, M. (1991) The papillomavirus E2 protein: a factor with many talents. *Trends biochem. Sci.*, **16**, 440–444

Hampton, G.M., Penny, L.A., Baergen, R.N., Larson, A., Brewer, C., Liao, S., Busby Earle, R.M., Williams, A.W., Steel, C.M. & Bird, C.C. (1994) Loss of heterozygosity in cervical carcinoma: subchromosomal localization of a putative tumor-suppressor gene to chromosome 11q22–q24. *Proc. natl Acad. Sci. USA*, **91**, 6953–6957

Han, R., Breitburd, F., Marche, P.N. & Orth, G. (1992) Linkage of regression and malignant conversion of rabbit viral papillomas to MHC class II genes. *Nature*, **356**, 66–68

Handley, J.M., Maw, R.D., Bingham, E.A., Horner, T., Bharucha, H., Swann, A., Lawther, H. & Dinsmore, W.W. (1993) Anogenital warts in children. *Clin. exp. Dermatol.*, **18**, 241–247

Harper, J.W., Adami, G.R., Wei, N., Keyomarsi, K. & Elledge, S.J. (1993) The p21 Cdk-interacting protein Cip1 is a potent inhibitor of G1 cyclin-dependent kinases. *Cell*, **75**, 805–816

Hashida, T. & Yasumoto, S. (1991) Induction of chromosome abnormalities in mouse and human epidermal keratinocytes by the human papillomavirus type 16 E7 oncogene. *J. gen. Virol.*, **72**, 1569–1577

Hatch, K.D., Shingleton, H.M., Orr, J.W., Jr, Gore, H. & Soong, S.-J. (1985) Role of endocervical curettage in colposcopy. *Obstet. Gynecol.*, **65**, 403–408

Hatch, K.D., Schneider, A. & Abdel-Nour, M.W. (1995) An evaluation of human papillomavirus testing for intermediate and high-risk types as triage prior to coloscopy. *Am. J. Obstet. Gynecol.*, **172**, 1150–1157

Hawley-Nelson, P., Vousden, K.H., Hubbert, N.L., Lowy, D.R. & Schiller, J.T. (1989) HPV16 E6 and E7 proteins cooperate to immortalize human foreskin keratinocytes. *EMBO J.*, **8**, 3905–3910

Hawthorn, R.J., Murdoch, J.B., MacLean, A.B. & Mackie, R.M. (1988) Langerhans' cells and subtypes of human papillomavirus in cervical intraepithelial neoplasia. *Br. med. J.*, **297**, 643–646

Hayashi, N., Furihata, M., Ohtsuki, Y. & Ueno, H. (1994) Search for accumulation of p53 protein and detection of human papillomavirus genomes in sebaceous gland carcinoma of the eyelid. *Virchows Arch.*, **424**, 503–509

Hayward, M.L.R., Baird, P.J. & Meischke, H.R.C. (1993) Filiform viral squamous papillomas on sheep. *Vet. Rec.*, **132**, 86–88

Healy, G.B., Gelber, R.D., Trowbridge, A.L., Grundfast, K.M., Ruben, R.J. & Price, K.N. (1988) Treatment of recurrent respiratory papillomatosis with human leukocyte interferon. Results of a multicenter randomized clinical trial. *N. Engl. J. Med.*, **319**, 401–407

Heck, D.V., Yee, C.L., Howley, P.M. & Münger, K. (1992) Efficiency of binding the retinoblastoma protein correlates with the transforming capacity of the E7 oncoproteins of the human papillomaviruses. *Proc. natl Acad. Sci. USA*, **89**, 4442–4446

Hegde, R.S., Grossman, S.R., Laimins, L.A. & Sigler, P.B. (1992) Crystal structure at 1.7 Å of the bovine papillomavirus-1 E2 DNA-binding domain bound to its DNA target. *Nature*, **359**, 505–512

Hei, T.K., Piao, C.Q., Willey, J.C., Thomas, S. & Hall, E.J. (1994) Malignant transformation of human bronchial epithelial cells by radon-simulated alpha-particles. *Carcinogenesis*, **15**, 431–437

Heino, P., Goldman, S., Lagerstedt, U. & Dillner, J. (1993) Molecular and serological studies of human papillomavirus among patients with anal epidermoid carcinoma. *Int. J. Cancer*, **53**, 377–381

Heinzel, P.A., Chan, S.-Y., Ho, L., O'Connor, M., Balaram, P., Campo, M.S., Fujinaga, K., Kiviat, N., Kuypers, J., Pfister, H., Steinberg, B.M., Tay, S.-K., Villa, L.L. & Bernard, H.-U. (1995) Variation of human papillomavirus type 6 (HPV-6) and HPV-11 genomes samples throughout the world. *J. clin. Microbiol.*, **33**, 1746–1754

Helland, A., Børresen, A.L., Kaern, J., Rønningen, K.S. & Thorsby, E. (1992) HLA antigens and cervical carcinoma (Letter to the Editor). *Nature*, **356**, 23

Helland, A., Holm, R., Kristensen, G., Kaern, J., Karlsen, F., Trope, C., Nesland, J.M. & Børresen, A.-L. (1993) Genetic alterations of the TP53 gene, p53 protein expression and HPV infection in primary cervical carcinomas. *J. Pathol.*, **171**, 105–114

Hellberg, D., Nilsson, S., Grad, A., Hongxiu, J., Fuju, C., Syrjänen, S. & Syrjänen, K. (1993) Behavior of cervical intraepithelial neoplasia (CIN) associated with various human papillomavirus (HPV) types. *Arch. Gynecol. Obstet.*, **252**, 119–128

Henry, M.J., Stanley, M.W., Cruikshank, S. & Carson, L. (1989) Association of human immunodeficiency virus-induced immunosuppression with human papillomavirus infection and cervical intraepithelial neoplasia. *Am. J. Obstet. Gynecol.*, **160**, 352–353

Hepburn, D.J., Divakar, D., Bailey, R.R. & Macdonald, K.J.S. (1994) Cutaneous manifestations of renal transplantation in a New Zealand population. *N. Z. med. J.*, **107**, 497–499

Hermonat, P.L. (1994) Adeno-associated virus inhibits human papillomavirus type 16: a viral interaction implicated in cervical cancer. *Cancer Res.*, **54**, 2278–2281

Herrero, R., Brinton, L.A., Reeves, W.C., Brenes, M.M., Tenorio, F., de Britton, R.C., Gaitán, E., Montalván, P., García, M. & Rawls, W.E. (1990) Risk factors for invasive carcinoma of the uterine cervix in Latin America. *Bull. Pan Am. Health Org.*, **24**, 263–283

Herrero, R., Brinton, L.A., Reeves, W.C., Brenes, M.M., de Britton, R.C., Gaitán, E. & Tenorio, F. (1992) Screening for cervical cancer in Latin America: a case–control study. *Int. J. Epidemiol.*, **21**, 1050–1056

Higgins, G.D., Uzelin, D.M., Phillips, G.E., Pieterse, A.S. & Burrell, C.J. (1991a) Differing characteristics of human papillomavirus RNA-positive and RNA-negative anal carcinomas. *Cancer*, **68**, 561–567

Higgins, G.D., Davy, M., Roder, D., Uzelin, D.M., Phillips, G.E. & Burrell, C.J. (1991b) Increased age and mortality associated with cervical carcinomas negative for human papillomavirus RNA. *Lancet*, **338**, 910–913

Higgins, G.D., Phillips, G.E., Smith, L.A., Uzelin, D.M. & Burrell, C.J. (1992a) High prevalence of human papillomavirus transcripts in all grades of cervical intraepithelial glandular neoplasia. *Cancer*, **70**, 136–146

Higgins, G.D., Uzelin, D.M., Phillips, G.E., Villa, L.L. & Burrell, C.J. (1992b) Differing prevalence of human papillomavirus RNA in penile dysplasias and carcinomas may reflect differing etiologies. *Am. J. clin. Pathol.*, **97**, 272–278

Hilders, C.G., Houbiers, J.G.A., van Ravenswaay Claasen, H.H., Veldhuizen, R.W. & Fleuren, G.J. (1993) Association between HLA-expression and infiltration of immune cells in cervical carcinoma. *Lab. Invest.*, **69**, 651–659

Hilders, C.G., Houbiers, J.G., Krul, E.J. & Fleuren, G.J. (1994) The expression of histocompatibility-related leukocyte antigens in the pathway to cervical carcinoma. *Am. J. clin. Pathol.*, **101**, 5–12

Hildesheim, A., Mann, V., Brinton, L.A., Szklo, M., Reeves, W.C. & Rawls, W.E. (1991) Herpes simplex virus type 2: a possible interaction with human papillomavirus types 16/18 in the development of invasive cervical cancer. *Int. J. Cancer,* **49**, 335–340

Hildesheim, A., Gravitt, P., Schiffman, M.H., Kurman, R.J., Barnes, W., Jones, S., Tchabo, J.-G., Brinton, L.A., Copeland, C., Epp, J. & Manos, M.M. (1993) Determinants of genital human papillomavirus infection in low-income women in Washington, D.C. *Sex. transm. Dis.,* **20**, 279–284

Hildesheim, A., Schiffman, M.H., Gravitt, P.E., Glass, A.G., Greer, C.E., Zhang, T., Scott, D.R., Rush, B.B., Lawler, P., Sherman, M.E., Kurman, R.J. & Manos, M.M. (1994) Persistence of type-specific human papillomavirus infection among cytologically normal women. *J. infect. Dis.,* **169**, 235–240

Hines, J.F., Ghim, S.J., Christensen, N.D., Kreider, J.W., Barnes, W.A., Schlegel, R. & Jenson, A.B. (1994) Role of conformational epitopes expressed by human papillomavirus major capsid proteins in the serologic detection of infection and prophylactic vaccination. *Gynecol. Oncol.,* **55**, 13–20

Hinselmann, H. (1925) Improvement of possibility of inspection of vulva, vagina and cervix uteri. *München Med. Wschr.,* **77**, 1733 (in German)

Hiorns, L.R., Scholefield, J.H., Palmer, J.G., Shepherd, N.A. & Kerr, I.B. (1990) Ki-*ras* oncogene mutations in non-HPV-associated anal carcinoma. *J. Pathol.,* **161**, 99–103

Hippeläinen, M.I., Syrjänen, S., Hippeläinen, M., Koskela, H., Pulkkinen, J., Saarikoski, S. & Syrjänen, K. (1993) Prevalence and risk factors of genital human papillomavirus (HPV) infections in healthy males: a study on Finnish conscripts. *Sex. transmiss. Dis.,* **20**, 321–328

Hippeläinen, M.I., Yliskoski, M., Syrjänen, S., Saastamoinen, J., Hippeläinen, M., Saarikoski, S. & Syrjanen, K. (1994) Low concordance of genital human papillomavirus (HPV) lesions and viral types in HPV-infected women and their male sexual partners. *Sex. transmiss. Dis.,* **21**, 76–82

Hirschowitz, L., Raffle, A.E., Mackenzie, E.F. & Hughes, A.O. (1992) Long term follow up of women with borderline cervical smear test results: effects of age and viral infection on progression to high grade dyskaryosis. *Br. med. J.,* **304**, 1209–1212

Ho, L., Tay, S.-K., Chan, S.-Y. & Bernard, H.-U. (1993a) Sequence variants of human papillomavirus type 16 from couples suggest sexual transmission with low infectivity and polyclonality in genital neoplasia. *J. infect. Dis.,* **168**, 803–809

Ho, L., Chan, S.-Y., Burk, R.D., Das, B.C., Fujinaga, K., Icenogle, J.P., Kahn, T., Kiviat, N., Lancaster, W., Mavromara-Nazos, P., Labropoulou, V., Mitrani-Rosenbaum, S., Norrild, B., Pillai, M.R., Stoerker, J., Syrjaenen, K., Syrjaenen, S., Tay, S.-K., Villa, L.L., Wheeler, C.M., Williamson, A.L. & Bernard, H.-U. (1993b) The genetic drift of human papillomavirus type 16 is a means of reconstructing prehistoric viral spread and the movement of ancient human populations. *J. Virol.,* **67**, 6413–6423

Ho, G.Y., Burk, R.D., Fleming, I. & Klein, R.S. (1994) Risk of genital human papillomavirus infection in women with human immunodeficiency virus-induced immunosuppression. *Int. J. Cancer,* **56**, 788–792

Höckenström, T., Jonassen, F., Knutsson, F., Löwhagen, G.-B. & Rådberg, T. (1987) High prevalence of cervical dysplasia in female consorts of men with genital warts. *Acta derm. venereol. (Stockh.),* **67**, 511–516

Holladay, E.B. & Gerald, W.L. (1993) Viral gene detection in oral neoplasms using the polymerase chain reaction. *Am. J. clin. Pathol.,* **100**, 36–40

Hollstein, M., Sidransky, D., Vogelstein, B. & Harris, C.C. (1991) p53 Mutations in human cancers. *Science,* **253**, 49–53

Holly, E.A. & Palefsky, J.M. (1993) Factors related to risk of penile cancer: new evidence from a study in the Pacific Northwest. *J. natl Cancer Inst.*, **85**, 2–4

Höpfl, R.M., Sandbichler, M., Sepp, N., Heim, K., Müller-Holzner, E., Wartusch, B., Dapunt, O., Jochmus-Kudielka, L., ter-Meulen, J. & Gissmann, L. (1991) Skin test for HPV type 16 proteins in cervical intraepithelial neoplasia. *Lancet*, **337**, 373–374

Höpfl, R.M., Christensen, N.D., Angell, M.G. & Kreider, J.W. (1993) Skin test to assess immunity against cottontail rabbit papillomavirus antigens in rabbits with progressing papillomas or after papilloma regression. *J. invest. Dermatol.*, **101**, 227–231

Hoppe-Seyler, F. & Butz, K. (1993) Repression of endogenous p53 transactivation function in HeLa cervical carcinoma cells by human papillomavirus type 16 E6, human mdm-2, and mutant p53. *J. Virol.*, **67**, 3111–3117

Hørding, U., Daugaard, S., Iversen, A.K., Knudsen, J., Bock, J.E. & Norrild, B. (1991a) Human papillomavirus type 16 in vulvar carcinoma, vulvar intraepithelial neoplasia, and associated cervical neoplasia. *Gynecol. Oncol.*, **42**, 22–26

Hørding, U., Daugaard, S., Bock, J.E., Sebbelov, A.M. & Norrild, B. (1991b) HPV 11, 16 and 18 DNA sequences in cervical swabs from women with cervical dysplasia: prevalence and associated risk of progression. *Eur. J. Obstet. Gynecol. reprod. Biol.*, **40**, 43–48

Hørding, U., Teglbjaerg, C.S., Visfeldt, J. & Bock, J.E. (1992) Human papillomavirus types 16 and 18 in adenocarcinoma of the uterine cervix. *Gynecol. Oncol.*, **46**, 313–316

Hørding, U., Kringsholm, B., Andreasson, B., Visfeldt, J., Daugaard, S. & Bock, J.E. (1993) Human papillomavirus in vulvar squamous-cell carcinoma and in normal vulvar tissues: a search for a possible impact of HPV on vulvar cancer prognosis. *Int. J. Cancer*, **55**, 394–396

Horwitz, B.H., Weinstat, D.L. & DiMaio, D. (1989) Transforming activity of a 16-amino-acid segment of the bovine papillomavirus E5 protein linked to random sequences of hydrophobic amino acids. *J. Virol.*, **63**, 4515–4519

Hoshikawa, T., Nakajima, T., Uhara, H., Gotoh, M., Shimosato, Y., Tsutsumi, K., Ono, I. & Ebihara, S. (1990) Detection of human papillomavirus DNA in laryngeal squamous cell carcinomas by polymerase chain reaction. *Laryngoscope*, **100**, 647–650

Howes, K.A., Ransom, N., Papermaster, D.S., Lasudry, J.G., Albert, D.M. & Windle, J.J. (1994) Apoptosis or retinoblastoma: alternative fates of photoreceptors expressing the HPV-16 E7 gene in the presence or absence of p53. *Genes Dev.*, **8**, 1300–1310

Hsieh, C.-Y., Lee, S.-C. & Huang, S.-C. (1988) Presence and expression of human papillomavirus types 16 and 18 DNA sequences in cervical carcinomas. *Asia-Oceania J. Obstet. Gynaecol.*, **14**, 87–95

Hubbert, N.L., Sedman, S.A. & Schiller, J.T. (1992) Human papillomavirus type 16 E6 increases the degradation rate of p53 in human keratinocytes. *J. Virol.*, **66**, 6237–6241

Hubert, W.G. & Lambert, P.F. (1993) The 23-kilodalton E1 phosphoprotein of bovine papillomavirus type 1 is nonessential for stable plasmid replication in murine C127 cells. *J. Virol.*, **67**, 2932–2937

Hudson, J.B., Bedell, M.A., McCance, D.J. & Laimins, L.A. (1990) Immortalization and altered differentiation of human keratinocytes *in vitro* by the E6 and E7 open reading frames of human papillomavirus type 18. *J. Virol.*, **64**, 519–526

Hughes, R.G., Norval, M. & Howie, S.E.M. (1988) Expression of major histocompatibility class II antigens by Langerhans' cells in cervical intraepithelial neoplasia. *J. clin. Pathol.*, **41**, 253–259

Hughes, R.G., Neill, W.A. & Norval, M. (1989) Papillomavirus and c-*myc* antigen expression in normal and neoplastic cervical epithelium. *J. clin. Pathol.*, **42**, 46–51

REFERENCES

Huibregtse, J.M., Scheffner, M. & Howley, P.M. (1991) A cellular protein mediates association of p53 with the E6 oncoprotein of human papillomavirus types 16 or 18. *EMBO J.*, **10**, 4129–4135

Huibregtse, J.M., Scheffner, M. & Howley, P.M. (1993) Cloning and expression of the cDNA for E6-AP, a protein that mediates the interaction of the human papillomavirus E6 oncoprotein with p53. *Mol. cell. Biol.*, **13**, 775–784

Hurlin, P.J., Kaur, P., Smith, P.P., Perez-Reyes, N., Blanton, R.A. & McDougall, J.K. (1991) Progression of human papillomavirus type 18-immortalized human keratinocytes to a malignant phenotype. *Proc. natl Acad. Sci. USA*, **88**, 570–574

Hwang, J.-Y., Lin, B.-Y., Tang, F.-M. & Yu, W.C.Y. (1992) Tamoxifen stimulates human papillomavirus type 16 gene expression and cell proliferation in a cervical cancer cell line. *Cancer Res.*, **52**, 6848–6852

Hwang, E.-S., Riese, D.J., II, Settleman, J., Nilson, L.A., Honig, J., Flynn, S. & DiMaio, D. (1993) Inhibition of cervical carcinoma cell line proliferation by the introduction of a bovine papillomavirus regulatory gene. *J. Virol.*, **67**, 3720–3729

IARC (1986) *IARC Monographs on the Evaluation of the Carcinogenic Risk of Chemicals to Humans*, Vol. 38, *Tobacco Smoking*, Lyon

IARC (1987a) *IARC Monographs on the Evaluation of Carcinogenic Risks of Chemicals to Humans*, Suppl. No. 7, *Overall Evaluations of Carcinogenicity: An Updating of* IARC Monographs *Volumes 1–42*, Lyon, p. 66

IARC (1987b) *IARC Monographs on the Evaluation of Carcinogenic Risks of Chemicals to Humans*, Suppl. No. 7, *Overall Evaluations of Carcinogenicity: An Updating of* IARC Monographs *Volumes 1–42*, Lyon, pp. 284–285

IARC (1987c) *IARC Monographs on the Evaluation of Carcinogenic Risks of Chemicals to Humans*, Suppl. No. 7, *Overall Evaluations of Carcinogenicity: An Updating of* IARC Monographs *Volumes 1–42*, Lyon, pp. 135–136

IARC (1987d) *IARC Monographs on the Evaluation of Carcinogenic Risks of Chemicals to Humans*, Suppl. No. 7, *Overall Evaluations of Carcinogenicity: An Updating of* IARC Monographs *Volumes 1–42*, Lyon, pp. 248–250

IARC (1987e) *IARC Monographs on the Evaluation of Carcinogenic Risks of Chemicals to Humans*, Suppl. No. 7, *Overall Evaluations of Carcinogenicity: An Updating of* IARC Monographs *Volumes 1–42*, Lyon, pp. 119–120

IARC (1987f) *IARC Monographs on the Evaluation of Carcinogenic Risks of Chemicals to Humans*, Suppl. No. 7, *Overall Evaluations of Carcinogenicity: An Updating of* IARC Monographs *Volumes 1–42*, Lyon, p. 71

IARC (1992) *IARC Monographs on the Evaluation of Carcinogenic Risks of Chemicals to Humans*, Vol. 55, *Solar and Ultraviolet Radiation*, Lyon

IARC (1994a) *IARC Monographs on the Evaluation of Carcinogenic Risks of Chemicals to Humans*, Vol. 59, *Hepatitis Viruses*, Lyon, pp. 165–221

IARC (1994b) *IARC Monographs on the Evaluation of Carcinogenic Risks of Chemicals to Humans*, Vol. 59, *Hepatitis Viruses*, Lyon, pp. 45–164

Ibrahim, G.K., Gravitt, P.E., Dittrich, K.L., Ibrahim, S.N., Melhus, O., Anderson, S.M. & Robertson, C.N. (1992) Detection of human papillomavirus in the prostate by polymerase chain reaction and in situ hybridization. *J. Urol.*, **148**, 1822–1826

Icenogle, J.P., Sathya, P., Miller, D.L., Tucker, R.A. & Rawls, W.E. (1991) Nucleotide and amino acid sequence variation in the L1 and E7 open reading frames of human papillomavirus type 6 and type 16. *Virology*, **184**, 101–107

Iftner, T., Oft, M., Bohm, S., Wilczynksi, S.P. & Pfister, H. (1992) Transcription of the E6 and E7 genes of human papillomavirus type 6 in anogenital condylomata is restricted to undifferentiated cell layers of the epithelium. *J. Virol.*, **66**, 4639–4646

Ikenberg, H., Gissmann, L., Gross, G., Grussendorf-Conen, E.I. & zur Hausen, H. (1983) Human papillomavirus type-16-related DNA in genital Bowen's disease and in Bowenoid papulosis. *Int. J. Cancer*, **32**, 563–565

Ikenberg, H., Schwörer, D. & Pfleiderer, A. (1988) Detection of human papilloma virus (HPV) DNA in vulvar cancers. *Geburtsh. Frauenheilk.*, **48**, 776–780 (in German)

Ikenberg, H., Runge, M., Goppinger, A. & Pfleiderer, A. (1990) Human papillomavirus DNA in invasive carcinoma of the vagina. *Obstet. Gynecol.*, **76**, 432–438

Imai, Y., Matsushima, Y., Sugimura, T. & Terada, M. (1991) Purification and characterization of human papillomavirus type 16 E7 protein with preferential binding capacity to the underphosphorylated form of retinoblastoma gene product. *J. Virol.*, **65**, 4966–4972

Inaba, Y., Egawa, K., Yoshimura, K. & Ono, T. (1993) Demonstration of HPV type 1 DNA in a wart with Bowenoid histologic changes. *Am. J. Dermatopath.*, **15**, 172–175

Ingoldby, C.J., McWhinney, N.A., Wachtel, E. & Castro, J.E. (1980) Serial urinary and cervical cytological studies in women undergoing renal transplantation. *J. clin. Pathol.*, **33**, 990–992

Ishibashi, T., Matsushima, S., Tsunokawa, Y., Asai, M., Nomura, Y., Sugimura, T. & Terada, M. (1990) Human papillomavirus DNA in squamous cell carcinoma of the upper aerodigestive tract. *Arch. Otolaryngol. Head Neck Surg.*, **116**, 294–298

Ishiji, T., Lace, M.J., Parkkinen, S., Anderson, R.D., Haugen, T.H., Cripe, T.P., Xiao, J.-H., Davidson, I., Chambon, P. & Turek, L.P. (1992) Transcriptional enhancer factor (TEF)-1 and its cell-specific co-activator activate human papillomavirus-16 E6 and E7 oncogene transcription in keratinocytes and cervical carcinoma cells. *EMBO J.*, **11**, 2271–2281

Ishiwatari, H., Hayasaka, N., Inoue, H., Yutsudo, M. & Hakura, A. (1994) Degradation of p53 only is not sufficient for the growth stimulatory effect of human papillomavirus 16 E6 oncoprotein in human embryonic fibroblasts. *J. med. Virol.*, **44**, 243–249

Iwasaka, T., Ohuchida, M., Matsuo, N., Yokoyama, M., Fukuda, K., Hara, K., Fukuyama, K., Hori, K. & Sugimori, H. (1993) Correlation between HPV positivity and state of the p53 gene in cervical carcinoma cell lines. *Gynecol. Oncol.*, **48**, 104–109

Iwasawa, A., Kumamoto, Y. & Fujinaga, K. (1993) Detection of human papillomavirus deoxyribonucleic acid in penile carcinoma by polymerase chain reaction and in situ hybridization. *J. Urol.*, **149**, 59–63

Jablonska, S., Orth, G., Obalek, S. & Croissant, O. (1985) Cutaneous warts: clinical, histologic, and virologic correlations. *Clin. Dermatol.*, **3**, 71–82

Jablonska, S. & Majewski, S. (1994) Epidermodysplasia verruciformis: immunological and clinical aspects. *Current Topics Microbiol. Immunol.*, **186**, 157–175

Jackson, M.E., Campo, M.S. & Gaukroger, J.M. (1993) Cooperation between papillomavirus and chemical cofactors in oncogenesis. *Crit. Rev. Oncogen.*, **4**, 277–291

Jacobs, M.V., de Roda Husman, A.M., van den Brule, A.J.C., Snijders, P.J.F., Meijer, C.J.L.M. & Walboomers, J.M.M. (1995) Group specific differentiation between high- and low-risk human papillomavirus genotypes by general primers-mediated polymerase chain reaction and two cocktails of oligonucleotide-probes. *J. clin. Microbiol.*, **33**, 901–905

Jacyk, W.K. & de Villiers, E.-M. (1993) Epidermodysplasia verruciformis in Africans. *Int. J. Dermatol.*, **32**, 806–810

Jacyk, W.K., Dreyer, L. & de Villiers, E.-M. (1993a) Seborrheic keratoses of black patients with epidermodysplasia verruciformis contain homan papillomavirus DNA. *Am. J. Dermatopathol.*, **15**, 1–6

Jacyk, W.K., Hazelhurst, J.A., Dreyer, L. & Coccia-Portugal, M.A. (1993b) Epidermodysplasia verruciformis and malignant thymoma. *Clin. exp. Dermatol.*, **18**, 89–91

Jarrett, W.F.H. (1978) Transformation of warts to malignancy in alimentary carcinoma in cattle. *Bull. Cancer (Paris)*, **65**, 191–194

Jarrett, W.F.H. (1985) The natural history of bovine papillomavirus infections. In: Klein, G., ed., *Advances in Viral Oncology*, New York, Raven Press, pp. 83–101

Jarrett, W.F.H., McNeil, P.E., Grimshaw, W.T.R., Selman, I.E. & McIntyre, W.I.M. (1978a) High incidence area of cattle cancer with a possible interaction between an environmental carcinogen and a papilloma virus. *Nature*, **274**, 215–217

Jarrett, W.F.H., Murphy, J., O'Neil, B.W. & Laird, H.M. (1978b) Virus-induced papillomas of the alimentary tract of cattle. *Int. J. Cancer*, **22**, 323–328

Jarrett, W.F.H., Campo, M.S., O'Neil, B.W., Laird, H.M. & Coggins, L.W. (1984a) A novel bovine papillomavirus (BPV-6) causing true epithelial papillomas of the mammary gland skin: a member of a proposed new BPV subgroup. *Virology*, **136**, 255–264

Jarrett, W.F.H., Campo, M.S., Blaxter, M.L., O'Neil, B.W., Laird, H.M., Moar, M.H. & Sartirana, M.L. (1984b) Alimentary fibropapilloma in cattle: a spontaneous tumor, nonpermissive for papillomavirus replication. *J. natl Cancer Inst.*, **73**, 499–504

Jarrett, W.F.H., Smith, K.T., O'Neil, B.W., Gaukroger, J.M., Chandrachud, L.M., Grindlay, G.J., McGarvie, G.M. & Campo, M.S. (1991) Studies on vaccination against papillomaviruses: prophylactic and therapeutic vaccination with recombinant structural proteins. *Virology*, **184**, 33–42

Jenison, S.A., Yu, X.-P., Valentine, J.M. & Galloway, D.A. (1989) Human antibodies react with an epitope of the human papillomavirus type 6b L1 open reading frame which is distinct from the type-common epitope. *J. Virol.*, **63**, 809–818

Jenison, S.A., Yu, X.-P., Valentine, J.M., Koutsky, L.A., Christiansen, A.E., Beckmann, A.M. & Galloway, D.A. (1990) Evidence of prevalent genital-type human papillomavirus infections in adults and children. *J. infect. Dis.*, **162**, 60–69

Jenison, S.A., Yu, X.-P., Valentine, J.M. & Galloway, D.A. (1991) Characterization of human antibody-reactive epitopes encoded by human papillomavirus types 16 and 18. *J. Virol.*, **65**, 1208–1218

Jenson, A.B., Rosenthal, J.D., Olson, C., Pass, F., Lancaster, W.D. & Shah, K.V. (1980) Immunologic relatedness of papillomaviruses from different species. *J. natl Cancer Inst.*, **64**, 495–500

Jenson, A.B., Kurman, R.J. & Lancaster, W.D. (1985) Detection of papillomavirus common antigens in lesions of skin and mucosa. *Clin. Dermatol.*, **3**, 56–63

Jenson, A.B., Lim, P., Ghim, S., Cowsert, L., Olson, C., Lim, L.-Y., Farquhar, C. & Pilacinski, W. (1991) Identification of linear epitopes of the BPV-1 L1 protein recognized by sera of infected or immunized animals. *Pathobiology*, **59**, 396–403

Jeon, S. & Lambert, P.F. (1995) Integration of human papillomavirus type 16 DNA into the human genome leads to increased stability of E6 and E7 mRNAs: implications for cervical carcinogenesis. *Proc. natl Acad. Sci. USA*, **92**, 1654–1658

Jeon, S., Allen-Hoffmann, B. L. & Lambert, P.F. (1995) Integration of human papillomavirus type 16 into the human genome correlates with a selective growth advantage of cells. *J. Virol.*, **69**, 2989–2997

Jewers, R.J., Hildebrandt, P., Ludlow, J.W., Kell, B. & McCance, D.J. (1992) Regions of human papillomavirus type 16 E7 oncoprotein required for immortalization of human keratinocytes. *J. Virol.*, **66**, 1329–1335

Jha, P.K.S., Beral, V., Peto, J., Hack, S., Hermon, C., Deacon, J., Mant, D., Chilvers, C., Vessey, M.P., Pike, M.C., Müller, M. & Gissmann, L. (1993) Antibodies to human papillomavirus and to other genital infectious agents and invasive cervical cancer risk. *Lancet*, **341**, 1116–1118

Ji, H.X., Syrjänen, S., Syrjänen, K., Wu, A.R. & Chang, F.J. (1990) In situ hybridization analysis of HPV DNA in cervical precancer and cervical cancers from China. *Arch. Gynecol. Obstet.*, **247**, 21–29

Jiko, K., Tsuda, H., Sato, S. & Hirohashi, S. (1994) Pathogenetic significance of p53 and c-Ki-*ras* gene mutations and human papillomavirus DNA integration in adenocarcinoma of the uterine cervix and uterine isthmus. *Int. J. Cancer*, **59**, 601–606

Jochmus-Kudielka, I., Schneider, A., Braun, R., Kimmig, R., Koldovsky, U., Schneweis, K.E., Seedorf, K. & Gissmann, L. (1989) Antibodies against the human papillomavirus type 16 early proteins in human sera: correlation of anti-E7 reactivity with cervical cancer. *J. natl Cancer Inst.*, **81**, 1698–1704

Jochmus-Kudielka, I., Bouwes Bavinck, J.N., Claas, F.H., Schneider, A., Van der Woude, F.J. & Gissmann, L. (1992) Seroreactivity against HPV 16 E4 and E7 proteins in renal transplant recipients and pregnant women (Letter to the Editor). *J. invest. Dermatol.*, **98**, 389–390

Johnson, J.E., Dehaeck, C.M., Soeters, R. & Williamson, A.-L. (1991) Typing and molecular characterization of human papillomaviruses in genital warts from South African women. *J. med. Virol.*, **33**, 39–42

Johnson, T.L., Kim, W., Plieth, D.A. & Sarkar, F.H. (1992a) Detection of HPV 16/18 DNA in cervical adenocarcinoma using polymerase chain reaction (PCR) methodology. *Mod. Pathol.*, **5**, 35–40

Johnson, J.C., Burnett, A.F., Willet, G.D., Young, M.A. & Doniger, J. (1992b) High frequency of latent and clinical human papillomavirus cervical infections in immunocompromised human immunodeficiency virus-infected women. *Obstet. Gynecol.*, **79**, 321–327

Johnson, D.G., Cress, W.D., Jakoi, L. & Nevins, J.R. (1994) Oncogenic capacity of the E2F1 gene. *Proc. natl Acad. Sci. USA*, **91**, 12823–12827

Jones, R.W., Park, J.S., McLean, M.R. & Shah, K.V. (1990a) Human papillomavirus in women with vulvar intraepithelial neoplasia III. *J. reprod. Med.*, **35**, 1124–1126

Jones, R.E., Wegrzyn, R.J., Patrick, D.R., Balishin, N.L., Vuocolo, G.A., Riemen, M.W., Defeo-Jones, D., Garsky, V.M., Heimbrook, D.C. & Oliff, A. (1990b) Identification of HPV-16 E7 peptides that are potent antagonists of E7 binding to the retinoblastoma suppressor protein. *J. biol. Chem.*, **265**, 12782–12785

Jones, M.H., Koi, S., Fujimoto, I., Hasumi, K., Kato, K. & Nakamura, Y. (1994) Allelotype of uterine cancer by analysis of RFLP and microsatellite polymorphisms: frequent loss of heterozygosity on chromosome arms 3p, 9q, 10q, and 17p. *Genes Chromosomes Cancer*, **9**, 119–123

Judd, R., Zaki, S.R., Coffield, L.M. & Evatt, B.L. (1991) Human papillomavirus type 6 detected by the polymerase chain reaction in invasive sinonasal papillary squamous cell carcinoma. *Arch. Pathol. Lab. Med.*, **115**, 1150–1153

Junge, R.E., Sundberg, J.P. & Lancaster, W.D. (1984) Papillomas and squamous cell carcinomas of horses. *J. Am. vet. Med. Assoc.*, **185**, 656–659

Kadish, A., Burk, R., Kress, Y., Calderin, S. & Romney, S.L. (1986) Human papillomavirus of different types in precancerous lesions of the uterine cervix: histologic, immunocytochemical and ultrastructural studies. *Hum. Pathol.*, **17**, 384–392

Kadish, A.S., Hagan, R.J., Ritter, D.B., Goldberg, G.L., Romney, S.L., Kanetsky, P.A., Beiss, B.K. & Burk, R.D. (1992) Biologic characteristics of specific human papillomavirus types predicted from morphology of cervical lesions. *Hum. Pathol.*, **23**, 1262–1269

Kadish, A.S., Romney, S.L., Ledwidge, R., Tindle, R., Fernando, G.J.P., Zee, S.Y., Van Ranst, M.A. & Burk, R.D. (1994) Cell-mediated immune responses to E7 peptides of human papillomavirus (HPV) type 16 are dependent on the HPV type infecting the cervix whereas serological reactivity is not type-specific. *J. gen. Virol.*, **75**, 2277–2284

Kaelbling, M., Burk, R.D., Atkin, N.B., Johnson, A.B. & Klinger, H.P. (1992) Loss of heterozygosity on chromosome 17p and mutant p53 in HPV-negative cervical carcinomas. *Lancet*, **340**, 140–142

Kahn, T., Schwarz, E. & zur Hausen, H. (1986) Molecular cloning and characterization of the DNA of a new human papillomavirus (HPV 30) from a laryngeal carcinoma. *Int. J. Cancer*, **37**, 61–65

Kanda, R., Tanigaki, T., Kitano, Y., Yoshikawa, K., Yutsudo, M. & Hakura, A. (1989) Types of human papillomavirus isolated from Japanese patients with epidermodysplasia verruciformis. *Br. J. Dermatol.*, **121**, 463–469

Kanda, T., Onda, T., Zanma, S., Yasugi, T., Furuno, A., Watanabe, S., Kawana, T., Sugase, M., Ueda, K., Sonoda, T., Suzuki, S., Yamashiro, T., Yoshikawa, H. & Yoshiike, K. (1992) Independent association of antibodies against human papillomavirus type 16 E1/E4 and E7 proteins with cervical cancer. *Virology*, **190**, 724–732

Kanetsky, P.A., Mandelblatt, J., Richart, R. & Gammon, M. (1992) Risk factors for cervical cancer in a black, elderly population: preliminary findings. *Ethn. Dis.*, **2**, 337–342

Karlen, S. & Beard, P. (1993) Identification and characterization of novel promoters in the genome of human papillomavirus type 18. *J. Virol.*, **67**, 4296–4306

Karlsen, F., Rabbitts, P.H., Sundresan, V. & Hagmar, B. (1994) PCR-RFLP studies on chromosome 3p in formaldehyde-fixed, paraffin-embedded cervical cancer tissues. *Int. J. Cancer*, **58**, 787–792

Kashima, H.K., Leventhal, B., Mounts, P. & Papilloma Study Group (1985) Scoring system to assess severity and course in recurrent respiratory papillomatosis in papillomaviruses. Molecular and clinical aspects. In: Howley, P.M. & Broker, T.R., eds, *UCLA Symposia on Molecular and Cellular Biology*, Vol. 32, New York, NY, Alan R. Liss, pp. 125–136

Kashima, H.K., Wu, T.C., Mounts, P., Heffner, D., Cachay, A. & Hyams, V. (1988) Carcinoma ex-papilloma: histologic and virologic studies in whole-organ sections of the larynx. *Laryngoscope*, **98**, 619–624

Kashima, H.K., Kutcher, M., Kessis, T., Levin, L.S., de Villiers, E.-M. & Shah, K.V. (1990) Human papillomavirus in squamous cell carcinoma, leukoplakia, lichen planus, and clinically normal epithelium of the oral cavity. *Ann. Otol. Rhinol. Laryngol.*, **99**, 55–61

Kashima, H.K., Shah, F., Lyles, A., Glackin, R., Muhammad, N., Turner, L., Van Zandt, S., Whitt, S. & Shah, K.V. (1992a) A comparison of risk factors in juvenile-onset and adult-onset recurrent respiratory papillomatosis. *Laryngoscope*, **102**, 9–13

Kashima, H.K., Kessis, T., Hruban, R.H., Wu, T.C., Zinreich, S.J. & Shah, K.V. (1992b) Human papillomavirus in sinonasal papillomas and squamous cell carcinoma. *Laryngoscope*, **102**, 973–976

Kashima, H.K., Mounts, P., Leventhal, B. & Hruban, R.H. (1993) Sites of predilection in recurrent respiratory papillomatosis. *Ann. Otol. Rhinol. Laryngol.*, **102**, 580–583

Kasperbauer, J.L., O'Halloran, G.L., Espy, M.J., Smith, T.F. & Lewis, J.E. (1993) Polymerase chain reaction (PCR) identification of human papillomavirus (HPV) DNA in verrucous carcinoma of the larynx. *Laryngoscope*, **103**, 416–420

Kast, W.M., Brandt, R.M.P., Drijfhout, J.W. & Melief, C.J.M. (1993) Human leukocyte antigen-A2.1 restricted candidate cytotoxic T lymphocyte epitopes of human papillomavirus type 16 E6 and E7 proteins identified by using the processing-defective human cell line T2. *J. Immunother.*, **14**, 115–120

Kast, W.M., Brandt, R.M., Sidney, J., Drijfhout, J.W., Kubo, R.T., Grey, H.M., Melief, C.J. & Sette, A. (1994) Role of HLA-A motifs in identification of potential CTL epitopes in human papillomavirus type 16 E6 and E7 proteins. *J. Immunol.*, **152**, 3904–3912

Kataja, V., Syrjänen, K., Mäntyjärvi, R., Väyrynen, M., Syrjänen, S., Saarikoski, S., Parkkinen, S., Yliskoski, M., Salonen, J.T. & Castren, O. (1989) Prospective follow-up of cervical HPV infections: life table analysis of histopathological, cytological and colposcopic data. *Eur. J. Epidemiol.*, **5**, 1–7

Kataja, V., Syrjänen, K., Syrjänen, S., Mäntyjärvi, R., Yliskoski, M., Saarikoski, S. & Salonen, J.T. (1990) Prospective follow-up of genital HPV infections: survival analysis of the HPV typing data. *Eur. J. Epidemiol.*, **6**, 9–14

Kataoka, A. & Yakushiji, M. (1990) Detection and typing of human papillomavirus infection of uterine cervix in young women by non-isotopic subgenomic probes on Southern blot — a report of studies in Sweden. *Kurume med. J.*, **37**, 195–201

Kataoka, A., Claesson, U., Hansson, B.G., Eriksson, M. & Lindh, E. (1991) Human papillomavirus infection of the male diagnosed by Southern-blot hybridization and polymerase chain reaction: comparison between urethra samples and penile biopsy samples. *J. med. Virol.*, **33**, 159–164

Kato, N. & Ueno, H. (1992) Two cases of plantar epidermal cyst associated with human papillomavirus. *Clin. exp. Dermatol.*, **17**, 252–256

Kato, I., Santamaria, M., Alonso de Ruiz, P., Aristizabal, N., Bosch, F.X., de Sanjosé, S. & Muñoz, N. (1995) Inter-observer variation in cytological and histological diagnoses of cervical neoplasia and its epidemiologic implication. *J. clin. Epidemiol.*, **48**, 1167–1174

Kaufman, R.H., Bornstein, J., Gordon, A.N., Adam, E., Kaplan, A.L. & Adler-Storthz, K. (1987) Detection of human papillomavirus DNA in advanced epithelial ovarian carcinoma. *Gynecol. Oncol.*, **27**, 340–349

Kaufman, R.H., Bornstein, J., Adam, E., Burek, J., Tessin, B. & Adler-Storthz, K. (1988) Human papillomavirus and herpes simplex virus in vulvar squamous cell carcinoma in situ. *Am. J. Obstet. Gynecol.*, **158**, 862–871

Kaur, P. & McDougall, J.K. (1988) Characterization of primary human keratinocytes transformed by human papillomavirus type 18. *J. Virol.*, **62**, 1917–1924

Kawashima, M., Jablonska, S., Favre, M., Obalek, S., Croissant, O. & Orth, G. (1986) Characterization of a new type of human papillomavirus found in a lesion of Bowen's disease of the skin. *J. Virol.*, **57**, 688–692

Kawashima, M., Favre, M., Obalek, S., Jablonska, S. & Orth, G. (1990) Premalignant lesions and cancers of the skin in the general population: evaluation of the role of human papillomaviruses. *J. invest. Dermatol.*, **95**, 537–542

Keefe, M., Al-Ghamdi, A., Coggon, D., Maitland, N.J., Egger, P., Keefe, C.J., Carey, A. & Sanders, C.M. (1994a) Cutaneous warts in butchers. *Br. J. Dermatol.*, **130**, 9–14

Keefe, M., Al-Ghamdi, A., Coggon, D., Maitland, N.J., Egger, P., Keefe, C.J., Carey, A. & Sanders, C.M. (1994b) Butchers' warts: no evidence for person to person transmission of HPV 7. *Br. J. Dermatol.*, **130**, 15–17

Keen, N., Elston, R. & Crawford, L. (1994) Interaction of the E6 protein of human papillomavirus with cellular proteins. *Oncogene*, **9**, 1493–1499

Keijser, K.G.G., Kenemans, P., van der Zanden, P.H.T.H., Schijf, C.P.T., Vooijs, G.P. & Rolland, R. (1992) Diathermy loop excision in the management of cervical intraepithelial neoplasia: diagnosis and treatment in one procedure. *Am. J. Obstet. Gynecol.*, **166**, 1281–1287

Kennedy, I.M., Haddow, J.K. & Clements, J.B. (1991) A negative regulatory element in the human papillomavirus type 16 genome acts at the level of late mRNA stability. *J. Virol.*, **65**, 2093–2097

Kenter, G.G., Cornelisse, C.J., Jiwa, N.M., Aartsen, E.J., Hermans, J., Mooi, W., Heintz, A.P. & Fleuren, G.J. (1993) Human papillomavirus type 16 in tumor tissue of low-stage squamous carcinoma of the uterine cervix in relation to ploidy grade and prognosis. *Cancer*, **71**, 397–401

Kerley, S.W., Persons, D.L. & Fishback, J.L. (1991) Human papillomavirus and carcinoma of the urinary bladder. *Mod. Pathol.*, **4**, 316–319

Kern, S.E., Kinzler, K.W., Bruskin, A., Jarosz, D., Friedman, P., Prives, C. & Vogelstein, B. (1991) Identification of p53 as a sequence-specific DNA-binding protein. *Science*, **252**, 1708–1711

Kessis, T.D., Slebos, R.J., Nelson, W.G., Kastan, M.B., Plunkett, B.S., Han, S.M., Lörincz, A.T., Hedrick, L. & Cho, K.R. (1993a) Human papillomavirus 16 E6 expression disrupts the p53-mediated cellular response to DNA damage. *Proc. natl Acad. Sci. USA*, **90**, 3988–3992

Kessis, T.D., Slebos, R.J., Han, S.M., Shah, K., Bosch, X.F., Muñoz, N., Hedrick, L. & Cho, K.R. (1993b) p53 Gene mutations and MDM2 amplification are uncommon in primary carcinomas of the uterine cervix. *Am. J. Pathol.*, **143**, 1398–1405

Kettler, A.H., Rutledge, M., Tschen, J.A. & Buffone, G. (1990) Detection of human papillomavirus in nongenital Bowen's disease by in situ DNA hybridization. *Arch. Dermatol.*, **126**, 777–781

Kharsany, A.B.M., Hoosen, A.A., Moodley, J., Bagaratee, J. & Gouws, E. (1993) The association between sexually transmitted pathogens and cervical intra-epithelial neoplasia in a developing community. *Genitourin. Med.*, **69**, 357–360

Kienzler, J.L., Lemoine, M.T., Orth, G., Jibard, N., Blanc, D., Laurent, R. & Agache, P. (1983) Humoral and cell-mediated immunity to human papillomavirus type 1 (HPV-1) in human warts. *Br. J. Dermatol.*, **108**, 665–672

Kihana, T., Tsuda, H., Teshima, S., Nomoto, K., Tsugane, S., Sonoda, T., Matsuura, S. & Hirohashi, S. (1994) Prognostic significance of the overexpression of c-*erb*B-2 protein in adenocarcinoma of the uterine cervix. *Cancer*, **73**, 148–153

Kim, M.S., Shin, K.-H., Baek, J.-H., Cherrick, H.M. & Park, N.-H. (1993a) HPV-16, tobacco-specific N-nitrosamine, and N-methyl-N'-nitro-N-nitrosoguanidine in oral carcinogenesis. *Cancer Res.*, **53**, 4811–4816

Kim, M.S., Li, S.-L., Bertolami, C.N., Cherrick, H.M. & Park, N.-H. (1993b) State of p53, Rb and DCC tumor suppressor genes in human oral cancer cell lines. *Anticancer Res.*, **13**, 1405–1413

Kim, Y.-I., Giuliano, A., Hatch, K.D., Schneider, A., Nour, M.A., Dallal, G.E., Selhub, J. & Mason, J.B. (1994) Global DNA hypomethylation increases progressively in cervical dysplasia and carcinoma. *Cancer*, **74**, 893–899

Kinghorn, G.R., McMillan, A., Mulcahy, F., Drake, S., Lacey, C. & Bingham, J.S. (1993) An open, comparative, study of the efficacy of 0.5% podophyllotoxin lotion and 25% podophyllotoxin solution in the treatment of condylomata acuminata in males and females. *Int. J. STD AIDS*, **4**, 194–199

Kinlen, L.J., Sheil, A.G.R., Peto, J. & Doll, R. (1979) Collaborative United Kingdom-Australasian study of cancer in patients treated with immunosuppressive drugs. *Br. med. J.*, **2**, 1461–1466

Kirby, A.J., Spiegelhalter, D.J., Day, N.E., Fenton, L., Swanson, K., Mann, E.M. & Macgregor, J.E. (1992) Conservative treatment of mild/moderate cervical dyskaryosis: long-term outcome. *Lancet*, **339**, 828–831

Kirgan, D., Manalo, P. & McGregor, B. (1990a) Immunohistochemical demonstration of human papilloma virus antigen in human colon neoplasms. *J. surg. Res.*, **48**, 397–402

Kirgan, D., Manalo, P., Hall, M. & McGregor, B. (1990b) Association of human papillomavirus and colon neoplasms. *Arch. Surg.*, **125**, 862–865

Kirnbauer, R., Booy, F., Cheng, N., Lowy, D.R. & Schiller, J.T. (1992) Papillomavirus L1 major capsid protein self-assembles into virus-like particles that are highly immunogenic. *Proc. natl Acad. Sci. USA*, **89**, 12180–12184

Kirnbauer, R., Taub, J., Greenstone, H., Roden, R., Dürst, M., Gissmann, L., Lowy, D.R. & Schiller, J.T. (1993) Efficient self-assembly of human papillomavirus type 16 L1 and L1-L2 into virus-like particles. *J. Virol.*, **67**, 6929–6936

Kirnbauer, R., Hubbert, N.L., Wheeler, C.M., Becker, T.M., Lowy, D.R. & Schiller, J.T. (1994) A virus-like particle enzyme-linked immunosorbent assay detects serum antibodies in a majority of women infected with human papillomavirus type 16. *J. natl Cancer Inst.*, **86**, 494–499

Kitamura, T., Yogo, Y., Ueki, T., Murakami, S. & Aso, Y. (1988) Presence of human papillomavirus type 16 genome in bladder carcinoma in situ of a patient with mild immunodeficiency. *Cancer Res.*, **48**, 7207–7211

Kitasato, H., Delius, H., zur Hausen, H., Sorger, K., Rösl, F. & de Villiers, E.-M. (1994) Sequence rearrangements in the upstream regulatory region of human papillomavirus type 6: are these involved in malignant transition? *J. gen. Virol.*, **75**, 1157–1162

Kiviat, N.B. & Koutsky, L.A. (1993) Specific human papillomavirus types as the causal agents of most cervical intraepithelial neoplasia: implications for current views and treatment. *J. natl Cancer Inst.*, **85**, 934–935

Kiviat, N.B., Koutsky, L.A., Paavonen, J.A., Galloway, D.A., Critchlow, C.W., Beckmann, A.M., McDougall, J.K., Peterson, M.L., Stevens, C.E., Lipinski, C.M. & Holmes, K.K. (1989) Prevalence of genital papillomavirus infection among women attending a college student health clinic or a sexually transmitted disease clinic. *J. infect. Dis.*, **159**, 293–302

Kiviat, N.B., Rompalo, A., Bowden, R., Galloway, D., Holmes, K.K., Corey, L., Roberts, P.L. & Stamm, W.E. (1990) Anal human papillomavirus infection among human immunodeficiency virus-seropositive and -seronegative men. *J. infect. Dis.*, **162**, 358–361

Kiviat, N.B., Critchlow, C.W. & Kurman, R.J. (1992) Reassessment of the morphological continuum of cervical intraepithelial lesions: does it reflect different stages in the progression to cervical carcinoma? In: Muñoz, N., Bosch, F.X., Shah, K.V. & Meheus, A., eds, *The Epidemiology of Cervical Cancer and Human Papillomavirus* (IARC Scientific Publications No. 119), Lyon, IARC, pp. 59–66

Kiviat, N.B., Critchlow, C.W., Holmes, K.K., Kuypers, J., Sayer, J., Dunphy, C., Surawicz, C., Kirby, P., Wood, R. & Daling, J.R. (1993) Association of anal dysplasia and human papillomavirus with immunosuppression and HIV infection among homosexual men. *AIDS*, **7**, 43–49

Kiyabu, M.T., Shibata, D., Arnheim, N., Martin, W.J. & Fitzgibbons, P.L. (1989) Detection of human papillomavirus in formalin-fixed, invasive squamous carcinomas using the polymerase chain reaction. *Am. J. surg. Pathol.*, **13**, 221–224

Kjaer, S.K. & Lynge, E. (1989) Incidence, prevalence and time trends of genital HPV infection determined by clinical examination and cytology. In: Muñoz, N., Bosch, F.X., Shah, K.V. & Meheus, A., eds, *The Epidemiology of Cervical Cancer and Human* Papillomavirus (IARC Scientific Publications No. 119), Lyon, IARC, pp. 113–124

Kjaer, S.K., de Villiers, E.-M., Haugaard, B.J., Christensen, R.B., Teisen, C., Møller, K.A., Poll, P., Jensen, H., Vestergaard, B.F., Lynge, E. & Jensen, O.M. (1988) Human papillomavirus, herpes simplex virus and cervical cancer incidence in Greenland and Denmark. A population-based cross-sectional study. *Int. J. Cancer*, **41**, 518–524

Kjaer, S.K., de Villiers, E.-M., Dahl, C., Engholm, G., Bock, J.E., Vestergaard, B.F., Lynge, E. & Jensen, O.M. (1991) Case–control study of risk factors for cervical neoplasia in Denmark. I: Role of the 'male factor' in women with one lifetime sexual partner. *Int. J. Cancer*, **48**, 39–44

Kjaer, S.K., Dahl, C., Engholm, G., Bock, J.E., Lynge, E. & Jensen, O.M. (1992) Case–control study of risk factors for cervical neoplasia in Denmark. II: Role of sexual activity, reproductive factors, and venereal infections. *Cancer Causes Control*, **3**, 339–348

Kjaer, S.K., de Villiers, E.-M., Caglayan, H., Svare, E., Haugaard, B.J., Engholm, G., Christensen, R.B., Møller, K.A., Poll, P., Jensen, H., Vestergaard, B.F., Lynge, E. & Jensen, O.M. (1993) Human papillomavirus, herpes simplex virus and other potential risk factors for cervical cancer in a high-risk area (Greenland) and a low-risk area (Denmark) — a second look. *Br. J. Cancer*, **67**, 830–837

Klein, R.S., Ho, G.Y., Vermund, S.H., Fleming, I. & Burk, R.D. (1994) Risk factors for squamous intraepithelial lesions on Pap smear in women at risk for human immunodeficiency virus infection. *J. infect. Dis.*, **170**, 1404–1409

Kleine, K., König, G., Kreuzer, J., Komitowski, D., zur Hausen, H. & Rösl, F. (1995) Expression of the JE (MCP-1) gene encoding the monocyte chemoattractant protein-1 results in partial tumor suppression of HeLa cells in nude mice. *Mol. Carcinog.* (in press)

Klemi, P.J., Joensuu, H., Siivonen, L., Virolainen, E., Syrjänen, S. & Syrjänen, K. (1989) Association of DNA aneuploidy with human papillomavirus-induced malignant transformation of sinonasal transitional papillomas. *Otolaryngol. Head Neck Surg.*, **100**, 563–567

Klingelhutz, A.J., Smith, P.P., Garrett, L.R. & McDougall, J.K. (1993) Alteration of the DCC tumor-suppressor gene in tumorigenic HPV-18 immortalized human keratinocytes transformed by nitrosomethylurea. *Oncogene*, **8**, 95–99

Kloster, B.E., Manias, D.A., Ostrow, R.S., Shaver, M.K., McPherson, S.W., Rangen, S.R.S., Uno, H. & Faras, A.J. (1988) Molecular cloning and characterization of the DNA of two papillomaviruses from monkeys. *Virology*, **166**, 30–40

Klug, A. & Finch, J.T. (1965) Structure of viruses of the papilloma-polyoma type 1. I. Human wart virus. *J. mol. Biol.*, **11**, 403–423

von Knebel-Doeberitz, M., Oltersdorf, T., Schwarz, E. & Gissmann, L. (1988) Correlation of modified human papillomavirus early gene expression with altered growth properties in C4-1 cervical carcinoma cells. *Cancer Res.*, **48**, 3780–3786

von Knebel-Doeberitz, M., Bauknecht, T., Bartsch, D. & zur Hausen, H. (1991) Influence of chromosomal integration on glucocorticoid-regulated transcription of growth-stimulating papillomavirus genes E6 and E7 in cervical carcinoma cells. *Proc. natl Acad. Sci. USA*, **88**, 1411–1415

von Knebel-Doeberitz, M., Rittmüller, C., zur Hausen, H. & Dürst, M. (1992) Inhibition of tumorigenicity of cervical cancer cells in nude mice by HPV E6-E7 anti-sense RNA (Letter to the Editor). *Int. J. Cancer*, **51**, 831–834

von Knebel-Doeberitz, M., Rittmüller, C., Aengeneyndt, F., Jansen-Dürr, P. & Spitkovsky, D. (1994) Reversible repression of papillomavirus oncogene expression in cervical carcinoma cells: consequences for the phenotype and E6-p53 and E7-pRB interactions. *J. Virol.*, **68**, 2811–2821

Knobler, R.M., Schneider, S., Neumann, R.A., Bodemer, W., Radlwimmer, B., Aberer, E., Söltz-Szöts, J. & Gebhart, W. (1989) DNA dot-blot hybridization implicates human papillomavirus type 11-DNA in epithelioma cuniculatum. *J. med. Virol.*, **29**, 33–37

Knowles, M.A. (1992) Human papillomavirus sequences are not detectable by Southern blotting or general primer-mediated polymerase chain reaction in transitional cell tumours of the bladder. *Urol. Res.*, **20**, 297–301

Köchel, H.G., Monazahian, M., Sievert, K., Höhne, M., Thomssen, C., Teichmann, A., Arendt, P. & Thomssen, R. (1991) Occurrence of antibodies to L1, L2, E4 and E7 gene products of human papillomavirus types 6b, 16 and 18 among cervical cancer patients and controls. *Int. J. Cancer*, **48**, 682–688

Kock, K.F. & Johansen, P. (1987) Prevalence of condylomatous atypia and human papilloma virus antigen in cervical biopsies in 1972 and 1983. *Acta obstet. gynecol. scand.*, **66**, 111–115

Koi, M., Morita, H., Yamada, H., Satoh, H., Barrett, J.C. & Oshimura, M. (1989) Normal human chromosome 11 suppresses tumorigenicity of human cervical tumor cell line SiHa. *Mol. Carcinog.*, **2**, 12–21

Komly, C.A., Breitburd, F., Croissant, O. & Streeck, R.E. (1986) The L2 open reading frame of human papillomavirus type 1a encodes a minor structural protein carrying type-specific antigens. *J. Virol.*, **60**, 813–816

Kondoh, G., Murata, Y., Aozasa, K., Yutsudo, M. & Hakura, A. (1991) Very high incidence of germ cell tumorigenesis (seminomagenesis) in human papillomavirus type 16 transgenic mice. *J. Virol.*, **65**, 3335–3339

Koss, L.G. (1992) *Diagnostic Cytology and Its Histopathologic Bases*, 4th Ed., Philadelphia, J.B. Lippincott Co.

Koss, L.G. & Durfee, G.R. (1955) Cytological changes preceding the appearance of in situ carcinoma of the uterine cervix. *Cancer*, **8**, 295–301

Kottmeier, H.L. (1961) Evolution and treatment of epitheliomas. *Rev. fr. Gynécol. Obstét.*, **56**, 821–826 (in French)

Koulos, J., Symmans, F., Chumas, J. & Nuovo, G. (1991) Human papillomavirus detection in adenocarcinoma of the anus. *Mod. Pathol.*, **4**, 58–61

Koutsky, L.A. & Kiviat, N.B. (1993) Genital infectious agents and invasive cervical cancer (Letter to the Editor). *Lancet*, **342**, 184–185

Koutsky, L.A., Galloway, D.A. & Holmes, K.K. (1988) Epidemiology of genital human papillomavirus infection. *Epidemiol. Rev.*, **10**, 122–163

Koutsky, L.A., Holmes, K.K., Critchlow, C.W., Stevens, C.E., Paavonen, J., Beckmann, A.M., DeRouen, T.A., Galloway, D.A., Vernon, D. & Kiviat, N.B. (1992) A cohort study of the risk of cervical intraepithelial neoplasia grade 2 or 3 in relation to papillomavirus infection. *N. Engl. J. Med.*, **327**, 1272–1278

Krchnák, V., Vágner, J., Suchánková, A., Krcmár, M., Ritterová, L. & Vonka, V. (1990) Synthetic peptides derived from E7 region of human papillomavirus type 16 used as antigens in ELISA. *J. gen. Virol.*, **71**, 2719–2724

Krchnák, V., Pistek, T., Vágner, J., Suchánková, A., Kanka, J., Ritterová, L. & Vonka, V. (1993) Identification of seroreactive epitopes of human papillomavirus type 18 E7 protein by synthetic peptides. *Acta virol.*, **37**, 395–402

Krebs, H.-B. (1991) Treatment of genital condylomata with topical 5-fluorouracil. *Dermatol. Clin.*, **9**, 333–341

Krebs, H.-B. & Helmkamp, B.F. (1991) Chronic ulcerations following topical therapy with 5-fluorouracil for vaginal human papillomavirus-associated lesions. *Obstet. Gynecol.*, **78**, 205–208

Kreider, J.W. (1980) Neoplastic progression of the Shope rabbit papilloma. In: Essex, M., Todaro, G. & zur Hausen, H., eds, *Viruses in Naturally Occurring Cancers*, Cold Spring Harbor, CSH Press, pp. 283–299

Kreider, J.W., Howett, M.K., Lill, N.L., Bartlett, G.L., Zaino, R.J., Sedlacek, T.V. & Martel, R. (1986) In vivo transformation of human skin with human papillomavirus type 11 from condylomata acuminata. *J. Virol.*, **59**, 369–376

Kreiss, J.K., Kiviat, N.B., Plummer, F.A., Roberts, P.L., Waiyaki, P., Ngugi, E. & Holmes, K.K. (1992) Human immunodeficiency virus, human papillomavirus, and cervical intraepithelial neoplasia in Nairobi prostitutes. *Sex. transm. Dis.*, **19**, 54–59

Kremsdorf, D., Favre, M., Jablonska, S., Obalek, S., Rueda, L.A., Lutzner, M.A., Blanchet-Bardon, C., van Voorst Vader, P.C. & Orth, G. (1984) Molecular cloning and characterization of the genomes of nine newly recognized human papillomavirus types associated with epidermodysplasia verruciformis. *J. Virol.*, **52**, 1013–1018

Kripke, M.L. & Morison, W.L. (1985) Modulation of immune function by UV radiation. *J. invest. Dermatol.*, **85** (Suppl. 1), S62–S66

Kristiansen, E., Jenkins, A., Kristensen, G., Ask, E., Kaern, J., Abeler, V., Lindqvist, B.H., Trope, C. & Kristiansen, B.E. (1994a) Human papillomavirus infection in Norwegian women with cervical cancer. *Acta pathol. microbiol. immunol. scand.*, **102**, 122–128

Kristiansen, E., Jenkins, A. & Holm, R. (1994b) Coexistence of episomal and integrated HPV16 DNA in squamous cell carcinoma of the cervix. *J. clin. Pathol.*, **47**, 253–256 von Krogh, G. (1981) Podophyllotoxin for condylomata acuminata eradication. Clinical and experimental comparative studies on Podophyllum lignans, colchicine and 5-fluorouracil. *Acta derm. venereol. (Stockh.)*, **Suppl. 98**, 1–48

Krone, M.R., Kiviat, N.B. & Koutsky, L.A. (1995) The epidemiology of cervical neoplasia. In: Jordan, J., Richart, R. & Luesley, D., eds, *Intraepithelial Neoplasia of the Female Lower Genital Tract*, Edinburgh, Churchill Livingston (in press)

Kulski, J.K., Howard, M.J. & Pixley, E.C. (1987) DNA sequences of human papillomavirus types 11, 16 or 18 in invasive cervical carcinoma of Western Australian women. *Immunol. Cell Biol.*, **65**, 77–84

Kulski, J.K., Demeter, T., Rakoczy, P., Sterrett, G.F. & Pixley, E.C. (1989) Human papillomavirus coinfections of the vulva and uterine cervix. *J. med. Virol.*, **27**, 244–251

Kulski, J.K., Demeter, T., Mutavdzic, S., Sterrett, G.F., Mitchell, K.M. & Pixley, E.C. (1990) Survey of histologic specimens of human cancer for human papillomavirus types 6/11/16/18 by filter in situ hybridization. *Am. J. clin. Pathol.*, **94**, 566–570

Kurman, R.J., Schiffman, M.H., Lancaster, W.D., Reid, R., Jenson, A.B., Temple, G.F. & Lörincz, A.T. (1988) Analysis of individual human papillomavirus types in cervical neoplasia: a possible role for type 18 in rapid progression. *Am. J. Obstet. Gynecol.*, **159**, 293–296

Kurman, R.J,. Henson, D.E., Herbst, A.L., Noller, K.L. & Schiffman, M.H. for the 1992 National Cancer Institute Workshop (1994) Interim guidelines for the management of abnormal cervical cytology. *J. Am. med. Assoc.*, **271**, 1866–1869

Kurvinen, K., Tervahauta, A., Syrjänen, S., Chang, F. & Syrjänen, K. (1994) The state of the p53 gene in human papillomavirus (HPV)-positive and HPV-negative genital precancer lesions and carcinomas as detected by single strand conformation polymorphism analysis and sequencing. *Anticancer Res.*, **14**, 177–181

Labropoulou, V., Balamotis, A., Tosca, A., Rotola, A. & Mavromara-Nazos, P. (1994) Typing of human papillomaviruses in condylomata acuminata from Greece. *J. med. Virol.*, **42**, 259–263

Lacey, M., Alpert, S. & Hanahan, D. (1986) Bovine papillomavirus genome elicits skin tumours in transgenic mice. *Nature*, **322**, 609–612

Laga, M., Icenogle, J.P., Marsella, R., Manoka, A.T., Nzila, N., Ryder, R.W., Vermund, S.H., Heyward, W.L., Nelson, A. & Reeves, W.C. (1992) Genital papillomavirus infection and cervical dysplasia — opportunistic complications of HIV infection. *Int. J. Cancer*, **50**, 45–48

Lai, C.-H., Wang, C.-Y., Lin, C.-Y. & Pao, C.C. (1994) Detection of human papillomavirus RNA in ovarian and endometrial carcinomas by reverse transcription/polymerase chain reaction. *Gynecol. obstet. Invest.*, **38**, 276–280

Lam, E.W., Morris, J.D., Davies, R., Crook, T., Watson, R.J. & Vousden, K.H. (1994) HPV16 E7 oncoprotein deregulates B-*myb* expression: correlation with targeting of p107/E2F complexes. *EMBO J.*, **13**, 871–878

Lambert, P.F. (1991) Minireview. Papillomavirus DNA replication. *J. Virol.*, **65**, 3417–3420

Lambert, P.F., Baker, C.C. & Howley, P.M. (1988) The genetics of bovine papillomavirus type 1. *Annu. Rev. Genet.*, **22**, 235–258

Lambert, P.F., Pan, H., Pitot, H.C., Liem, A., Jackson, M. & Griep, A.E. (1993) Epidermal cancer associated with expression of human papillomavirus type 16 E6 and E7 oncogenes in the skin of transgenic mice. *Proc. natl Acad. Sci. USA*, **90**, 5583–5587

Lamberti, C., Morrissey, L.C., Grossman, S.R. & Androphy, E.J. (1990) Transcriptional activation by the papillomavirus E6 zinc finger oncoprotein. *EMBO J.*, **9**, 1907–1913

Lambropoulos, A.F., Agorastos, T., Frangoulides, R., Karahaliou, R., Bontis, J. & Dozi-Vassiliades, I. (1994) Detection of human papillomavirus using the polymerase chain reaction and typing for HPV 16 and 18 in the cervical smears of Greek women. *J. med. Virol.*, **43**, 228–230

Lancaster, W.D. & Olson, C. (1978) Demonstration of two distinct classes of bovine papilloma virus. *Virology*, **89**, 372–379

Lancaster, W.D., Olson, C. & Meinke, W. (1977) Bovine papilloma virus: presence of virus-specific DNA sequences in naturally occurring equine tumors. *Proc. natl Acad. Sci. USA*, **74**, 524–528

Lane, D.P. (1992) Cancer: p53, guardian of the genome. *Nature*, **358**, 15–16

Lane, D.P. & Crawford, L.V. (1979) T-antigen is bound to a host protein in SV40-transformed cells. *Nature*, **278**, 261–263

Lass, J.H., Grove, A.S., Papale, J.J., Albert, D.M., Jenson, A.B. & Lancaster, W.D. (1983) Detection of human papillomavirus DNA sequences in conjunctival papilloma. *Am. J. Ophthalmol.*, **96**, 670–674

Lauer, S.A., Malter, J.S. & Meier, J.R. (1990) Human papillomavirus type 18 in conjunctival intraepithelial neoplasia. *Am. J. Ophthalmol.*, **110**, 23–27

Laurent, S., Frances, V. & Bastin, M. (1995) Intrachromosomal recombination mediated by the polyomavirus large T antigen. *Virology*, **206**, 227–233

Lavi, S. (1982) Carcinogen-mediated amplification of specific DNA sequences. *J. cell. Biochem.*, **18**, 149–156

Law, C.L., Qassim, M., Thompson, C.H., Rose, B.R., Grace, J., Morris, B.J. & Cossart, Y.E. (1991) Factors associated with clinical and sub-clinical anal human papillomavirus infection in homosexual men. *Genitourin. Med.*, **67**, 92–98

Lawlor, G.J., Jr, Ammann, A.J., Wright, W.C., Jr., La Franchi, S.H., Bilstrom, D. & Stiehm, E.R. (1974) The syndrome of cellular immunodeficiency with immunoglobulins. *J. Pediatr.*, **84**, 183–192

Leake, J.F., Woodruff, J.D., Searle, C., Daniel, R., Shah, K.V. & Currie, J.L. (1989) Human papillomavirus and epithelial ovarian neoplasia. *Gynecol. Oncol.*, **34**, 268–273

Le Cann, P., Coursaget, P., Iochmann, S. & Touze, A. (1994) Self-assembly of human papillomavirus type 16 capsids by expression of the L1 protein in insect cells. *FEMS Microbiol. Lett.*, **117**, 269–274

Lechner, M.S., Mack, D.H., Finicle, A.B., Crook, T., Vousden, K.H. & Laimins, L.A. (1992) Human papillomavirus E6 proteins bind p53 *in vivo* and abrogate p53-mediated repression of transcription. *EMBO J.*, **11**, 3045–3052

Lee, K.R., Howard, P., Heintz, N.H. & Collins, C.C. (1993) Low prevalence of human papillomavirus types 16 and 18 in cervical adenocarcinoma *in situ*, invasive adenocarcinoma, and glandular dysplasia by polymerase chain reaction. *Mod. Pathol.*, **6**, 433–437

Lee, Y.Y., Wilczynski, S.P., Chumakov, A., Chih, D. & Koeffler, H.P. (1994) Carcinoma of the vulva: HPV and p53 mutations. *Oncogene*, **9**, 1655–1659

Leechanachai, P., Banks, L., Moreau, F. & Matlashewski, G. (1992) The E5 gene from human papillomavirus type 16 is an oncogene which enhances growth factor-mediated signal transduction to the nucleus. *Oncogene*, **7**, 19–25

Lehn, H., Ernst, T.M. & Sauer, G. (1984) Transcription of episomal papillomavirus DNA in human condylomata acuminata and Burke-Loewentein tumor. *J. gen. Virol.*, **65**, 2003–2010

Lehn, H., Villa, L.L., Marziona, F., Hilgarth, M., Hillemans, H.G. & Sauer, G. (1988) Physical state and biological activity of human papillomavirus genomes in precancerous lesions of the female genital tract. *J. gen. Virol.*, **69**, 187–196

Lehtinen, M., Parkkonen, P., Niemelä, J. & Paavonen, J. (1990) Demonstration of evolutionary differences between conserved antigenic epitopes in the minor nucleocapsid protein of human papillomavirus types 6b, 16 and 18. *Biochem. biophys. Res. Commun.*, **172**, 1378–1383

Lehtinen, M., Leminen, A., Kuoppala, T., Tiikkainen, M., Lehtinen, T., Lehtovirta, P., Punnonen, R., Vesterinen, E. & Paavonen, J. (1992) Pre- and posttreatment serum antibody responses to HPV 16 E2 and HSV 2 ICP8 proteins in women with cervical carcinoma. *J. med. Virol.*, **37**, 180–186

Leminen, A., Paavonen, J., Vesterinen, E., Wahlström, T., Rantala, I. & Lehtinen, M. (1991) Human papillomavirus types 16 and 18 in adenocarcinoma of the uterine cervix. *Am. J. clin. Pathol.*, **95**, 647–652

Leonardi, C.L., Zhu, W.Y., Kinsey, W.H. & Penneys, N.S. (1991a) Trichilemmomas are not associated with HPV DNA. *J. cutan. Pathol.*, **18**, 193–197

Leonardi, C.L., Zhu, W.Y., Kinsey, W.H. & Penneys, N.S. (1991b) Epidermolytic acanthoma does not contain HPV DNA. *J. cutan. Pathol.*, **18**, 103–105

Leventhal, B.G., Kashima, H.K., Weck, P.W., Mounts, P., Whisnant, J.K., Clark, K.L., Cohen, S., Dedo, H.H., Donovan, D.J., Fearon, B.W., Gardiner, L.J., Lusk, R.P., Muntz, H.R., Richardson, M.A., Singleton, G.T., Yonkers, A.J. & Wold, D. (1988) Randomized surgical adjuvant trial of interferon alfa-n1 in recurrent papillomatosis. *Arch. Otolaryngol. Head Neck Surg.*, **114**, 1163–1169

Levine, A.J., Harper, J., Hilborne, L., Rosenthal, D.L., Weismeier, E. & Haile, R.W. (1993) HPV DNA and the risk of squamous intraepithelial lesions of the uterine cervix in young women. *Am. J. clin. Pathol.*, **100**, 6–11

Lewandowsky, F. & Lutz, W. (1922) One case of skin cancer undescribed until now (epidermodysplasia verruciformis). *Arch. Dermatol. Syphilol.*, **141**, 193–203 (in German)

Lewensohn-Fuchs, I., Wester, D., Bistoletti, P., Elfgren, K., Ohlman, S., Dillner, J. & Dalianis, T. (1993) Serological responses to human papillomavirus type 16 antigens in women before and after renal transplantation. *J. med. Virol.*, **40**, 188–192

Ley, C., Bauer, H.M., Reingold, A., Schiffman, M.H., Chambers, J.C., Tashiro, C.J. & Manos, M.M. (1991) Determinants of genital human papillomavirus infection in young women. *J. natl Cancer Inst.*, **83**, 997–1003

Li, J.-Y., Li, F.P., Blot, W.J., Miller, R.W. & Fraumeni, J.F., Jr (1982) Correlation between cancers of the uterine cervix and penis in China. *J. natl Cancer Inst.*, **69**, 1063–1065

Li, C.C.H., Shah, K.V., Seth, A. & Gilden, R.V. (1987) Identification of the human papillomavirus type 6b L1 open reading frame protein in condylomata and corresponding antibodies in human sera. *J. Virol.*, **61**, 2684–2690

Li, S.-L., Kim, M.S., Cherrick, H.M., Doniger, J. & Park, N.-H. (1992) Sequential combined tumorigenic effect of HPV-16 and chemical carcinogens. *Carcinogenesis*, **13**, 1981–1987

Liaw, K.-L., Hsing, A.W., Chen, C.-J., Schiffman, M.H., Zhang, T.Y., Hsieh, C.-Y., Greer, C.E., You, S.-L., Huang, T.W., Wu, T.-C., O'Leary, T.J., Seidman, J., Blot, W.J., Meinert, C.L. & Manos, M.M. (1995) Human papillomavirus and cervical neoplasia: a case–control study in Taiwan. *Int. J. Cancer*, **62**, 565–571

Lichy, J.H., Modi, W.S., Seuanez, H.N. & Howley, P.M. (1992) Identification of a human chromosome 11 gene which is differentially regulated in tumorigenic and nontumorigenic somatic cell hybrids of HeLa cells. *Cell Growth Differ.*, **3**, 541–548

Lim, P.S., Jenson, A.B., Cowsert, L., Nakai, Y., Lim, L.Y., Jin, X.W. & Sundberg, J.P. (1990) Distribution and specific identification of papillomavirus major capsid protein epitopes by immunocytochemistry and epitope scanning of synthetic peptides. *J. infect. Dis.*, **162**, 1263–1269

Lim-Tan, S.K., Yoshikawa, H., Sng, I.T.Y., de Villiers, E.-M., zur Hausen, H., Ho, T.H. & Yoong, T. (1988) Human papillomavirus in dysplasia and carcinoma of the cervix in Singapore. *Pathology*, **20**, 317–319

Lin, Y.-L., Borenstein, L.A., Selvakumar, R., Ahmed, R. & Wettstein, F.O. (1992) Effective vaccination against papilloma development by immunization with L1 or L2 structural protein of cottontail rabbit papillomavirus. *Virology*, **187**, 612–619

Lin, Y.-L., Borenstein, L.A., Ahmed, R. & Wettstein, F.O. (1993) Cottontail rabbit papillomavirus L1 protein-based vaccines: protection is achieved only with a full-length, nondenatured product. *J. Virol.*, **67**, 4154–4162

Lindeberg, H. & Elbrønd, O. (1991) Malignant tumours in patients with a history of multiple laryngeal papillomas: the significance of irradiation. *Clin. Otolaryngol.*, **16**, 149–151

Lindh, E., Chua, K.-L., Kataoka, A., Bistoletti, P., Groff, D. & Hjerpe, A. (1992) Detection of human papillomavirus (HPV) using dot blot and Southern blot, hybridizing with a mixture of seven probes. *Acta pathol. microbiol. immunol. scand.*, **100**, 301–308

Lindholm, I., Murphy, J., O'Neil, B.W., Campo, M.S. & Jarrett, W.F.H. (1984) Papillomas of the teats and udder of cattle and their causal viruses. *Vet. Rec.*, **115**, 574–577

Linzer, D.I.H. & Levine, A.J. (1979) Characterization of a 54K dalton cellular SV40 tumor antigen present in SV40-transformed cells and uninfected embryonal carcinoma cells. *Cell*, **17**, 43–52

Lippman, S.M., Donovan, D.T., Frankenthaler, R.A., Weber, R.S., Earley, C.L., Hong, W.K. & Goepfert, H. (1994) 13-*cis*-Retinoic acid plus interferon-α2a in recurrent respiratory papillomatosis. *J. natl Cancer Inst.*, **86**, 859–861

Livingstone, L.R., White, A., Sprouse, J., Livanos, E., Jacks, T. & Tlsty, T.D. (1992) Altered cell cycle arrest and gene amplification potential accompany loss of wild-type p53. *Cell*, **70**, 923–935

Lo, K.-W., Mok, C.-H., Chung, G., Huang, D.P., Wong, F., Chan, M., Lee, J.C.K. & Tsao, S.-W. (1992) Presence of p53 mutations in human cervical carcinomas associated with HPV-33 infection. *Anticancer Res.*, **12**, 1989–1994

Loke, S.L., Ma, L., Wong, M., Srivastava, G., Lo, I. & Bird, C.C. (1990) Human papillomavirus in oesophageal squamous cell carcinoma. *J. clin. Pathol.*, **43**, 909–912

Löning, T., Riviere, A., Henke, R.-P., von Preyss, S. & Dörner, A. (1988) Penile/anal condylomas and squamous cell cancer: a HPV DNA hybridization study. *Virchows Arch. A*, **413**, 491–498

Lookingbill, D.P., Kreider, J.W., Howett, M.K., Olmstead, P.M. & Conner, G.H. (1987) Human papillomavirus type 16 in bowenoid papulosis, intraoral papillomas, and squamous cell carcinoma of the tongue. *Arch. Dermatol.*, **123**, 363–368

Lopes, A., Morgan, P., Murdoch, J., Piura, B. & Monaghan, J.M. (1993) The case for conservative management of 'incomplete excision' of CIN after laser conization. *Gynecol. Oncol.*, **49**, 247–249

Lörincz, A.T., Temple, G.F., Kurman, R.J., Jenson, A.B. & Lancaster, W.D. (1987) Oncogenic association of specific human papillomavirus types with cervical neoplasia. *J. natl Cancer Inst.*, **79**, 671–677

Lörincz, A.T., Schiffman, M.H., Jaffurs, W.J., Marlow, J., Quinn, A.P. & Temple, G.F. (1990) Temporal associations of human papillomavirus infection with cervical cytologic abnormalities. *Am. J. Obstet. Gynecol.*, **162**, 645–651

Lörincz, A.T., Reid, R., Jenson, A.B., Greenberg, M.D., Lancaster, W. & Kurman, R.J. (1992) Human papillomavirus infection of the cervix: relative risk associations of 15 common anogenital types. *Obstet. Gynecol.*, **79**, 328–337

Low, S.-H., Thong, T.-W., Ho, T.-H., Lee, Y.-S., Morita, T., Singh, M., Yap, E.-H. & Chan, Y.-C. (1990) Prevalence of human papillomavirus types 16 and 18 in cervical carcinomas: a study by dot and Southern blot hybridization and the polymerase chain reaction. *Jpn J. Cancer Res.*, **81**, 1118–1123

Lu, J.Z.-J., Sun, Y.-N., Rose, R.C., Bonnez, W. & McCance, D.J. (1993) Two E2 binding sites (E2BS) alone or one E2BS plus an A/T-rich region are minimal requirements for the replication of the human papillomavirus type 11 origin. *J. Virol.*, **67**, 7131–7139

Luesley, D.M., Jordan, J.A., Woodman, C.B.J. *et al.* (1987) A retrospective review of adenocarcinoma-in-situ and glandular atypia of the uterine cervix. *Br. J. Obstet. Gynaecol.*, **94**, 699–703

Luesley, D.M., Cullimore, J., Redman, C.W.E., Lawton, F.G., Emens, J.M., Rollason, T.P., Williams, D.R. & Buxton, E.J. (1990) Loop diathermy excision of the cervical transformation zone in patients with abnormal cervical smears. *Br. med. J.*, **300**, 1690–1693

Luff, R.D. (1992) The Bethesda System for reporting cervical/vaginal cytologic diagnoses: report of the 1991 Bethesda Workshop. *Hum. Pathol.*, **23**, 719–721

Lungu, O., Sun, X.W., Felix, J,. Richart, R.M., Silverstein, S. & Wright, T.C., Jr (1992) Relationship of human papillomavirus type to grade of cervical intraepithelial neoplasia. *J. Am. med. Assoc.*, **267**, 2493–2496

Lungu, O., Sun, X.W., Wright, T.C., Jr, Ferenczy, A., Richart, R.M. & Silverstein, S. (1995) A polymerase chain reaction-enzyme-linked immunosorbent assay method for detecting human papillomavirus in cervical carcinomas and high-grade cervical cancer precursors. *Obstet. Gynecol.*, **85**, 337–341

Luthi, T.E. & Burk, R.D. (1993) Human papillomavirus and cervical intraepithelial neoplasia (Letter to the Editor). *J. natl Cancer Inst.*, **85**, 1868

Lutzner, M.A. (1978) Epidermodysplasia verruciformis. An autosomal recessive disease characterised by viral warts and skin cancer. A model for viral oncogenesis. *Bull. Cancer (Paris)*, **65**, 169–182

Lutzner, M.A. (1985) Papillomavirus lesions in immunodepression and immunosuppression. *Clin. Dermatol.*, **3**, 165–169

Lutzner, M.A. & Blanchet-Bardon, C. (1985) Epidermodysplasia verucciformis. *Curr. Probl. Dermatol.*, **13**, 164–185

Lutzner, M.A., Orth, G., Dutronquay, V., Ducasse, M.-F., Kreis, H. & Crosnier, J. (1983) Detection of human papillomavirus type 5 DNA in skin cancers of an immunosuppressed renal allograft recipient. *Lancet*, **ii**, 422–424

Lutzner, M.A., Blanchet-Bardon, C. & Orth, G. (1984) Clinical observations, virologic studies and treatment trials in patients with epidermodysplasia verruciformis, a disease induced by specific human papillomaviruses. *J. invest. Dermatol.*, **83**, S18–S25

MacLean, A.B., Lynn, K.L., Bailey, R.R., Swainson, C.P. & Walker, R.J. (1986) Colposcopic assessment of the lower genital tract in female renal transplant recipients. *Clin. Nephrol.*, **26**, 45–47

Macnab, J.C., Walkinshaw, S.A., Cordiner, J.W. & Clements, J.B. (1986) Human papillomavirus in clinically and histologically normal tissue of patients with genital cancer. *N. Engl. J. Med.*, **315**, 1052–1058

Maden, C., Beckmann, A.M., Thomas, D.B., McKnight, B., Sherman, K.J., Ashley, R.L., Corey, L. & Daling, J.R. (1992) Human papillomaviruses, herpes simplex viruses, and the risk of oral cancer in men. *Am. J. Epidemiol.*, **135**, 1093–1102

Maden, C., Sherman, K.J., Beckmann, A.M., Hislop, T.G., Teh, C.-Z., Ashley, R.L. & Daling, J.R. (1993) History of circumcision, medical conditions, and sexual activity and risk of penile cancer. *J. natl Cancer Inst.*, **85**, 19–24

Madreperla, S.A., Green, W.R., Daniel, R. & Shah, K.V. (1993) Human papillomavirus in primary epithelial tumors of the lacrimal sac. *Ophthalmology*, **100**, 569–573

Magee, K.L., Rapini, R.P., Duvic, M. & Adler-Storthz, K. (1989) Human papillomavirus associated with keratoacanthoma (Letter to the Editor). *Arch. Dermatol.*, **125**, 1587–1589

Maggwa, B.N., Hunter, D.J., Mbugua, S., Tukei, P. & Mati, J.K. (1993) The relationship between HIV infection and cervical intraepithelial neoplasia among women attending two family planning clinics in Nairobi, Kenya. *AIDS*, **7**, 733–738

Maiman, M., Tarricone, N., Vieira, J., Suarez, J., Serur, E. & Boyce, J.G. (1991) Colposcopic evaluation of human immunodeficiency virus-seropositive women. *Obstet. Gynecol.*, **78**, 84–88

Maiman, M., Fruchter, R.G., Serur, E., Levine, P.A., Arrastia, C.D. & Sedlis, A. (1993) Recurrent cervical intraepithelial neoplasia in human immunodeficiency virus-seropositive women. *Obstet. Gynecol.*, **82**, 170–174

Maitland, N.J., Cox, M.F., Lynas, C., Prime, S.S., Meanwell, C.A. & Scully, C. (1987) Detection of human papillomavirus DNA in biopsies of human oral tissue. *Br. J. Cancer*, **56**, 245–250

Malek, R.S., Goellner, J.R., Smith, T.F., Espy, M.J. & Cupp, M.R. (1993) Human papillomavirus infection and intraepithelial, *in situ*, and invasive carcinoma of penis. *Urology*, **42**, 159–170

Maloney, K.E., Wiener, J.S. & Walther, P.J. (1994) Oncogenic human papillomaviruses are rarely associated with squamous cell carcinoma of the bladder: evaluation by differential polymerase chain reaction. *J. Urol.*, **151**, 360–364

Malviya, V.K., Deppe, G., Pluszczynski, R. & Boike, G. (1987) Trichloroacetic acid in the treatment of human papillomavirus infection of the cervix without associated dysplasia. *Obstet. Gynecol.*, **70**, 72–74

Manavi, M., Czerwenka, K.F., Enzelsberger, H., Knogler, W., Seifert, M., Raimann, H., Reinold, E. & Kubista, E. (1992) Human papillomavirus (HPV) DNA infections of the uterine cervix. *Geburtsh. Frauenheilk.*, **52**, 283–286 (in German)

Mandal, D., Haye, K.R., Ray, T.K., Goorney, B.P., Stanbridge, C.M. & Corbitt, G. (1991) Prevalence of occult human papillomavirus infection, determined by cytology and DNA hybridization, in heterosexual men attending a genitourinary medicine clinic. *Int. J. STD AIDS*, **2**, 351–355

Mandelblatt, J., Richart, R., Thomas, L., Chauhan, P., Matseoane, S., Kanetsky, P., Traxler, M. & Lakin, P. (1992) Is human papillomavirus associated with cervical neoplasia in the elderly? *Gynecol. Oncol.*, **46**, 6–12

Mandelson, M.T., Jenison, S.A., Sherman, K.J., Valentine, J.M., McKnight, B., Daling, J.R. & Galloway, D.A. (1992) The association of human papillomavirus antibodies with cervical cancer risk. *Cancer Epidemiol. Biomarkers Prev.*, **1**, 281–286

Manias, D.A., Ostrow, R.S., McGlennen, R.C., Estensen, R.D. & Faras, A.J. (1989) Characterization of integrated human papillomavirus type 11 DNA in primary and metastatic tumors from a renal transplant recipient. *Cancer Res.*, **49**, 2514–2519

Mann, V.M., De Lao, S.L., Brenes, M., Brinton, L.A., Rawls, J.A., Green, M., Reeves, W.C. & Rawls, W.E. (1990) Occurrence of IgA and IgG antibodies to select peptides representing human papillomavirus type 16 among cervical cancer cases and controls. *Cancer Res.*, **50**, 7815–7819

Manos, M.M., Ting, T., Wright, D.K., Lewis, A.J., Broker, T.R. & Wolinsky, S.M. (1989) The use of polymerase chain reaction amplification for the detection of genital human papillomaviruses. *Cancer Cells mol. Diagnost. hum. Cancer*, **7**, 209–214

Marcante, M.L. & Venuti, A. (1991) Human papillomavirus DNA as a possible index of invasiveness in female genital tract carcinomas. *Eur. J. Cancer*, **27**, 187–190

Margall, N., Matias-Guiu, X., Chillon, M., Coll, P., Alejo, M., Nunes, V., Quilez, M., Rabella, N., Prats, G. & Prat, J. (1993) Detection of human papillomavirus 16 and 18 DNA in epithelial lesions of the lower genital tract by in situ hybridization and polymerase chain reaction: cervical scrapes are not substitutes for biopsies. *J. clin. Microbiol.*, **31**, 924–930

Marin, J., Ursic Vrscaj, M. & Erzen, M. (1994) Detection of human papillomaviruses (HPV-16,18) in cervical smears by in situ hybridization. *Isr. J. med. Sci.*, **30**, 448–450

Martin, R.G. & Chou, J.Y. (1975) Simian virus 40 functions required for the establishment and maintenance of malignant transformation. *J. Virol.*, **15**, 599–612

Martin, P., Vass, W.C., Schiller, J.T., Lowy, D.R. & Velu, T.J. (1989) The bovine papillomavirus E5 transforming protein can stimulate the transforming activity of EGF and CSF-1 receptors. *Cell*, **59**, 21–32

Masih, A.S., Stoler, M.H., Farrow, G.M. & Johansson, S.L. (1993) Human papillomavirus in penile squamous cell lesions: a comparison of an isotopic RNA and two commercial nonisotopic DNA in situ hybridization methods. *Arch. Pathol. Lab. Med.*, **117**, 302-307

Masood, S., Rhatigan, R.M., Powell, S., Thompson, J. & Rodenroth, N. (1991) Human papillomavirus in prostatic cancer: no evidence found by in situ DNA hybridization. *South. med. J.*, **84**, 235-236

Massing, A.M. & Epstein, W.L. (1963) Natural history of warts. A two-year study. *Arch. Dermatol.*, **87**, 306–310

Matas, A.J., Simmons, R.L., Kjellstrand, C.M., Buselmeier, T.J. & Najarian, J.S. (1975) Increased incidence of malignancy during chronic renal failure. *Lancet*, **i**, 883–886

Matlashewski, G., Banks, L., Wu-Liao, J., Spence, P., Pim, D. & Crawford, L. (1986a) The expression of human papillomavirus type 18 E6 protein in bacteria and the production of anti-E6 antibodies. *J. gen. Virol.*, **67**, 1909–1916

Matlashewski, G., Banks, L., Pim, D. & Crawford, L. (1986b) Analysis of human p53 proteins and mRNA levels in normal and transformed cells. *Eur. J. Biochem.*, **154**, 665–672

Matlashewski, G., Schneider, J., Banks, L., Jones, N., Murray, A. & Crawford, L. (1987) Human papillomavirus type 16 DNA cooperates with activated ras in transforming primary cells. *EMBO J.*, **6**, 1741–1746

Matsukura, T. & Sugase, M. (1995) Identification of genital human papillomaviruses in cervical biopsy specimens: segregation of specific virus types in specific clinicopathologic lesions. *Int. J. Cancer*, **61**, 13–22

Matsukura, T., Koi, S. & Sugase, M. (1989) Both episomal and integrated forms of human papillomavirus type 16 are involved in invasive cervical cancers. *Virology*, **172**, 63–72

Matsuo, N., Iwasaka, T., Hayashi, Y., Hara, K., Mvula, M. & Sugimori, H. (1993) Polymerase chain reaction analysis of human papillomavirus in adenocarcinoma and adenosquamous carcinoma of the uterine cervix. *Int. J. Gynaecol. Obstet.*, **41**, 251–256

Matulic, M. & Soric, J. (1994) Papillomavirus genomes in human cervical carcinoma: analysis of their integration and transcriptional activity. *Neoplasma*, **41**, 95–100

Matz, B., Schlehofer, J.R., zur Hausen, H., Huber, B. & Fanning, F. (1985) HSV- and chemical carcinogenesis-induced amplification of SV40 DNA sequences in transformed cells is cell-line dependent. *Int. J.Cancer*, **35**, 521–525

May, M., Dong, X.-P., Beyer Finkler, E., Stubenrauch, F., Fuchs, P.G. & Pfister, H. (1994) The E6/E7 promoter of extrachromosomal HPV16 DNA in cervical cancers escapes from cellular repression by mutation of target sequences for YY1. *EMBO J.*, **13**, 1460–1466

Mayor, H.D., Drake, S., Stahmann, J. & Mumford, D.M. (1976) Antibodies to adeno-associated satellite virus and herpes simplex in sera from cancer patients and normal adults. *Amer. J. Obstet. Gynecol.*, **126**, 100–104

McBride, A.A., Romanczuk, H. & Howey, P.M. (1991) The papillomavirus E2 regulatory proteins. *J. biol. Chem.*, **266**, 18411–18414

McCance, D.J., Campion, M.J., Clarkson, P.K., Chesters, P.M., Jenkins, D. & Singer, A. (1985) Prevalence of human papillomavirus type 16 DNA sequences in cervical intraepithelial neoplasia and invasive carcinoma of the cervix. *Br. J. Obstet. Gynaecol.*, **92**, 1101–1105

McCance, D.J., Kalache, A., Ashdown, K., Andrade, L., Menezes, F., Smith, P. & Doll, R. (1986) Human papillomavirus types 16 and 18 in carcinomas of the penis from Brazil. *Int. J. Cancer*, **37**, 55–59

McCance, D.J., Kopan, R., Fuchs, E. & Laimins, L.A. (1988) Human papillomavirus type 16 alters human epithelial cell differentiation *in vitro*. *Proc. natl Acad. Sci. USA*, **85**, 7169–7173

McDonnell, J.M., McDonnell, P.J., Mounts, P., Wu, T.-C. & Green, W.R. (1986) Demonstration of papillomavirus capsid antigen in human conjunctival neoplasia. *Arch. Ophthalmol.*, **104**, 1801–1805

McDonnell, P.J., McDonnell, J.M., Kessis, T., Green, W.R. & Shah, K.V. (1987) Detection of human papillomavirus type 6/11 DNA in conjunctival papillomas by in situ hybridization with radioactive probes. *Hum. Pathol.*, **18**, 1115–1119

McDonnell, J.M., Mayr, A.J. & Martin, W.J. (1989a) DNA of human papillomavirus type 16 in dysplastic and malignant lesions of the conjunctiva and cornea. *N. Engl. J. Med.*, **320**, 1442–1446

McDonnell, J.M., McDonnell, P.J., Stout, W.C. & Martin, W.J. (1989b) Human papillomavirus DNA in a recurrent squamous carcinoma of the eyelid. *Arch. Ophthalmol.*, **107**, 1631–1634

McDonnell, J.M., McDonnell, P.J. & Sun, Y.Y. (1992) Human papillomavirus DNA in tissues and ocular surface swabs of patients with conjunctival epithelial neoplasia. *Invest. Ophthalmol. vis. Sci.*, **33**, 184–189

McDougall, J.K. (1994) Immortalization and transformation of human cells by human papillomavirus. *Curr. Top. Microbiol. Immunol.*, **186**, 101–119

McGlennen, R.C., Adams, G.L., Lewis, C.M., Faras, A.J. & Ostrow, R.S. (1993) Pilot trial of ribavirin for the treatment of laryngeal papillomatosis. *Head Neck*, **15**, 504–513

McGrae, J.D. (1993) Multiple Bowen's disease of the fingers associated with human papillomavirus type 16. *Int. J. Dermatol.*, **32**, 104–107

McGregor, B., Byrne, P., Kirgan, D., Albright, J., Manalo, P. & Hall, M. (1993) Confirmation of the association of human papillomavirus with human colon cancer. *Am. J. Surg.*, **166**, 738–740

McGregor, J.M., Farthing, A., Crook, T., Yu, C.C.-W., Dublin, E.A., Levison, D.A. & MacDonald, D.M. (1994) Posttransplant skin cancer: a possible role for p53 gene mutation but not for oncogenic human papillomaviruses. *J. Am. Acad. Dermatol.*, **30**, 701–706

McIndoe, W.A., McLean, M.R., Jones, R.W. & Mullins, P.R. (1984) The invasive potential of carcinoma *in situ* of the cervix. *Obstet. Gynecol.*, **64**, 451–458

McIntyre, M.C., Frattini, M.G., Grossman, S.R. & Laimins, L.A. (1993) Human papillomavirus type 18 E7 protein requires intact Cys-X-X-Cys motifs for zinc binding, dimerization, and transformation but not for Rb binding. *J. Virol.*, **67**, 3142–3150

McKenzie, J., King, A., Hare, J., Fulford, T., Wilson, B. & Stanley, M. (1991) Immunocytochemical characterization of large granular lymphocytes in normal cervix and HPV associated disease. *J. Pathol.*, **165**, 75–80

McLean, C.S., Sterling, J.S., Mowat, J., Nash, A.A. & Stanley, M.A. (1993) Delayed-type hypersensitivity response to the human papillomavirus type 16 E7 protein in a mouse model. *J. gen. Virol.*, **74**, 239–245

McLellan, R., Buscema, J., Guerrero, E., Shah, K.V., Woodruff, J.D. & Currie, J.L. (1990) Investigation of ovarian neoplasia of low malignant potential for human papillomavirus. *Gynecol. Oncol.*, **38**, 383–385

McNicol, P.J. & Dodd, J.G. (1990) Detection of papillomavirus DNA in human prostatic tissue by Southern blot analysis. *Can. J. Microbiol.*, **36**, 359–362

McNicol, P.J. & Dodd, J.G. (1991) High prevalence of human papillomavirus in prostate tissues. *J. Urol.*, **145**, 850–853

McNicol, P.J., Guijon, F.B., Paraskevas, M. & Brunham, R.C. (1989) Comparison of filter in situ deoxyribonucleic acid hybridization with cytologic, colposcopic, and histopathologic examination for detection of human papillomavirus infection in women with cervical intraepithelial neoplasia. *Am. J. Obstet. Gynecol.*, **160**, 265–270

Meanwell, C.A., Cox, M.F., Blackledge, G. & Maitland, N.J. (1987) HPV 16 DNA in normal and malignant cervical epithelium: implications for the aetiology and behaviour of cervical neoplasia. *Lancet*, **i**, 703–707

Meekin, G.E., Sparrow, M.J., Fenwicke, R.J. & Tobias, M. (1992) Prevalence of genital human papillomavirus infection in Wellington women. *Genitourin. Med.*, **68**, 228–232

Meguenni, S., El-Mehdaoui, S., Bandoui, D., Bouguermouh, A., Allouache, A., Bendib, A., Chouiter, A., Djenaoui, T., Lalliam, N., Bouhadef, A. & Bouhadjar, H. (1992) Detection of human papillomavirus (H.P.V.) DNA in genital lesions using molecular hybridization. *Arch. Inst. Pasteur Algér.*, **58**, 291–297 (in French)

Meisels, A. & Fortin, R. (1976) Condylomatous lesions of the cervix and vagina. I. Cytologic paterns. *Acta cytol.*, **20**, 505–509

Meisels, A. & Morin, C. (1981) Human papillomavirus and cancer of the uterine cervix. *Gynecol. Oncol.*, **12**, S111–S123

Melbye, M. & Sprøgel, P. (1991) Aetiological parallel between anal cancer and cervical cancer. *Lancet*, **338**, 657–659

Melbye, M., Njelesani, E.K., Bayley, A., Mukelabai, K., Manuwele, J.K., Bowa, F.J., Clayden, S.A., Levin, A., Blattner, W.A., Weiss, R.A., Tedder, R. & Biggar, R.J. (1986) Evidence for heterosexual transmission and clinical manifestations of human immunodeficiency virus infection and related conditions in Lusaka, Zambia. *Lancet*, **ii**, 1113–1115

Melbye, M., Palefsky, J., Gonzales, J., Ryder, L.P., Nielsen, H., Bergmann, O., Pindborg, J. & Biggar, R.J. (1990) Immune status as a determinant of human papillomavirus detection and its association with anal epithelial abnormalities. *Int. J. Cancer*, **46**, 203–206

Melbye, M., Rabkin, C., Frisch, M. & Biggar, R.J. (1994a) Changing patterns of anal cancer incidence in the United States, 1940–1989. *Am. J. Epidemiol.*, **139**, 772–780

Melbye, M., Cote, T.R., Kessler, L., Gail, M. & Biggar, R.J. & The AIDS/Cancer Working Group (1994b) High incidence of anal cancer among AIDS patients. *Lancet*, **343**, 636–639

Melchers, W., de Mare, S., Kuitert, E., Galama, J., Walboomers, J. & van den Brule, A.J.C. (1993) Human papillomavirus and cutaneous warts in meat handlers. *J. clin. Microbiol.*, **31**, 2547–2549

Melillo, R.M., Helin, K., Lowy, D.R. & Schiller, J.T. (1994) Positive and negative regulation of cell proliferation by E2F1-1: influence of protein level and human papillomavirus oncoproteins. *Mol. cell. Biol.*, **14**, 8241–8249

Melkert, P.W.J., Hopman, E., van den Brule, A.J.C., Risse, E.K.J., van Diest, P.J., Bleker, O.P., Helmerhorst, T., Schipper, M.E.I., Meijer, C.J.L.M. & Walboomers, J.M.M. (1993) Prevalence of HPV in cytomorphologically normal cervical smears, as determined by the polymerase chain reaction, is age-dependent. *Int. J. Cancer*, **53**, 919–923

Melton, J.L. & Rasmussen, J.E. (1991) Clinical manifestations of human papillomavirus infection in nongenital sites. *Dermatol. Clin.*, **9**, 219–233

Meneguzzi, G., Kieny, M.P., Lecocq, J.-P., Chambon, P., Cuzin, F. & Lathe, R. (1990) Vaccinia recombinants expressing early bovine papilloma virus (BPV1) proteins: retardation of BPV1 tumour development. *Vaccine*, **8**, 199–204

Meneguzzi, G., Cerni, C., Kieny, M.P. & Lathe, R. (1991) Immunization against human papillomavirus type 16 tumor cells with recombinant vaccinia viruses expressing E6 and E7. *Virology*, **181**, 62–69

Menendez Velasquez, J.F., Gonzalez Sanchez, J.L., Rodriguez de Santiago, J.D. & Muñoz Reyes, R. & Uriza, R.B. (1993) Treatment of cervical infection of HPV by trichloroacetic acid. *Ginecol. Obst. Méx.*, **61**, 48–51 (in Spanish)

Meng, X.-J., Sun, Y., Chen, M.-H., Liu, Z.-H., Zhang, Y.-X., Li, X.-Z., Li, K., Han, R.-C., Si, J.-Y., Hu, L.-Y. & Zeng, W.-K. (1989) Viral etiology of cervical carcinoma. Human papilloma virus and herpes simplex virus type 2. *Chin. med. J.*, **102**, 94–99

ter Meulen, J., Eberhardt, H.C., Luande, J., Mgaya, H.N., Chang-Claude, J., Mtiro, H., Mhina, M., Kashaija, P., Ockert, S., Yu, X., Meinhardt, G., Gissmann, L. & Rawlita, M. (1992) Human papillomavirus (HPV) infection, HIV infection and cervical cancer in Tanzania, East Africa. *Int. J. Cancer*, **51**, 515–521

Mevorach, R.A., Cos, L.R., di Sant'Agnese, P.A. & Stoler, M. (1990) Human papillomavirus type 6 in grade I transitional cell carcinoma of the urethra. *J. Urol.*, **143**, 126–128

Meyer, M.P., Carbonell, R.I., Mauser, N.A., Kanbour, A.I. & Amortegui, A.J. (1993) Detection of human papillomavirus in cervical swab samples by ViraPap and in cervical biopsy specimens by in situ hybridization. *Am. J. clin. Pathol.*, **100**, 12–17

Mietz, J.A., Unger, T., Huibregtse, J.M. & Howley, P.M. (1992) The transcriptional transactivation function of wild-type p53 is inhibited by SV40 large T-antigen and by HPV-16 E6 oncoprotein. *EMBO J.*, **11**, 5013–5020

Milde-Langosch, K., Schreiber, C., Becker, G., Löning, T. & Stegner, H.-E. (1993) Human papillomavirus detection in cervical adenocarcinoma by polymerase chain reaction. *Hum. Pathol.*, **24**, 590–594

Miller, A.B. (1992) *Cervical Cancer Screening Programmes: Managerial Guidelines*, Geneva, World Health Organization

Mincheva, A., Gissmann, L. & zur Hausen, H. (1987) Chromosomal integration sites of human papillomavirus DNA in three cervical cancer cell lines mapped by in situ hybridization. *Med. Microbiol. Immunol. (Berl.)*, **176**, 245–256

Mitchell, H., Drake, M. & Medley, G. (1986) Prospective evaluation of risk of cervical cancer after cytological evidence of human papilloma virus infection. *Lancet*, **i**, 573–575

Mitra, A.B., Murty, V.V.V.S., Li, R.G., Pratap, M., Luthra, U.K. & Chaganti, R.S.K. (1994) Allelotype analysis of cervical carcinoma. *Cancer Res.*, **54**, 4481–4487

Mitrani-Rosenbaum, S., Gal, D., Friedman, M., Kitron, N., Tsvieli, R., Mordel, N. & Anteby, S.O. (1988) Papillomaviruses in lesions of the lower genital tract in Israeli patients. *Eur. J. Cancer clin. Oncol.*, **24**, 725–731

Mittal, R., Pater, A. & Pater, M.M. (1993a) Multiple human papillomavirus type 16 glucocorticoid response elements functional for transformation, transient expression, and DNA-protein interactions. *J. Virol.*, **67**, 5656–5659

Mittal, R., Tsutsumi, K., Pater, A. & Pater, M.M. (1993b) Human papillomavirus type 16 expression in cervical keratinocytes: role of progesterone and glucocorticoid hormones. *Obstet. Gynecol.*, **81**, 5–12

Moar, M.H. & Jarrett, W.F.H. (1985) A cutaneous fibropapilloma from a red deer (*Cervus elaphus*) associated with a papillomavirus. *Intervirology*, **24**, 108–118

Moar, M.H., Campo, M.S., Laird, H.M. & Jarrett, W.F.H. (1981) Unintegrated viral DNA sequences in a hamster tumor induced by bovine papilloma virus. *J. Virol.*, **39**, 945–949

Moar, M.H., Jarrett, W.F.H. & O'Neil, B.W. (1986) Viral DNA sequences detected in a hamster liposarcoma induced by bovine papillomavirus type 4. *J. gen. Virol.*, **67**, 187–190

Mohr, I.J., Clark, R., Sun, S., Androphy, E.J., MacPherson, P. & Botchan, M.R. (1990) Targeting the E1 replication protein to the papillomavirus origin of replication by complex formation with the E2 transactivator. *Science*, **250**, 1694–1699

Monsonego, J., Magdelenat, H., Catalan, F., Coscas, Y., Zerat, L. & Sastre, X. (1991) Estrogen and progesterone receptors in cervical human papillomavirus related lesions. *Int. J. Cancer*, **48**, 533–539

Monsonego, J., Zerat, L., Catalan, F. & Coscas, Y. (1993) Genital human papillomavirus infections: correlation of cytological, colposcopic and histological features with viral types in women and their male partners. *Int. J. STD AIDS*, **4**, 13–20

Montz, F.J., Monk, B.J., Fowler, J.M. & Nguyen, L. (1992) Natural history of the minimally abnormal Papanicolaou smear. *Obstet. Gynecol.*, **80**, 385–388

Morelli, A.E., Belardi, G., DiPaola, G., Paredes, A. & Fainboim, L. (1994) Cellular subsets and epithelial ICAM-1 and HLA-DR expression in human papillomavirus infection of the vulva. *Acta derm. venereol. (Stockh).*, **74**, 45–50

Moreno, V., Muñoz, N., Bosch, F.X., de Sanjosé, S., Gonzalez, L.C., Tafur, L., Gili, M., Izarzugaza, I., Navarro, C., Vergara, A., Viladiu, P., Ascunce, N. & Shah, K.V. (1995) Risk factors for progression of cervical intraepithelial neoplasm grade III to invasive cervical cancer. *Cancer Epidemiol. Biomarkers Prev.*, **4**, 459–467

Moreno-Lopez, J., Pettersson, U., Dinter, Z. & Philipson, L. (1981) Characterization of a papilloma virus from the European elk (EEPV). *Virology*, **112**, 589–595

Moreno-Lopez, J., Ahola, H., Stenlund, A., Osterhaus, A. & Pettersson, U. (1984) Genome of an avian papillomavirus. *J. Virol.*, **51**, 872–875

Moreno-Lopez, J., Ahola, H., Eriksson, A., Bergman, P. & Pettersson, U. (1987) Reindeer papillomavirus transforming properties correlate with a highly conserved E5 region. *J. Virol.*, **61**, 3394–3400

Moriyama, N., Nagase, Y., Ueki, T., Hosaka, Y., Higashihara, E., Murahashi, I. & Aso, Y. (1990) In situ hybridization study of human papillomavirus from the penile cancer. *Nippon Hinyokika Gakkai Zasshi*, **81**, 1706–1710 (in Japanese)

Morris, H.B., Gatter, K.C., Pulford, K., Haynes, P., Charnock, M., Taylor-Papadimitriou, J., Lane, E.B. & Mason, D.Y. (1983) Cervical wart virus infection, intraepithelial neoplasia and carcinoma; an immunohistological study using a panel of monoclonal antibodies. *Br. J. Obstet. Gynaecol.*, **90**, 1069–1081

Morrison, E.A. (1994) Natural history of cervical infection with human papillomaviruses. *Clin. infect. Dis.*, **18**, 172–180

Morrison, E.A., Ho, G.Y., Vermund, S.H., Goldberg, G.L., Kadish, A.S., Kelley, K.F. & Burk, R.D. (1991) Human papillomavirus infection and other risk factors for cervical neoplasia: a case–control study. *Int. J. Cancer*, **49**, 6–13

Moscicki, A.-B. (1992) Human papillomavirus infections. *Adv. Pediatr.*, **39**, 257–281

Moscicki, A.-B., Palefsky, J., Gonzales, J. & Schoolnik, G.K. (1990) Human papillomavirus infection in sexually active adolescent females: prevalence and risk factors. *Pediatr. Res.*, **28**, 507–513

Moscicki, A.-B., Broering, J., Powell, K., Klein, J., Clayton, L., Smith, G., Boero, S., Darragh, T.M., Brescia, R.J. & Palefsky, J. (1993) Comparison between colposcopic, cytologic, and histologic findings in women positive and negative for human papillomavirus DNA. *J. adolesc. Health*, **14**, 74–79

Mose Larsen, P., Storgaard, L. & Fey, S.J. (1987) Proteins present in bovine papillomavirus particles. *J. Virol.*, **61**, 3596–3601

Moy, R.L. & Quan, M.B. (1991) The presence of HPV 16 in squamous-cell carcinoma of the proximal finger and reconstruction with a bilobed transposition flap. *J. dermatol. Surg. Oncol.*, **17**, 171–175

Moy, R.L., Eliezri, Y.D., Nuovo, G.J., Zitelli, J.A., Bennett, R.G. & Silverstein, S. (1989) Human papillomavirus type 16 DNA in periungual squamous cell carcinomas. *J. Am. med. Assoc.*, **261**, 2669–2673

Moyret-Lalle, C., Marcais, C., Jacquemier, J., Moles, J.-P., Daver, A., Soret, J.-Y., Jeanteur, P., Ozturk, M. & Theillet, C. (1995) *ras, p53* And HPV status in benign and malignant prostate tumors. *Int. J. Cancer*, **64**, 124–129

Müller, M., Gausepohl, H., de Martynoff, G., Frank, R., Brasseur, R. & Gissmann, L. (1990) Identification of seroreactive regions of the human papillomavirus type 16 protein E4, E6, E7 and L1. *J. gen. Virol.*, **71**, 2709–2717

Müller, M., Viscidi, R.P., Sun, Y., Guerrero, E., Hill, P.M., Shah, F., Bosch, F.X., Muñoz, N., Gissmann, L. & Shah, K.V. (1992) Antibodies to HPV-16 E6 and E7 proteins as markers for HPV-16-associated invasive cervical cancer. *Virology*, **187**, 508–514

Müller, M., Gissmann, L., Cristiano, R.J., Sun, X.-Y., Frazer, I.H., Jenson, A.B., Alonso, A., Zentgraf, H. & Zhou, J. (1995a) Papillomavirus capsid binding and uptake by cells from different tissues and species. *J. Virol.*, **69**, 948–954

Müller, M., Viscidi, R.P., Ulken, V., Bouwes Bavinck, J.N., Hill, P.M., Fisher, S.G., Reid, R., Muñoz, N., Schneider, A., Shah, K.V. & Gissmann, L. (1995b) Antibodies to the E4, E6, and E7 proteins of human papillomavirus (HPV) type 16 in patients with HPV-associated diseases and in the normal population. *J. invest. Dermatol.,* **104**, 138–141

Münger, K. & Phelps, W.C. (1993) The human papillomavirus E7 protein as a transforming and transactivating factor. *Biochim. biophys. Acta,* **1155**, 111–123

Münger, K., Phelps, W.C., Bubb, V., Howley, P.M. & Schlegel, R. (1989a) The E6 and E7 genes of the human papillomavirus type 16 together are necessary and sufficient for transformation of primary human keratinocytes. *J. Virol.,* **63**, 4417–4421

Münger, K., Werness, B.A., Dyson, N., Phelps, W.C., Harlow, E. & Howley, P.M. (1989b) Complex formation of human papillomavirus E7 proteins with the retinoblastoma tumor suppressor gene product. *EMBO J.,* **8**, 4099–4105

Muñoz, N. & Bosch, F.X. (1992) HPV and cervical neoplasia: review of case–control and cohort studies. In: Muñoz, N., Bosch, F.X., Shah, K.V. & Meheus, A., eds, *The Epidemiology of Cervical Cancer and Human* Papillomavirus (IARC Scientific Publications No. 119), Lyon, IARC, pp. 251–261

Muñoz, N., Bosch, X. & Kaldor, J.M. (1988) Does human papillomavirus cause cervical cancer? The state of the epidemiological evidence. *Br. J. Cancer,* **57**, 1–5

Muñoz, N., Cardis, E. & Teuchmann, S. (1990) Comparative epidemiological aspects of oro-genital cancers. In: Monsonego, J., ed., *Papillomaviruses in Human Pathology. Recent Progress in Epidermoid Precancers* (Serono Symposia Publication Vol. 78), New York, Raven Press, pp. 1–12

Muñoz, N., Bosch, F.X., de Sanjosé, S., Tafur, L., Izarzugaza, I., Gili, M., Viladiu, P., Navarro, C., Martos, C., Ascunce, N., Gonzalez, L.C., Kaldor, J.M., Guerrero, E., Lörincz, A., Santamaria, M. de Ruiz, P. A., Aristizabal, N. & Shah, K.V. (1992) The causal link between human papillomavirus and invasive cervical cancer: a population-based case–control study in Colombia and Spain. *Int. J. Cancer,* **52**, 743–749

Muñoz, N., Bosch, F.X., de Sanjosé, S., Vergara, A., del Moral, A., Muñoz, M.T., Tafur, L., Gili, M., Izarzugaza, I., Viladiu, P., Navarro, C., Alonso de Ruiz, Aristizabal, N., Santamaria, M., Orfila, J., Daniel, R.W., Guerrero, E. & Shah, K.V. (1993) Risk factors for cervical intraepithelial neoplasia grade III/carcinoma *in situ* in Spain and Colombia. *Cancer Epidemiol. Biomarkers Prev.,* **2**, 423–431

Muñoz, N., Bosch, F.X., de Sanjosé, S. & Shah, K.V. (1994) The role of HPV in the etiology of cervical cancer. *Mutat. Res.,* **305**, 293–301

Muñoz, N., Crawford, L. & Couraget, P. (1995) HPV vaccines for cervical neopasia. *Lancet,* **345**, 249

Myers, G., Bernard H.-U., Delius, H., Favre, M., Icenogel, J., Van Ranst, M. & Wheeler, C., eds (1994) *Human Papillomaviruses 1994: A compilation and Analysis of Nucleic Acid and Amino Acid Sequences,* Los Alamos, NM, Los Alamos National Laboratory

Nahass, G.T., Blauvert, A., Leonardi, C.L. & Penneys, N.S. (1992) BCC of the scrotum: report of three cases and review of the literature. *J. Am. Acad. Dermatol.,* **26**, 574–578

Nahmias, A., Josey, W., Naib, Z.M., Luce, C.F. & Guest, B.A. (1970) Antibodies to *Herpesvirus hominis* types 1 and 2 in humans. II. Women with cervical cancer. *Am. J. Epidemiol.,* **91**, 547–552

Nakazawa, A., Inoue, M., Saito, J., Sasagawa, T., Ueda, G. & Tanizawa, O. (1992) Detection of human papillomavirus types 16 and 18 in the exfoliated cervical cells using the polymerase chain reaction. *Int. J. Gynaecol. Obstet.,* **37**, 13–18

Nasiell, K., Roger, V. & Nasiell, M. (1986) Behavior of mild cervical dysplasia during long-term follow-up. *Obstet. Gynecol.,* **67**, 665–669

Nasseri, M., Hirochika, R., Broker, T.R. & Chow, L.T. (1987) A human papilloma virus type 11 transcript encoding an $E_1{\wedge}E_4$ protein. *Virology,* **159**, 433–439

National Cancer Institute Workshop (1989) The 1988 Bethesda System for reporting cervical/vaginal cytologic diagnoses. *J. Am. med. Assoc.,* **262**, 931–934

Negrini, B.P., Schiffman, M.H., Kurman, R.J., Barnes, W., Lannom, L., Malley, K., Brinton, L.A., Delgado, G., Jones, S., Tchabo, J.G. & Lancaster, W.D. (1990) Oral contraceptive use, human papillomavirus infection, and risk of early cytological abnormalities of the cervix. *Cancer Res.,* **50**, 4670–4675

Neil, S.M., Lessana-Liebowitch, M., Pelisse, M. & Moyal-Barracco, M. (1990) Lichen sclerosus, invasive squamous cell carcinoma, and human papillomavirus (Letter to the Editor). *Am. J. Obstet. Gynecol.,* **162**, 1633–1644

Nevins, J.R. (1992) E2F: a link between the Rb tumor suppressor protein and viral oncoproteins. *Science,* **258**, 424–429

Newfield, L., Goldsmith, A., Bradlow, H.L. & Auborn, K. (1993) Estrogen metabolism and human papillomavirus-induced tumors of the larynx: chemo-prophylaxis with indole-3-carbinol. *Anticancer Res.,* **13**, 337–341

Ngan, H.Y.S., Stanley, M., Liu, S.S. & Ma, H.K. (1994) HPV and p53 in cervical cancer. *Genitourin. Med.,* **70**, 167–170

Nicklin, J.L., Wright, R.G., Bell, J.R., Samaratunga, H., Cox, N.C. & Ward, B.G. (1991) A clinicopathological study of adenocarcinoma *in situ* of the cervix. The influence of cervical HPV infection and other factors, and the role of conservative surgery. *Aust. N. Z. J. Obstet. Gynaecol.,* **31**, 179–183

Niedobitek, G., Pitteroff, S., Herbst, H., Shepherd, P., Finn, T., Anagnostopoulos, I. & Stein, H. (1990) Detection of human papillomavirus type 16 DNA in carcinomas of the palatine tonsil. *J. clin. Pathol.,* **43**, 918–921

Nindl, I., Benitez-Bribiesca, L., Berumen, J., Farmanara, N., Fisher, S., Gross, G., Lopez-Carillo, L., Müller, M., Tommasino, M., Vazquez-Curiel, A. & Gissmann, L. (1994) Antibodies against linear and conformational epitopes of the human papillomavirus (HPV) type 16 E6 and E7 oncoproteins in sera of cervical cancer patients. *Arch. Virol.,* **137**, 341–353

Nishikawa, A., Fukushima, M., Shimada, M., Yamakawa, Y., Shimano, S., Kato, I. & Fujinaga, K. (1991) Relatively low prevalence of human papillomavirus 16, 18 and 33 DNA in the normal cervices of Japanese women shown by polymerase chain reaction. *Jpn J. Cancer Res.,* **82**, 532–538

Noble-Topham, S.E., Fliss, D.M., Hartwick, W.J., McLachlin, C.M., Freeman, J.L., Noyek, A.M. & Andrulis, I.L. (1993) Detection and typing of human papillomavirus in verrucous carcinoma of the oral cavity using the polymerase chain reaction. *Arch. Otolaryngol. Head Neck Surg.,* **119**, 1299–1304

Noel, J.C., Penny, M.O., Goldschmidt, D., Verhest, A., Heenen, M. & de Dobbeleer, G. (1993) Human papillomavirus type 1 DNA in verrucous carcinoma of the leg. *J. Am. Acad. Dermatol.,* **29**, 1036–1038

Nonnenmacher, B., Hubbert, N.L., Kirnbauer, R., Shah, K.V., Muñoz, N., Bosch, F.X., de Sanjosé, S., Viscidi, R., Lowry, D.R. & Schiller, J.T. (1995) Serologic response to human papillomavirus type 16 (HPV-16) virus-like particles in HPV-16 DNA-positive invasive cervical cancer and cervical intraepithelial neoplasia grade III patients and controls from Colombia and Spain. *J. infect. Dis.* (in press)

Nordin, P., Stenquist, B. & Hansson, B.G. (1994) Joint occurrence of human papillomavirus type 16 DNA in Bowen's disease on a finger and in dysplasia of the vulva and the uterine cervix (Letter to the Editor). *Br. J. Dermatol.*, **131**, 740

Northfelt, D.W. & Palefsky, J.M. (1992) Human papillomavirus-associated anogenital neoplasia in persons with HIV infection. *AIDS clin. Rev.*, 241–259

Norval, M., Michie, J.R., Apps, M.V., Head, K.W. & Else, R.E. (1985) Rumen papillomas in sheep. *Vet. Microbiol.*, **10**, 219–229

Nuovo, G. (1991) Evidence against a role for human papillomavirus in colon neoplasms (Letter to the Editor). *Arch. Surg.*, **126**, 656

Nuovo, G., Friedman, D. & Richart, R.M. (1990) In-situ hybridization analysis of human papillomavirus DNA segregation patterns in lesions of the female genital tract. *Gynecol. Oncol.*, 36, 256–262

Nuovo, G.J., MacConnell, P., Forde, A. & Delvenne, P. (1991a) Detection of human papillomavirus DNA in formalin-fixed tissues by in situ hybridization after amplification by polymerase chain reaction. *Am. J. Pathol.*, **139**, 847–854

Nuovo, G.J., Darfler, M.M., Impraim, C.C. & Bromley, S.E. (1991b) Occurrence of multiple types of human papillomavirus in genital tract lesions. Analysis by in situ hybridization and the polymerase chain reaction. *Am. J. Pathol.*, **138**, 53–58

Nuovo, G.J., Delvenne, P., MacConnell, P., Chalas, E., Neto, C. & Mann, W.J. (1991c) Correlation of histology and detection of human papillomavirus DNA in vulvar cancers. *Gynecol. Oncol.*, **43**, 275–280

Obalek, S., Favre, M., Jablonska, S., Szymanczyk, J. & Orth, G. (1988) Human papillomavirus type 2-associated basal cell carcinoma in two immunosuppressed patients. *Arch. Dermatol.*, **124**, 930–934

Obalek, S., Misiewicz, J., Jablonska, S., Favre, M. & Orth, G. (1993) Childhood condyloma acuminatum: association with genital and cutaneous human papillomaviruses. *Pediatr. Dermatol.*, **10**, 101–106

O'Banion, M.K., Reichmann, M.E. & Sundberg, J.P. (1986) Cloning and characterization of an equine cutaneous papillomavirus. *Virology*, **152**, 100–109

O'Banion, M.K., Sundberg, J.P., Shima, A.L. & Reichmann, M.E. (1987) Venereal papilloma and papillomavirus in a colobus monkey (*Colobus guereza*). *Intervirology*, **28**, 232–237

Ocadiz, R., Sauceda, R., Cruz, M., Graef, A.M. & Gariglio, P. (1987) High correlation between molecular alterations of the c-*myc* oncogene and carcinoma of the uterine cervix. *Cancer Res.*, **47**, 4173–4177

Odrich, M.G., Jakobiec, F.A., Lancaster, W.D., Kenyon, K.R., Kelly, L.D., Kornmehl, E.W., Steinert, R.F., Grove, A.S., Jr, Shore, J.W., Gregoire, L. & Albert, D.M. (1991) A spectrum of bilateral squamous conjunctival tumors associated with human papillomavirus type 16. *Ophthalmology*, **98**, 628–635

Odunsi, K., Terry, G., Ho, L., Bell, J., Cuzick, J. & Ganesan, T.S. (1995) Association between HLA DQB1 * 03 and cervical intra-epithelial neoplasia. *Mol. Med.*, **1**, 161–171

Ogunbiyi, O.A., Scholefield, J.H., Robertson, G., Smith, J.H.F., Sharp, F. & Rogers, K. (1994a) Anal human papillomavirus infection and squamous neoplasia in patients with invasive vulvar cancer. *Obstet. Gynecol.*, **83**, 212–216

Ogunbiyi, O.A., Scholefield, J.H., Raftery, A.T., Smith, J.H., Duffy, S., Sharp, F. & Rogers, K. (1994b) Prevalence of anal human papillomavirus infection and intraepithelial neoplasia in renal allograft recipients. *Br. J. Surg.*, **81**, 365–367

Ogura, H., Watanabe, S., Fukushima, K., Masuda, Y., Fujiwara, T. & Yabe, Y. (1993) Human papillomavirus DNA in squamous cell carcinomas of the respiratory and upper digestive tracts. *Jpn. J. clin. Oncol.*, **23**, 221–225

Ohta, M., Casanova, H., Mizuno, K., Kaseki, H., Niwa, K. & Ishiko, H. (1991) Epidemiologic background and changes in patients infected with human papilloma virus. *Nippon Sanka Fujinka Gakkai Zasshi*, **43**, 479–484 (in Japanese)

Okabayashi, M., Angeli, M.G., Christensen, N.D. & Kreider, J.W. (1991) Morphometric analysis and identification of infiltrating leucocytes in regressing and progressing Shope rabbit papillomas. *Int. J. Cancer*, **49**, 919–923

Okada, Y., Yahata, G., Takeuchi, S., Seidoh, T. & Tanaka, K. (1989) A correlation between the expression of CD 8 antigen and specific cytotoxicity of tumor-infiltrating lymphocytes. *Jpn J. Cancer Res.*, **80**, 249–256

Okagaki, T., Tase, T., Twiggs, L.B. & Carson, L.F. (1989) Histogenesis of cervical adenocarcinoma with reference to human papillomavirus-18 as a carcinogen. *J. reprod. Med.*, **34**, 639–644

Olson, C. (1987) Animal papillomas: historical perspectives. In: Selzman, N.P. & Howley, P.M., eds, *The Papillomaviruses*, New York, Plenum Press, pp. 39–66

Olson, C., Jr & Cook, R.H. (1951) Cutaneous sarcoma-like lesions of the horse caused by the agent of bovine papilloma. *Proc. Soc. exp. biol. Med.*, **27**, 281–284

Olson, C., Pamukcu, A.M., Brobst, D.F., Kowalczyk, T., Satter, E.J. & Price, J.M. (1959) A urinary bladder tumor induced by a bovine cutaneous papilloma agent. *Cancer Res.*, **19**, 779–783

Olson, C., Pamukcu, A.M. & Brobst, D.F. (1965) Papilloma-like virus from bovine urinary bladder tumors. *Cancer Res.*, **25**, 840–849

Olson, C., Gordon, D.E., Robl, M.G. & Lee, K.P. (1969) Oncogenicity of bovine papilloma virus. *Arch. environ. Health.*, **19**, 827–837

Onda, T., Kanda, T., Zanma, S., Yasugi, T., Watanabe, S., Kawana, T., Ueda, K., Yoshikawa, H., Taketani, Y. & Yoshiike, K. (1993) Association of the antibodies against human papillomavirus 16 E4 and E7 proteins with cervical cancer positive for human papillomavirus DNA. *Int. J. Cancer*, **54**, 624–628

Ong, C.-K., Chan, S.-Y., Campo, M.S., Fujinaga, K., Mavromara-Nazos, P., Labropoulou, V., Pfister, H., Tay, S.-K., ter Meulen, J., Villa, L.L. & Bernard, H.-U. (1993) Evolution of human papillomavirus type 18: an ancient phylogenetic root in Africa and intratype diversity reflect coevolution with human ethnic groups. *J. Virol.*, **67**, 6424–6431

Oriel, J.D. (1971) Natural history of genital warts. *Br. J. vener. Dis.*, **47**, 1–13

Orth, G. (1986) Epidermodysplasia verruciformis: a model for understanding the oncogenicity of human papillomaviruses In: *Papillomaviruses* (Ciba Foundation Symposium 120), New York, John Wiley & Sons, pp. 157–174

Orth, G., Jablonska, S., Jarzabeck-Chorzelska, M., Obalek, S., Rzesa, G., Favre, M. & Croissant, O. (1979) Characteristics of the lesions and risk of malignant conversion associated with the type of human papillomavirus involved in epidermodysplasia verruciformis. *Cancer Res.*, **39**, 1074–1082

Orth, G., Jablonska, S., Favre, M., Croissant, O., Obalek, S., Jarzabek-Chorzelska, M. & Jibard, N. (1981) Identification of papillomaviruses in butchers' warts. *J. invest. Dermatol.*, **76**, 97–102

Oshima, J., Steinmann, K.E., Campisi, J. & Schlegel, R. (1993) Modulation of cell growth, $p34^{cdc2}$ and cyclin A levels by SV-40 large T antigen. *Oncogene*, **8**, 2987–2993

Osterhaus, A.D.M.E., Ellens, D.J. & Horzinek, M.C. (1977) Identification and characterization of a papillomavirus from birds (Fringillidae). *Intervirology*, **8**, 351–359

Östör, A.G. (1993) Natural history of cervical intraepithelial neoplasia: a critical review. *Int. J. gynecol. Pathol.*, **12**, 186–192

Ostrow, R.S., Krzyzek, R., Pass, F. & Faras, A.J. (1981) Identification of a novel human papilloma virus in cutaneous warts of meathandlers. *Virology*, **108**, 21–27

Ostrow, R.S., Bender, M., Nimura, M., Seki, T., Kawashima, M., Pass, F. & Faras, A. (1982) Human papillomavirus DNA in cutaneous primary and metastasized squamous cell carcinomas from patients with epidermodysplasia verruciformis. *Proc. natl Acad. Sci. USA*, **79**, 1634–1638

Ostrow, R.S., Manias, D.A., Fong, W.J., Zachow, K.R. & Faras, A.J. (1987a) A survey of human cancers for human papillomavirus DNA by filter hybridization. *Cancer*, **59**, 429–434

Ostrow, R.S., Manias, D., Mitchell, A.J., Stawowy, L. & Faras, A.J. (1987b) Epidermodysplasia verruciformis. A case associated with primary lymphatic dysplasia, depressed cell-mediated immunity, and Bowen's disease containing human papillomavirus 16 DNA. *Arch. Dermatol.*, **123**, 1511–1516

Ostrow, R.S., Manias, D.A., Clark, B.A., Fukushima, M., Okagaki, T., Twiggs, L.B. & Faras, A.J. (1988) The analysis of carcinomas of the vagina for human papillomavirus DNA. *Int. J. gynecol. Pathol.*, **7**, 308–314

Ostrow, R.S., Shaver, M.K., Turnquist, S., Viksnins, A., Bender, M., Vance, C., Kaye, V. & Faras, A.J. (1989a) HPV 16 DNA in a cutaneous invasive cancer. *Arch. Dermatol.*, **125**, 666–669

Ostrow, R.S., Zachow, K.R., Shaver, M.K. & Faras, A.J. (1989b) Human papillomavirus type 27: detection of a novel human papillomavirus in common warts of a renal transplant recipient. *J. Virol.*, **63**, 4904–4906

Ostrow, R.S., McGlennen, R.C., Shaver, M.K., Kloster, B.E., Houser, D. & Faras, A.J. (1990) A rhesus monkey model for sexual transmission of a papillomavirus isolated from a squamous cell carcinoma. *Proc. natl Acad. Sci. USA*, **87**, 8170–8174

Ostrow, R.S., LaBresh, K.V. & Faras, A.J. (1991) Characterization of the complete RhPV 1 genomic sequence and an integration locus from a metastatic tumor. *Virology*, **181**, 424–429

Ostrow, R.S., Forslund, K.M., McGlennen, R.C., Shaw, D.P., Schlievert, P.M., Ussery, M.A., Huggins, J.W. & Faras, A.J. (1992) Ribavirin mitigates wart growth in rabbits at early stages of infection with cottontail rabbit papillomavirus. *Antiviral Res.*, **17**, 99–113

Ostrow, R.S., Coughlin, S.M., McGlennen, R.C., Johnson, A.N., Ratterree, M.S., Scheffler, J., Yaegashi, N., Galloway, D.A. & Faras, A.J. (1995) Serological and molecular evidence of rhesus papillomavirus type 1 infections in tissues from geographically distinct institutions. *J. gen. Virol.*, **76**, 293–299

Ostwald, C., Müller P., Barten, M., Rutsatz, K., Sonnenburg, M., Milde-Langosch, K. & Löning, T. (1994) Human papillomavirus DNA in oral squamous cell carcinomas and normal mucosa. *J. oral Pathol. Med.*, **23**, 220–225

Otten, N., von Tscharner, C., Lazary, S., Antczak, D.F. & Gerber, H. (1993) DNA of bovine papillomavirus type 1 and 2 in equine sarcoids: PCR detection and direct sequencing. *Arch. Virol.*, **132**, 121–131

Oyesanya, O.A., Amerasinghe, C. & Manning, E.A. (1993a) A comparison between loop diathermy conization and cold-knife conization for management of cervical dysplasia associated with unsatisfactory colposcopy. *Gynecol. Oncol.*, **50**, 84–88

Oyesanya, O.A., Amerasinghe, C.N. & Manning, E.A. (1993b) Outpatient excisional management of cervical intraepithelial neoplasia. A prospective, randomized comparison between loop diathermy excision and laser excisional conization. *Am. J. Obstet. Gynecol.*, **168**, 485–488

Paez, C.G., Yaegashi, N., Sato, S. & Yajima, A. (1993) Prevalence of serum IgG antibodies for the E7 and L2 proteins of human papillomavirus type 16 in cervical cancer patients and controls. *Tohoku J. exp. Med.*, **170**, 113–121

Pagano, R., Chanen, W., Rome, R.M. & Johnstone, N.R. (1987) The significance of human papilloma virus atypia ('wart virus infection') found alone on cervical cytology screening. *Aust. N. Z. J. Obstet. Gynaecol.*, **27**, 136–139

Pagano, M., Dürst, M., Joswig, S., Draetta, G. & Jansen-Dürr, P. (1992) Binding of the human E2F transcription factor to the retinoblastoma protein but not to cyclin A is abolished in HPV-16-immortalized cells. *Oncogene*, **7**, 1681–1686

Palefsky, J.M. (1991) Human papillomavirus-associated anogenital neoplasia and other solid tumors in human immunodeficiency virus-infected individuals. *Current Opinion Oncol.*, **3**, 881–885

Palefsky, J.M. (1994) Anal human papillomavirus infection and anal cancer in HIV-positive individuals: an emerging problem. *AIDS*, **8**, 283–295

Palefsky, J.M., Gonzales, J., Greenblatt, R.M., Ahn, D.K. & Hollander, H. (1990) Anal intraepithelial neoplasia and anal papillomavirus infection among homosexual males with group IV HIV disease. *J. Am. med. Assoc.*, **263**, 2911–2916

Palefsky, J.M., Holly, E.A., Gonzales, J., Berline, J., Ahn, D.K. & Greenspan, J.S. (1991) Detection of human papillomavirus DNA in anal intraepithelial neoplasia and anal cancer. *Cancer Res.*, **51**, 1014–1019

Palefsky, J.M., Holly, E.A., Gonzales, J., Lamborn, K. & Hollander, H. (1992) Natural history of anal cytologic abnormalities and papillomavirus infection among homosexual men with group IV HIV disease. *J. acquir. immune Defic. Syndr.*, **5**, 1258–1265

Palefsky, J.M., Shiboski, S. & Moss, A. (1994) Risk factors for anal human papillomavirus infection and anal cytologic abnormalities in HIV-positive and HIV-negative homosexual men. *J. acquir. immune Defic. Syndr.*, **7**, 599–606

Palmer, J.G., Scholefield, J.H., Coates, P.J., Shepherd, N.A., Jass, J.R., Crawford, L.V. & Northover, J.M.A. (1989) Anal cancer and human papillomaviruses. *Dis. Colon Rectum*, **32**, 1016–1022

Pamukcu, A.M. (1963) Epidemiologic studies on urinary bladder tumors in Turkish cattle. *Ann. N. Y. Acad. Sci.*, **108**, 938–947

Pan, H. & Griep, A.E. (1994) Altered cell cycle regulation in the lens of HPV-16 E6 or E7 transgenic mice: implications for tumor suppressor gene function in development. *Genes Dev.*, **8**, 1285–1299

Pao, C.C., Lai, C.-H., Wu, S.-Y., Young, K.-C., Chang, P.-L. & Soong, Y.-K. (1989) Detection of human papillomaviruses in exfoliated cervicovaginal cells by in situ DNA hybridization analysis. *J. clin. Microbiol.*, **27**, 168-173

Pao, C.C., Lin, C.-Y., Maa, J.-S., Lai, C.-H., Wu, S.-Y. & Soong, Y.-K. (1990) Detection of human papillomaviruses in cervicovaginal cells using polymerase chain reaction. *J. infect. Dis.*, **161**, 113-115

Pao, C.C., Kao, S.M., Tang, G.C., Lee, K., Si, J. & Ruan, S. (1994a) Prevalence of human papillomavirus DNA sequences in an area with very high incidence of cervical carcinoma. *Br. J. Cancer*, **70**, 694-696

Pao, C.C., Kao, S.M., Chen, J.H., Tang, G.C., Chang, P.Y. & Tan, T.T. (1994b) State of mutational alterations of p53 and retinoblastoma susceptibility genes in papillomavirus-negative small cell cervical carcinomas. *J. surg. Oncol.*, **57**, 87-93

Papanicolaou, G.N. & Traut, H.F. (1943) *Diagnosis of Uterine Cancer by the Vaginal Smear*, New York, The Commonwealth Fund

Paquette, R.L., Lee, Y.Y., Wilczynski, S.P., Karmakar, A., Kizaki, M., Miller, C.W. & Koeffler, H.P. (1993) Mutations of p53 and human papillomavirus infection in cervical carcinoma. *Cancer*, **72**, 1272-1280

Parham, P. (1994) Evolution of class I HLA antigen presenting molecules. In: Stanley, M.A., ed., *Immunology of Human Papillomaviruses*, New York, Plenum, pp. 161-172

Park, J.S., Jones, R.W., McLean, M.R., Currie, J.L., Woodruff, J.D., Shah, K.V. & Kurman, R.J. (1991) Possible etiologic heterogeneity of vulvar intraepithelial neoplasia: a correlation of pathologic characteristics with human papillomavirus detection by in situ hybridization and polymerase chain reaction. *Cancer*, **67**, 1599-1607

Park, D.S., Selvey, L.A., Kelsall, S.R. & Frazer, I.H. (1993) Human papillomavirus type 16 E6, E7 and L1 and type 18 E7 proteins produced by recombinant baculoviruses. *J. virol. Meth.*, **45**, 303-318

Park, D.J., Wilczynski, S.P., Paquette, R.L., Miller, C.W. & Koeffler, H.P. (1994) p53 Mutations in HPV-negative cervical carcinoma. *Oncogene*, **9**, 205-210

Parry, G., Byrne, M., Morse, A., Coleman, D.V., Taylor-Robinson, D. & Malcolm, A.D.B. (1990) Human papillomavirus infection of the cervix — the results of a prospective study. In: Howley, P.M. & Broker, T.R., eds, *Papillomaviruses*, New York, Wiley-Liss, pp. 13-20

Pasetto, N., Sesti, F., De Santis, L., Piccione, E., Novelli, G. & Dallapiccola, B. (1992) The prevalence of HPV16 DNA in normal and pathological cervical scrapes using the polymerase chain reaction. *Gynecol. Oncol.*, **46**, 33-36

Pater, M.M. & Pater, A. (1991) RU486 inhibits glucocorticoid hormone-dependent oncogenesis by human papillomavirus type 16 DNA. *Virology*, **183**, 799-802

Pater, M.M., Hughes, G.A., Hyslop, D.E., Nakshatri, H. & Pater, A. (1988) Glucocorticoid-dependent oncogenic transformation by type 16 but not type 11 human papilloma virus DNA. *Nature*, **335**, 832-835

Pater, A., Bayatpour, M. & Pater, M.M. (1990) Oncogenic transformation by human papillomavirus type 16 deoxyribonucleic acid in the presence of progesterone or progestins from oral contraceptives. *Am. J. Obstet. Gynecol.*, **162**, 1099-1103

Paterson-Brown, S., Chappatte, O.A., Clark, S.K., Wright, A., Maxwell, P., Taub, N.A. & Raju, K.S. (1992) The significance of cone biopsy resection margins. *Gynecol. Oncol.*, **46**, 182-185

Patrick, D.R., Oliff, A. & Heimbrook, D.C. (1994) Identification of a novel retinoblastoma gene product binding site on human papillomavirus type 16 E7 protein. *J. biol. Chem.*, **269**, 6842–6850

Pecoraro, G., Lee, M., Morgan, D. & Defendi, V. (1991) Evolution of in vitro transformation and tumorigenesis of HPV 16 and HPV 18 immortalized primary cervical epithelial cells. *Am. J. Pathol.*, **138**, 1–8

Pei, X.F., Gorman, P.A. & Watt, F.M. (1991) Two strains of human keratinocytes transfected with HPV16 DNA: comparison with the normal parental cells. *Carcinogenesis*, **12**, 277–284

Pei, X.F., Meck, J.M., Greenhalgh, D. & Schlegel, R. (1993) Cotransfection of HPV-18 and *v-fos* DNA induces tumorigenicity of primary human keratinocytes. *Virology*, **196**, 855–860

Pélisson, I., Chardonnet, Y., Euvrard, S. & Schmitt, D. (1994) Immunohistochemical detection of p53 protein in cutaneous lesions from transplant recipients harbouring human papillomavirus DNA. *Virchows Arch.*, **424**, 623–630

Peng, H.Q., Liu, S.L., Mann, V., Rohan, T. & Rawls, W. (1991) Human papillomavirus types 16 and 33, herpes simplex virus type 2 and other risk factors for cervical cancer in Sichuan Province, China. *Int. J. Cancer*, **47**, 711–716

Peng, X., Olson, R.O., Christian, C.B., Lang, C.M. & Kreider, J.W. (1993) Papillomas and carcinomas in transgenic rabbits carrying EJ-*ras* DNA and cottontail rabbit papillomavirus DNA. *J. Virol.*, **67**, 1698–1701

Penn, I. (1986) Cancers of the anogenital region in renal transplant recipients: analysis of 65 cases. *Cancer*, **58**, 611–616

Pereira-Smith, O.M. & Smith, J.R. (1981) Expression of SV40 T antigen in finite life-span hybrids of normal and SV40-transformed fibroblasts. *Somatic Cell Genet.*, **7**, 411–421

Pérez-Ayala, M., Ruiz-Cabello, F., Esteban, F., Concha, A., Redondo, M., Oliva, M.R., Cabrera, T. & Garrido, F. (1990) Presence of HPV 16 sequences in laryngeal carcinomas. *Int. J. Cancer*, **46**, 8–11

Peters, R.K., Thomas, D., Hagan, D.G., Mack, T.M. & Henderson, B.E. (1986) Risk factors for invasive cervical cancer among Latinas and non-Latinas in Los Angeles County. *J. natl Cancer Inst.*, **77**, 1063–1077

Petersen, C.S., Sjølin, K.-E., Rosman, N. & Lindeberg, H. (1994) Lack of human papillomavirus DNA in carcinoma cuniculatum (Letter to the Editor). *Acta derm. venereol. (Stockh.)*, **74**, 231–232

Petry, K.U., Scheffel, D., Bode, U., Gabrysiak, T., Köchel, H., Kupsch, E., Glaubitz, M., Niesert, S., Kühnle, H. & Schedel, I. (1994) Cellular immunodeficiency enhances the progression of human papillomavirus-associated cervical lesions. *Int. J. Cancer*, **57**, 836–840

Petti, L., Nilson, L.A. & DiMaio, D. (1991) Activation of the platelet-derived growth factor receptor by the bovine papillomavirus E5 transforming protein. *EMBO J.*, **10**, 845–855

Pfister, H. (1987) Human papillomaviruses and genital cancer. *Adv. Cancer Res.*, **48**, 113–147

Pfister, H. & Fuchs, P.G. (1994) Anatomy, taxonomy and evolution of papillomaviruses. *Intervirology*, **37**, 143–149

Pfister, H. & Haneke, E. (1984) Demonstration of human papillomavirus type 2 DNA in Bowen's disease. *Arch. dermatol. Res.*, **276**, 123–125

Pfister, H. & zur Hausen, H. (1978) Characterization of proteins of human papilloma viruses (HPV) and antibody response to HPV 1. *Med. Microbiol. Immunol. (Berl.)*, **166**, 13–19

Pfister, H., Gissmann, L. & zur Hausen, H. (1977) Partial characterization of the proteins of human papillomaviruses (HPV) 1-3. *Virology*, **83**, 131–137

Pfister, H., Linz, U., Gissmann, L., Huchthausen, B., Hoffmann, D. & zur Hausen, H. (1979a) Partial characterization of a new type of bovine papilloma viruses. *Virology,* **96**, 1–8

Pfister, H., Huchthausen, B., Gross, G. & zur Hausen, H. (1979b) Seroepidemiologic studies of bovine papillomavirus infections. *J. natl Cancer Inst.,* **62**, 1423–1425

Pfister, H., Nurnberger, F., Gissmann, L. & zur Hausen, H. (1981a) Characterization of a human papillomavirus from epidermodysplasia verruciformis lesions of a patient from Upper-volta. *Int. J. Cancer,* **27**, 645–650

Pfister, H., Fink, B. & Thomas, C. (1981b) Extrachromosomal bovine papillomavirus type 1 DNA in hamster fibromas and fibrosarcomas. *Virology,* **115**, 414–418

Pfister, H., Hettich, I., Runne, U., Gissmann, L. & Chilf, G.N. (1983a) Characterization of human papillomavirus type 13 from focal epithelial hyperplastic neck lesion. *J. Virol.,* **47**, 363–366

Pfister, H., Gassenmaier, A., Nürnberger, F. & Stuttgen, G. (1983b) Human papillomavirus 5-DNA in a carcinoma of an epidermodysplasia verruciformis patient infected with various human papillomavirus types. *Cancer Res.,* **43**, 1436–1441

Phelps, W.C., Yee, C.L., Münger, K. & Howley, P.M. (1988) The human papillomavirus type 16 E7 gene encodes transactivation and transformation functions similar to those of adenovirus E1A. *Cell,* **53**, 539–547

Phelps, W.C., Bagchi, S., Barnes, J.A., Raychaudhuri, P., Kraus, V., Münger, K., Howley, P.M. & Nevins, J.R. (1991) Analysis of *trans* activation by human papillomavirus type 16 E7 and adenovirus 12S E1A suggests a common mechanism. *J. Virol.,* **65**, 6922–6930

Phelps, W.C., Münger, K., Yee, C.L., Barnes, J.A. & Howley, P.M. (1992) Structure-function analysis of the human papillomavirus type 16 E7 oncoprotein. *J. Virol.,* **66**, 2418–2427

Phillips, D.H. & Ni Shé, M. (1993) Smoking-related DNA adducts in human cervical biopsies. In: Phillips, D.H., Castegnaro, M. & Bartsch, H., eds., *Postlabelling Methods for the Detection of DNA Damage* (IARC Scientific Publications No. 124), Lyon, IARC, pp. 327–330

Pich, A., Margaria, E., Ghiringhello, B. & Navone, R. (1992) In situ hybridization for human papillomavirus as a method of predicting the evolution of cervical intraepithelial neoplasia. *Arch. Gynecol. Obstet.,* **252**, 11–19

Pierceall, W.E., Goldberg, L.H. & Ananthaswamy, H.N. (1991) Presence of human papilloma virus type 16 DNA sequences in human nonmelanoma skin cancers. *J. invest. Dermatol.,* **97**, 880–884

Pietenpol, J.A., Tokino, T., Thiagalingam, S., El-Deiry, W.S., Kinzler, K.W. & Vogelstein, B. (1994) Sequence-specific transcriptional activation is essential for growth suppression by p53. *Proc. natl Acad. Sci. USA,* **91**, 1998–2002

Pilotti, S., Rotola, A., D'Amato, L., Di Luca, D., Shah, K.V., Cassai, E. & Rilke, F. (1990) Vulvar carcinomas: search for sequences homologous to human papillomavirus and herpes simplex virus DNA. *Mod. Pathol.,* **3**, 442–448

Pim, D., Collins, M. & Banks, L. (1992) Human papillomavirus type 16 E5 gene stimulates the transforming activity of the epidermal growth factor receptor. *Oncogene,* **7**, 27–32

Pirisi, L., Yasumoto, S., Feller, M., Doniger, J. & DiPaolo, J.A. (1987) Transformation of human fibroblasts and keratinocytes with human papillomavirus type 16 DNA. *J. Virol.,* **61**, 1061–1066

Pirisi, L., Creek, K.E., Doniger, J. & DiPaolo, J.A. (1988) Continuous cell lines with altered growth and differentiation properties originate after transfection of human keratinocytes with human papillomavirus type 16 DNA. *Carcinogenesis,* **9**, 1573–1579

Planner, R.S. & Hobbs, J.B. (1988) Intraepithelial and invasive neoplasia of the vulva in association with human papillomavirus infection. *J. reprod. Med.*, **33**, 503–509

Poljak, M. & Cerar, A. (1993) Human papillomavirus type 16 DNA in oesophageal squamous cell carcinoma. *Anticancer Res.*, **13**, 2113–2116

Popescu, N.C. & DiPaolo, J.A. (1990) Integration of human papillomavirus 16 DNA and genomic rearrangements in immortalized human keratinocyte lines. *Cancer Res.*, **50**, 1316–1323

Popescu, N.C., Zimonjic, D. & DiPaolo, J.A. (1989) Viral integration, fragile sites and proto-oncogenes in human neoplasia. *Human Genet.*, **84**, 383–386

Popper, H.H., El-Shabrawi, Y., Wöckel, W., Höfler, G., Kenner, L., Jüttner-Smolle, F.M. & Pongratz, M.G. (1994) Prognostic importance of human papilloma virus typing in squamous cell papilloma of the bronchus: comparison of in situ hybridization and the polymerase chain reaction. *Hum. Pathol.*, **25**, 1191–1197

Porreco, R., Penn, I., Droegemueller, W., Greer, B. & Makowski, E. (1975) Gynecologic malignancies in immunosuppressed organ homograft recipients. *Obstet. Gynecol.*, **45**, 359–364

Premoli-de-Percoco, G., Galindo, I., Ramirez, J.L., Perrone, M. & Rivera, H. (1993) Detection of human papillomavirus-related oral verruca vulgaris among venezuelans. *J. oral Pathol. Med.*, **22**, 113–116

Prendiville, W., Cullimore, J. & Norman, S. (1989) Large loop excision of the transformation zone (LLETZ). A new method of management for women with cervical intraepithelial neoplasia. *Br. J. Obstet. Gynaecol.*, **96**, 1054–1060

Price, M.L., Tidman, M.J., Fagg, N.L.K., Palmer, T.J. & MacDonald, D.M. (1988) Distinctive epidermal atypia in immunosuppression-associated cutaneous malignancy. *Histopathology*, **13**, 89–94

Purdie, K.J., Sexton, C.J., Proby, C.M., Glover, M.T., Williams, A.T., Stables, J.N. & Leigh, I.M. (1993) Malignant transformation of cutaneous lesions in renal allograft patients: a role for human papillomavirus. *Cancer Res.*, **53**, 5328–5333

Purola, E. & Savia, E. (1977) Cytology of gynecologic condyloma acuminatum. *Acta cytol.*, **21**, 26–31

Pyrhönen, S. & Neuvonen, E. (1978) The occurrence of human wart virus antibodies in dogs, pigs and cattle. *Arch. Virol.*, **57**, 297–305

Qin, X.-Q., Livingston, D.M., Kaelin, W.G., Jr & Adams, P.D. (1994) Deregulated transcription factor E2F-1 expression leads to S-phase entry and p53-mediated apoptosis. *Proc. natl Acad. Sci. USA*, **91**, 10918–10922

Querci della Rovere, G., Oliver, R.T.D., McCance, D.J. & Castro, J.E. (1988) Development of bladder tumour containing HPV type 11 DNA after renal transplantation. *Br. J. Urol.*, **62**, 36–38

Rabkin, C.S. & Blattner, W.A. (1991) HIV infection and cancers other than non-Hodgkin lymphoma and Kaposi's sarcoma. *Cancer Surv.*, **10**, 151–160

Rabkin, C.S., Biggar, R.J., Melbye, M. & Curtis, R.E. (1992) Second primary cancers following anal and cervical carcinoma: evidence of shared etiologic factors. *Am. J. Epidemiol.*, **136**, 54–58

Rabkin, C.S., Biggar, R.J., Baptiste, M.S., Abe, T., Kohler, B.A. & Nasca, P.C. (1993) Cancer incidence trends in women at high risk of human immunodeficiency virus (HIV) infection. *Int. J. Cancer*, **55**, 208–212

Rasmussen, K.A. (1958) Verrucae plantares: symptomology and epidemiology. *Acta derm.-venereol.*, **38** (Suppl. 39), 1–146

Rawls, W.E., Laurel, D., Melnick, J.L., Glicksman, J.M. & Kaufman, R.H. (1968) A search for viruses in smegma, premalignant and early malignant cervical tissues. The isolation of herpesviruses with distinct antigen properties. *Am. J. Epidemiol.*, **87**, 647–656

Reagan, J.W. & Hamonic, M.J. (1956) The cellular pathology in carcinoma *in situ*: a cytohistopathologic correlation. *Cancer*, **9**, 385–402

Reeves, W.C., Caussy, D., Brinton, L.A., Brenes, M.M., Montalvan, P., Gomez, B., de Britton, R.C., Morice, E., Gaitan, E. & De Lao, S.L. (1987) Case–control study of human papillomaviruses and cervical cancer in Latin America. *Int. J. Cancer*, **40**, 450–454

Reeves, W.C., Brinton, L.A., Garcia, M., Brenes, M.M., Herrero, R., Gaitán, E., Tenorio, F., de Britton, R.C. & Rawls, W.E. (1989) Human papillomavirus infection and cervical cancer in Latin America. *N. Engl. J. Med.*, **320**, 1437–1441

Reichman, R.C., Oakes, D., Bonnez, W., Brown, D., Reid Mattison, H., Bailey-Farchione, A., Stoler, M.H., Demeter, L.M., Tyring, S.K., Miller, L., Whitley, R., Carveth, H., Weidner, M., Krueger, G. & Choi, A. (1990) Treatment of condyloma acuminatum with three different interferon-α preparations administered parenterally: a double-blind, placebo-controlled trial. *J. infect. Dis.*, **162**, 1270–1276

Reid, S.W.J. & Smith, K.T. (1992) The equine sarcoid: detection of papillomaviral DNA in sarcoid tumours by use of consensus primers and the polymerase chain reaction. In: Plowright, W., Rossdale, P.D. & Wade, J.F., eds, *Equine Infectious Disease VI*, Newmarket, R & W Publications, pp. 297–300

Reid, R., Stanhope, C.R., Herschman, B.R., Booth, E., Phibbs, G.D. & Smith, J.P. (1982) Genital warts and cervical cancer. I: Evidence of an association between subclinical papillomavirus infection and cervical malignancy. *Cancer*, **50**, 377–387

Reid, R., Elfont, E.A., Zirkin, R.M. & Fuller, T.A. (1985) Superficial laser vulvectomy. II: The anatomic and biophysical principles permitting accurate control over the depth of dermal destruction with the carbon dioxide laser. *Am. J. Obstet. Gynecol.*, **152**, 261–271

Reid, R., Greenberg, M.D., Lörincz, A.T., Daoud, Y., Pizzuti, D. & Stoler, M. (1990) Superficial laser vulvectomy. IV: Extended laser vaporization and adjunctive 5-fluorouracil therapy of human papillomavirus-associated vulvar disease. *Obstet. Gynecol.*, **76**, 439–448

Reid, R., Greenberg, M.D., Pizzuti, D.J., Omoto, K.H., Rutledge, L.H. & Soo, W. (1992) Superficial laser vulvectomy. V: Surgical debulking is enhanced by adjuvant systemic interferon. *Am. J. Obstet. Gynecol.*, **166**, 815–820

Reid, S.W.J., Smith, K.T. & Jarrett, W.F.H. (1994) Detection, cloning and characterisation of papillomaviral DNA present in sarcoid tumours of *Equus asinus*. *Vet. Rec.*, **135**, 430–432

Remmink, A.J., Walboomers, J.M.M., Helmerhorst, T.J.M., Voorhorst, F.J., Rozendaal, L., Risse, E.K.J., Meijer, C.J.L.M. & Kenemans, P. (1995) The presence of persistent high-risk HPV genotypes in dysplastic cervical lesions is associated with progressive disease: natural history up to 36 months. *Int. J. Cancer*, **61**, 306–311

Reszka, A.A., Sundberg, J.P. & Reichmann, M.E. (1991) In vitro transformation and molecular characterization of Colobus monkey venereal papillomavirus DNA. *Virology*, **181**, 787–792

Richart, R.M. (1973) Cervical intraepithelial neoplasia: a review. In: Sommers, S.C., ed., *Pathology Annual*, East Norwalk, CT, Appleton-Century-Crofts, pp. 301–328

Richart, R.M. (1987) Causes and management of cervical intraepithelial neoplasia. *Cancer*, **60**, 1951–1959

Richart, R.M. (1990) A modified terminology for cervical intraepithelial neoplasia. *Obstet. Gynecol.*, **75**, 131–133

Richart, R.M. & Barron, B.A. (1969) A follow-up study of patients with cervical dysplasia. *Am. J. Obstet. Gynecol.*, **105**, 386–393

Richart, R.M. & Wright, T.C. (1994) The histology of lower anogenital tract neoplasia. In: Singer, A. & Monaghan, J.M., eds, *Lower Genital Tract Precancer: Colposcopy, Pathology, and Treatment*, Oxford, Blackwell Scientific Publications, pp. 2–9

Richart, R.M., Fu, Y.S. & Winkler, B. (1992) Pathology of cervical squamous and glandular intraepithelial neoplasia. In: Coppleson, M., ed., *Gynecologic Oncology*, 2nd Ed., New York, Churchill Livingstone, pp. 557–570

Ries, L.A.G., Miller, B.A., Hankey, B.F., Kosary, C.L., Harras, A. & Edwards, B.K., eds (1994) *SEER Cancer Statistics Review, 1973–1991: Tables and Graphs* (NIH Pub. No. 94-2789), Bethesda, MD, National Cancer Institute

Rihkanen, H., Aaltonen, L.-M. & Syrjänen, S.M. (1993) Human papillomavirus in laryngeal papillomas and in adjacent normal epithelium. *Clin. Otolaryngol.*, **18**, 470–474

Rihkanen, H., Peltomaa, J. & Syrjänen, S. (1994) Prevalence of human papillomavirus (HPV) DNA in vocal cords without laryngeal papillomas. *Acta otolaryngol. (Stockh.)*, **114**, 348–351

Riou, G., Barrois, M., Tordjman, I., Dutronquay, V. & Orth, G. (1984) Detection of papillomavirus genomes and evidence for amplification of the oncogenes c-*myc* and c-Ha-*ras* in invasive squamous cell carcinomas of the uterine cervix. *C. R. Acad. Sci. Paris*, **299**, 575–580 (in French)

Riou, G., Barrois, M., Sheng, Z.M., Duvillard, P. & Lhomme, C. (1988) Somatic deletions and mutations of c-Ha-*ras* gene in human cervical cancers. *Oncogene*, **3**, 329–333

Riou, G., Favre, M., Jeannel, D., Bourhis, J., Le Doussal, V. & Orth, G. (1990) Association between poor prognosis in early-stage invasive cervical carcinomas and non-detection of HPV DNA. *Lancet*, **335**, 1171–1174

Riou, G., Lê, M.G., Favre, M., Jeannel, D., Bourhis, J. & Orth, G. (1992) Human papillomavirus-negative status and c-*myc* gene overexpression: independent prognostic indicators of distant metastasis for early-stage invasive cervical cancers. *J. natl Cancer Inst.*, **84**, 1525–1526

Roberts, J.M. & Weintraub, H. (1986) Negative control of DNA replication in composite SV40-bovine papilloma virus plasmids. *Cell*, **46**, 741–752

Roberts, S., Ashmole, I., Johnson, G.D., Kreider, J.W. & Gallimore, P.H. (1993) Cutaneous and mucosal human papillomavirus E4 proteins form intermediate filament-like structures in epithelial cells. *Virology*, **197**, 176–187

Robertson, J.H., Woodend, B.E., Crozier, E.H. & Hutchinson, J. (1988) Risk of cervical cancer associated with mild dyskaryosis. *Br. med. J.*, **297**, 18–21

de Roda Husman, A.-M., Walboomers, J.M.M., Meijer, C.J.L.M., Risse, E.K.J., Schipper, M.E.I., Helmerhorst, T.M., Bleker, O.P., Delius, H., van den Brule, A.J.C. & Snijders, P.J.F. (1994) Analysis of cytomorphologically abnormal cervical scrapes for the presence of 27 mucosotropic human papillomavirus genotypes, using polymerase chain reaction. *Int. J. Cancer*, **56**, 802–806

de Roda Husman, A.-M., Walboomers, J.M.M., van den Brule, A.J.C., Meijer, C.J.L.M. & Snijders, P.J.F. (1995) The use of general primers GP5 and GP6 elongated at their 3′ ends with adjacent highly conserved sequences improves human papillomavirus detection by PCR. *J. gen. Virol.*, **76**, 1057–1062

Roden, R.B., Kirnbauer, R., Jenson, A.B., Lowy, D.R. & Schiller, J.T. (1994a) Interaction of papillomaviruses with the cell surface. *J. Virol.*, **68**, 7260–7266

Roden, R.B., Weissinger, E.M., Henderson, D.W., Booy, F., Kirnbauer, R., Mushinski, J.F., Lowy, D.R. & Schiller, J.T. (1994b) Neutralization of bovine papillomavirus by antibodies to L1 and L2 capsid proteins. *J. Virol.*, **68**, 7570–7574

Roggenbuck, B., Larsen, P.M., Fey, S.J., Bartsch, D., Gissmann, L. & Schwarz, E. (1991) Human papillomavirus type 18 E6*, E6, and E7 protein synthesis in cell-free translation systems and comparison of E6 and E7 in vitro translation products to proteins immunoprecipitated from human epithelial cells. *J. Virol.*, **65**, 5068–5072

Roman, A. & Fife, K. (1986) Human papillomavirus DNA associated with foreskins of normal newborns. *J. infect. Dis.*, **153**, 855–861

Romanczuk, H. & Howley, P.M. (1992) Disruption of either the *E1* or the *E2* regulatory gene of human papillomavirus type 16 increases viral immortalization capacity. *Proc. natl Acad. Sci. USA*, **89**, 3159–3163

Romanczuk, H., Thierry, F. & Howley, P.M. (1990) Mutational analysis of cis elements involved in E2 modulation of human papillomavirus type 16 P_{97} and type 18 P_{105} promoters. *J. Virol.*, **64**, 2849–2859

Romanczuk, H., Villa, L.L., Schlegel, R. & Howley, P.M. (1991) The viral transcriptional regulatory region upstream of the *E6* and *E7* genes is a major determinant of the differential immortalization activities of human papillomavirus types 16 and 18. *J. Virol.*, **65**, 2739–2744

Roncalli, M., Sideri, M., Giè, P. & Servida, E. (1988) Immunophenotypic analysis of the transformation zone of human cervix. *Lab. Invest.*, **58**, 141–149

Rose, R.C., Bonnez, W., Strike, D.G. & Reichman, R.C. (1990) Expression of the full-length products of the human papillomavirus type 6b (HPV-6b) and HPV-11 L2 open reading frames by recombinant baculovirus, and antigenic comparisons with HPV-11 whole virus particles. *J. gen. Virol.*, **71**, 2725–2729

Rose, R.C., Bonnez, W., Reichman, R.C. & Garcea, R.L. (1993) Expression of human papillomavirus type 11 L1 protein in insect cells: in vivo and in vitro assembly of virus-like particles. *J. Virol.*, **67**, 1936–1944

Rose, R.C., Reichman, R.C. & Bonnez, W. (1994a) Human papillomavirus (HPV) type 11 recombinant virus-like particles induce the formation of neutralizing antibodies and detect HPV-specific antibodies in human sera. *J. gen. Virol.*, **75**, 2075–2079

Rose, R.C., Bonnez, W., Da Rin, C., McCance, D.J. & Reichman, R.C. (1994b) Serological differentiation of human papillomavirus types 11, 16 and 18 using recombinant virus-like particles. *J. gen. Virol.*, **75**, 2445–2449

Rosemberg, S.K. (1991) Sexually transmitted papillomaviral infection in men. An update. *Dermatol. Clin.*, **9**, 317–331

Rosenberger, G. (1971) Nature, manifestations, cause and control of chronic enzootic haematuria in cattle. *Vet. Med. Rev.*, **2/3**, 189–206

Rosenfeld, W.D., Vermund, S.H., Wentz, S.J. & Burk, R.D. (1989) High prevalence rate of human papillomavirus infection and association with abnormal Papanicolaou smears in sexually active adolescents. *Am. J. Dis. Child.*, **143**, 1443–1447

Rösl, F., Dürst, M. & zur Hausen, H. (1988) Selective suppression of human papillomavirus transcription in non-tumorigenic cells by 5-azacytidine. *EMBO J.*, **7**, 1321–1328

Rösl, F., Achtstätter, T., Bauknecht, T., Hutter, K.-J., Futterman, G. & zur Hausen, H. (1991) Extinction of the HPV 18 upstream regulatory region in cervical carcinoma cells after fusion with non-tumorigenic human keratinocytes under non-selective conditions. *EMBO J.*, **10**, 1337–1345

Rösl, F., Arab, A., Klevenz, B. & zur Hausen, H. (1993) The effect of DNA methylation on gene regulation of human papillomaviruses. *J. gen. Virol.*, **74**, 791–801

Rösl, F., Lengert, M., Albrecht, J., Kleine, K., Zawatzky, R., Schraven, F. & zur Hausen, H. (1994) Differential regulation of the JE gene encoding the monocyte chemoattractant protein (MCP-1) in cervical carcinoma cells and derived hybrids. *J. Virol.*, **68**, 2142–2150

Rotenberg, M.O., Chow, L.T. & Broker, T.R. (1989) Characterization of rare human papillomavirus type 11 mRNAs coding for regulatory and structural proteins, using the polymerase chain reaction. *Virology*, **172**, 489–497

Roth, E.J., Kurz, B., Liang, L., Hansen, C.L., Dameron, C.T., Winge, D.R. & Smotkin, D. (1992) Metal thiolate coordination in the E7 proteins of human papilloma virus 16 and cottontail rabbit papilloma virus as expressed in *Escherichia coli*. *J. biol. Chem.*, **267**, 16390–16395

Rotola, A., Monini, P., Di Luca, D., Savioli, A., Simone, R., Secchiero, P., Reggiani, A. & Cassai, E. (1992) Presence and physical state of HPV DNA in prostate and urinary-tract tissues. *Int. J. Cancer*, **52**, 359–365

Rotteleur, G., Riboulet, J.L., Vanlerberghe, K., Pollet, M., Lemaire, B. & Brunetaud, J.M. (1986) Management of vulvar condylomata acuminata with argon laser. *Lasers surg. Med.*, **6**, 119–122

Rous, P. & Beard, J.W. (1934) A virus-induced mammalian growth with the characters of a tumour (the Shope rabbit papilloma). 1. The growth on implantation within a favourable host. *J. exp. Med.*, **60**, 701–722

Rous, P. & Friedewald, W.F. (1944) The effect of chemical carcinogens on virus-induced rabbit papilloma. *J. exp. Med.*, **79**, 511–537

Rous, P. & Kidd, J.G. (1938) The carcinogenic effect of a papilloma virus on the tarred skin of rabbits. I. Description of the phenomenon. *J. exp. Med.*, **67**, 399–427

Rowson, K.E.K. & Mahy, B.W.J. (1967) Human papova (wart) virus. *Bacteriol. Rev.*, **31**, 110–131

Rübben, A., Krones, R., Schwetschenau, B. & Grussendorf-Conen, E.-I. (1993) Common warts from immunocompetent patients show the same distribution of human papillomavirus types as common warts from immunocompromised patients. *Br. J. Dermatol.*, **128**, 264–270

Rüdlinger, R., Smith, I.W., Bunney, M.H. & Hunter, J.A. (1986) Human papillomavirus infections in a group of renal transplant recipients. *Br. J. Dermatol.*, **115**, 681–692

Rüdlinger, R., Bunney, M.H., Grob, R. & Hunter, J.A.A. (1989a) Warts in fish handlers. *Br. J. Dermatol.*, **120**, 375–381

Rüdlinger, R., Grob, R., Yu, Y.X. & Schnyder, U.W. (1989b) HPV 35 positive bowenoid papulosis of the anogenital area and concurrent HPV-35 positive verruca with bowenoid dysplasia of the periungual area. *Arch. Dermatol.*, **125**, 655–659

Rueda, L.A. & Rodriguez, G. (1976) Human warts after HPV. Clinical, histological and ultrastructural correlation. *Med. Cut. I.L.A.*, **2**, 113–136 (in Spanish)

Rusk, D., Sutton, G.P., Look, K.Y. & Roman, A. (1991) Analysis of invasive squamous cell carcinoma of the vulva and vulvar intraepithelial neoplasia for the presence of human papillomavirus DNA. *Obstet. Gynecol.*, **77**, 918–922

Rylander, E., Ruusuvaara, L., Almströmer, M.W., Evander, M. & Wadell, G. (1994) The absence of vaginal human papillomavirus 16 DNA in women who have not experienced sexual intercourse. *Obstet. Gynecol.*, **83**, 735–737

Sadovnikova, E., Zhu, X., Collins, S.M., Zhou, J., Vousden, K., Crawford, L., Beverley, P. & Stauss, H.J. (1994) Limitations of predictive motifs revealed by cytotoxic T lymphocyte epitope mapping of the human papilloma virus E7 protein. *Int. Immunol.*, **6**, 289–296

Saiki, R.K.,Gelfand, D.H., Stoffel, S., Scharf, S.J,. Higuchi, R., Horn, G.T., Mullis, K.B. & Erlich, H.A. (1988) Primer-directed enzymatic amplification of DNA with a thermostable DNA polymerase. *Science*, **239**, 487–491

Saito, J., Fukuda, T., Nakatani, H., Sumiyoshi, M., Kinoshita, M., Ikeda, M. & Noda, K. (1992) Detection of human papillomavirus DNA in the normal cervices of Japanese women by the dot-blot (Vira Pap™) method. *Asia-Oceania J. Obstet. Gynaecol.*, **18**, 283–287

Saltzstein, D.R., Orihuela, E., Kocurek, J.N., Payne, D.A., Chan, T.-S. & Tyring, S.K. (1993) Failure of the polymerase chain reaction (PCR) to detect human papilloma virus (HPV) in transitional cell carcinoma of the bladder. *Anticancer Res.*, **13**, 423–425

Sandler, A.B., Vande Pol, S.B. & Spalholz, B.A. (1993) Repression of bovine papillomavirus type 1 transcription by the E1 replication protein. *J. Virol.*, **67**, 5079–5087

Sang, B.C. & Barbosa, M.S. (1992a) Single amino acid substitutions in 'low-risk' human papillomavirus (HPV) type 6 E7 protein enhance features characteristic of the 'high-risk' HPV E7 oncoproteins. *Proc. natl Acad. Sci. USA*, **89**, 8063–8067

Sang, B.C. & Barbosa, M.S. (1992b) Increased E6/E7 transcription in HPV 18-immortalized human keratinocytes results from inactivation of E2 and additional cellular events. *Virology*, **189**, 448–455

de Sanjosé, S., Palacio, V., Tafur, L., Vazquez, S., Espitia, V., Vazquez, F., Koman, G., Muñoz, N. & Bosch, F.X. (1993) Prostitution, HIV and cervical neoplasia: a survey in Spain and Colombia. *Cancer Epidemiol. Biomarkers Prev.*, **2**, 531–535

de Sanjosé, S., Muñoz, N., Bosch, F.X., Reimann, K., Pedersen, N.S., Orfila, J., Ascunce, N., González, L.C., Tafur, L., Gili, M., Lette, I., Viladiu, P., Tormo, M.J., Moreo, P., Shah, K.V. & Wahren, B. (1994) Sexually transmitted agents and cervical neoplasia in Colombia and Spain. *Int. J. Cancer*, **56**, 358–363

Saragoni, A., Medri, L., Bacci, F., Padovani, F., Sabattini, E., Nanni, O. & Gaudio, M. (1992) Value of the in situ hybridization technique in the diagnosis of human papilloma virus infections of the uterine cervix: correlations between the human papilloma virus type and the morphological features. *Pathologica*, **84**, 57–66 (in Italian)

Sarkar, S., Verma, K., Kaur, H. & Seth, P. (1992a) Detection of human papilloma virus types 16 and 18 DNA in cervical lesions of Indian women using in situ hybridization. *Indian J. med. Res.*, **96**, 356–360

Sarkar, F.H., Miles, B.J., Plieth, D.H. & Crissman, J.D. (1992b) Detection of human papillomavirus in squamous neoplasm of the penis. *J. Urol.*, **147**, 389–392

Sarkar, F.H., Sakr, W.A., Li, Y.-W., Sreepathi, P. & Crissman, J.D. (1993) Detection of human papillomavirus (HPV) DNA in human prostatic tissues by polymerase chain reaction (PCR). *Prostate*, **22**, 171–180

Sasagawa, T., Inoue, M., Tanizawa, O., Yutsudo, M. & Hakura, A. (1992a) Identification of antibodies against human papillomavirus type 16 E6 and E7 proteins in sera of patients with cervical neoplasias. *Jpn J. Cancer Res.*, **83**, 705–713

Sasagawa, T., Inoue, M., Inoue, H., Yutsudo, M., Tanizawa, O. & Hakura, A. (1992b) Induction of uterine cervical neoplasias in mice by human papillomavirus type 16 E6/E7 genes. *Cancer Res.*, **52**, 4420–4426

Sassolas, B., Bourbigot, B., Plantin, P., Le Roy, J.P. & Guillet, G. (1991) Papillomavirus type II skin infection associated with spinocellular carcinoma in a kidney transplant recipient (Letter to the Editor). *Presse méd.*, **20**, 563–564 (in French)

Sasson, I.M., Haley, J., Hoffmann, D., Wynder, E.L., Hellberg, D. & Nilsson, S. (1985) Cigarette smoking and neoplasia of the uterine cervix: smoke constituents in cervical mucus. *N. Engl. J. Med.*, **312**, 315–316

Sato, H., Watanabe, S., Furuno, A. & Yoshiike, K. (1989a) Human papillomavirus type 16 E7 protein expressed in *Escherichia coli* and monkey COS-1 cells: immunofluorescence detection of the nuclear E7 protein. *Virology*, **170**, 311–315

Sato, H., Furuno, A. & Yoshiike, K. (1989b) Expression of human papillomavirus type 16 E7 gene induces DNA synthesis of rat 3Y1 cells. *Virology*, **168**, 195–199

Sau, P., McMarlin, S.L., Sperling, L.C. & Katz, R. (1994) Bowen's disease of the nail bed and periungual area: a clinicopathologic analysis of seven cases. *Arch. Dermatol.*, **130**, 204–209

Saxon, P.J., Srivatsan, E.S. & Stanbridge, E.J. (1986) Introduction of human chromosome 11 via microcell transfer controls tumorigenic expression of HeLa cells. *EMBO J.*, **5**, 3461–3466

Schäfer, A., Friedmann, W., Mielke, M., Schwartlander, B. & Koch, M.A. (1991) The increased frequency of cervical dysplasia-neoplasia in women infected with the human immunodeficiency virus is related to the degree of immunosuppression. *Am. J. Obstet. Gynecol.*, **164**, 593–599

Scheffner, M., Werness, B.A., Huibregtse, J.M., Levine, A.J. & Howley, P.M. (1990) The E6 oncoprotein encoded by human papillomavirus types 16 and 18 promotes the degradation of p53. *Cell*, **63**, 1129–1136

Scheffner, M., Münger, K., Byrne, J.C. & Howley, P.M. (1991) The state of the p53 and retinoblastoma genes in human cervical carcinoma cell lines. *Proc. natl Acad. Sci. USA*, **88**, 5523–5527

Scheffner, M., Huibregtse, J.M., Vierstra, R.D. & Howley, P.M. (1993) The HPV-16 E6 and E6-AP complex functions as a ubiquitin-protein ligase in the ubiquitination of p53. *Cell*, **75**, 495–505

Scheffner, M., Nuber, U. & Huibregtse, J.M. (1995) Protein ubiquitination involving an E1-E2-E3 enzyme ubiquitin thioester cascade. *Nature*, **373**, 81–83

Scheurlen, W., Stremlau, A., Gissmann, L., Hohn, D., Zenner, H.P. & zur Hausen, H. (1986a) Rearranged HPV 16 molecules in an anal and in a laryngeal carcinoma. *Int. J. Cancer*, **38**, 671–676

Scheurlen, W., Gissmann, L., Gross, G. & zur Hausen, H. (1986b) Molecular cloning of two new HPV types (HPV 37 and HPV 38) from a keratoacanthoma and a malignant melanoma. *Int. J. Cancer*, **37**, 505–510

Schiffman, M.H. (1992a) Validation of hybridization assays: correlation of filter *in situ*, dot blot and PCR and Southern blot. In: Muñoz, N., Bosch, F.X., Shah, K.V. & Meheus, A., eds, *The Epidemiology of Human Papillomavirus and Cervical Cancer* (IARC Scientific Publications No. 119), Lyon, IARC, pp. 169–179

Schiffman, M.H. (1992b) Recent progress in defining the epidemiology of human papillomavirus infection and cervical neoplasia. *J. natl Cancer Inst.*, **84**, 394–398

Schiffman, M.H. (1994) Epidemiology of cervical human papillomavirus infections. *Curr. Top. Microbiol. Immunol.*, **196**, 54–81

Schiffman, M.H. & Schatzkin, A. (1994) Test reliability is critically important to molecular epidemiology: an example from studies of human papillomavirus infection and cervical neoplasia. *Cancer Res.*, **54**, S1944–S1947

Schiffman, M.H., Haley, N.J., Felton, J.S., Andrews, A.W., Kaslow, R.A., Lancaster, W.D., Kurman, R.J., Brinton, L.A., Lannom, L.B. & Hoffmann, D. (1987) Biochemical epidemiology of cervical neoplasia: measuring cigarette smoke constituents in the cervix. *Cancer Res.*, **47**, 3886–3888

Schiffman, M.H., Bauer, H.M., Hoover, R.N., Glass, A.G., Cadell, D.M., Rush, B.B., Scott, D.R., Sherman, M.E., Kurman, R.J. & Wacholder, S. (1993) Epidemiologic evidence showing that human papillomavirus infection causes most cervical intraepithelial neoplasia. *J. natl Cancer Inst.*, **85**, 958–964

Schiffman, M.H., Kiviat, N.B., Burk, R.D., Shah, K.V., Daniel, R.W., Lewis, R., Kupers, J., Manos, M.M., Scott, D.R., Sherman, M.E., Kurman, R.J., Stoler, M.H., Glass, A.G., Rush, B.B., Mielzynska, I. & Lörincz, A.T. (1995) Accuracy and interlaboratory reliability of human papillomavirus DNA testing using Hybrid Capture. *J. clin. Microbiol.*, **33**, 545–550

Schlegel, R., Phelps, W.C., Zhang, Y.L. & Barbosa, M. (1988) Quantitative keratinocyte assay detects two biological activities of human papillomavirus DNA and identifies viral types associated with cervical carcinoma. *EMBO J.*, **7**, 3181–3187

Schlehofer, J.R., Gissmann, L., Matz, B. & zur Hausen, H. (1983a) Herpes simplex virus induced amplification of SV40 sequences in transformed Chinese hamster cells. *Int. J. Cancer*, **32**, 99–103

Schlehofer, J.R., Heilbronn, R., Georg-Fries, B. & zur Hausen, H. (1983b) Inhibition of initiator-induced SV40 gene amplification in SV40-transformed Chinese hamster cells by infection with a defective papovavirus. *Int. J. Cancer*, **32**, 591–595

Schmitt, J., Schlehofer, J.R., Mergener, K., Gissmann, L. & zur Hausen, H. (1989) Amplification of bovine papillomavirus DNA by N-methyl-N'-nitro-N-nitrosoguanidine, ultraviolet irradiation, or infection with herpes simplex virus. *Virology*, **172**, 73–81

Schmitt, A., Harry, J.B., Rapp, B., Wettstein, F.O. & Iftner, T. (1994) Comparison of the properties of the E6 and E7 genes of low- and high-risk cutaneous papillomaviruses reveals strongly transforming and high Rb-binding activity for the E7 protein of the low-risk human papillomavirus type 1. *J. Virol.*, **68**, 7051–7059

Schneider, A. (1994) Natural history of genital papillomavirus infections. *Intervirology*, **37**, 201–214

Schneider, V., Kay, S. & Lee, H.M. (1983) Immunosuppression as a high-risk factor in the development of condyloma acuminatum and squamous neoplasia of the cervix. *Acta cytol.*, **27**, 220–224

Schneider, A., Papendick, U., Gissmann, L. & de Villiers, E.-M. (1987a) Interferon treatment of human genital papillomavirus infection: importance of viral type. *Int. J. Cancer*, **40**, 610–614

Schneider, A., de Villiers, E.-M. & Schneider, V. (1987b) Multifocal squamous neoplasia of the female genital tract: significance of human papillomavirus infection of the vagina after hysterectomy. *Obstet. Gynecol.*, **70**, 294–298

Schneider, A., Meinhardt, G., Kirchmayr, R. & Schneider, V. (1991) Prevalence of human papillomavirus genomes in tissues from the lower genital tract as detected by molecular in situ hybridization. *Int. J. gynecol. Pathol.*, **10**, 1–14

Schneider, A., Grubert, T., Kirchmayr, R., Wagner, D., Papendick, U. & Schlunck, G. (1995) Efficacy trial of topically administered interferon gamma-1β gel in comparison to laser treatment in cervical intraepithelial neoplasia. *Arch. Gynecol. Obstet.*, **256**, 75–83

Schneider-Maunoury, S., Croissant, O., Orth, G. (1987) Integration of human papillomavirus type 16 DNA sequences: a possible early event in the progression of genital tumors. *J. Virol.*, **61**, 3295–3298

Scholefield, J.H., Sonnex, C., Talbot, I.C., Palmer, J.G., Whatrup, C., Mindel, A. & Northover, J.M.A. (1989) Anal and cervical intraepithelial neoplasia: possible parallel. *Lancet*, **ii**, 765–769

Scholefield, J.H., McIntyre, P., Palmer, J.G., Coates, P.J., Shepherd, N.A. & Northover, J.M. (1990a) DNA hybridisation of routinely processed tissue for detecting HPV DNA in anal squamous cell carcinomas over 40 years. *J. clin. Pathol.*, **43**, 133–136

Scholefield, J.H., Palmer, J.G., Shepherd, N.A., Love, S., Miller, K.J. & Northover, J.M. (1990b) Clinical and pathological correlates of HPV type 16 DNA in anal cancer. *Int. J. colorect. Dis.*, **5**, 219–222

Scholefield, J.H., Kerr, I.B., Shepherd, N.A., Miller, K.J., Bloomfield, R. & Northover, J.M. (1991) Human papillomavirus type 16 DNA in anal cancers from six different countries. *Gut*, **32**, 674–676

Scholefield, J.H., Hickson, W.G., Smith, J.H., Rogers, K. & Sharp, F. (1992) Anal intraepithelial neoplasia: part of a multifocal disease process. *Lancet*, **340**, 1271–1273

Schottlander, J. & Kermauner, F. (1912) Monograph on carcinoma of the uterus. Study on morphology, evolution and growth. Contribution to the clinics of the disease, Berlin, S. Karger (in German)

Schrager, L.K., Friedland, G.H., Maude, D., Schreiber, K., Adachi, A., Pizzuti, D.J., Koss, L.G. & Klein, R.S. (1989) Cervical and vaginal squamous cell abnormalities in women infected with human immunodeficiency virus. *J. acquir. immune Defic. Syndr.*, **2**, 570–575

Schwarz, E., Freese, U.K., Gissmann, L., Mayer, W., Roggenbuck, B., Stremlau, A. & zur Hausen, H. (1985) Structure and transcription of human papillomavirus sequences in cervical carcinoma cells. *Nature*, **314**, 111–114

Scully, C., Prime, S. & Maitland, N. (1985) Papillomaviruses: their possible role in oral disease. *Oral Surg. oral Med. oral Pathol.*, **60**, 166–174

Searle, P.F., Thomas, D.P., Faulkner, K.B. & Tinsley, J.M. (1994) Stomach cancer in transgenic mice expressing human papillomavirus type 16 early region genes from a keratin promoter. *J. gen. Virol.*, **75**, 1125–1137

Sebbelov, A.M., Kjørstad, K.E., Abeler, V.M. & Norrild, B. (1991) The prevalence of human papillomavirus type 16 and 18 DNA in cervical cancer in different age groups: a study on the incidental cases of cervical cancer in Norway in 1983. *Gynecol. Oncol.*, **41**, 141–148

Sebbelov, A.M., Svendsen, C., Jensen, H., Kjaer, S.K. & Norrild, B. (1994) Prevalence of HPV in premalignant and malignant cervical lesions in Greenland and Denmark: PCR and in situ hybridization analysis on archival material. *Res. Virol.*, **145**, 83–92

Seck, A.C., Faye, M.A., Critchlow, C.W., Mbaye, A.D., Kuypers, J., Woto-Gaye, G., Langley, C., De, E.B., Holmes, K.K. & Kiviat, N.B. (1994) Cervical intraepithelial neoplasia and human papillomavirus infection among Senegalese women seropositive for HIV-1 or HIV-2 or seronegative for HIV. *Int. J. STD AIDS*, **5**, 189–193

Sedlacek, T.V., Lindheim, S., Eder, C. Hasty, L., Woodland, M., Ludomirsky, A. & Rando, R.F. (1989) Mechanism for human papillomavirus transmission at birth. *Am. J. Obstet. Gynecol.*, **161**, 55–59

Sedman, S.A., Barbosa, M.S., Vass, W.C., Hubbert, N.L., Haas, J.A., Lowy, D.R. & Schiller, J.T. (1991) The full-length E6 protein of human papillomavirus type 16 has transforming and trans-activating activities and cooperates with E7 to immortalize keratinocytes in culture. *J. Virol.*, **65**, 4860–4866

Sedman, S.A., Hubbert, N.L., Vass, W.C., Lowy, D.R. & Schiller, J.T. (1992) Mutant p53 can substitute for human papillomavirus type 16 E6 in immortalization of human keratinocytes but does not have E6-associated *trans*-activation or transforming activity. *J. Virol.*, **66**, 4201–4208

Seedorf, K., Oltersdorf, T., Krämmer, G. & Röwekamp, W. (1987) Identification of early proteins of the human papilloma viruses type 16 (HPV 16) and type 18 (HPV 18) in cervical carcinoma cells. *EMBO J.*, **6**, 139–144

Segers, P., Haesen, S., Amy, J.-J., De Sutter, P., Van Dam, P. & Kirsch-Volders, M. (1994) Detection of premalignant stages in cervical smears with a biotinylated probe for chromosome 1. *Cancer Genet. Cytogenet.*, **75**, 120–129

Sekine, H., Fuse, A., Tada, A., Maeda, S. & Simizu, B. (1988) Expression of human papillomavirus type 6b E2 gene product with DNA-binding activity in insect (*Bombyx mori*) cells using a baculovirus expression vector. *Gene*, **65**, 187–193

Selvakumar, R., Borenstein, L.A., Lin, Y.-L., Ahmed, R. & Wettstein, F.O. (1994) T-cell response to cottontail rabbit papillomavirus structural proteins in infected rabbits. *J. Virol.*, **68**, 4043–4048

Selvakumar, R., Borenstein, L.A., Lin, Y.L., Ahmed, R. & Wettstein, F.O. (1995) Immunization with nonstructural proteins E1 and E2 of cottontail rabbit papillomavirus stimulates regression of virus-induced papillomas. *J. Virol.*, **69**, 602–605

Selvey, L.A., Dunn, L.A., Tindle, R.W., Park, D.S. & Frazer, I.H. (1994) Human papillomavirus (HPV) type 18 E7 protein is a short-lived steroid-inducible phosphoprotein in HPV-transformed cell lines. *J. gen. Virol.*, **75**, 1647–1653

Seo, Y.-S., Müller, F., Lusky, M. & Hurwitz, J. (1993) Bovine papilloma virus (BPV)-encoded E1 protein contains multiple activities required for BPV DNA replication. *Proc. natl Acad. Sci. USA*, **90**, 702–706

Serfling, U., Ciancio, G., Zhu, W.-Y., Leonardi, C. & Penneys, N.S. (1992) Human papillomavirus and herpes virus DNA are not detected in benign and malignant prostatic tissue using the polymerase chain reaction. *J. Urol.*, **148**, 192–194

Seshadri, L., Oomman, M., Hemalatha, K. & Jairaj, P. (1991) Cervical intraepithelial neoplasia and human papilloma virus infection. *Indian J. Cancer*, **28**, 27–32

Sevin, B.-U., Ford, J.H., Girtanner, R.D., Hoskins, W.J., Ng, A.B.P., Nordqvist, S.R.B. & Averette, H.E. (1979) Invasive cancer of the cervix after cryosurgery. *Obstet. Gynecol.*, **53**, 465–471

Shadan, F.F. & Villarreal, L.P. (1993) Coevolution of persistently infecting small DNA viruses and their hosts linked to host-interactive regulatory domains. *Proc. natl Acad. Sci. USA*, **90**, 4117–4121

Shah, K.V. & Gissmann, L. (1989) Experimental evidence on oncogenicity of papillomaviruses. In: Muñoz, N., Bosch, F.X. & Jensen, O.M., eds, *Human Papillomavirus and Cervical Cancer* (IARC Scientific Publications No. 94), Lyon, IARC, pp. 105–111

Shah, K.V. & Howley, P.M. (1992) Papillomaviruses. In: Lennette, E.H., ed., *Laboratory Diagnosis of Viral Infection*, 2nd Ed., Marcel Dekker, Inc., pp. 591–612

Shah, K.V. & Howley, P.M. (1996) Chapter 66. Papillomaviruses. In: Fields, B.N., Knipe, D.M., & Howley, P.M., eds, *Field Virology*, New York, Raven Press (in press)

Shah, K., Kashima, H., Polk, B.F., Shah, F., Abbey, H. & Abramson, A. (1986) Rarity of cesarean delivery in cases of juvenile-onset respiratory papillomatosis. *Obstet. Gynecol.*, **68**, 795–799

Shah, K.V., Daniel, R.W., Simons, J.W. & Vogelstein, B. (1992) Investigation of colon cancers for human papillomavirus genomic sequences by polymerase chain reaction. *J. surg. Oncol.*, **51**, 5–7

Shamanin, V., Glover, M., Rausch, C., Proby, C., Leigh, I.M., zur Hausen, H. & de Villiers, E.-M. (1994a) Specific types of human papillomavirus found in benign proliferations and carcinomas of the skin in immunosuppressed patients. *Cancer Res.*, **54**, 4610–4613

Shamanin, V., Delius, H. & de Villiers, E.-M. (1994b) Development of a broad spectrum PCR assay for papillomaviruses and its application in screening lung cancer biopsies. *J. gen. Virol.*, **75**, 1149–1156

Sharma, B.K., Nelson, J.W., Smith, C.C. & Aurelian, L. (1994) Detection of *LA-1* oncogene in paraffin embedded cervical cancer tissues by polymerase chain reaction. *Int. J. Oncol.*, **4**, 23–28

Shen, C.-Y., Ho, M.-S., Chang, S.-F., Yen, M.-S., Ng, H.-T., Huang, E.-S. & Wu, C.-W. (1993) High rate of concurrent genital infections with human cytomegalovirus and human papillomaviruses in cervical cancer patients. *J. infect. Dis.*, **168**, 449–452

Shepherd, P.S., Tran, T.T., Rowe, A.J., Cridland, J.C., Comerford, S.A., Chapman, M.G. & Rayfield, L.S. (1992) T cell responses to the human papillomavirus type 16 E7 protein in mice of different haplotypes. *J. gen. Virol.*, **73**, 1269–1274

Shepherd, P.S., Rowe, A.J., Cridland, J.C., Chapman, M.G., Luxton, J.C. & Rayfield, L.S. (1994) An immunodominant region in HPV 16 L1 identified by T cell responses in patients in cervical dysplasias. In: Stanley, M.A., eds, *Immunology of Human Papillomaviruses*, New York, Plenum, pp. 233–241

Sherman, L. & Alloul, N. (1992) Human papillomavirus type 16 expresses a variety of alternatively spliced mRNAs putatively encoding the E2 protein. *Virology*, **191**, 953–959

Sherman, K.J., Daling, J.R., Chu, J., Weiss, N.S., Ashley, R.L. & Corey, L. (1991) Genital warts, other sexually transmitted diseases, and vulvar cancer. *Epidemiology*, **2**, 257–262

Sherman, M.E., Schiffman, M.H., Lörincz, A.T., Manos, M.M., Scott, D.R., Kurman, R.J., Kiviat, N.B., Stoler, M., Glass, A.G. & Rush, B.B. (1994) Toward objective quality assurance in cervical cytopathology. Correlation of cytopathological diagnoses with detection of high-risk human papillomavirus types. *Am. J. clin. Pathol.*, **102**, 182–187

Shibutani, Y.F., Schoenberg, M.P., Carpiniello, V.L. & Malloy, T.R. (1992) Human papillomavirus associated with bladder cancer. *Urology*, **40**, 15–17

Shindoh, M., Sawada, Y., Kohgo, T., Amemiya, A. & Fujinaga, K. (1992) Detection of human papillomavirus DNA sequences in tongue squamous-cell carcinoma utilizing the polymerase chain reaction method. *Int. J. Cancer*, **50**, 167–171

Shope, R.E. & Hurst, E.W. (1933) Infectious papillomatosis of rabbits. *J. exp. Med.*, **58**, 607–624

Shoultz D.A., Kiviat, N.B., Kuypers, J.M., Hughes, J.P., Lee, S.-K., Adam, D. & Koutsky, L.A. (1994) Determinants of persistent genital HPV infection among young women (Abstract). *Proceedings of the 13th International Papillomavirus Conference, Amsterdam, October 8–12 1994*

Shroyer, K.R., Kim, J.G., Manos, M.M., Greer, C.E., Pearlman, N.W. & Franklin, W.A. (1992) Papillomavirus found in anorectal squamous carcinoma, not in colon adenocarcinoma. *Arch. Surg.*, **127**, 741–744

Shroyer, K.R., Greer, R.O., Fankhouser, C.A., McGuirt, W.F. & Marshall, R. (1993) Detection of human papillomavirus DNA in oral verrucous carcinoma by polymerase chain reaction. *Mod. Pathol.*, **6**, 669–672

Si, J.Y., Lee, K., Han, R., Zhang, W., Tan, B.B., Song, G.X., Liu, S., Chen, L.F., Zhao, W.M., Jia, L.P., Mai, Y., Zeng, Y., Zhou, Y., Wang, Y., Ling, J., Sun, Y., Meng, X., Yu, Z. & Pu, L. (1991) A research for the relationship between human papillomavirus and human uterine cervical carcinoma. I. The identification of viral genome and subgenomic sequences in biopsies of Chinese patients. *J. Cancer Res. clin. Oncol.*, **117**, 454–459

Sibbet, G.J. & Campo, M.S. (1990) Multiple interactions between cellular factors and the non-coding region of human papillomavirus type 16. *J. gen. Virol.*, **71**, 2699–2707

Sibbet, G.J., Cuthill, S. & Campo, M.S. (1995) The enhancer in the long control region of human papillomavirus type 16 is up-regulated by PEF-1 and down-regulated by Oct-1. *J. Virol.*, **69** (in press)

Siegsmund, M., Wayss, K. & Amtmann, E. (1991) Activation of latent papillomavirus genomes by chronic mechanical irritation. *J. gen. Virol.*, **72**, 2787–2789

Sigurgeirsson, B., Lindelöf, B. & Eklund, G. (1991) Condylomata acuminata and risk of cancer: an epidemiological study. *Br. med. J.*, **303**, 341–344

Sillman, F.H. & Sedlis, A. (1991) Anogenital papillomavirus infection and neoplasia in immunodeficient women: an update. *Dermatol.-Clin.*, **9**, 353–369

Sinclair, A.L., Nouri, A.M., Oliver, R.T., Sexton, C. & Dalgleish, A.G. (1993) Bladder and prostate cancer screening for human papillomavirus by polymerase chain reaction: conflicting results using different annealing temperatures. *Br. J. biomed. Sci.*, **50**, 350–354

Singh, P., Wong, S.H. & Hong, W. (1994) Overexpression of E2F-1 in rat embryo fibroblasts leads to neoplastic transformation. *EMBO J.*, **13**, 3329–3338

Smith, G. van S. & Pemberton, F.A. (1934) The picture of very early carcinoma of the uterine cervix. *Surg. Gynecol. Obstet.*, **59**, 1–8

Smith, P.G., Kinlen, L.J., White, G.C., Adelstein, A.M. & Fox, A.J. (1980) Mortality of wives of men dying with cancer of the penis. *Br. J. Cancer*, **41**, 422–428

Smith, P.P., Bryant, E.M., Kaur, P. & McDougall, J.K. (1989) Cytogenetic analysis of eight human papillomavirus immortalized human keratinocyte cell lines. *Int. J. Cancer*, **44**, 1124–1131

Smith, S.E., Davis, I.C., Leshin, B., Fleischer, A.B., Jr, White, W.L. & Feldman, S.R. (1993) Absence of human papillomavirus in squamous cell carcinomas of nongenital skin from immunocompromised renal transplant patients. *Arch. Dermatol.*, **129**, 1585–1588

Smits, H.L., Raadsheer, E., Rood, I., Mehendale, S., Slater, R.M., van der Noordaa, J. & ter Schegget, J. (1988) Induction of anchorage-independent growth of human embryonic fibroblasts with a deletion in the short arm of chromosome 11 by human papillomavirus type 16 DNA. *J. Virol.*, **62**, 4538–4543

Smits, H.L., Tieben, L.M., Tjong-A-Hung, S.P., Jebbink, M.F., Minnaar, R.P., Jansen, C.L. & ter Schegget, J. (1992a) Detection and typing of human papillomaviruses present in fixed and stained archival cervical smears by a consensus polymerase chain reaction and direct sequence analysis allow the identification of a broad spectrum of human papillomavirus types. *J. gen. Virol.*, **73**, 3263–3268

Smits, P.H.M., Smits, H.L., Minnaar, R.P., Hemmings, B.A., Mayer-Jaekel, R.E., Schuurman, R., van der Noordaa, J. & ter Schegget, J. (1992b) The 55 kDa regulatory subunit of protein phosphatase 2A plays a role in the activation of the HPV 16 long control region in human cells with a deletion in the short arm of chromosome 11. *EMBO J.*, **11**, 4601–4606

Snijders, P.J.F., van den Brule, A.J.C., Schrijnemakers, H.F.J., Snow, G., Meijer, C.J.L.M. & Walboomers, J.M.M. (1990) The use of general primers in the polymerase chain reaction permits the detection of a broad spectrum of human papillomavirus genotypes. *J. gen. Virol.*, **71**, 173–181

Snijders, P.J.F., Meijer, C.J.L.M., van den Brule, A.J.C., Schrijnemakers, H.F.J., Snow, G.B. & Walboomers, J.M.M. (1992a) Human papilloma virus (HPV) type 16 and 33 E6/E7 region transcripts in tonsillar carcinomas can originate from both integrated and episomal HPV-DNA. *J. gen. Virol.*, **73**, 2059–2066

Snijders, P.J.F., Cromme, F.V., van den Brule, A.J., Schrijnemakers, H.F., Snow, G.B., Meijer, C.J. & Walboomers, J.M. (1992b) Prevalence and expression of human papillomavirus in tonsillar carcinomas, indicating a possible viral etiology. *Int. J. Cancer*, **51**, 845–850

Snijders, P.J.F., van den Brule, A.J.C., Meijer, C.J.L.M. & Walboomers, J.M.M. (1994a) Papillomaviruses and cancer of the upper digestive and respiratory tracts. *Cur. Top. Microbiol. Immunol.*, **186**, 177–198

Snijders, P.J.F., Steenbergen, R.D.M., Top, B., Scott, S.D., Meijer, C.J.L.M. & Walboomers, J.M.M. (1994b) Analysis of p53 status in tonsillar carcinomas associated with human papillomavirus. *J. gen. Virol.*, **75**, 2769–2775

Soler, C., Chardonnet, Y., Allibert, P., Euvrard, S., Mandrand, B. & Thivolet, J. (1992) Detection of multiple types of human papillomavirus in a giant condyloma from a grafted patient: analysis by immunohistochemistry, in situ hybridisation, Southern blot and polymerase chain reaction. *Virus Res.*, **23**, 193–208

Soler, C., Chardonnet, Y., Allibert, P., Euvrard, S., Schmitt, D. & Mandrand, B. (1993) Detection of mucosal human papillomavirus types 6/11 in cutaneous lesions from transplant recipients. *J. invest. Dermatol.*, **101**, 286–291

Solomon, D. (1989) The 1988 Bethesda system for reporting cervical/vaginal cytological diagnoses. *J. Am. med. Assoc.*, **262**, 931–934

Somers, K.D., Cartwright, S.L. & Schechter, G.L. (1990) Human papillomavirus DNA in squamous cell carcinoma of the larynx and tongue (Abstract). *Proc. Annu. Meet. Am. Assoc. Cancer Res.*, **31**, A1932

Soutter, W.P. & Fletcher, A. (1994) Invasive cancer of the cervix in women with mild dyskaryosis followed up cytologically. *Br. med. J.*, **308**, 1421–1423

Spalholz, B.A., McBride, A.A., Sarafi, T. & Quintero, J. (1993) Binding of bovine papillomavirus E1 to the origin is not sufficient for DNA replication. *Virology*, **193**, 201–212

Spitkovsky, D., Steiner, P., Lukas, J., Lees, E., Pagano, M., Schulze, A., Joswig, S., Picard, D., Tommasino, M., Eilers, M. & Janden-Dürr., P. (1994) Modulation of cyclin gene expression by adenovirus E1A in a cell line with E1A-dependent conditional proliferation. *J. Virol.*, **68**, 2206–2214

Spradbrow, P.B. (1987) Immune response to papillomavirus infection. In: Syrjanen, K., Gissmann, L. & Koss, L.G., eds, *Papillomaviruses and Human Disease*, Berlin, Springer Verlag, pp. 334–370

Spradbrow, P.B. & Hoffmann, D. (1980) Bovine ocular squamous cell carcinoma. *Vet. Bull.*, **50**, 449–459

Spradbrow, P.B., Samuel, J.L., Kelly, W.R. & Wood, A.L. (1987) Skin cancer and papillomaviruses in cattle. *J. comp. Pathol.*, **97**, 469–479

Sprecher-Goldberger, S., Thiry, L., Lefèbvre, W., Dekegel, D. & de Halleux, F. (1971) Complement-fixation antibodies to adeno-associated viruses, adenoviruses, cytomegaloviruses and herpes simplex viruses in patients with tumors and in control individuals. *Am. J. Epidemiol.*, **94**, 351–358

Sreekantaiah, C., De Braekeleer, M. & Haas, O. (1991) Cytogenetic findings in cervical carcinoma: a statistical approach. *Cancer Genet. Cytogenet.*, **53**, 75–81

Stacey, S.N., Bartholomew, J.S., Ghosh, A., Stern, P.L., Mackett, M. & Arrand, J.R. (1992) Expression of human papillomavirus type 16 E6 protein by recombinant baculovirus and use for detection of anti-E6 antibodies in human sera. *J. gen. Virol.*, **73**, 2337–2345

Stacey, S.N., Ghosh, A., Bartholomew, J.S., Tindle, R.W., Stern, P.L., Mackett, M. & Arrand, J.R. (1993) Expression of human papillomavirus type 16 E7 protein by recombinant baculovirus and use for the detection of E7 antibodies in sera from cervical carcinoma patients. *J. med. Virol.*, **40**, 14–21

Stanley, M.A. & Sarkar, S. (1994) Genetic changes in cervical carcinoma. *Papillomavirus Rep.*, **5**, 141–147

Stanley, M.A., Browne, H.M., Appleby, M. & Minson, A.C. (1989) Properties of a non-tumorigenic human cervical keratinocyte cell line. *Int. J. Cancer*, **43**, 672–676

Stanley, M., Coleman, N. & Chambers, M. (1994) The host response to lesions induced by human papillomavirus. In: *Vaccines Against Virally Induced Cancers* (Ciba Foundation Symposium 187), Chichester, John Wiley & Sons, pp. 21–44

Stanley, M.A., Chambers, M.A. & Coleman, N. (1995) Chapter 11. Immunology of human papillomavirus infection. In: Mindel, A., ed., *Genital Warts. Human Papillomavirus Infection*, London, Edward Arnold, pp. 252–270

Stark, L.A., Arends, M.J., McLaren, K.M., Benton, E.C., Shahidullah, H., Hunter, J.A. & Bird, C.C. (1994) Prevalence of human papillomavirus DNA in cutaneous neoplasms from renal allograft recipients supports a possible viral role in tumour promotion. *Br. J. Cancer*, **69**, 222–229

Steele, J.C. & Gallimore, P.H. (1990) Humoral assays of human sera to disrupted and nondisrupted epitopes of human papillomavirus type 1. *Virology*, **174**, 388–398

Steele, K., Shirodaria, P.V., Pfister, H., Pollock, B., Fuchs, P., Merrett, J.D., Irwin, W.G. & Simpson, D.I. (1988) A study of HPV 1, 2 and 4 antibody prevalence in patients presenting for treatment with cutaneous warts to general practitioners in N. Ireland. *Epidemiol. Infect.*, **101**, 537–546

Steele, J.C., Stankovic, T. & Gallimore, P.H. (1993) Production and characterization of human proliferative T-cell clones specific for human papillomavirus type 1 E4 protein. *J. Virol.*, **67**, 2799–2806

Steger, G., Olszewsky, M., Stockfleth, E. & Pfister, H. (1990) Prevalence of antibodies to human papillomavirus type 8 in human sera. *J. Virol.*, **64**, 4399–4406

Stehr-Green, P.A., Hewer, P., Meekin, G.E. & Judd, L.E. (1993) The aetiology and risk of factors for warts among poultry processing workers. *Int. J. Epidemiol.*, **22**, 294–298

Steinberg, B.M., Topp, W.C., Schneider, P.S. & Abramson, A.L. (1983) Laryngeal papillomavirus infection during clinical remission. *N. Engl. J. Med.*, **308**, 1261–1264

Stellato, G., Nieminen, P., Aho, H., Vesterinen, E., Vaheri, A. & Paavonen, J. (1992) Human papillomavirus infection of the female genital tract: correlation of HPV DNA with cytologic, colposcopic, and natural history findings. *Eur. J. gynaecol. Oncol.*, **13**, 262–267

REFERENCES

Stenlund, A., Moreno-Lopez, J., Ahola, H. & Pettersson, U. (1983) European elk papillomavirus: characterization of the genome, induction of tumors in animals, and transformation *in vitro*. *J. Virol.*, **48**, 370–376

Stenlund, A., Zabielski, J., Ahola, H., Moreno-Lopez, J. & Pettersson, U. (1985) Messenger RNAs from the transforming region of bovine papilloma virus type I. *J. mol. Biol.*, **182**, 541–554

Stenlund, A., Bream, G.L. & Botchan, M.R. (1987) A promoter with an internal regulatory domain is part of the origin of replication in BPV-1. *Science*, **236**, 1666–1671

Stern, P.L. & Duggan-Keen, M. (1994) MHC expression in the natural history of cervical cancer. In: Stern, P.L. & Stanley, M.A., eds, *Human Papillomaviruses and Cervical Cancer*, Oxford, Oxford University Press, pp. 162–176

Stirdivant, S.M., Huber, H.E., Patrick, D.R., Defeo-Jones, D., McAvoy, E.M., Garsky, V.M., Oliff, A. & Heimbrook, D.C. (1992) Human papillomavirus type 16 E7 protein inhibits DNA binding by the retinoblastoma gene product. *Mol. cell. Biol.*, **12**, 1905–1914

St Louis, M.E., Icenogle, J.P., Manzila, T., Kamenga, M., Ryder, R.W., Heyward, W.L. & Reeves, W.C. (1993) Genital types of papillomavirus in children of women with HIV-1 infection in Kinshasa, Zaire. *Int. J. Cancer*, **54**, 181–184

Stoler, M.H., Wolinsky, S.M., Whitbeck, A., Broker, T.R. & Chow, L.T. (1989) Differentiation-linked human papillomavirus types 6 and 11 transcription in genital condylomata revealed by in situ hybridization with message-specific RNA probes. *Virology*, **172**, 331–340

Stoler, M.H., Mills, S.E., Gersell, D.J. & Walker, A.N. (1991) Small-cell neuroendocrine carcinoma of the cervix. A human papillomavirus type 18-associated cancer. *Am. J. surg. Pathol.*, **15**, 28–32

Stoler, M.H., Rhodes, C.R., Whitbeck, A., Wolinsky, S.M., Chow, L.T. & Broker, T.R. (1992) Human papillomavirus type 16 and 18 gene expression in cervical neoplasias. *Hum. Pathol.*, **23**, 117–128

Stone, M.S., Noonan, C.A., Tschen, J. & Bruce, J. (1987) Bowen's disease of the feet. Presence of HPV 16 DNA in tumour tissue. *Arch. Dermatol.*, **123**, 1517–1520

Storey, A. & Banks, L. (1993) Human papillomavirus type 16 E6 gene cooperates with EJ-*ras* to immortalize primary mouse cells. *Oncogene*, **8**, 919–924

Storey, A., Pim, D., Murray, A., Osborn, K., Banks, L. & Crawford, L. (1988) Comparison of the in vitro transforming activities of human papillomavirus types. *EMBO J.*, **7**, 1815–1820

Storey, A., Almond, N., Osborn, K. & Crawford, L. (1990) Mutations of the human papillomavirus type 16 E7 gene that affect transformation, transactivation and phosphorylation by the E7 protein. *J. gen. Virol.*, **71**, 965–970

Straight, S.W., Hinkle, P.M., Jewers, R.J. & McCance, D.J. (1993) The E5 oncoprotein of human papillomavirus type 16 transforms fibroblasts and effects the downregulation of the epidermal growth factor receptor in keratinocytes. *J. Virol.*, **67**, 4521–4532

Straight, S.W., Herman, B. & McCance, D.J. (1995) The E5 oncoprotein of human papillomavirus type 16 inhibits the acidification of endosomes in human keratinocytes. *J. Virol.*, **69**, 3185–3192

Strang, G., Hickling, J.K., McIndoe, G.A.J., Howland, K., Wilkinson, D., Ikeda, H. & Rothbard, J.B. (1990) Human T cell responses to human papillomavirus type 16 L1 and E6 synthetic peptides: identification of T cell determinants, HLA-DR restriction and virus type specificity. *J. gen. Virol.*, **71**, 423–431

Stratton, P. & Ciacco, K.H. (1994) Cervical neoplasia in the patient with HIV infection. *Curr. Opin. Obstet. Gynecol.*, **6**, 86–91

Strauss, M. & Griffin, B.E. (1990) Cellular immortalization — an essential step or merely a risk factor in DNA virus-induced transformation ? *Cancer Cells*, **2**, 360–365

Stremlau, A., Gissmann, L., Ikenberg, H., Stark, M., Bannasch, P. & zur Hausen, H. (1985) Human papillomavirus type 16 related DNA in an anaplastic carcinoma of the lung. *Cancer*, **55**, 1737–1740

Strickler, H.D., Dillner, J., Schiffman, M.H., Eklund, C., Glass, A.G., Greer, C., Scott, D.R., Sherman, M.E., Kurman, R.J. & Manos, M. (1994) A seroepidemiologic study of HPV infection and incident cervical squamous intraepithelial lesions. *Viral Immunol.*, **7**, 169–177

Strickler, H.D., Rattray, C., Escoffery, C., Manns, A., Schiffman, M.H., Brown, C., Cranston, B., Hanchard, B., Palefsky, J.M. & Blattner, W.A. (1995) Human T-cell lymphotropic virus type 1 and severe neoplasia of the cervix in Jamaica. *Int. J. Cancer*, **61**, 23–26

Strike, D.G., Bonnez, W., Rose, R.C. & Reichman, R.C. (1989) Expression in *Escherichia coli* of seven DNA fragments comprising the complete L1 and L2 open reading frames of human papillomavirus type 6b and localization of the 'common antigen' region. *J. gen. Virol.*, **70**, 543–555

Stubenrauch, F. & Pfister, H. (1994) Low-affinity E2-binding site mediates downmodulation of E2 transactivation of the human papillomavirus type 8 late promoter. *J. Virol.*, **68**, 6959–6966

Stubenrauch, F., Malejczyk, J., Fuchs, P.G. & Pfister, H. (1992) Late promoter of human papillomavirus type 8 and its regulation. *J. Virol.*, **66**, 3485–3493

Su, L.-L. (1987) A study on the relationship between human papillomavirus infection and cervical carcinoma development. Immunoperoxidase localization of papillomavirus antigen in cervical tissue. *Chin. med. J. (Engl.)*, **100**, 750–752

Suchánková, A., Ritter, O., Hirsch, I., Krchnák, V., Kalos, Z., Hamsiková, E., Bricháček, B. & Vonka, V. (1990) Presence of antibody reactive with synthetic peptide derived from L2 open reading frame of human papillomavirus types 6b and 11 in human sera. *Acta virol. (Praha)*, **34**, 433–442

Suchánková, A., Ritterová, L., Krcmár, M., Krchnák, V., Vágner, J., Jochmus, I., Gissmann, L., Kanka, J. & Vonka, V. (1991) Comparison of ELISA and western blotting for human papillomavirus type 16 E7 antibody determination. *J. gen. Virol.*, **72**, 2577–2581

Suchánková, A., Krchnák, V., Vágner, J., Hamsiková, E., Krcmár, M., Ritterová, L. & Vonka, V. (1992) Epitope mapping of the human papillomavirus type 16 E4 protein by means of synthetic peptides. *J. gen. Virol.*, **73**, 429–432

Sun, T., Shah, K.V., Müller, M., Muñoz, N., Bosch, F.X. & Viscidi, R.P. (1994a) Comparison of peptide enzyme-linked immunosorbent assay and radioimmunoprecipitation assay with in vitro-translated proteins for detection of serum antibodies to human papillomavirus type 16 E6 and E7 proteins. *J. clin. Microbiol.*, **32**, 2216–2220

Sun, Y., Eluf-Neto, J., Bosch, F.X., Muñoz, N., Booth, M., Walboomers, J.M.M., Shah, K.V. & Viscidi, R.P. (1994b) Human papillomavirus-related serological markers of invasive cervical carcinoma in Brazil. *Cancer Epidemiol. Biomarkers Prev.*, **3**, 341–347

Sundberg, J.P. (1987) Papillomavirus infections in animals. In: Syrjaenen, K., Gissmann, L. & Koss, L.G., eds, *Papillomaviruses and Human Disease*, Berlin, Springer Verlag, pp. 40–103

Sundberg, J.P., Junge, R.E. & El Shazly, M.O. (1985) Oral papillomatosis in New Zealand white rabbits. *Am. J. vet. Res.*, **46**, 664–668

Sundberg, J.P., O'Banion, M.K., Shima, A., Knupp, C. & Reichmann, M.E. (1988) Papillomas and carcinomas associated with a papillomavirus in European harvest mice (*Micromys minutus*). *Vet. Pathol.*, **25**, 356–361

Sundberg, J.P., Reszka, A.A., Williams, E.S. & Reichmann, M.E. (1991) An oral papillomavirus that infected one coyote and three dogs. *Vet. Pathol.*, **28**, 87–88

Sundberg, J.P., Smith, E.K., Herron, A.J., Jenson, A.B., Burk, R.D. & Van Ranst, M. (1994) Involvement of canine oral papillomavirus in generalized oral and cutaneous verrucosis in a Chinese Shar Pei dog. *Vet. Pathol.*, **31**, 183–187

Surawicz, C.M., Kirby, P., Critchlow, C., Sayer, J., Dunphy, C. & Kiviat, N. (1993) Anal dysplasia in homosexual men: role of anoscopy and biopsy. *Gastroenterology*, **105**, 658–666

Suzuki, H., Sato, N., Kodama, T., Okano, T., Isaka, S., Shirasawa, H., Simizu, B. & Shimazaki, J. (1994) Detection of human papillomavirus DNA and state of p53 gene in Japanese penile cancer. *Jpn J. clin. Oncol.*, **24**, 1–6

Sverdrup, F. & Khan, S.A. (1994) Replication of human papillomavirus (HPV) DNAs supported by the HPV type 18 E1 and E2 proteins. *J. Virol.*, **68**, 505–509

Syed, T.A. & Lundin, S. (1993) Topical treatment of penile condylomata acuminata with podophyllotoxin 0.3% solution, 0.3% cream and 0.15% cream: a comparative open study. *Dermatology*, **187**, 30–33

Syrjänen, K.J. (1983) Human papillomavirus lesions in association with cervical dysplasias and neoplasias. *Obstet. Gynecol.*, **62**, 617–624

Syrjänen, K., Väyrynen, M., Castren, O., Mäntyjarvi, R., Pyrhonen, S. & Yliskoski, M. (1983) Morphological and immunohistochemical evidence of human papilloma virus (HPV) involvement in the dysplastic lesions of the uterine cervix. *Int. J. Gynaecol. Obstet.*, **21**, 261–269

Syrjänen, K., Väyrynen, M., Mäntyjarvi, R., Castren, O. & Saarikoski, S. (1986) Natural killer (NK) cells with HNK-1 phenotype in the cervical biopsies of women followed-up for human papillomavirus (HPV) lesions. *Acta obstet. gynecol. scand.*, **65**, 139–145

Syrjänen, S., Syrjänen, K., Mäntyjarvi, R., Collan, Y. & Karja, J. (1987a) Human papillomavirus DNA in squamous cell carcinomas of the larynx demonstrated by in situ DNA hybridization. *J. Otorhinolaryngol. relat. Spec.*, **49**, 175–186

Syrjänen, K., Mäntyjarvi, R., Väyrynen, M., Syrjänen, S., Parkkinen, S., Yliskoski, M., Saarikoski, S. & Castrén, O. (1987b) Human papillomavirus (HPV) infections involved in the neoplastic process of the uterine cervix as established by prospective follow-up of 513 women for two years. *Eur. J. gynaecol. Oncol.*, **8**, 5–16

Syrjänen, S.M., Syrjänen, K.J. & Happonen, R.P. (1988) Human papillomavirus (HPV) DNA sequences in oral precancerous lesions and squamous cell carcinoma demonstrated by in situ hybridization. *J. oral Pathol.*, **17**, 273–278

Syrjänen, K., Syrjänen, S., Kellokoski, J., Karja, J. & Mäntyjarvi, R. (1989) Human papillomavirus (HPV) type 6 and 16 DNA sequences in bronchial squamous cell carcinomas demonstrated by in situ DNA hybridization. *Lung*, **167**, 33–42

Szabó, I., Sepp, R., Nakamoto, K., Maeda, M., Sakamoto, H. & Uda, H. (1994) Human papillomavirus not found in squamous and large cell lung carcinomas by polymerase chain reaction. *Cancer*, **73**, 2740–2744

Tachezy, R., Hamsikova, E., Valvoda, J., Van Ranst, M., Betka, J., Burk, R.D. & Vonka, V. (1994) Antibody response to a synthetic peptide derived from the human papillomavirus type 6/11 L2 protein in recurrent respiratory papillomatosis: correlation between Southern blot hybridization, polymerase chain reaction, and serology. *J. med. Virol.*, **42**, 52–59

Tada, A., Fuse, A., Sekine, H., Simiru, B., Kondo, A. & Maeda, S. (1988) Expression of the E2 open reading frame of papillomaviruses BPV 1 and HPV 6b in silkworm by a bacilovirus vector. *Virus Res.*, **9**, 357–367

Tan, S.-H., Leong, L.E.-C., Walker, P.A. & Bernard, H.-U. (1994a) The human papillomavirus type 16 E2 transcription factor binds with low cooperativity to two flanking sites and represses the E6 promoter through displacement of Sp1 and TFIID. *J. Virol.*, **68**, 6411–6420

Tan, C.-H., Tachezy, R., Van Ranst, M., Chan, S.-Y., Bernard, H.-U. & Burk, R.D. (1994b) The *Mastomys natalensis* papillomavirus: nucleotide sequence, genome organization, and phylogenetic relationship of a rodent papillomavirus involved in tumorigenesis of cutaneous epithelia. *Virology*, **198**, 534–541

Tanaka, H., Tazaki, T., Hasuo, Y., Yakushiji, M. & Lindh, E. (1992) Detection of human papillomavirus (HPV) infections in Japanese women with and without abnormal cervical cytology by dot blot and Southern blot hybridization. *Kurume med. J.*, **39**, 95–103

Tang, C.-K., Shermeta, D.W. & Wood, C. (1978) Congenital condylomata acuminata (Short communication). *Am. J. Obstet. Gynecol.*, **131**, 912–913

Tanigaki, T., Kanda, R., Yutsudo, M. & Hakura, A. (1986) Epidemiological aspects of epidermodysplasia verruciformis in Japan. *Jpn J. Cancer Res.*, **77**, 896–900

Tarpey, I., Stacey, S., Hickling, J., Birley, H.D., Renton, A., McIndoe, A. & Davies, D.H. (1994) Human cytotoxic T lymphocytes stimulated by endogenously processed human papillomavirus type 11 E7 recognize a peptide containing a HLA-A2 (A*0201) motif. *Immunology*, **81**, 222–227

Tase, T., Okagaki, T., Clark, B.A., Manias, D.A., Ostrow, R.S., Twiggs, L.B. & Faras, A.J. (1988) Human papillomavirus types and localization in adenocarcinoma and adenosquamous carcinoma of the uterine cervix: a study by in situ DNA hybridization. *Cancer Res.*, **48**, 993–998

Tate, J.E., Mutter, G.L., Prasad, C.J., Berkowitz, R., Goodman, H. & Crum, C.P. (1994) Analysis of HPV-positive and -negative vulvar carcinomas for alterations in c-*myc*, Ha-, Ki-, and N-*ras* genes. *Gynecol. Oncol.*, **53**, 78–83

Taxy, J.B., Gupta, P.K., Gupta, J.W. & Shah, K.V. (1989) Anal cancer. Microscopic condyloma and tissue demonstration of human papillomavirus capsid antigen and viral DNA. *Arch. Pathol. Lab. Med.*, **113**, 1127–1131

Tay, S.K., Jenkins, D., Maddox, P., Campion, M. & Singer, A. (1987a) Subpopulations of Langerhans' cells in cervical neoplasia. *Br. J. Obstet. Gynaecol.*, **94**, 10–15

Tay, S.K., Jenkins, D., Maddox, P. & Singer, A. (1987b) Lymphocyte phenotypes in cervical intraepithelial neoplasia and human papillomavirus infection. *Br. J. Obstet. Gynaecol.*, **94**, 16–21

Teokharov, B.A. (1969) Non-gonococcal infections of the female genitalia. *Br. J. vener. Dis.*, **45**, 334–340

Tervahauta, A.I., Syrjänen, S.M., Väyrynen, M., Saastamoinen, J. & Syrjänen, K.J. (1993) Expression of p53 protein related to the presence of human papillomavirus (HPV) DNA in genital carcinomas and precancer lesions. *Anticancer Res.*, **13**, 1107–1111

Thanapatra, S., Karalak, A., Itiravivonge, P., Vongchanglor, S. & Koonnarn, K. (1992) Human papilloma virus infection in cervical cytology study. *J. med. Assoc. Thai.*, **75**, 393–398

Thankamani, V., Kumari, T.V. & Vasudevan, D.M. (1992a) Papilloma virus in cervical carcinoma: detection of viral antigen in cancer cells. *J. exp. Pathol.*, **6**, 41–53

Thankamani, V., Kumari, T.V. & Vasudevan, D.M. (1992b) Detection of herpes simplex virus type-2 DNA and human papilloma virus DNA sequences in cervical carcinoma tissue by molecular hybridization. *J. exp. Pathol.*, **6**, 55–64

Thierry, F. & Howley, P.M. (1991) Functional analysis of E2-mediated repression of the HPV18 P_{105} promoter. *New Biol.*, **3**, 90–100

Thierry, F. & Yaniv, M. (1987) The BPV1-E2 *trans*-acting protein can be either an activator or a repressor of the HPV18 regulatory region. *EMBO J.*, **6**, 3391–3397

Thierry, F., Spyrou, G., Yaniv, M. & Howley, P. (1992) Two AP1 sites binding JunB are essential for human papillomavirus type 18 transcription in keratinocytes. *J. Virol.*, **66**, 3740–3748

Thompson, G.H. & Roman, A. (1987) Expression of human papillomavirus type 6 E1, E2, L1 and L2 open reading frames in *Escherichia coli*. *Gene*, **56**, 289–295

Tidy, J., Vousden, K.H., Mason, P. & Farrell, P.J. (1989) A novel deletion within the upstream regulatory region of episomal human papillomavirus type 16. *J. gen. Virol.*, **70**, 999–1004

Tieben, L.M., ter Schegger, J., Minnaar, R.P., Bouwes Bavinck, J.N., Berkhout, R.J.M., Vermeer, B.J., Jebbink, M.F. & Smits, H.L. (1993) Detection of cutaneous and genital HPV types in clinical samples by PCR using consensus primers. *J. virol. Meth.*, **42**, 265–280

Tieben, L.M., Berkhout, R.J.M., Smits, H.L., Bouwes Bavinck, J.N., Vermeer, B.J., Bruijn, J.A., Van der Woude, F.J. & ter Schegget, J. (1994) Detection of epidermodysplasia verruciformis-like human papillomavirus types in malignant and premalignant skin lesions of renal transplant recipients. *Br. J. Dermatol.*, **131**, 226–230

Tilbrook, P.A., Greenoak, G.E., Reeve, V.E., Canfield, P.J., Gissmann, L., Gallagher, C.H. & Kulski, J.K. (1989) Identification of papillomaviral DNA sequences in hairless mouse tumours induced by ultraviolet irradiation. *J. gen. Virol.*, **70**, 1005–1009

Tilbrook, P.A., Sterrett, G. & Kulski, J.K. (1992) Detection of papillomaviral-like DNA sequences in premalignant and malignant perineal lesions of sheep. *Vet. Microbiol.*, **31**, 327–341

Tindle, R.W. & Frazer, I.H. (1994) Immune response to human papillomaviruses and the prospects for human papillomavirus-specific immunisation. *Curr. Top. Microbiol. Immunol.*, **186**, 217–253

Tindle, R.W., Fernando, G.J.P., Sterling, J.C. & Frazer, I.H. (1991) A "public" T-helper epitope of the E7 transforming protein of human papillomavirus 16 provides cognate help for several E7 B-cell epitopes from cervical cancer-associated human papillomavirus genotypes. *Proc. natl Acad. Sci. USA*, **88**, 5887–5891

Togawa, K., Jaskiewicz, K., Takahashi, H., Meltzer, S.J. & Rustgi, A.K. (1994) Human papillomavirus DNA sequences in esophagus squamous cell carcinoma. *Gastroenterology*, **107**, 128–136

Toh, Y., Kuwano, H., Tanaka, S., Baba, K., Matsuda, H., Sugimachi, K. & Mori, R. (1992) Detection of human papillomavirus DNA in esophageal carcinoma in Japan by polymerase chain reaction. *Cancer*, **70**, 2234–2238

Toki, T., Kurman, R.J., Park, J.S., Kessis, T., Daniel, R.W. & Shah, K.V. (1991) Probable nonpapillomavirus etiology of squamous cell carcinoma of the vulva in older women: a clinico-pathologic study using in situ hybridization and polymerase chain reaction. *Int. J. gynecol. Pathol.*, **10**, 107–125

Tomasini, C., Aloi, F. & Pippione, M. (1993) Seborrheic keratosis-like lesions in epidermodysplasia verruciformis. *J. cutan. Pathol.*, **20**, 237–241

Tomita, Y., Shirasawa, H. & Simizu, B. (1987a) Expression of human papillomavirus types 6b and 16 L1 open reading frames in Escherichia coli: detection of a 56,000-dalton polypeptide containing genus-specific (common) antigens. *J. Virol.*, **61**, 2389–2394

Tomita, Y., Shirasawa, H., Sekine, H. & Simizu, B. (1987b) Expression of the human papillomavirus type 6b L2 open reading frame in *Escherichia coli*: L2-β-galactosidase fusion proteins and their antigenic properties. *Virology*, **158**, 8–14

Tommasino, M., Contorni, M., Scarlato, V., Bugnoli, M., Maundrell, K. & Cavalieri, F. (1990) Synthesis, phosphorylation, and nuclear localization of human papillomavirus E7 protein in *Schizosaccharomyces pombe*. *Gene*, **93**, 265–270

Tommasino, M., Adamczewski, J.P., Carlotti, F., Barth, C.F., Manetti, R., Contorni, M., Cavalieri, F., Hunt, T. & Crawford, L. (1993) HPV16 E7 protein associates with the protein kinase $p33_{CDK2}$ and cyclin A. *Oncogene*, **8**, 195–202

Toolan, H.W. & Ledinko, N. (1968) Inhibition by H-1 virus of the incidence of tumors produced by adenovirus 12 in hamsters. *Virology*, **35**, 475–478

Tornesello, M.L., Buonaguro, F.M., Beth Giraldo, E., Kyalwazi, S.K. & Giraldo, G. (1992) Human papillomavirus (HPV) DNA in penile carcinomas and in two cell lines from high-incidence areas for genital cancers in Africa. *Int. J. Cancer*, **51**, 587–592

Torres, L.M., Cabrera, T., Concha, A., Oliva, M.R., Ruiz-Cabello, F. & Garrido, F. (1993) HLA class I expression and HPV-16 sequences in premalignant and malignant lesions of the cervix. *Tissue Antigens*, **41**, 65–71

Townsend, D.E., Richart, R.M., Marks, E. & Nielsen, J. (1981) Invasive cancer following outpatient evaluation and therapy for cervical disease. *Obstet. Gynecol.*, **57**, 145–149

Trenfield, K., Spradbrow, P.B. & Vanselow, B.A. (1990) Detection of papillomavirus DNA in precancerous lesions of the ears of sheep. *Vet. Microbiol.*, **25**, 103–116

Trenfield, K., Salmond, C.A., Pope, J.H. & Hardie, I.R. (1993) Southern blot analysis of skin biopsies for human papillomavirus DNA: renal allograft recipients in south-eastern Queensland. *Australas. J. Dermatol.*, **34**, 71–78

Tsuchiya, H., Tomita, Y., Shirasawa, H., Tanzawa, H., Sato, K. & Simizu, B. (1991) Detection of human papillomavirus in head and neck tumors with DNA hybridization and immunohistochemical analysis. *Oral Surg. oral Med. oral Pathol.*, **71**, 721–725

Tsuda, H. & Hirohashi, S. (1992) Frequent occurrence of p53 gene mutations in uterine cancers at advanced clinical stage and with aggressive histological phenotypes. *Jap. J. Cancer Res.*, **83**, 1184–1191

Tyan, Y.-S., Liu, S.-T., Ong, W.-R., Chen, M.-L., Shu, C.-H. & Chang, Y.-S. (1993) Detection of Epstein-Barr virus and human papillomavirus in head and neck tumors. *J. clin. Microbiol.*, **31**, 53–56

Ushikai, M., Fujiyoshi, T., Kono, M., Antrasena, S., Oda, H., Yoshida, H., Fukuda, K., Furuta, S., Hakura, A. & Sonoda, S. (1994) Detection and cloning of human papillomavirus DNA associated with recurrent respiratory papillomatosis in Thailand. *Jpn J. Cancer Res.*, **85**, 699–703

Vandenvelde, C. & Van Beers, D. (1993) High-risk genital papillomaviruses and degree of dysplastic changes in the cervix: a prospective study by fast multiplex polymerase chain reaction in Belgium. *J. med. Virol.*, **39**, 273–277

Van Ranst, M., Fuse, A., Sobis, H., De Meurichy, W., Syrjänen, S.M., Billiau, A. & Opdenakker, G. (1991) A papillomavirus related to HPV type 13 in oral focal epithelial hyperplasia in the pygmy chimpanzee. *J. oral Pathol. Med.*, **20**, 325–331

Van Ranst, M., Kaplan, J.B. & Burk, R.D. (1992a) Phylogenetic classification of human papillomaviruses: correlation with clinical manifestations. *J. gen. Virol.*, **73**, 2653–2660

Van Ranst, M., Fuse, A., Fiten, P., Beuken, E., Pfister, H., Burk, R.D. & Opdenakker, G. (1992b) Human papillomavirus type 13 and pygmy chimpanzee papillomavirus type 1: comparison of the genome organizations. *Virology*, **190**, 587–596

Van Ranst, M.A., Tachezy, R. & Burk, R.D. (1994) Human papillomavirus nucleotide sequences: what's in stock? *Papillomavirus Rep.*, **5**, 65–75

Vanselow, B.A. & Spradbrow, P.B. (1983) Squamous cell carcinoma of the vulva, hyperkeratosis and papillomaviruses in a ewe. *Aust. vet. J.*, **60**, 194–195

Vanselow, B.A., Spradbrow, P.B. & Jackson, A.R.B. (1982) Papillomaviruses, papillomas and squamous cell carcinomas in sheep. *Vet. Rec.*, **110**, 561–562

Varma, V.A., Sanchez-Lanier, M., Unger, E.R., Clark, C., Tickman, R., Hewan-Lowe, K., Chenggis, M.L. & Swan, D.C. (1991) Association of human papillomavirus with penile carcinoma: a study using polymerase chain reaction and in situ hybridization. *Hum. Pathol.*, **22**, 908–913

Venuti, A. & Marcante, M.L. (1989) Presence of human papillomavirus type 18 DNA in vulvar carcinomas and its integration into the cell genome. *J. gen. Virol.*, **70**, 1587–1592

Veress, G., Kónya, J., Csiky-Mészáros, T., Czeglédy, J. & Gergely, L. (1994) Human papillomavirus DNA and anti-HPV secretory IgA antibodies in cytologically normal cervical specimens. *J. med. Virol.*, **43**, 201–207

Vermund, S.H., Kelley, K.F., Klein, R.S., Feingold, A.R., Schreiber, K., Munk, G. & Burk, R.D. (1991) High risk of human papillomavirus infection and cervical squamous intraepithelial lesions among women with symptomatic human immunodeficiency virus infection. *Am. J. Obstet. Gynecol.*, **165**, 392–400

Vernon, S.D., Zaki, S.R. & Reeves, W.C. (1994) Localisation of HIV-1 to human papillomavirus associated cervical lesions (Letter to the Editor). *Lancet*, **344**, 954

Viac, J., Staquet, M.J., Miguet, M., Chabanon, M. & Thivolet, J. (1978) Specific immunity to human papilloma virus (HPV) in patients with genital warts. *Br. J. vener. Dis.*, **54**, 172–175

Viac, J., Guérin-Reverchon, I., Chardonnet, Y. & Brémond, A. (1990) Langerhans cells and epithelial cell modifications in cervical intraepithelial neoplasia: correlation with human papillomavirus infection. *Immunobiology*, **180**, 328–338

Viac, J., Chardonnet, Y., Euvrard, S., Chignol, M.C. & Thivolet, J. (1992) Langerhans cells, inflammation markers and human papillomavirus infections in benign and malignant epithelial tumors from transplant recipients. *J. Dermatol.*, **19**, 67–77

Villa, L.L. & Franco, E.L. (1989) Epidemiologic correlates of cervical neoplasia and risk of human papillomavirus infection in asymptomatic women in Brazil. *J. natl Cancer Inst.*, **81**, 332–340

Villa, L.L. & Lopez, A. (1986) Human papillomavirus DNA sequences in penile carcinomas in Brazil. *Int. J. Cancer*, **37**, 853–855

de Villiers, E.-M. (1989) Minireview. Heterogeneity of the human papillomavirus group. *J. Virol.*, **63**, 4898–4903

de Villiers, E.-M. (1994) Human pathogenic papillomavirus types: an update. *Curr. Top. Microbiol. Immunol.*, **186**, 1–12 de Villiers, E.-M., Neumann, C., Oltersdorf, T., Fierlbeck, G. & zur Hausen, H. (1986a) Butcher's wart virus (HPV 7) infections in non-butchers. *J. invest. Dermatol.*, **87**, 236–238

de Villiers, E.-M., Schneider, A., Gross, G. & zur Hausen, H. (1986b) Analysis of benign and malignant urogenital tumors for human papillomavirus infection by labelling cellular DNA. *Med. Microbiol. Immunol. Berl.*, **174**, 281–286

de Villiers, E.-M., Wagner, D., Schneider, A., Wesch, H., Munz, F., Miklaw, H. & zur Hausen, H. (1992) Human papillomavirus DNA in women without and with cytological abnormalities: results of a 5-year follow-up study. *Gynecol. Oncol.*, **44**, 33–39

Viscidi, R. & Shah, K.V. (1992) Immune response to genital tract infections with human papillomaviruses. In: Quinn, T.C., ed., *Sexually Transmitted Diseases*, New York, Raven Press, pp. 239–260

Viscidi, R.P., Sun, Y., Tsuzaki, B., Bosch, F.X., Muñoz, N. & Shah, K.V. (1993) Serologic response in human papillomavirus-associated invasive cervical cancer. *Int. J. Cancer*, **55**, 780–784

Volpers, C., Sapp, M., Komly, C.A., Richalet-Secordel, P. & Streeck, R.E. (1993) Development of type-specific and cross-reactive serological probes for the minor capsid protein of human papillomavirus type 33. *J. Virol.*, **67**, 1927–1935

Volpers, C., Schirmacher, P., Streeck, R.E. & Sapp, M. (1994) Assembly of the major and the minor capsid protein of human papillomavirus type 33 into virus-like particles and tubular structures in insect cells. *Virology*, **200**, 504–512

Volz, L.R., Carpiniello, V.L. & Malloy, T.R. (1994) Laser treatment of urethral condyloma: a five-year experience. *Urology*, **43**, 81–83

Vonka, V., Kanka, J., Hirsch, I., á, H., Krcmár, M., Suchánková, A., Rezácová, D., Broucek, J., Press, M., Domorázková, E., Svoboda, B., Havránková, A. & Jelinek, J. (1984) Prospective study on the relationship between cervical neoplasia and herpes-simplex-type-2 virus. II. Herpes-simplex-type-2 antibody presence in sera taken at enrollment. *Int. J. Cancer*, **33**, 61–66

van Voorst Vader, P.C., Orth, G., Dutronquay, V., Driessen, L., Eggink, H.F., Kallenberg, C. & The, T.H. (1986) Epidermodysplasia verruciformis. Skin carcinoma containing human papillomavirus type 5 DNA sequences and primary hepatocellular carcinoma associated with chronic hepatitis B virus infection in a patient. *Acta derm. venereol. (Stockh.)*, **66**, 231–236

van Voorst Vader, P.C., de Jong, M., Blanken, R., Kallenberg, C, Vermey, A. & Scheres, J. (1987) Epidermodysplasia verruciformis: Langerhans cells, immological effect of retinoid treatment and cytogenetics. *Arch. dermatol. Res.*, **279**, 366–373

Vousden, K.H., Doniger, J., DiPaolo, J.A. & Lowy, D.R. (1988) The E7 open reading frame of human papillomavirus type 16 encodes a transforming gene. *Oncogene Res.*, **3**, 167–175

Wagner, D., Ikenberg, H., Boehm, N. & Gissmann, L. (1984) Identification of human papillomavirus in cervical swabs by deoxyribonucleic acid in situ hybridization. *Obstet. Gynecol.*, **64**, 767–772

Walboomers, J.M.M., de Roda Husman, A.-M., van den Brule, A.J.C., Snijders, P.J.F. & Meijer, C.J.L.M. (1994) Detection of genital human papillomavirus infections: critical review of methods and prevalence studies in relation to cervical cancer. In: Stern, P.L. & Stanley, M.A., *Human Papillomaviruses and Cervical Cancer: Biology and Immunology*, Oxford, Oxford University Press, pp. 41–71

Waldeck, W., Rosl, F. & Zentgraf, H. (1984) Origin of replication in episomal bovine papilloma virus type 1 DNA isolated from transformed cells. *EMBO J.*, **3**, 2173–2178

REFERENCES

Walker, J., Bloss, J.D., Liao, S.-Y., Berman, M., Bergen, S. & Wilczynski, S.P. (1989) Human papillomavirus genotype as a prognostic indicator in carcinoma of the uterine cervix. *Obstet. Gynecol.*, **74**, 781–785

Wank, R. & Thomssen, C. (1991) High risk of squamous cell carcinoma of the cervix for women with HLA-DQw3. *Nature*, **352**, 723–725

Wank, R., ter Meulen, J., Luande, J., Eberhardt, H.-C. & Pawlita, M. (1993) Cervical intraepithelial neoplasia, cervical carcinoma, and risk for patients with HLA-DQB1*0602,*0301,*0303 alleles (Letter to the Editor). *Lancet*, **341**, 1215

Warhol, M.J. & Gee, B. (1989) The expression of histocompatibility antigen HLA-DR in cervical squamous epithelium infected with human papilloma virus. *Mod. Pathol.*, **2**, 101–104

Watanabe, S. & Yoshiike, K. (1988) Transformation of rat 3Y1 cells by human papillomavirus type-18 DNA. *Int. J. Cancer*, **41**, 896–900

Watanabe, S., Kanda, T., Sato, H., Furuno, A. & Yoshiike, K. (1990) Mutational analysis of human papillomavirus type 16 E7 functions. *J. Virol.*, **64**, 207–214

Watanabe, S., Ogura, H., Fukushima, K. & Yabe, Y. (1993) Comparison of Virapap filter hybridization with polymerase chain reaction and Southern blot hybridization methods for detection of human papillomavirus in tonsillar and pharyngeal cancers. *Eur. Arch. Otorhinolaryngol.*, **250**, 115–119

Watrach, A.M., Small, E. & Case, M.T. (1970) Canine papilloma: progression of oral papilloma to carcinoma. *J. natl Cancer Inst.*, **45**, 915–920

Watts, S.L., Brewer, E.E. & Fry, T.L. (1991) Human papillomavirus DNA types in squamous cell carcinomas of the head and neck. *Oral Surg. oral Med. oral Pathol.*, **71**, 701–707

Wazer, D.E., Liu, X.-L., Chu, Q., Gao, Q. & Band, V. (1995) Immortalisation of distinct human mammary epithelial cell types by human papillomavirus 16 E6 or E7. *Proc. natl Acad. Sci. USA*, **92**, 3687–3691

Weaver, M.G., Abdul-Karim, F.W., Dale, G., Sorensen, K. & Huang, Y.T. (1989) Detection and localization of human papillomavirus in penile condylomas and squamous cell carcinomas using in situ hybridization with biotinylated DNA viral probes. *Mod. Pathol.*, **2**, 94–100

Weaver, M.G., Abdul-Karim, F.W., Dale, G., Sorensen, K. & Huang, Y.T. (1990) Outcome in mild and moderate cervical dysplasias related to the presence of specific human papillomavirus types. *Mod. Pathol.*, **3**, 679–683

Wei, Z., Yazhou, S., Shunqian, J., Xiao, L., Lihua, M., Xiaohong, W., Ming, S., Airu, W., Xixia, W., Jianheng, S., Wenhua, Z., Zhiming, L., Shufan, L. & Fusheng, L. (1991) The association between cervical carcinoma and human papilloma virus (HPV) in Xiangyuan county. *Chin. med. Sci. J.*, **6**, 74–77

Weinberg, R.A. (1995) The retinoblastoma protein and cell cycle control. *Cell*, **81**, 323–330

Weintraub, S.J., Prater, C.A. & Dean, D.C. (1992) Retinoblastoma protein switches the E2F site from positive to negative element. *Nature*, **358**, 259–261

Weiss, L.K., Kau, T.Y., Sparks, B.T. & Swanson, G.M. (1994) Trends in cervical cancer incidence among young black and white women in metropolitan Detroit. *Cancer*, **73**, 1849–1854

Werness, B.A., Levine, A.J. & Howley, P.M. (1990) Association of human papillomavirus types 16 and 18 E6 proteins with p53. *Science*, **248**, 76–79

Wettstein, F.O. (1987) Cottontail rabbit (Shope) papillomavirus. In: Selzman, N.P. & Howley, P.M., eds, *The Papillomaviruses*, New York, Plenum Press, pp. 167–185

Wheeler, C.M., Parmenter, C.A., Hunt, W.C., Becker, T.M., Greer, C.E., Hildesheim, A. & Manos, M.M. (1993) Determinants of genital human papillomavirus infection among cytologically normal women attending the University of New Mexico student health center. *Sex. transm. Dis.*, **20**, 286–289

Whitaker, N.J., Kidston, E.L. & Reddel, R.R. (1992) Finite lifespan of hybrids formed by fusion of different simian virus 40-immortalized human cell lines. *J. Virol.*, **66**, 1202–1206

White, A.E., Livanos, E.M. & Tlsty, T.D. (1994) Differential disruption of genomic integrity and cell cycle regulation in normal human fibroblasts by the HPV oncoproteins. *Genes Dev.*, **8**, 666–677

Whiteley, P.F. & Oláh, K.S. (1990) Treatment of cervical intraepithelial neoplasia: experience with the low-voltage diathermy loop. *Am. J. Obstet. Gynecol.*, **162**, 1272–1277

Whyte, P., Buchkovich, K.J., Horowitz, J.M., Friend, S.H., Raybuck, M., Weinberg, R.A. & Harlow, E. (1988) Association between an oncogene and an anti-oncogene: the adenovirus E1A proteins bind to the retinoblastoma gene product. *Nature*, **334**, 124–129

Wideroff, L., Schiffman, M.H., Nonnenmacher, B., Hubbert, N., Kirnbauer, R., Greer, C.E., Lowy, D., Lorincz, A.T., Manos, M.M., Glass, A.G., Scott, D.R., Sherman, M.E., Kurman, R.J., Buckland, J., Tarone, R.E. & Schiller, J. (1995) Evaluation of HPV 16 virus-like paricle seroreactivity in an incident case–control study of cervical neoplasia. *J. inf. Dis.* (in press)

Wiener, J.S. & Walther, P.J. (1994) A high association of oncogenic human papillomaviruses with carcinomas of the female urethra: polymerase chain reaction-based analysis of multiple histological types. *J. Urol.*, **151**, 49–53

Wiener, J.S., Effert, P.J., Humphrey, P.A., Yu, L., Liu, E.T. & Walther, P.J. (1992a) Prevalence of human papillomavirus types 16 and 18 in squamous-cell carcinoma of the penis: a retrospective analysis of primary and metastatic lesions by differential polymerase chain reaction. *Int. J. Cancer*, **50**, 694–701

Wiener, J.S., Liu, E.T. & Walther, P.J. (1992b) Oncogenic human papillomavirus type 16 is associated with squamous cell cancer of the male urethra. *Cancer Res.*, **52**, 5018–5023

Wikström, A., Lidbrink, P., Johansson, B. & von Krogh, G. (1991) Penile human papillomavirus carriage among men attending Swedish STD clinics. *Int. J. STD AIDS*, **2**, 105–109

Wikström, A., Eklund, C., von Krogh, G., Lidbrink, P. & Dillner, J. (1992) Levels of immunoglobulin G antibodies against defined epitopes of the L1 and L2 capsid proteins of human papillomavirus type 6 are elevated in men with a history of condylomata acuminata. *J. clin. Microbiol.*, **30**, 1795–1800

Wilczynski, S.P., Walker, J., Liao, S.-Y., Bergen, S. & Berman, M. (1988a) Adenocarcinoma of the cervix associated with human papillomavirus. *Cancer*, **62**, 1331–1336

Wilczynski, S.P., Pearlman, L. & Walker, J. (1988b) Identification of HPV 16 early genes retained in cervical carcinomas. *Virology*, **166**, 624–627

Wilkinson, E.J. (1994) Premalignant and malignant tumors of the vulva. In: Kurman, R.J., ed., *Blaustein's Pathology of the Female Genital Tract*, 4th Ed., New York, Springer-Verlag, pp. 87–129

Willet, G.K., Kurman, R.J., Reid, R., Greenberg, M., Jenson, A.B. & Lorinez, A.T. (1989) Correlation of the histological appearance of intraepithelial neoplasia of the cervix with human papillomavirus types. *Int. J. gynecol. Pathol.*, **8**, 18–25

Willey, J.C., Hei, T.K., Piao, C.Q., Madrid, L., Willey, J.J., Apostolakos, M.J. & Hukku, B. (1993) Radiation-induced deletion of chromosomal regions containing tumor suppressor genes in human bronchial epithelial cells. *Carcinogenesis*, **14**, 1181–1188

Williams (1888) Cancer of the uterus. *Harveian Lectures for 1886*, London, H.K. Lewis

Williams, A.B., Darragh, T.M., Vranizan, K., Ochia, C., Moss, A.R. & Palefsky, J.M. (1994) Anal and cervical human papillomavirus infection and risk of anal and cervical epithelial abnormalities in human immunodeficiency virus-infected women. *Obstet. Gynecol.*, **83**, 205–211

Williamson, A.-L., Jaskiesicz, K. & Gunning, A. (1991) The detection of human papillomavirus in oesophageal lesions. *Anticancer Res.*, **11**, 263–265

Williamson, A.-L., Brink, N.S., Dehaeck, C.M.C., Ovens, S., Soerters, R. & Rybicki, E.P. (1994) Typing of human papillomaviruses in cervical carcinoma biopsies from Cape Town. *J. med. Virol.*, **43**, 231–237

Willis, G., Jennings, B., Ball, R.Y., New, N.E. & Gibson, I. (1993) Analysis of *ras* point mutations and human papillomavirus 16 and 18 in cervical carcinomata and their metastases. *Gynecol. Oncol.*, **49**, 359–364

Wilson, V.G. & Ludes-Meyers, J. (1991) A bovine papillomavirus E1-related protein binds specifically to bovine papillomavirus DNA. *J. Virol.*, **65**, 5314–5322

Wilson, V.G. & Ludes-Meyers, J. (1992) Partite expression of the bovine papillomavirus E1 open reading frame in *Escherichia coli*. *Biochim. biophys. Acta*, **1129**, 215–218

Wilson, C.A., Holmes, S.C., Campo, M.S., White, S.I., Tillman, D., Mackie, R.M. & Thomson, J. (1989) Novel variants of human papillomavirus type 2 in warts from immunocompromised individuals. *Br. J. Dermatol.*, **121**, 571–576

Winkelstein, W., Jr (1990) Smoking and cervical cancer — current status: a review. *Am. J. Epidemiol.*, **131**, 945–957

Winkler, B., Crum, C.P, Fujii, T., Ferenczy, A., Boon, M., Braun, L., Lancaster, W.D. & Richart, R.M. (1984) Koilocytotic lesions of the cervix. The relationship of mitotic abnormalities to the presence of papillomavirus antigens and nuclear DNA content. *Cancer*, **53**, 1081–1087

Wolber, R., Dupuis, B., Thiyagaratnam, P. & Owen, D. (1990) Anal cloacogenic and squamous carcinomas: comparative histologic analysis using in situ hybridization for human papillomavirus DNA. *Am. J. surg. Pathol.*, **14**, 176–182

Wong, Y.F., Wong, F.W.S., Cheung, T.H., Fung, H.Y.M., Chung, T., K.H., Lam, S.K., Tam, P.O.S. & Chang, A.M.Z. (1993) Frequent loss of heterozygosity on the short arm of chromosome 1 in cervical carcinoma. *Med. Sci. Res.*, **21**, 891–892

Woodruff, J.D., Braun, L., Cavalieri, R., Gupta, P., Pass, F. & Shah, K.V. (1980) Immunologic identification of papillomavirus antigen in condyloma tissues from the female genital tract. *Obstet. Gynecol.*, **56**, 727–732

Woods, K.V., Shillitoe, E.J., Spitz, M.R., Schantz, S.P. & Adler-Storthz, K. (1993) Analysis of human papillomavirus DNA in oral squamous cell carcinomas. *J. oral Pathol. Med.*, **22**, 101–108

Woods, C., LeFeuvre, C., Stewart, N. & Bacchetti, S. (1994) Induction of genomic instability in SV40 transformed human cells: sufficiency of the N-terminal 147 amino acids of large T antigen and role of pRB and p53. *Oncogene*, **9**, 2943–2950

Woodworth, C.D., Bowden, P.E., Doniger, J., Pirisi, L., Barnes, W., Lancaster, W.D. & DiPaolo, J.A. (1988) Characterization of normal human exocervical epithelial cells immortalized in vitro by papillomavirus types 16 and 18 DNA. *Cancer Res.*, **48**, 4620–4628

Wools, K., Bryan, J.T., Katz, B.P., Rodriguez, M., Davis, T. & Brown, D.R. (1994) Detection of human papillomavirus L1 protein in condylomata acuminata from various anatomical sites. *Sex. transmiss. Dis.*, **21**, 103–106

Wrede, D., Luqmani, Y.A., Coombes, R.C. & Vousden, K.H. (1992a) Short Communication. Absence of HPV 16 and 18 DNA in breast cancer. *Br. J. Cancer*, **65**, 891–894

Wrede, D., Tidy, J.A., Crook, T., Lane, D. & Vousden, K.H. (1992b) Expression of RB and p53 proteins in HPV-positive and HPV-negative cervical carcinoma cell lines. *Mol. Carcinog.*, **4**, 171–175

Wright, T.C., Jr & Richart, R.M. (1992) Pathogenesis and diagnosis of preinvasive lesions of the lower genital tract. In: Hoskins, W.J., Perez, C.A. & Young, R.C., eds, *Principles and Practices of Gynecologic Oncology*, Philadelphia, J.B. Lippincott, pp. 509–536

Wright, V.C. & Riopelle, M.A. (1984) Age at beginning of coitus versus chronological age as a basis for Papanicolaou smear screening: an analysis of 747 cases of preinvasive disease. *Am. J. Obstet. Gynecol.*, **149**, 824–830

Wright, T.C., Richart, R.M. & Ferency, A., eds (1992) *Electrosurgery for HPV-related Diseases of the Anogenital Tract*, New York, Arthur Vision

Wright, T.C., Jr, Ellerbrock, T.V., Chiasson, M.A., Van Devanter, N., Sun, X.-W. and the New York Cervical Disease Study (1994a) Cervical intraepithelial neoplasia in women infected with human immunodeficiency virus: prevalence, risk factors, and validity of Papanicolaou smears. *Obstet. Gynecol.*, **84**, 591–597

Wright, T.C., Ferenczy, A. & Kurman, R.J. (1994b) Carcinoma and other tumors of the cervix. In: Kurman, R.J., ed., *Blaustein's Pathology of the Female Genital Tract*, 4th Ed., New York, Springer-Verlag, pp. 279–326

Wu, E.W., Clemens, K.E., Heck, D.V. & Münger, K. (1993) The human papillomavirus E7 oncoprotein and the cellular transcription factor E2F bind to separate sites on the retinoblastoma tumor suppressor protein. *J. Virol.*, **67**, 2402–2407

Wu, X. & Levine, A.J. (1994) p53 and E2F-1 cooperate to mediate apoptosis. *Proc. natl Acad. Sci. USA*, **91**, 3602–3606

Xi, L.-F., Demers, G.W., Koutsky, L.A., Kiviat, N.B., Kuypers, J., Watts, D.H., Holmes, K.K., & Galloway, D.A. (1995) Analysis of human papillomavirus type 16 variants indicates establishment of persistent infection. *J. infect. Dis.* (in press)

Xiong, Y., Hannon, G.J., Zhang, H., Casso, D., Kobayashi, R. & Beach, D. (1993) p21 Is a universal inhibitor of cyclin kinases. *Nature*, **366**, 701–704

Yabe, Y., Tanimura, Y., Sakai, A., Hitsumoto, T. & Nohara, N. (1989) Molecular characteristics and physical state of human papillomavirus DNA change with progressing malignancy: studies in a patient with epidermodysplasia verruciformis. *Int. J. Cancer*, **43**, 1022–1028

Yaegashi, N., Jenison, S.A., Valentine, J.M., Dunn, M., Taichman, L.B., Baker, D.A. & Galloway, D.A. (1991) Characterization of murine polyclonal antisera and monoclonal antibodies generated against intact and denatured human papillomavirus type 1 virions. *J. Virol.*, **65**, 1578–1583

Yaegashi, N., Jenison, S.A., Batra, M. & Galloway, D.A. (1992) Human antibodies recognize multiple distinct type-specific and cross-reactive regions of the minor capsid proteins of human papillomavirus types 6 and 11. *J. Virol.*, **66**, 2008–2019

Yaegashi, N., Xi, L., Batra, M. & Galloway, D.A. (1993) Sequence and antigenic diversity in two immunodominant regions of the L2 protein of human papillomavirus types 6 and 16. *J. infect. Dis.*, **168**, 743–747

Yang, L., Mohr, I., Fouts, E., Lim, D.A., Nohaile, M. & Botchan, M. (1993) The E1 protein of bovine papilloma virus 1 is an ATP-dependent DNA helicase. *Proc. natl Acad. Sci. USA*, **90**, 5086–5090

Yasumoto, S., Burkhardt, A.L., Doniger, J. & DiPaolo, J.A. (1986) Human papillomavirus type 16 DNA-induced malignant transformation of NIH 3T3 cells. *J. Virol.*, **57**, 572–577

Yeudall, W.A. & Campo, M.S. (1991) Human papillomavirus DNA in biopsies of oral tissues. *J. gen. Virol.*, **72**, 173–176

Yliskoski, M., Cantell, K., Syrjänen, K. & Syrjänen, S. (1990) Topical treatment with human leukocyte interferon of HPV 16 infections associated with cervical and vaginal intraepithelial neoplasias. *Gynecol. Oncol.*, **36**, 353–357

Yliskoski, M., Syrjänen, K., Syrjänen, S., Saarikoski, S. & Nethersell, A. (1991) Systemic α-interferon (Wellferon) treatment of genital human papillomavirus (HPV) type 6, 11, 16, and 18 infections: double-blind, placebo-controlled trial. *Gynecol. Oncol.*, **43**, 55–60

Yokota, J., Tsukada, Y., Nakajima, T., Gotoh, M., Shimosato, Y., Mori, N., Tsunokawa, Y., Sugimura, T. & Terada, M. (1989) Loss of heterozygosity on the short arm of chromosome 3 in carcinoma of the uterine cervix. *Cancer Res.*, **49**, 3598–3601

Yokota, H., Yoshikawa, H., Shiromizu, K., Kawana, T. & Mizuno, M. (1990) Detection of human papillomavirus types 6/11, 16 and 18 in exfoliated cells from the uterine cervices of Japanese women with and without lesions. *Jpn J. Cancer Res.*, **81**, 896–901

Yorke, J.A., Heathcote, H.W. & Nold, A. (1978) Dynamics and control of the transmission of gonorrhea. *Sex transm. Dis.*, **5**, 51–56

Young, S.K. & Min, K.W. (1991) In situ DNA hybridization analysis of oral papillomas, leukoplakias, and carcinomas for human papillomavirus. *Oral Surg. oral Med. oral Pathol.*, **71**, 726–729

Young, F.I., Ward, L.M. & Brown, L.J. (1991) Absence of human papilloma virus in cervical adenocarcinoma determined by in situ hybridisation. *J. clin. Pathol.*, **44**, 340–341

Yousem, S.A., Ohori, N.P. & Sonmez Alpan, E. (1992) Occurrence of human papillomavirus DNA in primary lung neoplasms. *Cancer*, **69**, 693–697

Yutsudo, M., Tanigaki, T., Kanda, R., Sasagawa, T., Inoue, T., Jing, P., Hwang, Y.-I. & Hakura, A. (1994) Involvement of human papillomavirus type 20 in epidermodysplasia verruciformis skin carcinogenesis. *J. clin. Microbiol.*, **32**, 1076–1078

Zaki, S.R., Judd, R., Coffield, L.M., Greer, P., Rolston, F. & Evatt, B.L. (1992) Human papillomavirus infection and anal carcinoma. Retrospective analysis by in situ hybridization and the polymerase chain reaction. *Am. J. Pathol.*, **140**, 1345–1355

Zaninetti, P., Franceschi, S., Baccolo, M., Bonazzi, B., Gottardi, G. & Serraino, D. (1986) Characteristics of women under 20 with cervical intraepithelial neoplasia. *Int. J. Epidemiol.*, **15**, 477–482

Zeuss, M.S., Miller, C.S. & White, D.K. (1991) In situ hybridization analysis of human papillomavirus DNA in oral mucosal lesions. *Oral Surg. oral Med. oral Pathol.*, **71**, 714–720

Zhang, G. (1990) A study on the relationship between human papilloma virus (HPV) and cervical cancer. *Chin. J. Epidemiol.*, **11**, 31–33 (in Chinese)

Zhang, W.H., Wu, A.R., Li, J.X. & Lin, Y.C. (1987) Relation between human papillomavirus (HPV) and cancer of uterine cervix. *Chin. J. Oncol.*, **9**, 433–435 (in Chinese)

Zhang, W.H., Coppleson, M., Rose, B.R., Sorich, E.A., Nightingale, B.N., Thompson, C.H., Cossart, Y.E., Bannatyne, P.M., Elliott, P.M. & Atkinson, K.H. (1988) Papillomavirus and cervical cancer: a clinical and laboratory study. *J. med. Virol.*, **26**, 163–174

Zhou, J., Sun, X.-Y., Stenzel, D.J. & Frazer, I.H. (1991a) Expression of vaccinia recombinant HPV 16 L1 and L2 ORF proteins in epithelial cells is sufficient for assembly of HPV virion-like particles. *Virology*, **185**, 251–257

Zhou, J., Doorbar, J., Sun, X.-Y., Crawford, L.V., McLean, C.S. & Frazer, I.H. (1991b) Identification of the nuclear localization signal of human papillomavirus type 16 L1 protein. *Virology*, **185**, 625–632

Zhou, J., Sun, X.-Y. & Frazer, I.H. (1993) Glycosylation of human papillomavirus type 16 L1 protein. *Virology*, **194**, 210–218

Zhou, J., Sun, X.-Y., Louis, K. & Frazer, I.H. (1994) Interaction of human papillomavirus (HPV) type 16 capsid proteins with HPV DNA requires an intact L2 N-terminal sequence. *J. Virol.*, **68**, 619–625

Zhu, W.Y., Leonardi, C., Kinsey, W. & Penneys, N.S. (1991) Irritated seborrheic keratoses and benign verrucous acanthomas do not contain papillomavirus DNA. *J. cutan. Pathol.*, **18**, 449–452

Zhu, W.Y., Leonardi, C. & Penneys, N.S. (1993a) Polymerase chain reaction in detection of human papillomavirus DNA and types of condyloma acuminata. *Chin. med. J. (Engl.)*, **106**, 141–144

Zhu, W.Y., Leonardi, C., Blauvelt, A., Serfling, U. & Penneys, N.S. (1993b) Human papillomavirus DNA in the dermis of condyloma acuminatum. *J. cutan. Pathol.*, **20**, 447–450

zur Hausen, H. (1975) Oncogenic herpesviruses. *Biochim. biophys. Acta*, **417**, 25–53

zur Hausen, H. (1976) Condylomata acuminata and human genital cancer. *Cancer Res.*, **36**, 794

zur Hausen, H. (1982) Human genital cancer — synergism between two virus infections or synergism between a virus infection and initiating events ? *Lancet*, **ii**, 1370–1373

zur Hausen, H. (1983) Herpes simplex virus in human genital cancer. *Int. Rev. exp. Pathol.*, **25**, 307–326

zur Hausen, H. (1985) Genital papillomavirus infections. In: Rigby, P.W.J. & Wilkie, N.M., eds, *Viruses and Cancer*, Cambridge, Cambridge University Press, pp. 83–90

zur Hausen, H. (1986) Intracellular surveillance of persisting viral infections: human genital cancer resulting from deficient cellular control of papillomavirus gene expression. *Lancet*, **ii**, 489–491

zur Hausen, H. (1989) Papillomavirus in anogenital cancer: the dilemma of epidemiologic approaches. *J. natl Cancer Inst.*, **81**, 1680–1682

zur Hausen, H. (1990) The role of papillomaviruses in anogenital cancer. *Scand. J. infect. Dis.*, **69** (Suppl.), 107–111

zur Hausen, H. (1991) Human papillomaviruses in the pathogenesis of anogenital cancer. *Virology*, 184, 9–13

zur Hausen, H. (1994) Disrupted dichotomous intracellular control of human papillomavirus infection in cancer of the cervix. *Lancet*, **343**, 955–957

zur Hausen, H. & de Villiers, E.-M. (1994) Human papillomaviruses. *Annu. Rev. Microbiol.*, **48**, 427–447

SUPPLEMENTARY CORRIGENDA TO VOLUMES 1–63

Volume 60

p. 292	SLH	Sorsa *et al.* (1991)	*Replace* 2.5000 *with* 25.0000
p. 294	BHP	Christakopoulos *et al.* (1993)	*Replace* 45000.0000 *with* 45.0000
p. 466	SAO	Hachitani *et al.* (1981)	*Replace* 5000.0000 *with* 2300.0000
p. 466	SAO	Waegemaekers & Bensink (1984)	*Replace* 2300.0000 *with* 5000.0000

Volume 62

p. 370	para. 2	line 8	Replace mg/ml with µg/ml
p. 370	para. 2	line 9	Replace mg/ml with µg/ml
p. 371	last para.	1. (b)	Replace 10^3 mg/ml with 10^3 µg/ml
p. 372	first para.	line 2	Replace 4×10^5 with 4×10^{-5}

CUMULATIVE CROSS INDEX TO *IARC MONOGRAPHS ON THE EVALUATION OF CARCINOGENIC RISKS TO HUMANS*

The volume, page and year of publication are given. References to corrigenda are given in parentheses.

A

A-α-C	*40*, 245 (1986); *Suppl. 7*, 56 (1987)
Acetaldehyde	*36*, 101 (1985) (*corr. 42*, 263); *Suppl. 7*, 77 (1987)
Acetaldehyde formylmethylhydrazone (*see* Gyromitrin)	
Acetamide	*7*, 197 (1974); *Suppl. 7*, 389 (1987)
Acetaminophen (*see* Paracetamol)	
Acridine orange	*16*, 145 (1978); *Suppl. 7*, 56 (1987)
Acriflavinium chloride	*13*, 31 (1977); *Suppl. 7*, 56 (1987)
Acrolein	*19*, 479 (1979); *36*, 133 (1985); *Suppl. 7*, 78 (1987); *63*, 337 (1995)
Acrylamide	*39*, 41 (1986); *Suppl. 7*, 56 (1987); *60*, 389 (1994)
Acrylic acid	*19*, 47 (1979); *Suppl. 7*, 56 (1987)
Acrylic fibres	*19*, 86 (1979); *Suppl. 7*, 56 (1987)
Acrylonitrile	*19*, 73 (1979); *Suppl. 7*, 79 (1987)
Acrylonitrile-butadiene-styrene copolymers	*19*, 91 (1979); *Suppl. 7*, 56 (1987)
Actinolite (*see* Asbestos)	
Actinomycins	*10*, 29 (1976) (*corr. 42*, 255); *Suppl. 7*, 80 (1987)
Adriamycin	*10*, 43 (1976); *Suppl. 7*, 82 (1987)
AF-2	*31*, 47 (1983); *Suppl. 7*, 56 (1987)
Aflatoxins	*1*, 145 (1972) (*corr. 42*, 251); *10*, 51 (1976); *Suppl. 7*, 83 (1987); *56*, 245 (1993)
Aflatoxin B$_1$ (*see* Aflatoxins)	
Aflatoxin B$_2$ (*see* Aflatoxins)	
Aflatoxin G$_1$ (*see* Aflatoxins)	
Aflatoxin G$_2$ (*see* Aflatoxins)	
Aflatoxin M$_1$ (*see* Aflatoxins)	
Agaritine	*31*, 63 (1983); *Suppl. 7*, 56 (1987)
Alcohol drinking	*44* (1988)
Aldicarb	*53*, 93 (1991)
Aldrin	*5*, 25 (1974); *Suppl. 7*, 88 (1987)
Allyl chloride	*36*, 39 (1985); *Suppl. 7*, 56 (1987)
Allyl isothiocyanate	*36*, 55 (1985); *Suppl. 7*, 56 (1987)
Allyl isovalerate	*36*, 69 (1985); *Suppl. 7*, 56 (1987)
Aluminium production	*34*, 37 (1984); *Suppl. 7*, 89 (1987)

Amaranth	8, 41 (1975); *Suppl. 7*, 56 (1987)
5-Aminoacenaphthene	16, 243 (1978); *Suppl. 7*, 56 (1987)
2-Aminoanthraquinone	27, 191 (1982); *Suppl. 7*, 56 (1987)
para-Aminoazobenzene	8, 53 (1975); *Suppl. 7*, 390 (1987)
ortho-Aminoazotoluene	8, 61 (1975) (*corr.* 42, 254); *Suppl. 7*, 56 (1987)
para-Aminobenzoic acid	16, 249 (1978); *Suppl. 7*, 56 (1987)
4-Aminobiphenyl	1, 74 (1972) (*corr.* 42, 251); *Suppl. 7*, 91 (1987)
2-Amino-3,4-dimethylimidazo[4,5-*f*]quinoline (*see* MeIQ)	
2-Amino-3,8-dimethylimidazo[4,5-*f*]quinoxaline (*see* MeIQx)	
3-Amino-1,4-dimethyl-5*H*-pyrido[4,3-*b*]indole (*see* Trp-P-1)	
2-Aminodipyrido[1,2-*a*:3′,2′-*d*]imidazole (*see* Glu-P-2)	
1-Amino-2-methylanthraquinone	27, 199 (1982); *Suppl. 7*, 57 (1987)
2-Amino-3-methylimidazo[4,5-*f*]quinoline (*see* IQ)	
2-Amino-6-methyldipyrido[1,2-*a*:3′,2′-*d*]imidazole (*see* Glu-P-1)	
2-Amino-1-methyl-6-phenylimidazo[4,5-*b*]pyridine (*see* PhIP)	
2-Amino-3-methyl-9*H*-pyrido[2,3-*b*]indole (*see* MeA-α-C)	
3-Amino-1-methyl-5*H*-pyrido[4,3-*b*]indole (*see* Trp-P-2)	
2-Amino-5-(5-nitro-2-furyl)-1,3,4-thiadiazole	7, 143 (1974); *Suppl. 7*, 57 (1987)
2-Amino-4-nitrophenol	57, 167 (1993)
2-Amino-5-nitrophenol	57, 177 (1993)
4-Amino-2-nitrophenol	16, 43 (1978); *Suppl. 7*, 57 (1987)
2-Amino-5-nitrothiazole	31, 71 (1983); *Suppl. 7*, 57 (1987)
2-Amino-9*H*-pyrido[2,3-*b*]indole (*see* A-α-C)	
11-Aminoundecanoic acid	39, 239 (1986); *Suppl. 7*, 57 (1987)
Amitrole	7, 31 (1974); 41, 293 (1986) (*corr.* 52, 513; *Suppl. 7*, 92 (1987)
Ammonium potassium selenide (*see* Selenium and selenium compounds)	
Amorphous silica (*see also* Silica)	42, 39 (1987); *Suppl. 7*, 341 (1987)
Amosite (*see* Asbestos)	
Ampicillin	50, 153 (1990)
Anabolic steroids (*see* Androgenic (anabolic) steroids)	
Anaesthetics, volatile	11, 285 (1976); *Suppl. 7*, 93 (1987)
Analgesic mixtures containing phenacetin (*see also* Phenacetin)	*Suppl. 7*, 310 (1987)
Androgenic (anabolic) steroids	*Suppl. 7*, 96 (1987)
Angelicin and some synthetic derivatives (*see also* Angelicins)	40, 291 (1986)
Angelicin plus ultraviolet radiation (*see also* Angelicin and some synthetic derivatives)	*Suppl. 7*, 57 (1987)
Angelicins	*Suppl. 7*, 57 (1987)
Aniline	4, 27 (1974) (*corr.* 42, 252); 27, 39 (1982); *Suppl. 7*, 99 (1987)
ortho-Anisidine	27, 63 (1982); *Suppl. 7*, 57 (1987)
para-Anisidine	27, 65 (1982); *Suppl. 7*, 57 (1987)
Anthanthrene	32, 95 (1983); *Suppl. 7*, 57 (1987)
Anthophyllite (*see* Asbestos)	
Anthracene	32, 105 (1983); *Suppl. 7*, 57 (1987)
Anthranilic acid	16, 265 (1978); *Suppl. 7*, 57 (1987)
Antimony trioxide	47, 291 (1989)
Antimony trisulfide	47, 291 (1989)
ANTU (*see* 1-Naphthylthiourea)	

CUMULATIVE INDEX 383

Apholate	9, 31 (1975); *Suppl. 7*, 57 (1987)
Aramite"	5, 39 (1974); *Suppl. 7*, 57 (1987)
Areca nut (*see* Betel quid)	
Arsanilic acid (*see* Arsenic and arsenic compounds)	
Arsenic and arsenic compounds	*1*, 41 (1972); *2*, 48 (1973); 23, 39 (1980); *Suppl. 7*, 100 (1987)
Arsenic pentoxide (*see* Arsenic and arsenic compounds)	
Arsenic sulfide (*see* Arsenic and arsenic compounds)	
Arsenic trioxide (*see* Arsenic and arsenic compounds)	
Arsine (*see* Arsenic and arsenic compounds)	
Asbestos	2, 17 (1973) (*corr. 42*, 252); *14* (1977) (*corr. 42*, 256); *Suppl. 7*, 106 (1987) (*corr. 45*, 283)
Atrazine	53, 441 (1991)
Attapulgite	42, 159 (1987); *Suppl. 7*, 117 (1987)
Auramine (technical-grade)	*1*, 69 (1972) (*corr. 42*, 251); *Suppl. 7*, 118 (1987)
Auramine, manufacture of (*see also* Auramine, technical-grade)	*Suppl. 7*, 118 (1987)
Aurothioglucose	13, 39 (1977); *Suppl. 7*, 57 (1987)
Azacitidine	26, 37 (1981); *Suppl. 7*, 57 (1987); 50, 47 (1990)
5-Azacytidine (*see* Azacitidine)	
Azaserine	*10*, 73 (1976) (*corr. 42*, 255); *Suppl. 7*, 57 (1987)
Azathioprine	26, 47 (1981); *Suppl. 7*, 119 (1987)
Aziridine	9, 37 (1975); *Suppl. 7*, 58 (1987)
2-(1-Aziridinyl)ethanol	9, 47 (1975); *Suppl. 7*, 58 (1987)
Aziridyl benzoquinone	9, 51 (1975); *Suppl. 7*, 58 (1987)
Azobenzene	8, 75 (1975); *Suppl. 7*, 58 (1987)

B

Barium chromate (*see* Chromium and chromium compounds)	
Basic chromic sulfate (*see* Chromium and chromium compounds)	
BCNU (*see* Bischloroethyl nitrosourea)	
Benz[*a*]acridine	32, 123 (1983); *Suppl. 7*, 58 (1987)
Benz[*c*]acridine	3, 241 (1973); 32, 129 (1983); *Suppl. 7*, 58 (1987)
Benzal chloride (*see also* α-Chlorinated toluenes)	29, 65 (1982); *Suppl. 7*, 148 (1987)
Benz[*a*]anthracene	3, 45 (1973); 32, 135 (1983); *Suppl. 7*, 58 (1987)
Benzene	7, 203 (1974) (*corr. 42*, 254); 29, 93, 391 (1982); *Suppl. 7*, 120 (1987)
Benzidine	*1*, 80 (1972); 29, 149, 391 (1982); *Suppl. 7*, 123 (1987)
Benzidine-based dyes	*Suppl. 7*, 125 (1987)
Benzo[*b*]fluoranthene	3, 69 (1973); 32, 147 (1983); *Suppl. 7*, 58 (1987)
Benzo[*j*]fluoranthene	3, 82 (1973); 32, 155 (1983); *Suppl. 7*, 58 (1987)

Benzo[k]fluoranthene	32, 163 (1983); Suppl. 7, 58 (1987)
Benzo[ghi]fluoranthene	32, 171 (1983); Suppl. 7, 58 (1987)
Benzo[a]fluorene	32, 177 (1983); Suppl. 7, 58 (1987)
Benzo[b]fluorene	32, 183 (1983); Suppl. 7, 58 (1987)
Benzo[c]fluorene	32, 189 (1983); Suppl. 7, 58 (1987)
Benzofuran	63, 431 (1995)
Benzo[ghi]perylene	32, 195 (1983); Suppl. 7, 58 (1987)
Benzo[c]phenanthrene	32, 205 (1983); Suppl. 7, 58 (1987)
Benzo[a]pyrene	3, 91 (1973); 32, 211 (1983); Suppl. 7, 58 (1987)
Benzo[e]pyrene	3, 137 (1973); 32, 225 (1983); Suppl. 7, 58 (1987)
para-Benzoquinone dioxime	29, 185 (1982); Suppl. 7, 58 (1987)
Benzotrichloride (see also α-Chlorinated toluenes)	29, 73 (1982); Suppl. 7, 148 (1987)
Benzoyl chloride	29, 83 (1982) (corr. 42, 261); Suppl. 7, 126 (1987)
Benzoyl peroxide	36, 267 (1985); Suppl. 7, 58 (1987)
Benzyl acetate	40, 109 (1986); Suppl. 7, 58 (1987)
Benzyl chloride (see also α-Chlorinated toluenes)	11, 217 (1976) (corr. 42, 256); 29, 49 (1982); Suppl. 7, 148 (1987)
Benzyl violet 4B	16, 153 (1978); Suppl. 7, 58 (1987)
Bertrandite (see Beryllium and beryllium compounds)	
Beryllium and beryllium compounds	1, 17 (1972); 23, 143 (1980) (corr. 42, 260); Suppl. 7, 127 (1987); 58, 41 (1993)
Beryllium acetate (see Beryllium and beryllium compounds)	
Beryllium acetate, basic (see Beryllium and beryllium compounds)	
Beryllium-aluminium alloy (see Beryllium and beryllium compounds)	
Beryllium carbonate (see Beryllium and beryllium compounds)	
Beryllium chloride (see Beryllium and beryllium compounds)	
Beryllium-copper alloy (see Beryllium and beryllium compounds)	
Beryllium-copper-cobalt alloy (see Beryllium and beryllium compounds)	
Beryllium fluoride (see Beryllium and beryllium compounds)	
Beryllium hydroxide (see Beryllium and beryllium compounds)	
Beryllium-nickel alloy (see Beryllium and beryllium compounds)	
Beryllium oxide (see Beryllium and beryllium compounds)	
Beryllium phosphate (see Beryllium and beryllium compounds)	
Beryllium silicate (see Beryllium and beryllium compounds)	
Beryllium sulfate (see Beryllium and beryllium compounds)	
Beryl ore (see Beryllium and beryllium compounds)	
Betel quid	37, 141 (1985); Suppl. 7, 128 (1987)
Betel-quid chewing (see Betel quid)	
BHA (see Butylated hydroxyanisole)	
BHT (see Butylated hydroxytoluene)	
Bis(1-aziridinyl)morpholinophosphine sulfide	9, 55 (1975); Suppl. 7, 58 (1987)
Bis(2-chloroethyl)ether	9, 117 (1975); Suppl. 7, 58 (1987)
N,N-Bis(2-chloroethyl)-2-naphthylamine	4, 119 (1974) (corr. 42, 253); Suppl. 7, 130 (1987)
Bischloroethyl nitrosourea (see also Chloroethyl nitrosoureas)	26, 79 (1981); Suppl. 7, 150 (1987)
1,2-Bis(chloromethoxy)ethane	15, 31 (1977); Suppl. 7, 58 (1987)
1,4-Bis(chloromethoxymethyl)benzene	15, 37 (1977); Suppl. 7, 58 (1987)

Bis(chloromethyl)ether	4, 231 (1974) (corr. 42, 253); Suppl. 7, 131 (1987)
Bis(2-chloro-1-methylethyl)ether	41, 149 (1986); Suppl. 7, 59 (1987)
Bis(2,3-epoxycyclopentyl)ether	47, 231 (1989)
Bisphenol A diglycidyl ether (see Glycidyl ethers)	
Bisulfites (see Sulfur dioxide and some sulfites, bisulfites and metabisulfites)	
Bitumens	35, 39 (1985); Suppl. 7, 133 (1987)
Bleomycins	26, 97 (1981); Suppl. 7, 134 (1987)
Blue VRS	16, 163 (1978); Suppl. 7, 59 (1987)
Boot and shoe manufacture and repair	25, 249 (1981); Suppl. 7, 232 (1987)
Bracken fern	40, 47 (1986); Suppl. 7, 135 (1987)
Brilliant Blue FCF, disodium salt	16, 171 (1978) (corr. 42, 257); Suppl. 7, 59 (1987)
Bromochloroacetonitrile (see Halogenated acetonitriles)	
Bromodichloromethane	52, 179 (1991)
Bromoethane	52, 299 (1991)
Bromoform	52, 213 (1991)
1,3-Butadiene	39, 155 (1986) (corr. 42, 264 Suppl. 7, 136 (1987); 54, 237 (1992)
1,4-Butanediol dimethanesulfonate	4, 247 (1974); Suppl. 7, 137 (1987)
n-Butyl acrylate	39, 67 (1986); Suppl. 7, 59 (1987)
Butylated hydroxyanisole	40, 123 (1986); Suppl. 7, 59 (1987)
Butylated hydroxytoluene	40, 161 (1986); Suppl. 7, 59 (1987)
Butyl benzyl phthalate	29, 193 (1982) (corr. 42, 261); Suppl. 7, 59 (1987)
β-Butyrolactone	11, 225 (1976); Suppl. 7, 59 (1987)
γ-Butyrolactone	11, 231 (1976); Suppl. 7, 59 (1987)

C

Cabinet-making (see Furniture and cabinet-making)	
Cadmium acetate (see Cadmium and cadmium compounds)	
Cadmium and cadmium compounds	2, 74 (1973); 11, 39 (1976) (corr. 42, 255); Suppl. 7, 139 (1987); 58, 119 (1993)
Cadmium chloride (see Cadmium and cadmium compounds)	
Cadmium oxide (see Cadmium and cadmium compounds)	
Cadmium sulfate (see Cadmium and cadmium compounds)	
Cadmium sulfide (see Cadmium and cadmium compounds)	
Caffeic acid	56, 115 (1993)
Caffeine	51, 291 (1991)
Calcium arsenate (see Arsenic and arsenic compounds)	
Calcium chromate (see Chromium and chromium compounds)	
Calcium cyclamate (see Cyclamates)	
Calcium saccharin (see Saccharin)	
Cantharidin	10, 79 (1976); Suppl. 7, 59 (1987)
Caprolactam	19, 115 (1979) (corr. 42, 258); 39, 247 (1986) (corr. 42, 264); Suppl. 7, 390 (1987)
Captafol	53, 353 (1991)

Captan	*30*, 295 (1983); *Suppl. 7*, 59 (1987)
Carbaryl	*12*, 37 (1976); *Suppl. 7*, 59 (1987)
Carbazole	*32*, 239 (1983); *Suppl. 7*, 59 (1987)
3-Carbethoxypsoralen	*40*, 317 (1986); *Suppl. 7*, 59 (1987)
Carbon blacks	*3*, 22 (1973); *33*, 35 (1984); *Suppl. 7*, 142 (1987)
Carbon tetrachloride	*1*, 53 (1972); *20*, 371 (1979); *Suppl. 7*, 143 (1987)
Carmoisine	*8*, 83 (1975); *Suppl. 7*, 59 (1987)
Carpentry and joinery	*25*, 139 (1981); *Suppl. 7*, 378 (1987)
Carrageenan	*10*, 181 (1976) (*corr. 42*, 255); *31*, 79 (1983); *Suppl. 7*, 59 (1987)
Catechol	*15*, 155 (1977); *Suppl. 7*, 59 (1987)
CCNU (*see* 1-(2-Chloroethyl)-3-cyclohexyl-1-nitrosourea)	
Ceramic fibres (see Man-made mineral fibres)	
Chemotherapy, combined, including alkylating agents (*see* MOPP and other combined chemotherapy including alkylating agents)	
Chloral	*63*, 245 (1995)
Chloral hydrate	*63*, 245 (1995)
Chlorambucil	*9*, 125 (1975); *26*, 115 (1981) *Suppl. 7*, 144 (1987)
Chloramphenicol	*10*, 85 (1976); *Suppl. 7*, 145 (1987); *50*, 169 (1990)
Chlordane (*see also* Chlordane/Heptachlor)	*20*, 45 (1979) (*corr. 42*, 258)
Chlordane/Heptachlor	*Suppl. 7*, 146 (1987); *53*, 115 (1991)
Chlordecone	*20*, 67 (1979); *Suppl. 7*, 59 (1987)
Chlordimeform	*30*, 61 (1983); *Suppl. 7*, 59 (1987)
Chlorendic acid	*48*, 45 (1990)
Chlorinated dibenzodioxins (other than TCDD)	*15*, 41 (1977); *Suppl. 7*, 59 (1987)
Chlorinated drinking-water	*52*, 45 (1991)
Chlorinated paraffins	*48*, 55 (1990)
α-Chlorinated toluenes	*Suppl. 7*, 148 (1987)
Chlormadinone acetate (*see also* Progestins; Combined oral contraceptives)	*6*, 149 (1974); *21*, 365 (1979)
Chlornaphazine (*see* N,N-Bis(2-chloroethyl)-2-naphthylamine)	
Chloroacetonitrile (*see* Halogenated acetonitriles)	
para-Chloroaniline	*57*, 305 (1993)
Chlorobenzilate	*5*, 75 (1974); *30*, 73 (1983); *Suppl. 7*, 60 (1987)
Chlorodibromomethane	*52*, 243 (1991)
Chlorodifluoromethane	*41*, 237 (1986) (*corr. 51*, 483); *Suppl. 7*, 149 (1987)
Chloroethane	*52*, 315 (1991)
1-(2-Chloroethyl)-3-cyclohexyl-1-nitrosourea (*see also* Chloroethyl nitrosoureas)	*26*, 137 (1981) (*corr. 42*, 260); *Suppl. 7*, 150 (1987)
1-(2-Chloroethyl)-3-(4-methylcyclohexyl)-1-nitrosourea (*see also* Chloroethyl nitrosoureas)	*Suppl. 7*, 150 (1987)
Chloroethyl nitrosoureas	*Suppl. 7*, 150 (1987)
Chlorofluoromethane	*41*, 229 (1986); *Suppl. 7*, 60 (1987)

CUMULATIVE INDEX

Chloroform	*1*, 61 (1972); *20*, 401 (1979)
	Suppl. 7, 152 (1987)
Chloromethyl methyl ether (technical-grade) (*see also* Bis(chloromethyl)ether)	*4*, 239 (1974); *Suppl. 7*, 131 (1987)
(4-Chloro-2-methylphenoxy)acetic acid (*see* MCPA)	
1-Chloro-2-methylpropene	*63*, 315 (1995)
3-Chloro-2-methylpropene	*63*, 325 (1995)
Chlorophenols	*Suppl. 7*, 154 (1987)
Chlorophenols (occupational exposures to)	*41*, 319 (1986)
Chlorophenoxy herbicides	*Suppl. 7*, 156 (1987)
Chlorophenoxy herbicides (occupational exposures to)	*41*, 357 (1986)
4-Chloro-*ortho*-phenylenediamine	*27*, 81 (1982); *Suppl. 7*, 60 (1987)
4-Chloro-*meta*-phenylenediamine	*27*, 82 (1982); *Suppl. 7*, 60 (1987)
Chloroprene	*19*, 131 (1979); *Suppl. 7*, 160 (1987)
Chloropropham	*12*, 55 (1976); *Suppl. 7*, 60 (1987)
Chloroquine	*13*, 47 (1977); *Suppl. 7*, 60 (1987)
Chlorothalonil	*30*, 319 (1983); *Suppl. 7*, 60 (1987)
para-Chloro-*ortho*-toluidine and its strong acid salts (*see also* Chlordimeform)	*16*, 277 (1978); *30*, 65 (1983); *Suppl. 7*, 60 (1987); *48*, 123 (1990)
Chlorotrianisene (*see also* Nonsteroidal oestrogens)	*21*, 139 (1979)
2-Chloro-1,1,1-trifluoroethane	*41*, 253 (1986); *Suppl. 7*, 60 (1987)
Chlorozotocin	*50*, 65 (1990)
Cholesterol	*10*, 99 (1976); *31*, 95 (1983);
	Suppl. 7, 161 (1987)
Chromic acetate (*see* Chromium and chromium compounds)	
Chromic chloride (*see* Chromium and chromium compounds)	
Chromic oxide (*see* Chromium and chromium compounds)	
Chromic phosphate (*see* Chromium and chromium compounds)	
Chromite ore (*see* Chromium and chromium compounds)	
Chromium and chromium compounds	*2*, 100 (1973); *23*, 205 (1980);
	Suppl. 7, 165 (1987); *49*, 49 (1990)
	(*corr. 51*, 483)
Chromium carbonyl (*see* Chromium and chromium compounds)	
Chromium potassium sulfate (*see* Chromium and chromium compounds)	
Chromium sulfate (*see* Chromium and chromium compounds)	
Chromium trioxide (*see* Chromium and chromium compounds)	
Chrysazin (*see* Dantron)	
Chrysene	*3*, 159 (1973); *32*, 247 (1983);
	Suppl. 7, 60 (1987)
Chrysoidine	*8*, 91 (1975); *Suppl. 7*, 169 (1987)
Chrysotile (*see* Asbestos)	
CI Acid Orange 3	*57*, 121 (1993)
CI Acid Red 114	*57*, 247 (1993)
CI Basic Red 9	*57*, 215 (1993)
Ciclosporin	*50*, 77 (1990)
CI Direct Blue 15	*57*, 235 (1993)
CI Disperse Yellow 3 (see Disperse Yellow 3)	
Cimetidine	*50*, 235 (1990)
Cinnamyl anthranilate	*16*, 287 (1978); *31*, 133 (1983);
	Suppl. 7, 60 (1987)
CI Pigment Red 3	*57*, 259 (1993)

CI Pigment Red 53:1 (see D&C Red No. 9)
Cisplatin   26, 151 (1981); Suppl. 7, 170 (1987)
Citrinin   40, 67 (1986); Suppl. 7, 60 (1987)
Citrus Red No. 2   8, 101 (1975) (corr. 42, 254)
                                                                             Suppl. 7, 60 (1987)
Clofibrate   24, 39 (1980); Suppl. 7, 171 (1987)
Clomiphene citrate   21, 551 (1979); Suppl. 7, 172 (1987)
Clonorchis sinensis (infection with)   61, 121 (1994)
Coal gasification   34, 65 (1984); Suppl. 7, 173 (1987)
Coal-tar pitches (see also Coal-tars)   35, 83 (1985); Suppl. 7, 174 (1987)
Coal-tars   35, 83 (1985); Suppl. 7, 175 (1987)
Cobalt[III] acetate (see Cobalt and cobalt compounds)
Cobalt-aluminium-chromium spinel (see Cobalt and cobalt compounds)
Cobalt and cobalt compounds   52, 363 (1991)
Cobalt[II] chloride (see Cobalt and cobalt compounds)
Cobalt-chromium alloy (see Chromium and chromium compounds)
Cobalt-chromium-molybdenum alloys (see Cobalt and cobalt compounds)
Cobalt metal powder (see Cobalt and cobalt compounds)
Cobalt naphthenate (see Cobalt and cobalt compounds)
Cobalt[II] oxide (see Cobalt and cobalt compounds)
Cobalt[II,III] oxide (see Cobalt and cobalt compounds)
Cobalt[II] sulfide (see Cobalt and cobalt compounds)
Coffee   51, 41 (1991) (corr. 52, 513)
Coke production   34, 101 (1984); Suppl. 7, 176 (1987)
Combined oral contraceptives (see also Oestrogens, progestins   Suppl. 7, 297 (1987)
    and combinations)
Conjugated oestrogens (see also Steroidal oestrogens)   21, 147 (1979)
Contraceptives, oral (see Combined oral contraceptives;
    Sequential oral contraceptives)
Copper 8-hydroxyquinoline   15, 103 (1977); Suppl. 7, 61 (1987)
Coronene   32, 263 (1983); Suppl. 7, 61 (1987)
Coumarin   10, 113 (1976); Suppl. 7, 61 (1987)
Creosotes (see also Coal-tars)   35, 83 (1985); Suppl. 7, 177 (1987)
meta-Cresidine   27, 91 (1982); Suppl. 7, 61 (1987)
para-Cresidine   27, 92 (1982); Suppl. 7, 61 (1987)
Crocidolite (see Asbestos)
Crotonaldehyde   63, 373 (1995)
Crude oil   45, 119 (1989)
Crystalline silica (see also Silica)   42, 39 (1987); Suppl. 7, 341 (1987)
Cycasin   1, 157 (1972) (corr. 42, 251); 10,
                                                                             121 (1976); Suppl. 7, 61 (1987)
Cyclamates   22, 55 (1980); Suppl. 7, 178 (1987)
Cyclamic acid (see Cyclamates)
Cyclochlorotine   10, 139 (1976); Suppl. 7, 61 (1987)
Cyclohexanone   47, 157 (1989)
Cyclohexylamine (see Cyclamates)
Cyclopenta[cd]pyrene   32, 269 (1983); Suppl. 7, 61 (1987)
Cyclopropane (see Anaesthetics, volatile)
Cyclophosphamide   9, 135 (1975); 26, 165 (1981);
                                                                             Suppl. 7, 182 (1987)

D

2,4-D (*see also* Chlorophenoxy herbicides; Chlorophenoxy herbicides, occupational exposures to)	*15*, 111 (1977)
Dacarbazine	*26*, 203 (1981); *Suppl. 7*, 184 (1987)
Dantron	*50*, 265 (1990) (*corr. 59*, 257)
D&C Red No. 9	*8*, 107 (1975); *Suppl. 7*, 61 (1987); *57*, 203 (1993)
Dapsone	*24*, 59 (1980); *Suppl. 7*, 185 (1987)
Daunomycin	*10*, 145 (1976); *Suppl. 7*, 61 (1987)
DDD (*see* DDT)	
DDE (*see* DDT)	
DDT	*5*, 83 (1974) (*corr. 42*, 253); *Suppl. 7*, 186 (1987); *53*, 179 (1991)
Decabromodiphenyl oxide	*48*, 73 (1990)
Deltamethrin	*53*, 251 (1991)
Deoxynivalenol (*see* Toxins derived from *Fusarium graminearum, F. culmorum* and *F. crookwellense*)	
Diacetylaminoazotoluene	*8*, 113 (1975); *Suppl. 7*, 61 (1987)
N,N'-Diacetylbenzidine	*16*, 293 (1978); *Suppl. 7*, 61 (1987)
Diallate	*12*, 69 (1976); *30*, 235 (1983); *Suppl. 7*, 61 (1987)
2,4-Diaminoanisole	*16*, 51 (1978); *27*, 103 (1982); *Suppl. 7*, 61 (1987)
4,4'-Diaminodiphenyl ether	*16*, 301 (1978); *29*, 203 (1982); *Suppl. 7*, 61 (1987)
1,2-Diamino-4-nitrobenzene	*16*, 63 (1978); *Suppl. 7*, 61 (1987)
1,4-Diamino-2-nitrobenzene	*16*, 73 (1978); *Suppl. 7*, 61 (1987); *57*, 185 (1993)
2,6-Diamino-3-(phenylazo)pyridine (*see* Phenazopyridine hydrochloride)	
2,4-Diaminotoluene (*see also* Toluene diisocyanates)	*16*, 83 (1978); *Suppl. 7*, 61 (1987)
2,5-Diaminotoluene (*see also* Toluene diisocyanates)	*16*, 97 (1978); *Suppl. 7*, 61 (1987)
ortho-Dianisidine (*see* 3,3'-Dimethoxybenzidine)	
Diazepam	*13*, 57 (1977); *Suppl. 7*, 189 (1987)
Diazomethane	*7*, 223 (1974); *Suppl. 7*, 61 (1987)
Dibenz[*a,h*]acridine	*3*, 247 (1973); *32*, 277 (1983); *Suppl. 7*, 61 (1987)
Dibenz[*a,j*]acridine	*3*, 254 (1973); *32*, 283 (1983); *Suppl. 7*, 61 (1987)
Dibenz[*a,c*]anthracene	*32*, 289 (1983) (*corr. 42*, 262); *Suppl. 7*, 61 (1987)
Dibenz[*a,h*]anthracene	*3*, 178 (1973) (*corr. 43*, 261); *32*, 299 (1983); *Suppl. 7*, 61 (1987)
Dibenz[*a,j*]anthracene	*32*, 309 (1983); *Suppl. 7*, 61 (1987)
7*H*-Dibenzo[*c,g*]carbazole	*3*, 260 (1973); *32*, 315 (1983); *Suppl. 7*, 61 (1987)
Dibenzodioxins, chlorinated (other than TCDD) [*see* Chlorinated dibenzodioxins (other than TCDD)]	
Dibenzo[*a,e*]fluoranthene	*32*, 321 (1983); *Suppl. 7*, 61 (1987)
Dibenzo[*h,rst*]pentaphene	*3*, 197 (1973); *Suppl. 7*, 62 (1987)

Dibenzo[*a,e*]pyrene	*3*, 201 (1973); *32*, 327 (1983); Suppl. *7*, 62 (1987)
Dibenzo[*a,h*]pyrene	*3*, 207 (1973); *32*, 331 (1983); Suppl. *7*, 62 (1987)
Dibenzo[*a,i*]pyrene	*3*, 215 (1973); *32*, 337 (1983); Suppl. *7*, 62 (1987)
Dibenzo[*a,l*]pyrene	*3*, 224 (1973); *32*, 343 (1983); Suppl. *7*, 62 (1987)
Dibromoacetonitrile (*see* Halogenated acetonitriles)	
1,2-Dibromo-3-chloropropane	*15*, 139 (1977); *20*, 83 (1979); Suppl. *7*, 191 (1987)
Dichloroacetic acid	*63*, 271 (1995)
Dichloroacetonitrile (*see* Halogenated acetonitriles)	
Dichloroacetylene	*39*, 369 (1986); Suppl. *7*, 62 (1987)
ortho-Dichlorobenzene	*7*, 231 (1974); *29*, 213 (1982); Suppl. *7*, 192 (1987)
para-Dichlorobenzene	*7*, 231 (1974); *29*, 215 (1982); Suppl. *7*, 192 (1987)
3,3'-Dichlorobenzidine	*4*, 49 (1974); *29*, 239 (1982); Suppl. *7*, 193 (1987)
trans-1,4-Dichlorobutene	*15*, 149 (1977); Suppl. *7*, 62 (1987)
3,3'-Dichloro-4,4'-diaminodiphenyl ether	*16*, 309 (1978); Suppl. *7*, 62 (1987)
1,2-Dichloroethane	*20*, 429 (1979); Suppl. *7*, 62 (1987)
Dichloromethane	*20*, 449 (1979); *41*, 43 (1986); Suppl. *7*, 194 (1987)
2,4-Dichlorophenol (*see* Chlorophenols; Chlorophenols, occupational exposures to)	
(2,4-Dichlorophenoxy)acetic acid (*see* 2,4-D)	
2,6-Dichloro-*para*-phenylenediamine	*39*, 325 (1986); Suppl. *7*, 62 (1987)
1,2-Dichloropropane	*41*, 131 (1986); Suppl. *7*, 62 (1987)
1,3-Dichloropropene (technical-grade)	*41*, 113 (1986); Suppl. *7*, 195 (1987)
Dichlorvos	*20*, 97 (1979); Suppl. *7*, 62 (1987); *53*, 267 (1991)
Dicofol	*30*, 87 (1983); Suppl. *7*, 62 (1987)
Dicyclohexylamine (*see* Cyclamates)	
Dieldrin	*5*, 125 (1974); Suppl. *7*, 196 (1987)
Dienoestrol (*see also* Nonsteroidal oestrogens)	*21*, 161 (1979)
Diepoxybutane	*11*, 115 (1976) (*corr. 42*, 255); Suppl. *7*, 62 (1987)
Diesel and gasoline engine exhausts	*46*, 41 (1989)
Diesel fuels	*45*, 219 (1989) (*corr. 47*, 505)
Diethyl ether (*see* Anaesthetics, volatile)	
Di(2-ethylhexyl)adipate	*29*, 257 (1982); Suppl. *7*, 62 (1987)
Di(2-ethylhexyl)phthalate	*29*, 269 (1982) (*corr. 42*, 261); Suppl. *7*, 62 (1987)
1,2-Diethylhydrazine	*4*, 153 (1974); Suppl. *7*, 62 (1987)
Diethylstilboestrol	*6*, 55 (1974); *21*, 173 (1979) (*corr. 42*, 259); Suppl. *7*, 273 (1987)
Diethylstilboestrol dipropionate (*see* Diethylstilboestrol)	
Diethyl sulfate	*4*, 277 (1974); Suppl. *7*, 198 (1987); *54*, 213 (1992)

Diglycidyl resorcinol ether	*11*, 125 (1976); *36*, 181 (1985); Suppl. 7, 62 (1987)
Dihydrosafrole	*1*, 170 (1972); *10*, 233 (1976) Suppl. 7, 62 (1987)
1,8-Dihydroxyanthraquinone (*see* Dantron)	
Dihydroxybenzenes (*see* Catechol; Hydroquinone; Resorcinol)	
Dihydroxymethylfuratrizine	24, 77 (1980); Suppl. 7, 62 (1987)
Diisopropyl sulfate	54, 229 (1992)
Dimethisterone (*see also* Progestins; Sequential oral contraceptives	6, 167 (1974); *21*, 377 (1979))
Dimethoxane	*15*, 177 (1977); Suppl. 7, 62 (1987)
3,3'-Dimethoxybenzidine	*4*, 41 (1974); Suppl. 7, 198 (1987)
3,3'-Dimethoxybenzidine-4,4'-diisocyanate	*39*, 279 (1986); Suppl. 7, 62 (1987)
para-Dimethylaminoazobenzene	*8*, 125 (1975); Suppl. 7, 62 (1987)
para-Dimethylaminoazobenzenediazo sodium sulfonate	*8*, 147 (1975); Suppl. 7, 62 (1987)
trans-2-[(Dimethylamino)methylimino]-5-[2-(5-nitro-2-furyl)-vinyl]-1,3,4-oxadiazole	7, 147 (1974) (*corr. 42*, 253); Suppl. 7, 62 (1987)
4,4'-Dimethylangelicin plus ultraviolet radiation (*see also* Angelicin and some synthetic derivatives)	Suppl. 7, 57 (1987)
4,5'-Dimethylangelicin plus ultraviolet radiation (*see also* Angelicin and some synthetic derivatives)	Suppl. 7, 57 (1987)
2,6-Dimethylaniline	57, 323 (1993)
N,N-Dimethylaniline	57, 337 (1993)
Dimethylarsinic acid (*see* Arsenic and arsenic compounds)	
3,3'-Dimethylbenzidine	*1*, 87 (1972); Suppl. 7, 62 (1987)
Dimethylcarbamoyl chloride	*12*, 77 (1976); Suppl. 7, 199 (1987)
Dimethylformamide	47, 171 (1989)
1,1-Dimethylhydrazine	*4*, 137 (1974); Suppl. 7, 62 (1987)
1,2-Dimethylhydrazine	*4*, 145 (1974) (*corr. 42*, 253); Suppl. 7, 62 (1987)
Dimethyl hydrogen phosphite	48, 85 (1990)
1,4-Dimethylphenanthrene	*32*, 349 (1983); Suppl. 7, 62 (1987)
Dimethyl sulfate	*4*, 271 (1974); Suppl. 7, 200 (1987)
3,7-Dinitrofluoranthene	46, 189 (1989)
3,9-Dinitrofluoranthene	46, 195 (1989)
1,3-Dinitropyrene	46, 201 (1989)
1,6-Dinitropyrene	46, 215 (1989)
1,8-Dinitropyrene	*33*, 171 (1984); Suppl. 7, 63 (1987); 46, 231 (1989)
Dinitrosopentamethylenetetramine	*11*, 241 (1976); Suppl. 7, 63 (1987)
1,4-Dioxane	*11*, 247 (1976); Suppl. 7, 201 (1987)
2,4'-Diphenyldiamine	*16*, 313 (1978); Suppl. 7, 63 (1987)
Direct Black 38 (*see also* Benzidine-based dyes)	29, 295 (1982) (*corr. 42*, 261)
Direct Blue 6 (*see also* Benzidine-based dyes)	29, 311 (1982)
Direct Brown 95 (*see also* Benzidine-based dyes)	29, 321 (1982)
Disperse Blue 1	48, 139 (1990)
Disperse Yellow 3	*8*, 97 (1975); Suppl. 7, 60 (1987); 48, 149 (1990)
Disulfiram	*12*, 85 (1976); Suppl. 7, 63 (1987)
Dithranol	*13*, 75 (1977); Suppl. 7, 63 (1987)
Divinyl ether (*see* Anaesthetics, volatile)	
Dry cleaning	63, 33 (1995)

Dulcin   *12*, 97 (1976); *Suppl. 7*, 63 (1987)

E

Endrin   *5*, 157 (1974); *Suppl. 7*, 63 (1987)
Enflurane (*see* Anaesthetics, volatile)
Eosin   *15*, 183 (1977); *Suppl. 7*, 63 (1987)
Epichlorohydrin   *11*, 131 (1976) (*corr. 42*, 256);
                                                            Suppl. 7, 202 (1987)
1,2-Epoxybutane   *47*, 217 (1989)
1-Epoxyethyl-3,4-epoxycyclohexane (*see* 4-Vinylcyclohexene diepoxide)
3,4-Epoxy-6-methylcyclohexylmethyl-3,4-epoxy-6-methyl-   *11*, 147 (1976); *Suppl. 7*, 63 (1987)
  cyclohexane carboxylate
cis-9,10-Epoxystearic acid   *11*, 153 (1976); *Suppl. 7*, 63 (1987)
Erionite   *42*, 225 (1987); *Suppl. 7*, 203 (1987)
Ethinyloestradiol (*see also* Steroidal oestrogens)   *6*, 77 (1974); *21*, 233 (1979)
Ethionamide   *13*, 83 (1977); *Suppl. 7*, 63 (1987)
Ethyl acrylate   *19*, 57 (1979); *39*, 81 (1986);
                                                            Suppl. 7, 63 (1987)
Ethylene   *19*, 157 (1979); *Suppl. 7*, 63 (1987);
                                                            60, 45 (1994)
Ethylene dibromide   *15*, 195 (1977); *Suppl. 7*, 204 (1987)
Ethylene oxide   *11*, 157 (1976); *36*, 189 (1985)
                                                            (*corr. 42*, 263); *Suppl. 7*, 205
                                                            (1987); *60*, 73 (1994)
Ethylene sulfide   *11*, 257 (1976); *Suppl. 7*, 63 (1987)
Ethylene thiourea   *7*, 45 (1974); *Suppl. 7*, 207 (1987)
2-Ethylhexyl acrylate   *60*, 475 (1994)
Ethyl methanesulfonate   *7*, 245 (1974); *Suppl. 7*, 63 (1987)
N-Ethyl-*N*-nitrosourea   *1*, 135 (1972); *17*, 191 (1978);
                                                            Suppl. 7, 63 (1987)
Ethyl selenac (*see also* Selenium and selenium compounds) *12*, 107 (1976); *Suppl. 7*, 63 (1987)
Ethyl tellurac   *12*, 115 (1976); *Suppl. 7*, 63 (1987)
Ethynodiol diacetate (*see also* Progestins; Combined oral *6*, 173 (1974); *21*, 387 (1979)
  contraceptives)
Eugenol   *36*, 75 (1985); *Suppl. 7*, 63 (1987)
Evans blue   *8*, 151 (1975); *Suppl. 7*, 63 (1987)

F

Fast Green FCF   *16*, 187 (1978); *Suppl. 7*, 63 (1987)
Fenvalerate   *53*, 309 (1991)
Ferbam   *12*, 121 (1976) (*corr. 42*, 256);
                                                            Suppl. 7, 63 (1987)
Ferric oxide   *1*, 29 (1972); *Suppl. 7*, 216 (1987)
Ferrochromium (*see* Chromium and chromium compounds)
Fluometuron   *30*, 245 (1983); *Suppl. 7*, 63 (1987)
Fluoranthene   *32*, 355 (1983); *Suppl. 7*, 63 (1987)
Fluorene   *32*, 365 (1983); *Suppl. 7*, 63 (1987)

Fluorescent lighting (exposure to) (see Ultraviolet radiation)
Fluorides (inorganic, used in drinking-water)   27, 237 (1982); *Suppl. 7*, 208 (1987)
5-Fluorouracil   26, 217 (1981); *Suppl. 7*, 210 (1987)
Fluorspar (see Fluorides)
Fluosilicic acid (see Fluorides)
Fluroxene (see Anaesthetics, volatile)
Formaldehyde   *29*, 345 (1982); *Suppl. 7*, 211 (1987); 62, 217 (1995)
2-(2-Formylhydrazino)-4-(5-nitro-2-furyl)thiazole   *7*, 151 (1974) (*corr. 42*, 253); *Suppl. 7*, 63 (1987)
Frusemide (see Furosemide)
Fuel oils (heating oils)   *45*, 239 (1989) (*corr. 47*, 505)
Fumonisin B₁ (see Toxins derived from Fusarium moniliforme)
Fumonisin B₂ (see Toxins derived from Fusarium moniliforme)
Furan   *63*, 393 (1995)
Furazolidone   *31*, 141 (1983); *Suppl. 7*, 63 (1987)
Furfural   *63*, 409 (1995)
Furniture and cabinet-making   *25*, 99 (1981); *Suppl. 7*, 380 (1987)
Furosemide   *50*, 277 (1990)
2-(2-Furyl)-3-(5-nitro-2-furyl)acrylamide (see AF-2)
Fusarenon-X (see Toxins derived from *Fusarium graminearum*, *F. culmorum* and *F. crookwellense*)
Fusarenone-X (see Toxins derived from *Fusarium graminearum*, *F. culmorum* and *F. crookwellense*)
Fusarin C (see Toxins derived from *Fusarium moniliforme*)

G

Gasoline   45, 159 (1989) (corr. 47, 505)
Gasoline engine exhaust (see Diesel and gasoline engine exhausts)
Glass fibres (see Man-made mineral fibres)
Glass manufacturing industry, occupational exposures in   58, 347 (1993)
Glasswool (see Man-made mineral fibres)
Glass filaments (see Man-made mineral fibres)
Glu-P-1   *40*, 223 (1986); *Suppl. 7*, 64 (1987)
Glu-P-2   *40*, 235 (1986); *Suppl. 7*, 64 (1987)
L-Glutamic acid, 5-[2-(4-hydroxymethyl)phenylhydrazide] (see Agaritine)
Glycidaldehyde   *11*, 175 (1976); *Suppl. 7*, 64 (1987)
Glycidyl ethers   *47*, 237 (1989)
Glycidyl oleate   *11*, 183 (1976); *Suppl. 7*, 64 (1987)
Glycidyl stearate   *11*, 187 (1976); *Suppl. 7*, 64 (1987)
Griseofulvin   *10*, 153 (1976); *Suppl. 7*, 391 (1987)
Guinea Green B   *16*, 199 (1978); *Suppl. 7*, 64 (1987)
Gyromitrin   *31*, 163 (1983); *Suppl. 7*, 391 (1987)

H

Haematite   *1*, 29 (1972); *Suppl. 7*, 216 (1987)

Haematite and ferric oxide	*Suppl. 7*, 216 (1987)
Haematite mining, underground, with exposure to radon	*1*, 29 (1972); *Suppl. 7*, 216 (1987)
Hairdressers and barbers (occupational exposure as)	*57*, 43 (1993)
Hair dyes, epidemiology of	*16*, 29 (1978); *27*, 307 (1982);
Halogenated acetonitriles	*52*, 269 (1991)
Halothane (*see* Anaesthetics, volatile)	
HC Blue No. 1	*57*, 129 (1993)
HC Blue No. 2	*57*, 143 (1993)
α-HCH (*see* Hexachlorocyclohexanes)	
β-HCH (*see* Hexachlorocyclohexanes)	
γ-HCH (*see* Hexachlorocyclohexanes)	
HC Red No. 3	*57*, 153 (1993)
HC Yellow No. 4	*57*, 159 (1993)
Heating oils (*see* Fuel oils)	
Helicobacter pylori (infection with)	*61*, 177 (1994)
Hepatitis B virus	*59*, 45 (1994)
Hepatitis C virus	*59*, 165 (1994)
Hepatitis D virus	*59*, 223 (1994)
Heptachlor (*see also* Chlordane/Heptachlor)	*5*, 173 (1974); *20*, 129 (1979)
Hexachlorobenzene	*20*, 155 (1979); *Suppl. 7*, 219 (1987)
Hexachlorobutadiene	*20*, 179 (1979); *Suppl. 7*, 64 (1987)
Hexachlorocyclohexanes	*5*, 47 (1974); *20*, 195 (1979) (*corr. 42*, 258); *Suppl. 7*, 220 (1987)
Hexachlorocyclohexane, technical-grade (*see* Hexachlorocyclohexanes)	
Hexachloroethane	*20*, 467 (1979); *Suppl. 7*, 64 (1987)
Hexachlorophene	*20*, 241 (1979); *Suppl. 7*, 64 (1987)
Hexamethylphosphoramide	*15*, 211 (1977); *Suppl. 7*, 64 (1987)
Hexoestrol (*see* Nonsteroidal oestrogens)	
Human papillomaviruses	*64* (1995)
Hycanthone mesylate	*13*, 91 (1977); *Suppl. 7*, 64 (1987)
Hydralazine	*24*, 85 (1980); *Suppl. 7*, 222 (1987)
Hydrazine	*4*, 127 (1974); *Suppl. 7*, 223 (1987)
Hydrochloric acid	*54*, 189 (1992)
Hydrochlorothiazide	*50*, 293 (1990)
Hydrogen peroxide	*36*, 285 (1985); *Suppl. 7*, 64 (1987)
Hydroquinone	*15*, 155 (1977); *Suppl. 7*, 64 (1987)
4-Hydroxyazobenzene	*8*, 157 (1975); *Suppl. 7*, 64 (1987)
17α-Hydroxyprogesterone caproate (*see also* Progestins)	*21*, 399 (1979) (*corr. 42*, 259)
8-Hydroxyquinoline	*13*, 101 (1977); *Suppl. 7*, 64 (1987)
8-Hydroxysenkirkine	*10*, 265 (1976); *Suppl. 7*, 64 (1987)
Hypochlorite salts	*52*, 159 (1991)

I

Indeno[1,2,3-*cd*]pyrene	*3*, 229 (1973); *32*, 373 (1983); *Suppl. 7*, 64 (1987)
Inorganic acids (see Sulfuric acid and other strong inorganic acids, occupational exposures to mists and vapours from)	
Insecticides, occupational exposures in spraying and application of	*53*, 45 (1991)
IQ	*40*, 261 (1986); *Suppl. 7*, 64 (1987);

	56, 165 (1993)
Iron and steel founding	*34*, 133 (1984); *Suppl. 7*, 224 (1987)
Iron-dextran complex	*2*, 161 (1973); *Suppl. 7*, 226 (1987)
Iron-dextrin complex	*2*, 161 (1973) (*corr. 42*, 252); *Suppl. 7*, 64 (1987)
Iron oxide (*see* Ferric oxide)	
Iron oxide, saccharated (*see* Saccharated iron oxide)	
Iron sorbitol-citric acid complex	*2*, 161 (1973); *Suppl. 7*, 64 (1987)
Isatidine	*10*, 269 (1976); *Suppl. 7*, 65 (1987)
Isoflurane (*see* Anaesthetics, volatile)	
Isoniazid (*see* Isonicotinic acid hydrazide)	
Isonicotinic acid hydrazide	*4*, 159 (1974); *Suppl. 7*, 227 (1987)
Isophosphamide	*26*, 237 (1981); *Suppl. 7*, 65 (1987)
Isoprene	*60*, 215 (1994)
Isopropanol	*15*, 223 (1977); *Suppl. 7*, 229 (1987)
Isopropanol manufacture (strong-acid process) (*see* also Isopropanol; Sulfuric acid and other strong inorganic acids, occupational exposures to mists and vapours from)	*Suppl. 7*, 229 (1987)
Isopropyl oils	*15*, 223 (1977); *Suppl. 7*, 229 (1987)
Isosafrole	*1*, 169 (1972); *10*, 232 (1976); *Suppl. 7*, 65 (1987)

J

Jacobine	*10*, 275 (1976); *Suppl. 7*, 65 (1987)
Jet fuel	*45*, 203 (1989)
Joinery (*see* Carpentry and joinery)	

K

Kaempferol	*31*, 171 (1983); *Suppl. 7*, 65 (1987)
Kepone (*see* Chlordecone)	

L

Lasiocarpine	*10*, 281 (1976); *Suppl. 7*, 65 (1987)
Lauroyl peroxide	*36*, 315 (1985); *Suppl. 7*, 65 (1987)
Lead acetate (*see* Lead and lead compounds)	
Lead and lead compounds	*1*, 40 (1972) (*corr. 42*, 251); *2*, 52, 150 (1973); *12*, 131 (1976); *23*, 40, 208, 209, 325 (1980); *Suppl. 7*, 230 (1987)
Lead arsenate (*see* Arsenic and arsenic compounds)	
Lead carbonate (*see* Lead and lead compounds)	
Lead chloride (*see* Lead and lead compounds)	
Lead chromate (*see* Chromium and chromium compounds)	
Lead chromate oxide (*see* Chromium and chromium compounds)	
Lead naphthenate (*see* Lead and lead compounds)	

Lead nitrate (see Lead and lead compounds)
Lead oxide (see Lead and lead compounds)
Lead phosphate (see Lead and lead compounds)
Lead subacetate (see Lead and lead compounds)
Lead tetroxide (see Lead and lead compounds)

Leather goods manufacture	25, 279 (1981); Suppl. 7, 235 (1987)
Leather industries	25, 199 (1981); Suppl. 7, 232 (1987)
Leather tanning and processing	25, 201 (1981); Suppl. 7, 236 (1987)
Ledate (see also Lead and lead compounds)	12, 131 (1976)
Light Green SF	16, 209 (1978); Suppl. 7, 65 (1987)
d-Limonene	56, 135 (1993)

Lindane (see Hexachlorocyclohexanes)
Liver flukes (see Clonorchis sinensis, Opisthorchis felineus and Opisthorchis viverrini)

The lumber and sawmill industries (including logging)	25, 49 (1981); Suppl. 7, 383 (1987)
Luteoskyrin	10, 163 (1976); Suppl. 7, 65 (1987)
Lynoestrenol (see also Progestins; Combined oral contraceptives)	21, 407 (1979)

M

Magenta	4, 57 (1974) (corr. 42, 252); Suppl. 7, 238 (1987); 57, 215 (1993)
Magenta, manufacture of (see also Magenta)	Suppl. 7, 238 (1987); 57, 215 (1993)
Malathion	30, 103 (1983); Suppl. 7, 65 (1987)
Maleic hydrazide	4, 173 (1974) (corr. 42, 253); Suppl. 7, 65 (1987)
Malonaldehyde	36, 163 (1985); Suppl. 7, 65 (1987)
Maneb	12, 137 (1976); Suppl. 7, 65 (1987)
Man-made mineral fibres	43, 39 (1988)
Mannomustine	9, 157 (1975); Suppl. 7, 65 (1987)
Mate	51, 273 (1991)
MCPA (see also Chlorophenoxy herbicides; Chlorophenoxy herbicides, occupational exposures to)	30, 255 (1983)
MeA-α-C	40, 253 (1986); Suppl. 7, 65 (1987)
Medphalan	9, 168 (1975); Suppl. 7, 65 (1987)
Medroxyprogesterone acetate	6, 157 (1974); 21, 417 (1979) (corr. 42, 259); Suppl. 7, 289 (1987)

Megestrol acetate (see also Progestins; Combined oral contraceptives)

MeIQ	40, 275 (1986); Suppl. 7, 65 (1987); 56, 197 (1993)
MeIQx	40, 283 (1986); Suppl. 7, 65 (1987); 56, 211 (1993)
Melamine	39, 333 (1986); Suppl. 7, 65 (1987)
Melphalan	9, 167 (1975); Suppl. 7, 239 (1987)
6-Mercaptopurine	26, 249 (1981); Suppl. 7, 240 (1987)
Mercuric chloride (see Mercury and mercury compounds)	
Mercury and mercury compounds	58, 239 (1993)
Merphalan	9, 169 (1975); Suppl. 7, 65 (1987)
Mestranol (see also Steroidal oestrogens)	6, 87 (1974); 21, 257 (1979) (corr. 42, 259)

Metabisulfites (*see* Sulfur dioxide and some sulfites, bisulfites
    and metabisulfites)
Metallic mercury (*see* Mercury and mercury compounds)
Methanearsonic acid, disodium salt (*see* Arsenic and arsenic compounds)
Methanearsonic acid, monosodium salt (*see* Arsenic and arsenic
    compounds
Methotrexate   *26*, 267 (1981); *Suppl. 7*, 241 (1987)
Methoxsalen (*see* 8-Methoxypsoralen)
Methoxychlor   *5*, 193 (1974); *20*, 259 (1979);
                                                                               Suppl. 7, 66 (1987)

Methoxyflurane (*see* Anaesthetics, volatile)
5-Methoxypsoralen   *40*, 327 (1986); *Suppl. 7*, 242 (1987)
8-Methoxypsoralen (*see also* 8-Methoxypsoralen plus ultraviolet   *24*, 101 (1980)
    radiation)
8-Methoxypsoralen plus ultraviolet radiation   *Suppl. 7*, 243 (1987)
Methyl acrylate   *19*, 52 (1979); *39*, 99 (1986);
                                                                               Suppl. 7, 66 (1987)

5-Methylangelicin plus ultraviolet radiation (*see also* Angelicin
    and some synthetic derivatives)   *Suppl. 7*, 57 (1987)
2-Methylaziridine   *9*, 61 (1975); *Suppl. 7*, 66 (1987)
Methylazoxymethanol acetate   *1*, 164 (1972); *10*, 131 (1976);
                                                                               Suppl. 7, 66 (1987)

Methyl bromide   *41*, 187 (1986) (*corr. 45*, 283);
                                                                               Suppl. 7, 245 (1987)
Methyl carbamate   *12*, 151 (1976); *Suppl. 7*, 66 (1987)
Methyl-CCNU [*see* 1-(2-Chloroethyl)-3-(4-methylcyclohexyl)-
    1-nitrosourea]
Methyl chloride   *41*, 161 (1986); *Suppl. 7*, 246 (1987)
1-, 2-, 3-, 4-, 5- and 6-Methylchrysenes   *32*, 379 (1983); *Suppl. 7*, 66 (1987)
N-Methyl-*N*,4-dinitrosoaniline   *1*, 141 (1972); *Suppl. 7*, 66 (1987)
4,4′-Methylene bis(2-chloroaniline)   *4*, 65 (1974) (*corr. 42*, 252);
                                                                               Suppl. 7, 246 (1987); *57*, 271 (1993)
4,4′-Methylene bis(*N*,*N*-dimethyl)benzenamine   *27*, 119 (1982); *Suppl. 7*, 66 (1987)
4,4′-Methylene bis(2-methylaniline)   *4*, 73 (1974); *Suppl. 7*, 248 (1987)
4,4′-Methylenedianiline   *4*, 79 (1974) (*corr. 42*, 252);
                                                                               39, 347 (1986); *Suppl. 7*, 66 (1987)
4,4′-Methylenediphenyl diisocyanate   *19*, 314 (1979); *Suppl. 7*, 66 (1987)
2-Methylfluoranthene   *32*, 399 (1983); *Suppl. 7*, 66 (1987)
3-Methylfluoranthene   *32*, 399 (1983); *Suppl. 7*, 66 (1987)
Methylglyoxal   *51*, 443 (1991)
Methyl iodide   *15*, 245 (1977); *41*, 213 (1986);
                                                                               Suppl. 7, 66 (1987)

Methylmercury chloride (*see* Mercury and mercury compounds)
Methylmercury compounds (*see* Mercury and mercury compounds)
Methyl methacrylate   *19*, 187 (1979); *Suppl. 7*, 66 (1987);
                                                                               60, 445 (1994)

Methyl methanesulfonate   *7*, 253 (1974); *Suppl. 7*, 66 (1987)
2-Methyl-1-nitroanthraquinone   *27*, 205 (1982); *Suppl. 7*, 66 (1987)
N-Methyl-*N*′-nitro-*N*-nitrosoguanidine   *4*, 183 (1974); *Suppl. 7*, 248 (1987)
3-Methylnitrosaminopropionaldehyde [*see* 3-(*N*-Nitrosomethylamino)-
    propionaldehyde]

3-Methylnitrosaminopropionitrile [see 3-(N-Nitrosomethylamino)-
    propionitrile]
4-(Methylnitrosamino)-4-(3-pyridyl)-1-butanal-[see 4-(N-Nitrosomethyl-
    amino)-4-(3-pyridyl)-1-butanal]
4-(Methylnitrosamino)-1-(3-pyridyl)-1-butanone [see 4-(-Nitrosomethyl-
    amino)-1-(3-pyridyl)-1-butanone]

N-Methyl-N-nitrosourea	*1*, 125 (1972); *17*, 227 (1978); *Suppl. 7*, 66 (1987)
N-Methyl-N-nitrosourethane	*4*, 211 (1974); *Suppl. 7*, 66 (1987)
N-Methylolacrylamide	*60*, 435 (1994)
Methyl parathion	*30*, 131 (1983); *Suppl. 7*, 392 (1987)
1-Methylphenanthrene	*32*, 405 (1983); *Suppl. 7*, 66 (1987)
7-Methylpyrido[3,4-c]psoralen	*40*, 349 (1986); *Suppl. 7*, 71 (1987)
Methyl red	*8*, 161 (1975); *Suppl. 7*, 66 (1987)
Methyl selenac (see also Selenium and selenium compounds)	*12*, 161 (1976); *Suppl. 7*, 66 (1987)
Methylthiouracil	*7*, 53 (1974); *Suppl. 7*, 66 (1987)
Metronidazole	*13*, 113 (1977); *Suppl. 7*, 250 (1987)
Mineral oils	*3*, 30 (1973); *33*, 87 (1984) (corr. *42*, 262); *Suppl. 7*, 252 (1987)
Mirex	*5*, 203 (1974); *20*, 283 (1979) (corr. *42*, 258); *Suppl. 7*, 66 (1987)
Mitomycin C	*10*, 171 (1976); *Suppl. 7*, 67 (1987)
MNNG [see N-Methyl-N'-nitro-N-nitrosoguanidine]	
MOCA [see 4,4'-Methylene bis(2-chloroaniline)]	
Modacrylic fibres	*19*, 86 (1979); *Suppl. 7*, 67 (1987)
Monocrotaline	*10*, 291 (1976); *Suppl. 7*, 67 (1987)
Monuron	*12*, 167 (1976); *Suppl. 7*, 67 (1987); *53*, 467 (1991)
MOPP and other combined chemotherapy including alkylating agents	*Suppl. 7*, 254 (1987)
Morpholine	*47*, 199 (1989)
5-(Morpholinomethyl)-3-[(5-nitrofurfurylidene)amino]-2-oxazolidinone	*7*, 161 (1974); *Suppl. 7*, 67 (1987)
Mustard gas	*9*, 181 (1975) (corr. *42*, 254); *Suppl. 7*, 259 (1987)
Myleran (see 1,4-Butanediol dimethanesulfonate)	

N

Nafenopin	*24*, 125 (1980); *Suppl. 7*, 67 (1987)
1,5-Naphthalenediamine	*27*, 127 (1982); *Suppl. 7*, 67 (1987)
1,5-Naphthalene diisocyanate	*19*, 311 (1979); *Suppl. 7*, 67 (1987)
1-Naphthylamine	*4*, 87 (1974) (corr. *42*, 253); *Suppl. 7*, 260 (1987)
2-Naphthylamine	*4*, 97 (1974); *Suppl. 7*, 261 (1987)
1-Naphthylthiourea	*30*, 347 (1983); *Suppl. 7*, 263 (1987)
Nickel acetate (see Nickel and nickel compounds)	
Nickel ammonium sulfate (see Nickel and nickel compounds)	

Nickel and nickel compounds	2, 126 (1973) (*corr. 42*, 252); *11*, 75 (1976); *Suppl. 7*, 264 (1987) (*corr. 45*, 283); *49*, 257 (1990)
Nickel carbonate (*see* Nickel and nickel compounds)	
Nickel carbonyl (*see* Nickel and nickel compounds)	
Nickel chloride (*see* Nickel and nickel compounds)	
Nickel-gallium alloy (*see* Nickel and nickel compounds)	
Nickel hydroxide (*see* Nickel and nickel compounds)	
Nickelocene (*see* Nickel and nickel compounds)	
Nickel oxide (*see* Nickel and nickel compounds)	
Nickel subsulfide (*see* Nickel and nickel compounds)	
Nickel sulfate (*see* Nickel and nickel compounds)	
Niridazole	*13*, 123 (1977); *Suppl. 7*, 67 (1987)
Nithiazide	*31*, 179 (1983); *Suppl. 7*, 67 (1987)
Nitrilotriacetic acid and its salts	*48*, 181 (1990)
5-Nitroacenaphthene	*16*, 319 (1978); *Suppl. 7*, 67 (1987)
5-Nitro-*ortho*-anisidine	*27*, 133 (1982); *Suppl. 7*, 67 (1987)
9-Nitroanthracene	*33*, 179 (1984); *Suppl. 7*, 67 (1987)
7-Nitrobenz[*a*]anthracene	*46*, 247 (1989)
6-Nitrobenzo[*a*]pyrene	*33*, 187 (1984); *Suppl. 7*, 67 (1987); *46*, 255 (1989)
4-Nitrobiphenyl	*4*, 113 (1974); *Suppl. 7*, 67 (1987)
6-Nitrochrysene	*33*, 195 (1984); *Suppl. 7*, 67 (1987); *46*, 267 (1989)
Nitrofen (technical-grade)	*30*, 271 (1983); *Suppl. 7*, 67 (1987)
3-Nitrofluoranthene	*33*, 201 (1984); *Suppl. 7*, 67 (1987)
2-Nitrofluorene	*46*, 277 (1989)
Nitrofural	*7*, 171 (1974); *Suppl. 7*, 67 (1987); *50*, 195 (1990)
5-Nitro-2-furaldehyde semicarbazone (*see* Nitrofural)	
Nitrofurantoin	*50*, 211 (1990)
Nitrofurazone (*see* Nitrofural)	
1-[(5-Nitrofurfurylidene)amino]-2-imidazolidinone	*7*, 181 (1974); *Suppl. 7*, 67 (1987)
N-[4-(5-Nitro-2-furyl)-2-thiazolyl]acetamide	*1*, 181 (1972); *7*, 185 (1974); *Suppl. 7*, 67 (1987)
Nitrogen mustard	*9*, 193 (1975); *Suppl. 7*, 269 (1987)
Nitrogen mustard *N*-oxide	*9*, 209 (1975); *Suppl. 7*, 67 (1987)
1-Nitronaphthalene	*46*, 291 (1989)
2-Nitronaphthalene	*46*, 303 (1989)
3-Nitroperylene	*46*, 313 (1989)
2-Nitro-*para*-phenylenediamine (*see* 1,4-Diamino-2-nitrobenzene)	
2-Nitropropane	*29*, 331 (1982); *Suppl. 7*, 67 (1987)
1-Nitropyrene	*33*, 209 (1984); *Suppl. 7*, 67 (1987); *46*, 321 (1989)
2-Nitropyrene	*46*, 359 (1989)
4-Nitropyrene	*46*, 367 (1989)
N-Nitrosatable drugs	*24*, 297 (1980) (*corr. 42*, 260)
N-Nitrosatable pesticides	*30*, 359 (1983)
N'-Nitrosoanabasine	*37*, 225 (1985); *Suppl. 7*, 67 (1987)
N'-Nitrosoanatabine	*37*, 233 (1985); *Suppl. 7*, 67 (1987)

N-Nitrosodi-n-butylamine	4, 197 (1974); 17, 51 (1978); Suppl. 7, 67 (1987)
N-Nitrosodiethanolamine	17, 77 (1978); Suppl. 7, 67 (1987)
N-Nitrosodiethylamine	1, 107 (1972) (corr. 42, 251); 17, 83 (1978) (corr. 42, 257); Suppl. 7, 67 (1987)
N-Nitrosodimethylamine	1, 95 (1972); 17, 125 (1978) (corr. 42, 257); Suppl. 7, 67 (1987)
N-Nitrosodiphenylamine	27, 213 (1982); Suppl. 7, 67 (1987)
para-Nitrosodiphenylamine	27, 227 (1982) (corr. 42, 261); Suppl. 7, 68 (1987)
N-Nitrosodi-n-propylamine	17, 177 (1978); Suppl. 7, 68 (1987)
N-Nitroso-N-ethylurea (see N-Ethyl-N-nitrosourea)	
N-Nitrosofolic acid	17, 217 (1978); Suppl. 7, 68 (1987)
N-Nitrosoguvacine	37, 263 (1985); Suppl. 7, 68 (1987)
N-Nitrosoguvacoline	37, 263 (1985); Suppl. 7, 68 (1987)
N-Nitrosohydroxyproline	17, 304 (1978); Suppl. 7, 68 (1987)
3-(N-Nitrosomethylamino)propionaldehyde	37, 263 (1985); Suppl. 7, 68 (1987)
3-(N-Nitrosomethylamino)propionitrile	37, 263 (1985); Suppl. 7, 68 (1987)
4-(N-Nitrosomethylamino)-4-(3-pyridyl)-1-butanal	37, 205 (1985); Suppl. 7, 68 (1987)
4-(N-Nitrosomethylamino)-1-(3-pyridyl)-1-butanone	37, 209 (1985); Suppl. 7, 68 (1987)
N-Nitrosomethylethylamine	17, 221 (1978); Suppl. 7, 68 (1987)
N-Nitroso-N-methylurea (see N-Methyl-N-nitrosourea)	
N-Nitroso-N-methylurethane (see N-Methyl-N-nitrosourethane)	
N-Nitrosomethylvinylamine	17, 257 (1978); Suppl. 7, 68 (1987)
N-Nitrosomorpholine	17, 263 (1978); Suppl. 7, 68 (1987)
N'-Nitrosonornicotine	17, 281 (1978); 37, 241 (1985); Suppl. 7, 68 (1987)
N-Nitrosopiperidine	17, 287 (1978); Suppl. 7, 68 (1987)
N-Nitrosoproline	17, 303 (1978); Suppl. 7, 68 (1987)
N-Nitrosopyrrolidine	17, 313 (1978); Suppl. 7, 68 (1987)
N-Nitrososarcosine	17, 327 (1978); Suppl. 7, 68 (1987)
Nitrosoureas, chloroethyl (see Chloroethyl nitrosoureas)	
5-Nitro-ortho-toluidine	48, 169 (1990)
Nitrous oxide (see Anaesthetics, volatile)	
Nitrovin	31, 185 (1983); Suppl. 7, 68 (1987)
Nivalenol (see Toxins derived from Fusarium graminearum, F. culmorum and F. crookwellense)	
NNA [see 4-(N-Nitrosomethylamino)-4-(3-pyridyl)-1-butanal]	
NNK [see 4- (N-Nitrosomethylamino)-1-(3-pyridyl)-1-butanone]	
Nonsteroidal oestrogens (see also Oestrogens, progestins and combinations)	Suppl. 7, 272 (1987)
Norethisterone (see also Progestins; Combined oral contraceptives)	6, 179 (1974); 21, 461 (1979)
Norethynodrel (see also Progestins; Combined oral contraceptives)	6, 191 (1974); 21, 461 (1979) (corr. 42, 259)
Norgestrel (see also Progestins, Combined oral contraceptives)	6, 201 (1974); 21, 479 (1979)
Nylon 6	19, 120 (1979); Suppl. 7, 68 (1987)

O

Ochratoxin A	*10*, 191 (1976); *31*, 191 (1983) (*corr. 42*, 262); *Suppl. 7*, 271 (1987); *56*, 489 (1993)
Oestradiol-17β (*see also* Steroidal oestrogens)	*6*, 99 (1974); *21*, 279 (1979)
Oestradiol 3-benzoate (*see* Oestradiol-17β)	
Oestradiol dipropionate (*see* Oestradiol-17β)	
Oestradiol mustard	*9*, 217 (1975); *Suppl. 7*, 68 (1987)
Oestradiol-17β-valerate (*see* Oestradiol-17β)	
Oestriol (*see also* Steroidal oestrogens)	*6*, 117 (1974); *21*, 327 (1979); *Suppl. 7*, 285 (1987)
Oestrogen-progestin combinations (*see* Oestrogens, progestins and combinations)	
Oestrogen-progestin replacement therapy (*see also* Oestrogens, progestins and combinations)	*Suppl. 7*, 308 (1987)
Oestrogen replacement therapy (*see also* Oestrogens, progestins and combinations)	*Suppl. 7*, 280 (1987)
Oestrogens (*see* Oestrogens, progestins and combinations)	
Oestrogens, conjugated (*see* Conjugated oestrogens)	
Oestrogens, nonsteroidal (*see* Nonsteroidal oestrogens)	
Oestrogens, progestins and combinations	*6* (1974); *21* (1979); *Suppl. 7*, 272 (1987)
Oestrogens, steroidal (*see* Steroidal oestrogens)	
Oestrone (*see* also Steroidal oestrogens)	*6*, 123 (1974); *21*, 343 (1979) (*corr. 42*, 259)
Oestrone benzoate (*see* Oestrone)	
Oil Orange SS	*8*, 165 (1975); *Suppl. 7*, 69 (1987)
Opisthorchis felineus (infection with)	*61*, 121 (1994)
Opisthorchis viverrini (infection with)	*61*, 121 (1994)
Oral contraceptives, combined (*see* Combined oral contraceptives)	
Oral contraceptives, investigational (*see* Combined oral contraceptives)	
Oral contraceptives, sequential (*see* Sequential oral contraceptives)	
Orange I	*8*, 173 (1975); *Suppl. 7*, 69 (1987)
Orange G	*8*, 181 (1975); *Suppl. 7*, 69 (1987)
Organolead compounds (*see also* Lead and lead compounds)	*Suppl. 7*, 230 (1987)
Oxazepam	*13*, 58 (1977); *Suppl. 7*, 69 (1987)
Oxymetholone [*see also* Androgenic (anabolic) steroids]	*13*, 131 (1977)
Oxyphenbutazone	*13*, 185 (1977); *Suppl. 7*, 69 (1987)

P

Paint manufacture and painting (occupational exposures in)	*47*, 329 (1989)
Panfuran S (*see also* Dihydroxymethylfuratrizine)	*24*, 77 (1980); *Suppl. 7*, 69 (1987)
Paper manufacture (*see* Pulp and paper manufacture)	
Paracetamol	*50*, 307 (1990)
Parasorbic acid	*10*, 199 (1976) (*corr. 42*, 255); *Suppl. 7*, 69 (1987)
Parathion	*30*, 153 (1983); *Suppl. 7*, 69 (1987)
Patulin	10, 205 (1976); 40, 83 (1986);

	Suppl. 7, 69 (1987)
Penicillic acid	10, 211 (1976); Suppl. 7, 69 (1987)
Pentachloroethane	41, 99 (1986); Suppl. 7, 69 (1987)
Pentachloronitrobenzene (see Quintozene)	
Pentachlorophenol (see also Chlorophenols; Chlorophenols, occupational exposures to)	20, 303 (1979); 53, 371 (1991)
Permethrin	53, 329 (1991)
Perylene	32, 411 (1983); Suppl. 7, 69 (1987)
Petasitenine	31, 207 (1983); Suppl. 7, 69 (1987)
Petasites japonicus (see Pyrrolizidine alkaloids)	
Petroleum refining (occupational exposures in)	45, 39 (1989)
Some petroleum solvents	47, 43 (1989)
Phenacetin	13, 141 (1977); 24, 135 (1980); Suppl. 7, 310 (1987)
Phenanthrene	32, 419 (1983); Suppl. 7, 69 (1987)
Phenazopyridine hydrochloride	8, 117 (1975); 24, 163 (1980) (corr. 42, 260); Suppl. 7, 312 (1987)
Phenelzine sulfate	24, 175 (1980); Suppl. 7, 312 (1987)
Phenicarbazide	12, 177 (1976); Suppl. 7, 70 (1987)
Phenobarbital	13, 157 (1977); Suppl. 7, 313 (1987)
Phenol	47, 263 (1989) (corr. 50, 385)
Phenoxyacetic acid herbicides (see Chlorophenoxy herbicides)	
Phenoxybenzamine hydrochloride	9, 223 (1975); 24, 185 (1980); Suppl. 7, 70 (1987)
Phenylbutazone	13, 183 (1977); Suppl. 7, 316 (1987)
meta-Phenylenediamine	16, 111 (1978); Suppl. 7, 70 (1987)
para-Phenylenediamine	16, 125 (1978); Suppl. 7, 70 (1987)
Phenyl glycidyl ether (see Glycidyl ethers)	
N-Phenyl-2-naphthylamine	16, 325 (1978) (corr. 42, 257); Suppl. 7, 318 (1987)
ortho-Phenylphenol	30, 329 (1983); Suppl. 7, 70 (1987)
Phenytoin	13, 201 (1977); Suppl. 7, 319 (1987)
PhIP	56, 229 (1993)
Pickled vegetables	56, 83 (1993)
Picloram	53, 481 (1991)
Piperazine oestrone sulfate (see Conjugated oestrogens)	
Piperonyl butoxide	30, 183 (1983); Suppl. 7, 70 (1987)
Pitches, coal-tar (see Coal-tar pitches)	
Polyacrylic acid	19, 62 (1979); Suppl. 7, 70 (1987)
Polybrominated biphenyls	18, 107 (1978); 41, 261 (1986); Suppl. 7, 321 (1987)
Polychlorinated biphenyls	7, 261 (1974); 18, 43 (1978) (corr. 42, 258); Suppl. 7, 322 (1987)
Polychlorinated camphenes (see Toxaphene)	
Polychloroprene	19, 141 (1979); Suppl. 7, 70 (1987)
Polyethylene	19, 164 (1979); Suppl. 7, 70 (1987)
Polymethylene polyphenyl isocyanate	19, 314 (1979); Suppl. 7, 70 (1987)
Polymethyl methacrylate	19, 195 (1979); Suppl. 7, 70 (1987)
Polyoestradiol phosphate (see Oestradiol-17β)	
Polypropylene	19, 218 (1979); Suppl. 7, 70 (1987)
Polystyrene	19, 245 (1979); Suppl. 7, 70 (1987)

Polytetrafluoroethylene	*19*, 288 (1979); *Suppl. 7*, 70 (1987)
Polyurethane foams	*19*, 320 (1979); *Suppl. 7*, 70 (1987)
Polyvinyl acetate	*19*, 346 (1979); *Suppl. 7*, 70 (1987)
Polyvinyl alcohol	*19*, 351 (1979); *Suppl. 7*, 70 (1987)
Polyvinyl chloride	*7*, 306 (1974); *19*, 402 (1979); *Suppl. 7*, 70 (1987)
Polyvinyl pyrrolidone	*19*, 463 (1979); *Suppl. 7*, 70 (1987)
Ponceau MX	*8*, 189 (1975); *Suppl. 7*, 70 (1987)
Ponceau 3R	*8*, 199 (1975); *Suppl. 7*, 70 (1987)
Ponceau SX	*8*, 207 (1975); *Suppl. 7*, 70 (1987)
Potassium arsenate (*see* Arsenic and arsenic compounds)	
Potassium arsenite (*see* Arsenic and arsenic compounds)	
Potassium bis(2-hydroxyethyl)dithiocarbamate	*12*, 183 (1976); *Suppl. 7*, 70 (1987)
Potassium bromate	*40*, 207 (1986); *Suppl. 7*, 70 (1987)
Potassium chromate (*see* Chromium and chromium compounds)	
Potassium dichromate (*see* Chromium and chromium compounds)	
Prednimustine	*50*, 115 (1990)
Prednisone	*26*, 293 (1981); *Suppl. 7*, 326 (1987)
Procarbazine hydrochloride	*26*, 311 (1981); *Suppl. 7*, 327 (1987)
Proflavine salts	*24*, 195 (1980); *Suppl. 7*, 70 (1987)
Progesterone (*see also* Progestins; Combined oral contraceptives)	*6*, 135 (1974); *21*, 491 (1979) (*corr. 42*, 259)
Progestins (*see also* Oestrogens, progestins and combinations)	*Suppl. 7*, 289 (1987)
Pronetalol hydrochloride	*13*, 227 (1977) (*corr. 42*, 256); *Suppl. 7*, 70 (1987)
1,3-Propane sultone	*4*, 253 (1974) (*corr. 42*, 253); *Suppl. 7*, 70 (1987)
Propham	*12*, 189 (1976); *Suppl. 7*, 70 (1987)
β-Propiolactone	*4*, 259 (1974) (*corr. 42*, 253); *Suppl. 7*, 70 (1987)
n-Propyl carbamate	*12*, 201 (1976); *Suppl. 7*, 70 (1987)
Propylene	*19*, 213 (1979); *Suppl. 7*, 71 (1987); *60*, 161 (1994)
Propylene oxide	*11*, 191 (1976); *36*, 227 (1985) (*corr. 42*, 263); *Suppl. 7*, 328 (1987); *60*, 181 (1994)
Propylthiouracil	*7*, 67 (1974); *Suppl. 7*, 329 (1987)
Ptaquiloside (*see also* Bracken fern)	*40*, 55 (1986); *Suppl. 7*, 71 (1987)
Pulp and paper manufacture	*25*, 157 (1981); *Suppl. 7*, 385 (1987)
Pyrene	*32*, 431 (1983); *Suppl. 7*, 71 (1987)
Pyrido[3,4-*c*]psoralen	*40*, 349 (1986); *Suppl. 7*, 71 (1987)
Pyrimethamine	*13*, 233 (1977); *Suppl. 7*, 71 (1987)
Pyrrolizidine alkaloids (*see* Hydroxysenkirkine; Isatidine; Jacobine; Lasiocarpine; Monocrotaline; Retrorsine; Riddelliine; Seneciphylline; Senkirkine)	

Q

Quercetin (*see also* Bracken fern)	*31*, 213 (1983); *Suppl. 7*, 71 (1987)
para-Quinone	*15*, 255 (1977); *Suppl. 7*, 71 (1987)

Quintozene   5, 211 (1974); *Suppl. 7*, 71 (1987)

R

Radon   43, 173 (1988) (*corr. 45*, 283)
Reserpine   10, 217 (1976); 24, 211 (1980)
                                                       (*corr. 42*, 260); *Suppl. 7*, 330 (1987)
Resorcinol   15, 155 (1977); *Suppl. 7*, 71 (1987)
Retrorsine   10, 303 (1976); *Suppl. 7*, 71 (1987)
Rhodamine B   16, 221 (1978); *Suppl. 7*, 71 (1987)
Rhodamine 6G   16, 233 (1978); *Suppl. 7*, 71 (1987)
Riddelliine   10, 313 (1976); *Suppl. 7*, 71 (1987)
Rifampicin   24, 243 (1980); *Suppl. 7*, 71 (1987)
Rockwool (*see* Man-made mineral fibres)
The rubber industry   28 (1982) (*corr. 42*, 261); *Suppl. 7*,
                                                       332 (1987)
Rugulosin   40, 99 (1986); *Suppl. 7*, 71 (1987)

S

Saccharated iron oxide   2, 161 (1973); *Suppl. 7*, 71 (1987)
Saccharin   22, 111 (1980) (*corr. 42*, 259);
                                                       Suppl. 7, 334 (1987)
Safrole   *1*, 169 (1972); *10*, 231 (1976);
                                                       Suppl. 7, 71 (1987)
Salted fish   56, 41 (1993)
The sawmill industry (including logging) [*see* The lumber and
    sawmill industry (including logging)]
Scarlet Red   8, 217 (1975); *Suppl. 7*, 71 (1987)
Schistosoma haematobium (infection with)   *61*, 45 (1994)
Schistosoma japonicum (infection with)   *61*, 45 (1994)
Schistosoma mansoni (infection with)   *61*, 45 (1994)
Selenium and selenium compounds   9, 245 (1975) (*corr. 42*, 255);
                                                       Suppl. 7, 71 (1987)
Selenium dioxide (*see* Selenium and selenium compounds)
Selenium oxide (*see* Selenium and selenium compounds)
Semicarbazide hydrochloride   12, 209 (1976) (*corr. 42*, 256);
                                                       Suppl. 7, 71 (1987)
Senecio jacobaea L. (*see* Pyrrolizidine alkaloids)
Senecio longilobus (*see* Pyrrolizidine alkaloids)
Seneciphylline   *10*, 319, 335 (1976); *Suppl. 7*, 71
                                                       (1987)
Senkirkine   *10*, 327 (1976); *31*, 231 (1983);
                                                       Suppl. 7, 71 (1987)
Sepiolite   42, 175 (1987); *Suppl. 7*, 71 (1987)
Sequential oral contraceptives (*see also* Oestrogens, progestins   *Suppl. 7*, 296 (1987)
    and combinations)
Shale-oils   35, 161 (1985); *Suppl. 7*, 339 (1987)
Shikimic acid (*see also* Bracken fern)   40, 55 (1986); *Suppl. 7*, 71 (1987)

Shoe manufacture and repair (*see* Boot and shoe manufacture and repair)	
Silica (*see also* Amorphous silica; Crystalline silica)	*42*, 39 (1987)
Simazine	*53*, 495 (1991)
Slagwool (*see* Man-made mineral fibres)	
Sodium arsenate (*see* Arsenic and arsenic compounds)	
Sodium arsenite (*see* Arsenic and arsenic compounds)	
Sodium cacodylate (*see* Arsenic and arsenic compounds)	
Sodium chlorite	*52*, 145 (1991)
Sodium chromate (*see* Chromium and chromium compounds)	
Sodium cyclamate (*see* Cyclamates)	
Sodium dichromate (*see* Chromium and chromium compounds)	
Sodium diethyldithiocarbamate	*12*, 217 (1976); *Suppl. 7*, 71 (1987)
Sodium equilin sulfate (*see* Conjugated oestrogens)	
Sodium fluoride (*see* Fluorides)	
Sodium monofluorophosphate (*see* Fluorides)	
Sodium oestrone sulfate (*see* Conjugated oestrogens)	
Sodium *ortho*-phenylphenate (*see also* ortho-Phenylphenol)	*30*, 329 (1983); *Suppl. 7*, 392 (1987)
Sodium saccharin (*see* Saccharin)	
Sodium selenate (*see* Selenium and selenium compounds)	
Sodium selenite (*see* Selenium and selenium compounds)	
Sodium silicofluoride (*see* Fluorides)	
Solar radiation	*55* (1992)
Soots	*3*, 22 (1973); *35*, 219 (1985); *Suppl. 7*, 343 (1987)
Spironolactone	*24*, 259 (1980); *Suppl. 7*, 344 (1987)
Stannous fluoride (*see* Fluorides)	
Steel founding (*see* Iron and steel founding)	
Sterigmatocystin	*1*, 175 (1972); *10*, 245 (1976); *Suppl. 7*, 72 (1987)
Steroidal oestrogens (*see also* Oestrogens, progestins and combinations)	*Suppl. 7*, 280 (1987)
Streptozotocin	*4*, 221 (1974); *17*, 337 (1978); *Suppl. 7*, 72 (1987)
Strobaner (*see* Terpene polychlorinates)	
Strontium chromate (*see* Chromium and chromium compounds)	
Styrene	*19*, 231 (1979) (*corr. 42*, 258); *Suppl. 7*, 345 (1987); *60*, 233 (1994)
Styrene-acrylonitrile-copolymers	*19*, 97 (1979); *Suppl. 7*, 72 (1987)
Styrene-butadiene copolymers	*19*, 252 (1979); *Suppl. 7*, 72 (1987)
Styrene-7,8-oxide	*11*, 201 (1976); *19*, 275 (1979); *36*, 245 (1985); *Suppl. 7*, 72 (1987); *60*, 321 (1994)
Succinic anhydride	*15*, 265 (1977); *Suppl. 7*, 72 (1987)
Sudan I	*8*, 225 (1975); *Suppl. 7*, 72 (1987)
Sudan II	*8*, 233 (1975); *Suppl. 7*, 72 (1987)
Sudan III	*8*, 241 (1975); *Suppl. 7*, 72 (1987)
Sudan Brown RR	*8*, 249 (1975); *Suppl. 7*, 72 (1987)
Sudan Red 7B	*8*, 253 (1975); *Suppl. 7*, 72 (1987)
Sulfafurazole	*24*, 275 (1980); *Suppl. 7*, 347 (1987)
Sulfallate	*30*, 283 (1983); *Suppl. 7*, 72 (1987)

Sulfamethoxazole	*24*, 285 (1980); *Suppl. 7*, 348 (1987)
Sulfites (*see* Sulfur dioxide and some sulfites, bisulfites and metabisulfites)	
Sulfur dioxide and some sulfites, bisulfites and metabisulfites	*54*, 131 (1992)
Sulfur mustard (*see* Mustard gas)	
Sulfuric acid and other strong inorganic acids, occupational exposures to mists and vapours from	*54*, 41 (1992)
Sulfur trioxide	*54*, 121 (1992)
Sulphisoxazole (*see* Sulfafurazole)	
Sunset Yellow FCF	*8*, 257 (1975); *Suppl. 7*, 72 (1987)
Symphytine	*31*, 239 (1983); *Suppl. 7*, 72 (1987)

T

2,4,5-T (*see also* Chlorophenoxy herbicides; Chlorophenoxy herbicides, occupational exposures to)	*15*, 273 (1977)
Talc	*42*, 185 (1987); Suppl. 7, 349 (1987)
Tannic acid	*10*, 253 (1976) (*corr. 42*, 255); *Suppl. 7*, 72 (1987)
Tannins (*see* also Tannic acid)	*10*, 254 (1976); *Suppl. 7*, 72 (1987)
TCDD (*see* 2,3,7,8-Tetrachlorodibenzo-*para*-dioxin)	
TDE (*see* DDT)	
Tea	*51*, 207 (1991)
Terpene polychlorinates	*5*, 219 (1974); *Suppl. 7*, 72 (1987)
Testosterone (*see also* Androgenic (anabolic) steroids)	*6*, 209 (1974); *21*, 519 (1979)
Testosterone oenanthate (*see* Testosterone)	
Testosterone propionate (*see* Testosterone)	
2,2′,5,5′-Tetrachlorobenzidine	*27*, 141 (1982); *Suppl. 7*, 72 (1987)
2,3,7,8-Tetrachlorodibenzo-*para*-dioxin	*15*, 41 (1977); *Suppl. 7*, 350 (1987)
1,1,1,2-Tetrachloroethane	*41*, 87 (1986); *Suppl. 7*, 72 (1987)
1,1,2,2-Tetrachloroethane	*20*, 477 (1979); *Suppl. 7*, 354 (1987)
Tetrachloroethylene	*20*, 491 (1979); *Suppl. 7*, 355 (1987); *63*, 159 (1995)
2,3,4,6-Tetrachlorophenol (*see* Chlorophenols; Chlorophenols, occupational exposures to)	
Tetrachlorvinphos	*30*, 197 (1983); *Suppl. 7*, 72 (1987)
Tetraethyllead (*see* Lead and lead compounds)	
Tetrafluoroethylene	*19*, 285 (1979); *Suppl. 7*, 72 (1987)
Tetrakis(hydroxymethyl) phosphonium salts	*48*, 95 (1990)
Tetramethyllead (*see* Lead and lead compounds)	
Textile manufacturing industry, exposures in	*48*, 215 (1990) (*corr. 51*, 483)
Theobromine	*51*, 421 (1991)
Theophylline	*51*, 391 (1991)
Thioacetamide	*7*, 77 (1974); *Suppl. 7*, 72 (1987)
4,4′-Thiodianiline	*16*, 343 (1978); *27*, 147 (1982); *Suppl. 7*, 72 (1987)
Thiotepa	*9*, 85 (1975); *Suppl. 7*, 368 (1987); *50*, 123 (1990)
Thiouracil	*7*, 85 (1974); *Suppl. 7*, 72 (1987)
Thiourea	*7*, 95 (1974); *Suppl. 7*, 72 (1987)

CUMULATIVE INDEX

Thiram	*12*, 225 (1976); *Suppl. 7*, 72 (1987); *53*, 403 (1991)
Titanium dioxide	*47*, 307 (1989)
Tobacco habits other than smoking (*see* Tobacco products, smokeless)	
Tobacco products, smokeless	*37* (1985) (*corr. 42*, 263; *52*, 513); *Suppl. 7*, 357 (1987)
Tobacco smoke	*38* (1986) (*corr. 42*, 263); *Suppl. 7*, 357 (1987)
Tobacco smoking (*see* Tobacco smoke)	
ortho-Tolidine (*see* 3,3'-Dimethylbenzidine)	
2,4-Toluene diisocyanate (*see* also Toluene diisocyanates)	*19*, 303 (1979); *39*, 287 (1986)
2,6-Toluene diisocyanate (*see* also Toluene diisocyanates)	*19*, 303 (1979); *39*, 289 (1986)
Toluene	*47*, 79 (1989)
Toluene diisocyanates	*39*, 287 (1986) (*corr. 42*, 264); *Suppl. 7*, 72 (1987)
Toluenes, α-chlorinated (*see* α-Chlorinated toluenes)	
ortho-Toluenesulfonamide (*see* Saccharin)	
ortho-Toluidine	*16*, 349 (1978); *27*, 155 (1982); *Suppl. 7*, 362 (1987)
Toxaphene	*20*, 327 (1979); *Suppl. 7*, 72 (1987)
T-2 Toxin (*see* Toxins derived from *Fusarium sporotrichioides*)	
Toxins derived from *Fusarium graminearum, F. culmorum* and *F. crookwellense*	*11*, 169 (1976); *31*, 153, 279 (1983); *Suppl. 7*, 64, 74 (1987); *56*, 397 (1993)
Toxins derived from *Fusarium moniliforme*	*56*, 445 (1993)
Toxins derived from *Fusarium sporotrichioides*	*31*, 265 (1983); *Suppl. 7*, 73 (1987); *56*, 467 (1993)
Tremolite (*see* Asbestos)	
Treosulfan	*26*, 341 (1981); *Suppl. 7*, 363 (1987)
Triaziquone [*see* Tris(aziridinyl)-*para*-benzoquinone]	
Trichlorfon	*30*, 207 (1983); *Suppl. 7*, 73 (1987)
Trichlormethine	*9*, 229 (1975); *Suppl. 7*, 73 (1987); *50*, 143 (1990)
Trichloroacetic acid	*63*, 291 (1995)
Trichloroacetonitrile (*see* Halogenated acetonitriles)	
1,1,1-Trichloroethane	*20*, 515 (1979); *Suppl. 7*, 73 (1987)
1,1,2-Trichloroethane	*20*, 533 (1979); *Suppl. 7*, 73 (1987); *52*, 337 (1991)
Trichloroethylene	*11*, 263 (1976); *20*, 545 (1979); *Suppl. 7*, 364 (1987); *63*, 75 (1995)
2,4,5-Trichlorophenol (*see also* Chlorophenols; Chlorophenols occupational exposures to)	*20*, 349 (1979)
2,4,6-Trichlorophenol (*see also* Chlorophenols; Chlorophenols, occupational exposures to)	*20*, 349 (1979)
(2,4,5-Trichlorophenoxy)acetic acid (*see* 2,4,5-T)	
1,2,3-Trichloropropane	*63*, 223 (1995)
Trichlorotriethylamine-hydrochloride (*see* Trichlormethine)	
T$_2$-Trichothecene (*see* Toxins derived from *Fusarium sporotrichioides*)	
Triethylene glycol diglycidyl ether	*11*, 209 (1976); *Suppl. 7*, 73 (1987)
Trifluralin	*53*, 515 (1991)

4,4',6-Trimethylangelicin plus ultraviolet radiation (see also Angelicin and some synthetic derivatives)	Suppl. 7, 57 (1987)
2,4,5-Trimethylaniline	27, 177 (1982); Suppl. 7, 73 (1987)
2,4,6-Trimethylaniline	27, 178 (1982); Suppl. 7, 73 (1987)
4,5',8-Trimethylpsoralen	40, 357 (1986); Suppl. 7, 366 (1987)
Trimustine hydrochloride (see Trichlormethine)	
Triphenylene	32, 447 (1983); Suppl. 7, 73 (1987)
Tris(aziridinyl)-*para*-benzoquinone	9, 67 (1975); Suppl. 7, 367 (1987)
Tris(1-aziridinyl)phosphine-oxide	9, 75 (1975); Suppl. 7, 73 (1987)
Tris(1-aziridinyl)phosphine-sulphide (see Thiotepa)	
2,4,6-Tris(1-aziridinyl)-*s*-triazine	9, 95 (1975); Suppl. 7, 73 (1987)
Tris(2-chloroethyl) phosphate	48, 109 (1990)
1,2,3-Tris(chloromethoxy)propane	15, 301 (1977); Suppl. 7, 73 (1987)
Tris(2,3-dibromopropyl)phosphate	20, 575 (1979); Suppl. 7, 369 (1987)
Tris(2-methyl-1-aziridinyl)phosphine-oxide	9, 107 (1975); Suppl. 7, 73 (1987)
Trp-P-1	31, 247 (1983); Suppl. 7, 73 (1987)
Trp-P-2	31, 255 (1983); Suppl. 7, 73 (1987)
Trypan blue	8, 267 (1975); Suppl. 7, 73 (1987)
Tussilago farfara L. (see Pyrrolizidine alkaloids)	

U

Ultraviolet radiation	40, 379 (1986); 55 (1992)
Underground haematite mining with exposure to radon	1, 29 (1972); Suppl. 7, 216 (1987)
Uracil mustard	9, 235 (1975); Suppl. 7, 370 (1987)
Urethane	7, 111 (1974); Suppl. 7, 73 (1987)

V

Vat Yellow 4	48, 161 (1990)
Vinblastine sulfate	26, 349 (1981) (*corr.* 42, 261); Suppl. 7, 371 (1987)
Vincristine sulfate	26, 365 (1981); Suppl. 7, 372 (1987)
Vinyl acetate	19, 341 (1979); 39, 113 (1986); Suppl. 7, 73 (1987); 63, 443 (1995)
Vinyl bromide	19, 367 (1979); 39, 133 (1986); Suppl. 7, 73 (1987)
Vinyl chloride	7, 291 (1974); 19, 377 (1979) (*corr.* 42, 258); Suppl. 7, 373 (1987)
Vinyl chloride-vinyl acetate copolymers	7, 311 (1976); 19, 412 (1979) (*corr.* 42, 258); Suppl. 7, 73 (1987)
4-Vinylcyclohexene	11, 277 (1976); 39, 181 (1986) Suppl. 7, 73 (1987); 60, 347 (1994)
4-Vinylcyclohexene diepoxide	11, 141 (1976); Suppl. 7, 63 (1987); 60, 361 (1994)
Vinyl fluoride	39, 147 (1986); Suppl. 7, 73 (1987); 63, 467 (1995)
Vinylidene chloride	19, 439 (1979); 39, 195 (1986); Suppl. 7, 376 (1987)

Vinylidene chloride-vinyl chloride copolymers	19, 448 (1979) (corr. 42, 258); Suppl. 7, 73 (1987)
Vinylidene fluoride	39, 227 (1986); Suppl. 7, 73 (1987)
N-Vinyl-2-pyrrolidone	19, 461 (1979); Suppl. 7, 73 (1987)
Vinyl toluene	60, 373 (1994)

W

Welding	49, 447 (1990) (corr. 52, 513)
Wollastonite	42, 145 (1987); Suppl. 7, 377 (1987)
Wood dust	62, 35 (1995)
Wood industries	25 (1981); Suppl. 7, 378 (1987)

X

Xylene	47, 125 (1989)
2,4-Xylidine	16, 367 (1978); Suppl. 7, 74 (1987)
2,5-Xylidine	16, 377 (1978); Suppl. 7, 74 (1987)
2,6-Xylidine (see 2,6-Dimethylaniline)	

Y

Yellow AB	8, 279 (1975); Suppl. 7, 74 (1987)
Yellow OB	8, 287 (1975); Suppl. 7, 74 (1987)

Z

Zearalenone (see Toxins derived from *Fusarium graminearum*, *F. culmorum* and *F. crookwellense*)	
Zectran	12, 237 (1976); Suppl. 7, 74 (1987)
Zinc beryllium silicate (see Beryllium and beryllium compounds)	
Zinc chromate (see Chromium and chromium compounds)	
Zinc chromate hydroxide (see Chromium and chromium compounds)	
Zinc potassium chromate (see Chromium and chromium compounds)	
Zinc yellow (see Chromium and chromium compounds)	
Zineb	12, 245 (1976); Suppl. 7, 74 (1987)
Ziram	12, 259 (1976); Suppl. 7, 74 (1987); 53, 423 (1991)

PUBLICATIONS OF THE INTERNATIONAL AGENCY FOR RESEARCH ON CANCER
Scientific Publications Series

No. 1 **Liver Cancer**
1971; 176 pages (*out of print*)

No. 2 **Oncogenesis and Herpesviruses**
Edited by P.M. Biggs, G. de-Thé and L.N. Payne
1972; 515 pages (*out of print*)

No. 3 **N-Nitroso Compounds: Analysis and Formation**
Edited by P. Bogovski, R. Preussman and E.A. Walker
1972; 140 pages (*out of print*)

No. 4 **Transplacental Carcinogenesis**
Edited by L. Tomatis and U. Mohr
1973; 181 pages (*out of print*)

No. 5/6 **Pathology of Tumours in Laboratory Animals, Volume 1, Tumours of the Rat**
Edited by V.S. Turusov
1973/1976; 533 pages (*out of print*)

No. 7 **Host Environment Interactions in the Etiology of Cancer in Man**
Edited by R. Doll and I. Vodopija
1973; 464 pages (*out of print*)

No. 8 **Biological Effects of Asbestos**
Edited by P. Bogovski, J.C. Gilson, V. Timbrell and J.C. Wagner
1973; 346 pages (*out of print*)

No. 9 **N-Nitroso Compounds in the Environment**
Edited by P. Bogovski and E.A. Walker
1974; 243 pages (*out of print*)

No. 10 **Chemical Carcinogenesis Essays**
Edited by R. Montesano and L. Tomatis
1974; 230 pages (*out of print*)

No. 11 **Oncogenesis and Herpesviruses II**
Edited by G. de-Thé, M.A. Epstein and H. zur Hausen
1975; Part I: 511 pages
Part II: 403 pages (*out of print*)

No. 12 **Screening Tests in Chemical Carcinogenesis**
Edited by R. Montesano, H. Bartsch and L. Tomatis
1976; 666 pages (*out of print*)

No. 13 **Environmental Pollution and Carcinogenic Risks**
Edited by C. Rosenfeld and W. Davis
1975; 441 pages (*out of print*)

No. 14 **Environmental N-Nitroso Compounds. Analysis and Formation**
Edited by E.A. Walker, P. Bogovski and L. Griciute
1976; 512 pages (*out of print*)

No. 15 **Cancer Incidence in Five Continents, Volume III**
Edited by J.A.H. Waterhouse, C. Muir, P. Correa and J. Powell
1976; 584 pages (*out of print*)

No. 16 **Air Pollution and Cancer in Man**
Edited by U. Mohr, D. Schmähl and L. Tomatis
1977; 328 pages (*out of print*)

No. 17 **Directory of On-going Research in Cancer Epidemiology 1977**
Edited by C.S. Muir and G. Wagner
1977; 599 pages (*out of print*)

No. 18 **Environmental Carcinogens. Selected Methods of Analysis. Volume 1: Analysis of Volatile Nitrosamines in Food**
Editor-in-Chief: H. Egan
1978; 212 pages (*out of print*)

No. 19 **Environmental Aspects of N-Nitroso Compounds**
Edited by E.A. Walker, M. Castegnaro, L. Griciute and R.E. Lyle
1978; 561 pages (*out of print*)

No. 20 **Nasopharyngeal Carcinoma: Etiology and Control**
Edited by G. de-Thé and Y. Ito
1978; 606 pages (*out of print*)

No. 21 **Cancer Registration and its Techniques**
Edited by R. MacLennan, C. Muir, R. Steinitz and A. Winkler
1978; 235 pages (*out of print*)

No. 22 **Environmental Carcinogens. Selected Methods of Analysis. Volume 2: Methods for the Measurement of Vinyl Chloride in Poly(vinyl chloride), Air, Water and Foodstuffs**
Editor-in-Chief: H. Egan
1978; 142 pages (*out of print*)

No. 23 **Pathology of Tumours in Laboratory Animals. Volume II: Tumours of the Mouse**
Editor-in-Chief: V.S. Turusov
1979; 669 pages (*out of print*)

No. 24 **Oncogenesis and Herpesviruses III**
Edited by G. de-Thé, W. Henle and F. Rapp
1978; Part I: 580 pages, Part II: 512 pages (*out of print*)

Prices are subject to change without notice. Limited supplies of certain books marked '*out of print*' are available directly from IARC.

List of IARC Publications

No. 25 Carcinogenic Risk. Strategies for Intervention
Edited by W. Davis and C. Rosenfeld
1979; 280 pages (*out of print*)

No. 26 Directory of On-going Research in Cancer Epidemiology 1978
Edited by C.S. Muir and G. Wagner
1978; 550 pages (*out of print*)

No. 27 Molecular and Cellular Aspects of Carcinogen Screening Tests
Edited by R. Montesano, H. Bartsch and L. Tomatis
1980; 372 pages £30.00

No. 28 Directory of On-going Research in Cancer Epidemiology 1979
Edited by C.S. Muir and G. Wagner
1979; 672 pages (*out of print*)

No. 29 Environmental Carcinogens. Selected Methods of Analysis. Volume 3: Analysis of Polycyclic Aromatic Hydrocarbons in Environmental Samples
Editor-in-Chief: H. Egan
1979; 240 pages (*out of print*)

No. 30 Biological Effects of Mineral Fibres
Editor-in-Chief: J.C. Wagner
1980; Volume 1: 494 pages Volume 2: 513 pages (*out of print*)

No. 31 N-Nitroso Compounds: Analysis, Formation and Occurrence
Edited by E.A. Walker, L. Griciute, M. Castegnaro and M. Börzsönyi
1980; 835 pages (*out of print*)

No. 32 Statistical Methods in Cancer Research. Volume 1. The Analysis of Case-control Studies
By N.E. Breslow and N.E. Day
1980; 338 pages £18.00

No. 33 Handling Chemical Carcinogens in the Laboratory
Edited by R. Montesano *et al.*
1979; 32 pages (*out of print*)

No. 34 Pathology of Tumours in Laboratory Animals. Volume III. Tumours of the Hamster
Editor-in-Chief: V.S. Turusov
1982; 461 pages (*out of print*)

No. 35 Directory of On-going Research in Cancer Epidemiology 1980
Edited by C.S. Muir and G. Wagner
1980; 660 pages (*out of print*)

No. 36 Cancer Mortality by Occupation and Social Class 1851-1971
Edited by W.P.D. Logan
1982; 253 pages (*out of print*)

No. 37 Laboratory Decontamination and Destruction of Aflatoxins B_1, B_2, G_1, G_2 in Laboratory Wastes
Edited by M. Castegnaro *et al.*
1980; 56 pages (*out of print*)

No. 38 Directory of On-going Research in Cancer Epidemiology 1981
Edited by C.S. Muir and G. Wagner
1981; 696 pages (*out of print*)

No. 39 Host Factors in Human Carcinogenesis
Edited by H. Bartsch and B. Armstrong
1982; 583 pages (*out of print*)

No. 40 Environmental Carcinogens. Selected Methods of Analysis. Volume 4: Some Aromatic Amines and Azo Dyes in the General and Industrial Environment
Edited by L. Fishbein, M. Castegnaro, I.K. O'Neill and H. Bartsch
1981; 347 pages (*out of print*)

No. 41 N-Nitroso Compounds: Occurrence and Biological Effects
Edited by H. Bartsch, I.K. O'Neill, M. Castegnaro and M. Okada
1982; 755 pages (*out of print*)

No. 42 Cancer Incidence in Five Continents, Volume IV
Edited by J. Waterhouse, C. Muir, K. Shanmugaratnam and J. Powell
1982; 811 pages (*out of print*)

No. 43 Laboratory Decontamination and Destruction of Carcinogens in Laboratory Wastes: Some N-Nitrosamines
Edited by M. Castegnaro *et al.*
1982; 73 pages £7.50

No. 44 Environmental Carcinogens. Selected Methods of Analysis. Volume 5: Some Mycotoxins
Edited by L. Stoloff, M. Castegnaro, P. Scott, I.K. O'Neill and H. Bartsch
1983; 455 pages (*out of print*)

No. 45 Environmental Carcinogens. Selected Methods of Analysis. Volume 6: N-Nitroso Compounds
Edited by R. Preussmann, I.K. O'Neill, G. Eisenbrand, B. Spiegelhalder and H. Bartsch
1983; 508 pages (*out of print*)

No. 46 Directory of On-going Research in Cancer Epidemiology 1982
Edited by C.S. Muir and G. Wagner
1982; 722 pages (*out of print*)

No. 47 Cancer Incidence in Singapore 1968–1977
Edited by K. Shanmugaratnam, H.P. Lee and N.E. Day
1983; 171 pages (*out of print*)

No. 48 Cancer Incidence in the USSR (2nd Revised Edition)
Edited by N.P. Napalkov, G.F. Tserkovny, V.M. Merabishvili, D.M. Parkin, M. Smans and C.S. Muir
1983; 75 pages (*out of print*)

No. 49 Laboratory Decontamination and Destruction of Carcinogens in Laboratory Wastes: Some Polycyclic Aromatic Hydrocarbons
Edited by M. Castegnaro *et al.*
1983; 87 pages (*out of print*)

No. 50 Directory of On-going Research in Cancer Epidemiology 1983
Edited by C.S. Muir and G. Wagner
1983; 731 pages (*out of print*)

No. 51 Modulators of Experimental Carcinogenesis
Edited by V. Turusov and R. Montesano
1983; 307 pages (*out of print*)

List of IARC Publications

No. 52 **Second Cancers in Relation to Radiation Treatment for Cervical Cancer: Results of a Cancer Registry Collaboration**
Edited by N.E. Day and J.C. Boice, Jr
1984; 207 pages (*out of print*)

No. 53 **Nickel in the Human Environment**
Editor-in-Chief: F.W. Sunderman, Jr
1984; 529 pages (*out of print*)

No. 54 **Laboratory Decontamination and Destruction of Carcinogens in Laboratory Wastes: Some Hydrazines**
Edited by M. Castegnaro *et al.*
1983; 87 pages (*out of print*)

No. 55 **Laboratory Decontamination and Destruction of Carcinogens in Laboratory Wastes: Some N-Nitrosamides**
Edited by M. Castegnaro *et al.*
1984; 66 pages (*out of print*)

No. 56 **Models, Mechanisms and Etiology of Tumour Promotion**
Edited by M. Börzsönyi, N.E. Day, K. Lapis and H. Yamasaki
1984; 532 pages (*out of print*)

No. 57 **N-Nitroso Compounds: Occurrence, Biological Effects and Relevance to Human Cancer**
Edited by I.K. O'Neill, R.C. von Borstel, C.T. Miller, J. Long and H. Bartsch
1984; 1013 pages (*out of print*)

No. 58 **Age-related Factors in Carcinogenesis**
Edited by A. Likhachev, V. Anisimov and R. Montesano
1985; 288 pages (*out of print*)

No. 59 **Monitoring Human Exposure to Carcinogenic and Mutagenic Agents**
Edited by A. Berlin, M. Draper, K. Hemminki and H. Vainio
1984; 457 pages (*out of print*)

No. 60 **Burkitt's Lymphoma: A Human Cancer Model**
Edited by G. Lenoir, G. O'Conor and C.L.M. Olweny
1985; 484 pages (*out of print*)

No. 61 **Laboratory Decontamination and Destruction of Carcinogens in Laboratory Wastes: Some Haloethers**
Edited by M. Castegnaro *et al.*
1985; 55 pages (*out of print*)

No. 62 **Directory of On-going Research in Cancer Epidemiology 1984**
Edited by C.S. Muir and G. Wagner
1984; 717 pages (*out of print*)

No. 63 **Virus-associated Cancers in Africa**
Edited by A.O. Williams, G.T. O'Conor, G.B. de-Thé and C.A. Johnson
1984; 773 pages (*out of print*)

No. 64 **Laboratory Decontamination and Destruction of Carcinogens in Laboratory Wastes: Some Aromatic Amines and 4-Nitrobiphenyl**
Edited by M. Castegnaro *et al.*
1985; 84 pages (*out of print*)

No. 65 **Interpretation of Negative Epidemiological Evidence for Carcinogenicity**
Edited by N.J. Wald and R. Doll
1985; 232 pages (*out of print*)

No. 66 **The Role of the Registry in Cancer Control**
Edited by D.M. Parkin, G. Wagner and C.S. Muir
1985; 152 pages £10.00

No. 67 **Transformation Assay of Established Cell Lines: Mechanisms and Application**
Edited by T. Kakunaga and H. Yamasaki
1985; 225 pages (*out of print*)

No. 68 **Environmental Carcinogens. Selected Methods of Analysis. Volume 7. Some Volatile Halogenated Hydrocarbons**
Edited by L. Fishbein and I.K. O'Neill
1985; 479 pages (*out of print*)

No. 69 **Directory of On-going Research in Cancer Epidemiology 1985**
Edited by C.S. Muir and G. Wagner
1985; 745 pages (*out of print*)

No. 70 **The Role of Cyclic Nucleic Acid Adducts in Carcinogenesis and Mutagenesis**
Edited by B. Singer and H. Bartsch
1986; 467 pages (*out of print*)

No. 71 **Environmental Carcinogens. Selected Methods of Analysis. Volume 8: Some Metals: As, Be, Cd, Cr, Ni, Pb, Se, Zn**
Edited by I.K. O'Neill, P. Schuller and L. Fishbein
1986; 485 pages (*out of print*)

No. 72 **Atlas of Cancer in Scotland, 1975–1980. Incidence and Epidemiological Perspective**
Edited by I. Kemp, P. Boyle, M. Smans and C.S. Muir
1985; 285 pages (*out of print*)

No. 73 **Laboratory Decontamination and Destruction of Carcinogens in Laboratory Wastes: Some Antineoplastic Agents**
Edited by M. Castegnaro *et al.*
1985; 163 pages £13.50

No. 74 **Tobacco: A Major International Health Hazard**
Edited by D. Zaridze and R. Peto
1986; 324 pages £24.00

No. 75 **Cancer Occurrence in Developing Countries**
Edited by D.M. Parkin
1986; 339 pages £24.00

No. 76 **Screening for Cancer of the Uterine Cervix**
Edited by M. Hakama, A.B. Miller and N.E. Day
1986; 315 pages £31.50

No. 77 **Hexachlorobenzene: Proceedings of an International Symposium**
Edited by C.R. Morris and J.R.P. Cabral
1986; 668 pages (*out of print*)

No. 78 **Carcinogenicity of Alkylating Cytostatic Drugs**
Edited by D. Schmähl and J.M. Kaldor
1986; 337 pages (*out of print*)

No. 79 **Statistical Methods in Cancer Research. Volume III: The Design and Analysis of Long-term Animal Experiments**
By J.J. Gart, D. Krewski, P.N. Lee, R.E. Tarone and J. Wahrendorf
1986; 213 pages £23.50

List of IARC Publications

No. 80 Directory of On-going Research in Cancer Epidemiology 1986
Edited by C.S. Muir and G. Wagner
1986; 805 pages (*out of print*)

No. 81 Environmental Carcinogens: Methods of Analysis and Exposure Measurement. Volume 9: Passive Smoking
Edited by I.K. O'Neill, K.D. Brunnemann, B. Dodet and D. Hoffmann
1987; 383 pages £37.00

No. 82 Statistical Methods in Cancer Research. Volume II: The Design and Analysis of Cohort Studies
By N.E. Breslow and N.E. Day
1987; 404 pages £25.00

No. 83 Long-term and Short-term Assays for Carcinogens: A Critical Appraisal
Edited by R. Montesano, H. Bartsch, H. Vainio, J. Wilbourn and H. Yamasaki
1986; 575 pages £37.00

No. 84 The Relevance of N-Nitroso Compounds to Human Cancer: Exposure and Mechanisms
Edited by H. Bartsch, I.K. O'Neill and R. Schulte-Hermann
1987; 671 pages (*out of print*)

No. 85 Environmental Carcinogens: Methods of Analysis and Exposure Measurement. Volume 10: Benzene and Alkylated Benzenes
Edited by L. Fishbein and I.K. O'Neill
1988; 327 pages £42.00

No. 86 Directory of On-going Research in Cancer Epidemiology 1987
Edited by D.M. Parkin and J. Wahrendorf
1987; 676 pages (*out of print*)

No. 87 International Incidence of Childhood Cancer
Edited by D.M. Parkin, C.A. Stiller, C.A. Bieber, G.J. Draper, B. Terracini and J.L. Young
1988; 401 pages £35.00

No. 88 Cancer Incidence in Five Continents Volume V
Edited by C. Muir, J. Waterhouse, T. Mack, J. Powell and S. Whelan
1987; 1004 pages £58.00

No. 89 Method for Detecting DNA Damaging Agents in Humans: Applications in Cancer Epidemiology and Prevention
Edited by H. Bartsch, K. Hemminki and I.K. O'Neill
1988; 518 pages £50.00

No. 90 Non-occupational Exposure to Mineral Fibres
Edited by J. Bignon, J. Peto and R. Saracci
1989; 500 pages £52.50

No. 91 Trends in Cancer Incidence in Singapore 1968–1982
Edited by H.P. Lee, N.E. Day and K. Shanmugaratnam
1988; 160 pages (*out of print*)

No. 92 Cell Differentiation, Genes and Cancer
Edited by T. Kakunaga, T. Sugimura, L. Tomatis and H. Yamasaki
1988; 204 pages £29.00

No. 93 Directory of On-going Research in Cancer Epidemiology 1988
Edited by M. Coleman and J. Wahrendorf
1988; 662 pages (*out of print*)

No. 94 Human Papillomavirus and Cervical Cancer
Edited by N. Muñoz, F.X. Bosch and O.M. Jensen
1989; 154 pages £22.50

No. 95 Cancer Registration: Principles and Methods
Edited by O.M. Jensen, D.M. Parkin, R. MacLennan, C.S. Muir and R. Skeet
1991; 288 pages £28.00

No. 96 Perinatal and Multigeneration Carcinogenesis
Edited by N.P. Napalkov, J.M. Rice, L. Tomatis and H. Yamasaki
1989; 436 pages £52.50

No. 97 Occupational Exposure to Silica and Cancer Risk
Edited by L. Simonato, A.C. Fletcher, R. Saracci and T. Thomas
1990; 124 pages £24.00

No. 98 Cancer Incidence in Jewish Migrants to Israel, 1961–1981
Edited by R. Steinitz, D.M. Parkin, J.L. Young, C.A. Bieber and L. Katz
1989; 320 pages £37.00

No. 99 Pathology of Tumours in Laboratory Animals, Second Edition, Volume 1, Tumours of the Rat
Edited by V.S. Turusov and U. Mohr
740 pages £90.00

No. 100 Cancer: Causes, Occurrence and Control
Editor-in-Chief L. Tomatis
1990; 352 pages £25.50

No. 101 Directory of On-going Research in Cancer Epidemiology 1989/90
Edited by M. Coleman and J. Wahrendorf
1989; 818 pages £42.00

No. 102 Patterns of Cancer in Five Continents
Edited by S.L. Whelan, D.M. Parkin & E. Masuyer
1990; 162 pages £26.50

No. 103 Evaluating Effectiveness of Primary Prevention of Cancer
Edited by M. Hakama, V. Beral, J.W. Cullen and D.M. Parkin
1990; 250 pages £34.00

No. 104 Complex Mixtures and Cancer Risk
Edited by H. Vainio, M. Sorsa and A.J. McMichael
1990; 442 pages £40.00

No. 105 Relevance to Human Cancer of N-Nitroso Compounds, Tobacco Smoke and Mycotoxins
Edited by I.K. O'Neill, J. Chen and H. Bartsch
1991; 614 pages £74.00

No. 106 Atlas of Cancer Incidence in the Former German Democratic Republic
Edited by W.H. Mehnert, M. Smans, C.S. Muir, M. Möhner & D. Schön
1992; 384 pages £52.50

List of IARC Publications

No. 107 **Atlas of Cancer Mortality in the European Economic Community**
Edited by M. Smans, C.S. Muir and P. Boyle
1992; 280 pages £35.00

No. 108 **Environmental Carcinogens: Methods of Analysis and Exposure Measurement. Volume 11: Polychlorinated Dioxins and Dibenzofurans**
Edited by C. Rappe, H.R. Buser, B. Dodet and I.K. O'Neill
1991; 426 pages £47.50

No. 109 **Environmental Carcinogens: Methods of Analysis and Exposure Measurement. Volume 12: Indoor Air Contaminants**
Edited by B. Seifert, H. van de Wiel, B. Dodet and I.K. O'Neill
1993; 384 pages £45.00

No. 110 **Directory of On-going Research in Cancer Epidemiology 1991**
Edited by M. Coleman and J. Wahrendorf
1991; 753 pages £40.00

No. 111 **Pathology of Tumours in Laboratory Animals, Second Edition, Volume 2, Tumours of the Mouse**
Edited by V.S. Turusov and U. Mohr
1993; 776 pages; £90.00

No. 112 **Autopsy in Epidemiology and Medical Research**
Edited by E. Riboli and M. Delendi
1991; 288 pages £26.50

No. 113 **Laboratory Decontamination and Destruction of Carcinogens in Laboratory Wastes: Some Mycotoxins**
Edited by M. Castegnaro, J. Barek, J.-M. Frémy, M. Lafontaine, M. Miraglia, E.B. Sansone and G.M. Telling
1991; 64 pages £12.00

No. 114 **Laboratory Decontamination and Destruction of Carcinogens in Laboratory Wastes: Some Polycyclic Heterocyclic Hydrocarbons**
Edited by M. Castegnaro, J. Barek J. Jacob, U. Kirso, M. Lafontaine, E.B. Sansone, G.M. Telling and T. Vu Duc
1991; 50 pages £8.00

No. 115 **Mycotoxins, Endemic Nephropathy and Urinary Tract Tumours**
Edited by M. Castegnaro, R. Plestina, G. Dirheimer, I.N. Chernozemsky and H Bartsch
1991; 340 pages £47.50

No. 116 **Mechanisms of Carcinogenesis in Risk Identification**
Edited by H. Vainio, P.N. Magee, D.B. McGregor & A.J. McMichael
1992; 616 pages £69.00

No. 117 **Directory of On-going Research in Cancer Epidemiology 1992**
Edited by M. Coleman, J. Wahrendorf & E. Démaret
1992; 773 pages £44.50

No. 118 **Cadmium in the Human Environment: Toxicity and Carcinogenicity**
Edited by G.F. Nordberg, R.F.M. Herber & L. Alessio
1992; 470 pages £60.00

No. 119 **The Epidemiology of Cervical Cancer and Human Papillomavirus**
Edited by N. Muñoz, F.X. Bosch, K.V. Shah & A. Meheus
1992; 288 pages £29.50

No. 120 **Cancer Incidence in Five Continents, Volume VI**
Edited by D.M. Parkin, C.S. Muir, S.L. Whelan, Y.T. Gao, J. Ferlay & J.Powell
1992; 1080 pages £120.00

No. 121 **Trends in Cancer Incidence and Mortality**
M.P. Coleman, J. Estève, P. Damiecki, A. Arslan and H. Renard
1993; 806 pages, £120.00

No. 122 **International Classification of Rodent Tumours. Part 1. The Rat**
Editor-in-Chief: U. Mohr
1992/95; 10 fascicles of 60–100 pages, £120.00

No. 123 **Cancer in Italian Migrant Populations**
Edited by M. Geddes, D.M. Parkin, M. Khlat, D. Balzi and E. Buiatti
1993; 292 pages, £40.00

No. 124 **Postlabelling Methods for Detection of DNA Adducts**
Edited by D.H. Phillips, M. Castegnaro and H. Bartsch
1993; 392 pages; £46.00

No. 125 **DNA Adducts: Identification and Biological Significance**
Edited by K. Hemminki, A. Dipple, D. Shuker, F.F. Kadlubar, D. Segerbäck and H. Bartsch
1994; 480 pages; £52.00

No. 127 **Butadiene and Styrene: Assessment of Health Hazards**
Edited by M. Sorsa, K. Peltonen, H. Vainio and K. Hemminki
1993; 412 pages; £54.00

No. 128 **Statistical Methods in Cancer Research. Volume IV. Descriptive Epidemiology**
By J. Estève, E. Benhamou & L.Raymond
1994; 302 pages; £25.00

No. 129 **Occupational Cancer in Developing Countries**
Edited by N. Pearce, E. Matos, H. Vainio, P. Boffetta & M. Kogevinas
1994; 192 pages £20.00

No. 130 **Directory of On-going Research in Cancer Epidemiology 1994**
Edited by R. Sankaranarayanan, J. Wahrendorf and E. Démaret
1994; 792 pages, £46.00

No. 132 **Survival of Cancer Patients in Europe. The EUROCARE Study**
Edited by F. Berrino, M. Sant, A. Verdecchia, R. Capocaccia, T. Hakulinen and J. Estève
1994; 463 pages; £45.00

List of IARC Publications

IARC MONOGRAPHS ON THE EVALUATION OF CARCINOGENIC RISKS TO HUMANS

Volume 1 **Some Inorganic Substances, Chlorinated Hydrocarbons, Aromatic Amines, *N*-Nitroso Compounds, and Natural Products**
1972; 184 pages (*out of print*)

Volume 2 **Some Inorganic and Organometallic Compounds**
1973; 181 pages (*out of print*)

Volume 3 **Certain Polycyclic Aromatic Hydrocarbons and Heterocyclic Compounds**
1973; 271 pages (*out of print*)

Volume 4 **Some Aromatic Amines, Hydrazine and Related Substances, *N*-Nitroso Compounds and Miscellaneous Alkylating Agents**
1974; 286 pages Sw. fr. 18.–

Volume 5 **Some Organochlorine Pesticides**
1974; 241 pages (*out of print*)

Volume 6 **Sex Hormones**
1974; 243 pages (*out of print*)

Volume 7 **Some Anti-Thyroid and Related Substances, Nitrofurans and Industrial Chemicals**
1974; 326 pages (*out of print*)

Volume 8 **Some Aromatic Azo Compounds**
1975; 357 pages Sw. fr. 44.–

Volume 9 **Some Aziridines, *N*-, *S*- and *O*-Mustards and Selenium**
1975; 268 pages Sw.fr. 33.–

Volume 10 **Some Naturally Occurring Substances**
1976; 353 pages (*out of print*)

Volume 11 **Cadmium, Nickel, Some Epoxides, Miscellaneous Industrial Chemicals and General Considerations on Volatile Anaesthetics**
1976; 306 pages (*out of print*)

Volume 12 **Some Carbamates, Thiocarbamates and Carbazides**
1976; 282 pages Sw. fr. 41.-

Volume 13 **Some Miscellaneous Pharmaceutical Substances**
1977; 255 pages Sw. fr. 36.–

Volume 14 **Asbestos**
1977; 106 pages (*out of print*)

Volume 15 **Some Fumigants, The Herbicides 2,4-D and 2,4,5-T, Chlorinated Dibenzodioxins and Miscellaneous Industrial Chemicals**
1977; 354 pages (*out of print*)

Volume 16 **Some Aromatic Amines and Related Nitro Compounds – Hair Dyes, Colouring Agents and Miscellaneous Industrial Chemicals**
1978; 400 pages Sw. fr. 60.–

Volume 17 **Some *N*-Nitroso Compounds**
1978; 365 pages Sw. fr. 60.–

Volume 18 **Polychlorinated Biphenyls and Polybrominated Biphenyls**
1978; 140 pages Sw. fr. 24.–

Volume 19 **Some Monomers, Plastics and Synthetic Elastomers, and Acrolein**
1979; 513 pages (*out of print*)

Volume 20 **Some Halogenated Hydrocarbons**
1979; 609 pages (*out of print*)

Volume 21 **Sex Hormones (II)**
1979; 583 pages Sw. fr. 72.–

Volume 22 **Some Non-Nutritive Sweetening Agents**
1980; 208 pages Sw. fr. 30.–

Volume 23 **Some Metals and Metallic Compounds**
1980; 438 pages (*out of print*)

Volume 24 **Some Pharmaceutical Drugs**
1980; 337 pages Sw. fr. 48.–

Volume 25 **Wood, Leather and Some Associated Industries**
1981; 412 pages Sw. fr. 72.–

Volume 26 **Some Antineoplastic and Immunosuppressive Agents**
1981; 411 pages Sw. fr. 75.–

Volume 27 **Some Aromatic Amines, Anthraquinones and Nitroso Compounds, and Inorganic Fluorides Used in Drinking Water and Dental Preparations**
1982; 341 pages Sw. fr. 48.–

Volume 28 **The Rubber Industry**
1982; 486 pages Sw. fr. 84.–

Volume 29 **Some Industrial Chemicals and Dyestuffs**
1982; 416 pages Sw. fr. 72.–

Volume 30 **Miscellaneous Pesticides**
1983; 424 pages Sw. fr. 72.–

Volume 31 **Some Food Additives, Feed Additives and Naturally Occurring Substances**
1983; 314 pages Sw. fr. 66.–

Volume 32 **Polynuclear Aromatic Compounds, Part 1: Chemical, Environmental and Experimental Data**
1983; 477 pages Sw. fr. 88.–

Volume 33 **Polynuclear Aromatic Compounds, Part 2: Carbon Blacks, Mineral Oils and Some Nitroarenes**
1984; 245 pages (*out of print*)

Volume 34 **Polynuclear Aromatic Compounds, Part 3: Industrial Exposures in Aluminium Production, Coal Gasification, Coke Production, and Iron and Steel Founding**
1984; 219 pages Sw. fr. 53.–

Volume 35 **Polynuclear Aromatic Compounds, Part 4: Bitumens, Coal-tars and Derived Products, Shale-oils and Soots**
1985; 271 pages Sw. fr. 77.–

List of IARC Publications

Volume 36 Allyl Compounds, Aldehydes, Epoxides and Peroxides
1985; 369 pages Sw. fr. 77.–

Volume 37 Tobacco Habits Other than Smoking: Betel-quid and Areca-nut Chewing; and some Related Nitrosamines
1985; 291 pages Sw. fr. 77.–

Volume 38 Tobacco Smoking
1986; 421 pages Sw. fr. 83.–

Volume 39 Some Chemicals Used in Plastics and Elastomers
1986; 403 pages Sw. fr. 83.–

Volume 40 Some Naturally Occurring and Synthetic Food Components, Furocoumarins and Ultraviolet Radiation
1986; 444 pages Sw. fr. 83.–

Volume 41 Some Halogenated Hydrocarbons and Pesticide Exposures
1986; 434 pages Sw. fr. 83.–

Volume 42 Silica and Some Silicates
1987; 289 pages Sw. fr. 72.

Volume 43 Man-Made Mineral Fibres and Radon
1988; 300 pages Sw. fr. 72.–

Volume 44 Alcohol Drinking
1988; 416 pages Sw. fr. 83.

Volume 45 Occupational Exposures in Petroleum Refining; Crude Oil and Major Petroleum Fuels
1989; 322 pages Sw. fr. 72.–

Volume 46 Diesel and Gasoline Engine Exhausts and Some Nitroarenes
1989; 458 pages Sw. fr. 83.–

Volume 47 Some Organic Solvents, Resin Monomers and Related Compounds, Pigments and Occupational Exposures in Paint Manufacture and Painting
1989; 535 pages Sw. fr. 94.–

Volume 48 Some Flame Retardants and Textile Chemicals, and Exposures in the Textile Manufacturing Industry
1990; 345 pages Sw. fr. 72.–

Volume 49 Chromium, Nickel and Welding
1990; 677 pages Sw. fr. 105.-

Volume 50 Pharmaceutical Drugs
1990; 415 pages Sw. fr. 93.-

Volume 51 Coffee, Tea, Mate, Methylxanthines and Methylglyoxal
1991; 513 pages Sw. fr. 88.-

Volume 52 Chlorinated Drinking-water; Chlorination By-products; Some Other Halogenated Compounds; Cobalt and Cobalt Compounds
1991; 544 pages Sw. fr. 88.-

Volume 53 Occupational Exposures in Insecticide Application and some Pesticides
1991; 612 pages Sw. fr. 105.-

Volume 54 Occupational Exposures to Mists and Vapours from Strong Inorganic Acids; and Other Industrial Chemicals
1992; 336 pages Sw. fr. 72.-

Volume 55 Solar and Ultraviolet Radiation
1992; 316 pages Sw. fr. 65.-

Volume 56 Some Naturally Occurring Substances: Food Items and Constituents, Heterocyclic Aromatic Amines and Mycotoxins
1993; 600 pages Sw. fr. 95.-

Volume 57 Occupational Exposures of Hairdressers and Barbers and Personal Use of Hair Colourants; Some Hair Dyes, Cosmetic Colourants, Industrial Dyestuffs and Aromatic Amines
1993; 428 pages Sw. fr. 75.-

Volume 58 Beryllium, Cadmium, Mercury and Exposures in the Glass Manufacturing Industry
1993; 426 pages Sw. fr. 75.-

Volume 59 Hepatitis Viruses
1994; 286 pages Sw. fr. 65.-

Volume 60 Some Industrial Chemicals
1994; 560 pages Sw. fr. 90.-

Volume 61 Schistosomes, Liver Flukes and Helicobacter pylori
1994; 270 pages Sw. fr. 70.-

Volume 62 Wood Dust and Formaldehyde
1995; 406 pages Sw. fr. 80.–

Volume 63 Dry Cleaning, some Chlorinated Solvents and other Industrial Chemicals
1995; 558 pages Sw. fr. 90.–

Volume 64 Human Papilloma Viruses
1995; 409 pages Sw. fr. 80.–

Supplement No. 1
Chemicals and Industrial Processes Associated with Cancer in Humans (IARC Monographs, Volumes 1 to 20)
1979; 71 pages (out of print)

Supplement No. 2
Long-term and Short-term Screening Assays for Carcinogens: A Critical Appraisal
1980; 426 pages Sw. fr. 40.-

Supplement No. 3
Cross Index of Synonyms and Trade Names in Volumes 1 to 26
1982; 199 pages (out of print)

Supplement No. 4
Chemicals, Industrial Processes and Industries Associated with Cancer in Humans (IARC Monographs, Volumes 1 to 29)
1982; 292 pages (out of print)

Supplement No. 5
Cross Index of Synonyms and Trade Names in Volumes 1 to 36
1985; 259 pages (out of print)

Supplement No. 6
Genetic and Related Effects: An Updating of Selected IARC Monographs from Volumes 1 to 42
1987; 729 pages Sw. fr. 80.-

Supplement No. 7
Overall Evaluations of Carcinogenicity: An Updating of IARC Monographs Volumes 1-42
1987; 440 pages Sw. fr. 65.-

Supplement No. 8
Cross Index of Synonyms and Trade Names in Volumes 1 to 46
1990; 346 pages Sw. fr. 60.-

List of IARC Publications

IARC TECHNICAL REPORTS

No. 1 Cancer in Costa Rica
Edited by R. Sierra, R. Barrantes, G. Muñoz Leiva, D.M. Parkin, C.A. Bieber and N. Muñoz Calero
1988; 124 pages Sw. fr. 30.-

No. 2 SEARCH: A Computer Package to Assist the Statistical Analysis of Case-control Studies
Edited by G.J. Macfarlane, P. Boyle and P. Maisonneuve
1991; 80 pages (*out of print*)

No. 3 Cancer Registration in the European Economic Community
Edited by M.P. Coleman and E. Démaret
1988; 188 pages Sw. fr. 30.-

No. 4 Diet, Hormones and Cancer: Methodological Issues for Prospective Studies
Edited by E. Riboli and R. Saracci
1988; 156 pages Sw. fr. 30.-

No. 5 Cancer in the Philippines
Edited by A.V. Laudico, D. Esteban and D.M. Parkin
1989; 186 pages Sw. fr. 30.-

No. 6 La genèse du Centre International de Recherche sur le Cancer
Par R. Sohier et A.G.B. Sutherland
1990; 104 pages Sw. fr. 30.-

No. 7 Epidémiologie du cancer dans les pays de langue latine
1990; 310 pages Sw. fr. 30.-

No. 8 Comparative Study of Antismoking Legislation in Countries of the European Economic Community
Edited by A. Sasco, P. Dalla Vorgia and P. Van der Elst
1992; 82 pages Sw. fr. 30.-

No. 9 Epidemiologie du cancer dans les pays de langue latine
1991 346 pages Sw. fr. 30.-

No. 10 Manual for Cancer Registry Personnel
Edited by S. Whelan et al.
1995; 370 pages Sw. fr. 45.-

No. 11 Nitroso Compounds: Biological Mechanisms, Exposures and Cancer Etiology
Edited by I.K. O'Neill & H. Bartsch
1992; 149 pages Sw. fr. 30.-

No. 12 Epidémiologie du cancer dans les pays de langue latine
1992; 375 pages Sw. fr. 30.-

No. 13 Health, Solar UV Radiation and Environmental Change
By A. Kricker, B.K. Armstrong, M.E. Jones and R.C. Burton
1993; 216 pages Sw.fr. 30.-

No. 14 Epidémiologie du cancer dans les pays de langue latine
1993; 385 pages Sw. fr. 30.-

No. 15 Cancer in the African Population of Bulawayo, Zimbabwe, 1963–1977: Incidence, Time Trends and Risk Factors
By M.E.G. Skinner, D.M. Parkin, A.P. Vizcaino and A. Ndhlovu
1993; 123 pages Sw. fr. 30.-

No. 16 Cancer in Thailand, 1988–1991
By V. Vatanasapt, N. Martin, H. Sriplung, K. Vindavijak, S. Sontipong, S. Sriamporn, D.M. Parkin and J. Ferlay
1993; 164 pages Sw. fr. 30.-

No. 18 Intervention Trials for Cancer Prevention
By E. Buiatti
1994; 52 pages Sw. fr. 30.-

No. 19 Comparability and Quality Control in Cancer Registration
By D.M. Parkin, V.W. Chen, J. Ferlay, J. Galceran, H.H. Storm and S.L. Whelan
1994; 110 pages plus diskette Sw. fr. 40.-

No. 20 Epidémiologie du cancer dans les pays de langue latine
1994; 346 pages Sw. fr. 30.-

No. 21 ICD Conversion Programs for Cancer
By J. Ferlay
1994; 24 pages plus diskette Sw. fr. 30.-

No. 22 Cancer Incidence by Occupation and Industry in Tianjin, China, 1981–1987
By Q.S. Wang, P. Boffetta, M. Kogevinas and D.M. Parkin
1994; 96 pages Sw. fr. 30.–

No. 23 An Evaluation Programme for Cancer Preventive Agents
By B.W. Stewart
1995; 40 pages Sw. fr. 20.-

No. 24 Peroxisome Proliferation and its role in Carcinogenesis
Views and expert opinions of an IARC Working Group 7–11 December 1994
1995; 90 pages Sw. fr. 30.-

No. 25 Combined Analysis of Cancer Mortality in Nuclear Industry Workers in Canada, the United Kingdom and the United States
E. Cardis et al.
1995; 160 pages Sw. fr. 30.-

DIRECTORY OF AGENTS BEING TESTED FOR CARCINOGENICITY

(Until Vol. 13 Information Bulletin on the Survey of Chemicals Being Tested for Carcinogenicity)

No. 8 Edited by M.-J. Ghess, H. Bartsch and L. Tomatis
1979; 604 pages Sw. fr. 40.-

No. 9 Edited by M.-J. Ghess, J.D. Wilbourn, H. Bartsch and L. Tomatis
1981; 294 pages Sw. fr. 41.-

No. 10 Edited by M.-J. Ghess, J.D. Wilbourn and H. Bartsch
1982; 362 pages Sw. fr. 42.-

No. 11 Edited by M.-J. Ghess, J.D. Wilbourn, H. Vainio and H. Bartsch
1984; 362 pages Sw. fr. 50.-

No. 12 Edited by M.-J. Ghess, J.D. Wilbourn, A. Tossavainen and H. Vainio
1986; 385 pages Sw. fr. 50.-

No. 13 Edited by M.-J. Ghess, J.D. Wilbourn and A. Aitio 1988; 404 pages Sw. fr. 43.-

No. 14 Edited by M.-J. Ghess, J.D. Wilbourn and H. Vainio
1990; 370 pages Sw. fr. 45.-

No. 15 Edited by M.-J. Ghess, J.D. Wilbourn and H. Vainio
1992; 318 pages Sw. fr. 45.-

No. 16 Edited by M.-J. Ghess, J.D. Wilbourn and H. Vainio
1994; 294 pages Sw. fr. 50.-

List of IARC Publications

NON-SERIAL PUBLICATIONS

Alcool et Cancer
By A. Tuyns (in French only)
1978; 42 pages Fr. fr. 35.-

Cancer Morbidity and Causes of Death Among Danish Brewery Workers
By O.M. Jensen
1980; 143 pages Fr. fr. 75.-

Directory of Computer Systems Used in Cancer Registries
By H.R. Menck and D.M. Parkin
1986; 236 pages Fr. fr. 50.-

Facts and Figures of Cancer in the European Community
Edited by J. Estève, A. Kricker, J. Ferlay and D.M. Parkin
1993; 52 pages Sw. fr. 10.-

www.ingramcontent.com/pod-product-compliance
Ingram Content Group UK Ltd.
Pitfield, Milton Keynes, MK11 3LW, UK
UKHW051258180426
11947UKWH00020B/1776